D1572888

FEMALE PELVIC FLOOR DISORDERS

INVESTIGATION AND MANAGEMENT

FEMALE PELVIC FLOOR DISORDERS

INVESTIGATION AND MANAGEMENT

Edited by

J. THOMAS BENSON, MD, FACS, FACOG

Clinical Professor
Indiana University School of Medicine
Director of Obstetrics and Gynecology Education
Methodist Hospital of Indiana, Inc.
Indianapolis, Indiana

Norton Medical Books

W · W · Norton & Company
New York · London

The author wishes to acknowledge and thank the sculptor Heloise Crista for giving her permission to print the photograph on the cover of this book.

Impressed by the warmth, beauty, and spirit of Frank Lloyd Wright's work, Ms. Crista went to Taliesin, Wisconsin, to study his philosophy and architecture and to participate in the Taliesin Fellowship. In addition to her work as a sculptor, she also conducts correlation/dance programs; her dance training is evident in the strong flow and movement of her sculpture, which can be observed in the cover photograph of her sculpture, *Changing Woman*. This sculpture symbolizes the profound advances of women in today's culture and represents the book's intent to improve their care.

Copyright © 1992 by J. Thomas Benson

All rights reserved. Printed in the United States of America. The text and display of this book are composed in Sabon. Composition by ComCom. Manufacturing by Arcata Halliday. Book design by Jack Meserole.

Cover sculpture by Heloise Crista. Photograph by Arnold Roy.

DRUG DOSAGE

The authors and publishers have exerted every effort to insure that drug selection and dosage set forth in this text are in accord with current recommendations and practice at the time of publication. However, in view of ongoing research, changes in government regulations, and the constant flow of information relating to drug therapy and drug reactions, the reader is urged to check the package insert for each drug for any change in indications and dosage and for added warnings and precautions. This is particularly important when the recommended agent is a new and/or infrequently used drug.

First Edition

Library of Congress Cataloging-in-Publication Data

Investigation and management of female pelvic floor disorders /
[edited by] J. Thomas Benson.
    p. cm.
    Includes index.
    ISBN 0-393-71013-0
    1. Pelvis—Diseases. 2. Urinary incontinence. 3. Fecal
incontinence. 4. Urogynecolgy. 5. Generative organs, Female—
Diseases. I. Benson, J. Thomas.
    [DNLM: 1. Fecal Incontinence. 2. Pelvis—physiopathology.
3. Urinary Incontinence. 4. Urogential Diseases—diagnosis.
5. Urogenital Diseases—therapy. WJ 190 I62]
RG482.I58 1992
618.1—dc20
DGPO/DLC
for Library of Congress   91-31999
                                             CIP

W. W. Norton & Company, Inc., 500 Fifth Avenue, New York, N.Y. 10110
W. W. Norton & Company, Ltd., 10 Coptic Street, London WC1A 1PU

1 2 3 4 5 6 7 8 9 0

CONTENTS

CONTRIBUTORS

Andrew M. Agosta, MD

Director of Urogynecology/Assistant Program Director, Obstetrics and Gynecology Residency Program, Saginaw Cooperative Hospitals Inc.; Assistant Professor of Obstetrics and Gynecology, Michigan State University College of Human Medicine, Saginaw, Michigan *(Chapter 6)*

Rodney A. Appell, MD

Professor and Vice-Chairman of Urology/Director, Urodynamics Unit, Louisiana State University Medical Center, New Orleans, Louisiana *(Chapter 11D4)*

J. Thomas Benson, MD, FACS, FACOG

Clinical Professor, Indiana University School of Medicine; Director of Obstetrics and Gynecology Education, Methodist Hospital of Indiana, Indianapolis, Indiana *(Chapters 9A, 11D2, 12B, 13B, 13D, 16)*

Alfred E. Bent, MD

Head, Division of Urogynecology/Interim Coordinator, Residency Training, Greater Baltimore Medical Center, Baltimore, Maryland *(Chapter 11C1)*

Jerry S. Benzl, MD

Clinical Professor, University of California at Irvine, Irvine, California; Assistant Professor, Loma Linda University School of Medicine, Loma Linda, California *(Chapters 4B, 13C)*

Kathryn L. Burgio, PhD

Research Assistant Professor of Medicine, University of Pittsburgh School of Medicine, Pittsburgh, Pennsylvania *(Chapter 11C2)*

Hilary J. Cholhan, MD

Assistant Professor of Obstetrics-Gynecology/Director, Urogynecology Unit, University of Rochester Medical Center, Rochester, New York *(Chapter 11C1)*

Carolyn B. Coulam, MD

Director, Reproductive Immunology, Genetics and IVF Institute, Fairfax, Virginia *(Foreword)*

John O. L. DeLancey, MD

Assistant Professor of Obstetrics and Gynecology, University of Michigan School of Medicine, Ann Arbor, Michigan *(Chapter 2)*

Ananias C. Diokno, MD

Clinical Professor of Urology, University of Michigan Medical School Ann Arbor, Michigan; Chief of Urology, William Beaumont Hospital, Royal Oak, Michigan *(Chapter 11B)*

Bjarne Chr. Eriksen, MD, PhD

Consultant, Department of Gynecolgy and Obstetrics, Haugesund Hospital, Haugesund, Norway *(Chapter 11C3)*

J. Andrew Fantl, MD

Professor and Head, Section of Urogynecology, Department of Obstetrics and Gynecology, Medical College of Virginia, Richmond, Virginia *(Chapter 3)*

Scott A. Farrell, MD, FRCS(C)

Assistant Professor of Obstetrics and Gynecology, Dalhousie University, Halifax, Nova Scotia, Canada *(Chapter 11D1)*

M. M. Henry, MB, FRCS

Consulatant Surgeon, Central Middlesex Hospital; Senior Lecturer, Academic Surgical Unit, St. Mary's Hospital; Hon Consultant Surgeon, St. Mark's Hospital, London, England *(Chapters 5, 14B, 14D2)*

Jay B. Hollander, MD

Director of Medical Education/Attending Urologist, Department of Urology, William Beaumont Hospital, Royal Oak, Michigan *(Chapter 11B)*

Mickey M. Karram, MD, FACOG

Director, Urogynecology, Good Samaritan Hospital; Assistant Professor of Obstetrics and Gynecology, University of Cincinnati School of Medicine, Cincinnati, Ohio *(Chapter 8A)*

Frederick M. Kelvin, MD

Staff Radiologist, Methodist Hospital of Indiana, Inc.; Clinical Professor, Indiana University School of Medicine, Indianapolis, Indiana *(Chapter 7A1)*

Henry H. Lansman, MD

Professor of Clinical Obstetrics and Gynecology, University of Miami School of Medicine, Miami, Florida *(Chapter 1)*

Kenneth E. Levin, MD

Fellow in Colon and Rectal Surgery, Mayo Medical School, Mayo Clinic, and Mayo Foundation, Rochester, Minnesota *(Chapter 15)*

Vincent Lucente, MD

Physician in Charge of Urogynecology, Northshore University Hospital, Cornell Medical College, Manhasset, New York *(Chapter 7B)*

James H. MacLeod, MD, FACS, FRCS(C)

Former Clinical Instructor, Department of Surgery, Dalhousie Faculty of Medicine, Halifax, Nova Scotia, Canada; Former Clinical Instructor, Department of Surgery, University of Southern California School of Medicine, Los Angeles, California; Former Attending Surgeon, Intercommunity Presbyterian Hospital, Whittier, California. *(Chapter 14C)*

Victoria M. Maclin, MD

Assistant Professor of Obstetrics and Gynecology, Rush Presbyterian St. Lukes Medical Center, Chicago, Illinois; Director, Center for Fertility and Reproduction, Ingalls Memorial Hospital, Harvey, Illinois *(Chapter 4A)*

Elizabeth McClellan, RN

Incontinence Research Nurse, J. Thomas Benson, MD, Inc., Indianapolis, Indiana *(Chapter 14A)*

Debra A. Miller, MD

Clinical Instructor, Wright State University Integrated Obstetrics and Gynecology Residency Program, Dayton, Ohio *(Chapter 3)*

John J. Murray, MD

Staff Surgeon, Department of Colon and Rectal Surgery, Lahey Clinic Medical Center, Burlington, Massachusetts *(Chapter 14D1)*

David H. Nichols, MD, FACS, FACOG

Professor and Chairman, Department of Obstetrics and Gynecology, Brown University; Chief of Obstetrics and Gynecology, Women's and Infants' Hospital, Providence, Rhode Island *(Foreword)*

Peggy A. Norton, MD

Assistant Professor, Departments of Obstetrics and Gynecology and Urology, University of Utah School of Medicine, Salt Lake City, Utah; Recipient of a five-year Physician Scientist award from the NIH to study the role of connective tissue in genital prolapse *(Chapter 10)*

Donald R. Ostergard, MD, FACOG

Professor of Obstetrics and Gynecology, University of California at Irvine, Irvine, California; Associate Medical Director for Gynecology/Director, Division of Urogynecology, Women's Hospital, Long Beach Memorial Medical Center, Long Beach, California *(Chapter 11D1)*

John H. Pemberton, MD

Associate Professor of Surgery, Mayo Medical School, Mayo Clinic, and Mayo Foundation, Rochester, Minnesota *(Chapter 15)*

G. Byington Pratt, MD

Pediatric Radiologist/Chief, Pediatric Subsection, Radiology Department, Methodist Hospital of Indiana, Inc.; Medical Director, Ball State/Methodist Hospital X-ray Technology Program/Adjunct Professor of Radiology, Ball State University, Indianapolis, Indiana *(Chapter 7A2)*

N.W. Read, MA, MD, FRCP

Professor of Gastrointestinal Physiology and Nutrition, University of Sheffield, Sheffield, United Kingdom *(Chapter 8B)*

A. Cullen Richardson, MD

Associate Clinical Professor, Department of Gynecology and Obstetrics, Emory University School of Medicine, Atlanta, Georgia *(Chapters 2, 12A)*

Euan G. Robertson, MD

Associate Chairman of Gynecologic Services/Professor of Obstetrics and Gynecology, University of Miami School of Medicine, Miami, Florida *(Chapter 1)*

Jack R. Robertson, MD, FAOG, FACS

Clinical Professor of Obstetrics and Gynecology/Chief of Urogynecology, University of Nevada Medical School, Las Vegas, Nevada *(Chapters 11D5a, 11D5b)*

Barbara B. Sherwin, PhD

Associate Professor of Psychology and Obstetrics and Gynecology, McGill University; Codirector, McGill University Menopause Clinic; SMBD—Jewish General Hospital, Montreal, Quebec, Canada *(Chapter 13A)*

Giles W. Stevenson, MD

Professor and Chairman of Radiology, McMaster University, Hamilton, Ontario, Canada *(Chapter 7A1)*

W. M. Sun, PhD

Gatroenterology Research Fellow, Royal Adelaide Hospital, University of Adelaide, Adelaide, South Australia *(Chapter 8B)*

Emil A. Tanagho, MD

Professor and Chairman, Department of Urology, University of California School of Medicine, San Francisco, California *(Chapter 11D3)*

Henry A. Thiede, MD

Professor and Chairman, Department of Obstetrics and Gynecology, University of Rochester, Rochester, New York *(Chapter 11A)*

Geoffrey K. Turnbull, MD, FRCPC

Assistant Professor of Medicine/Active Staff Gastroenterologist, GI Unit, Camp Hill Medical Centre, Dalhousie University, Halifax, Nova Scotia, Canada *(Chapter 18)*

Malcolm C. Veidenheimer, MD

Staff Surgeon, Department of Colon and Rectal Surgery, Lahey Clinic Medical Center, Burlington, Massachusetts *(Chapter 14D1)*

D.W. Warrell, MD, FRCOG

Consultant Urological Gynecologist, St. Mary's Hospital, Manchester, England *(chapter 9B)*

Tiffany J. Williams, MD

Consultant, Section of Gynecologic Surgery, Mayo Clinic and Mayo Foundation; Professor of Obstetrics and Gynecology, Mayo Medical School, Rochester, Minnesota *(Chapter 17)*

FOREWORD

To help solve the problem of inadequate treatment for women with urinary incontinence and other pelvic floor disorders, Dr. Thomas Benson has organized this outstanding textbook on *Female Pelvic Floor Disorders: Investigation and Management*. He has utilized a group of distinguished contributors, each of them experts in their own field, to present new ideas regarding the etiology of pelvic floor disorders and how to apply them in patient care. The most exciting aspect of this book is the new concept of grouping all pelvic floor disorders, of which urinary incontinence is only one symptom. The term "pelvic floor" in this textbook refers to the pelvic diaphragm, sphincter mechanisms of the lower urinary tract, the upper and lower vaginal supports, and the internal and external anal sphincters. This concept allows a multidisciplinary approach to investigation and treatment of all pelvic floor disorders. The consolida-tion of knowledge gained from the medical subspecialties involved in managing various aspects of pelvic floor disorders will undoubtedly result in more effective patient management. To that end, this new textbook provides a complete contemporary source of basic and clinical aspects of pelvic floor disorders. It is directed toward undergraduate students, residents, fellows, and physicians of all specialties who treat patients with urinary or anal incontinence or other manifestations of pelvic floor relaxation. Because disorders of the pelvic floor are encountered with increasing frequency, and because its etiology, investigation, and treatment have gained new insights, this textbook is a welcome addition to reference libraries of students and physicians alike.

CAROLYN COULAM, MD

FOREWORD

Female pelvic floor disorders comprise a matrix of universal problems that threaten the quality of life for women of all ages throughout the world. Although the anatomic blueprint for pelvic structure and support probably has been constant for tens of thousands of years, the analysis of regular forces at work and their acquired and congenital malformations and malfunctions have been a subject of conjecture and opinion for many generations, with conclusions not always borne by fact.

The problems of defects of pelvic organ support and dysfunction are truly interdisciplinary, both in investigation and their solution. Dr. Benson has thoughtfully collected the views of many international contributors to this challenging subject. Their efforts have been pooled for the reader (in a mechanism of finding) in one volume that supplies current answers to questions that, individually, would require weeks of library research.

The spectrum of information in this intriguing volume progresses from diagnostic categories and considerations to the logical therapeutic responses geared toward restoration of patients' quality of life. This ambitious and exhaustive undertaking is a compendium of current thinking and a survey of the frontiers of future diagnosis, research, and therapy for these disorders that helps bring the reader up to date. The authors have taken commendably bold and exploratory steps toward the development of timely and useful interdisciplinary common denominators in the diagnosis, analysis, planning, and treatment of pelvic support defects.

DAVID H. NICHOLS, MD, FACS, FACOG

PREFACE

Many investigators and surgeons of the female pelvic floor, working independently in various parts of the world, are arriving at similar conclusions, which represent a revolution in the management of female pelvic floor defects. Recognition by careful, objective follow-up studies of excessive failure rates with heretofore standard treatment modalities is prompting a change from the compartmentalized approach to the female pelvic floor by various disciplines. Instead, a uniform consideration of the pelvic floor as an entity which, when defective, has interactive urinary, vaginal, and colorectal consequences is becoming apparent. The defects are multiple and all must be recognized and treated concomitantly to reduce the economic and emotional burdens of inadequate, partial, repeated therapies.

The evolutionary development and modern surgical anatomy of the pelvic floor will be explained, with descriptions of normal urinary, vaginal, and colorectal function. Investigation of pelvic floor dysfunction by clinical, radiologic, ultrasound, manometric, electrodiagnostic, and histologic means are presented in detail and attempts are made to consolidate the vast array of new insights into pelvic floor physiology fostered by such technologies.

Treatment considerations for pelvic floor disorders include medical, behavioral, and surgical aspects for the entire pelvic floor. Nonsurgical management of urinary, vaginal, and colorectal dysfunctions are thoroughly described.

Surgical therapies are outlined with emphasis on the need for the pelvic floor surgeon to:

1. Identify *all* the defects present in each patient and correct each defect precisely, anatomically, and at the same surgical setting;
2. Learn the surgical anatomy of the pelvic floor and operate in the "spaces" to reduce morbidity;
3. Be able to tailor the surgery to the individual patient and not tailor the patient to a given surgical procedure; and,
4. Carefully and objectively follow patients postoperatively to be aware of our failures and thus to improve our surgical efforts.

Particular highlights include psychosocial features of pelvic floor dysfunction and expanded clinical examination employing current technologies. An in-depth presentation of neurologic factors is given as neuromuscular factors are now recognized as being the common denominator in dysfunction of all compartments of the female pelvic floor.

J. Thomas Benson, M.D.

ACKNOWLEDGMENTS

It is a pleasure to acknowledge the assistance of Ms. Brenda Kester of Methodist Hospital Medical Media Production who has prepared many of the illustrations, Ms. Gina Hasz and Ms. Kris Ritter for their secretarial functions, Ms. Elizabeth McClellan for technical coordination, Ms. Regina Dahlgren (Norton Medical Books) and my beautiful wife, Susan, for editing guidance.

PART I

Anatomy and Physiology

CHAPTER 1

Evolution of the Pelvic Floor

Henry H. Lansman   Euan G. Robertson

INTRODUCTION

The development of upright posture in the human has been the dominant factor in the evolution of the pelvic floor. Anthropologists remind us that quadruped mammals have similar bones, muscles, and organs and yet are not prone to the problems that confront the human female as a result of the stress of gravity on the pelvic floor. The physiologic adaptation to the altered environment caused Keith[1] in 1912 (cited by Paramore[2] in 1918) to remark "when the power for easy mainte- nance was established, the body structure had been so altered in adaptation . . . that it rendered possible the erect posture by standing . . . and when terrestrial life became common then the ultimate and free pose of man on his feet was assured." But at what cost to the female? She delivers babies with large heads who have the abil- ity to continue learning for the rest of their lives. The birth process puts pressure on the supportive structures of the viscera within the pelvic cavity; then the final insult, menopause, leads to progressive weakening of the structural supports and ultimate prolapse of the visceral parts, incontinence, and embarrassment. This is in part caused by anatomical and physiological factors, but is amplified by greater life expectancy partly caused by advancements in modern medicine.

Any gynecologist who performs reconstructive sur- gery for prolapse of the pelvic viscera through the pelvic floor aperture must be familiar with the anatomy and physiology of the normal pelvis. He or she should be aware that no matter what the age of the patient, one of the most important concepts in reparative surgery is the maintenance of sexual competence. Obliteration of the vagina is no longer an acceptable mode of treat- ment. Many of our elderly patients regard the ability to retain sexual function as one of the most important facets of later life. In order to devise operative proce- dures that will create a functional vagina in patients with severe deterioration of support mechanisms, we must determine the full extent of the weakness of the supporting structures and if they are not utilizable, de- termine what other tissues can be used to reconstruct the pelvic floor. In order to do this, study of the evolu- tion of the mammalian pelvis will provide us with many valuable clues about potential repair procedures. Let us therefore trace the formation of pelvic structures from their earliest forms prior to man's migration onto land, the migration that necessitated the development of mus- cles and ligaments that could withstand the effects of gravity.

MARINE LIFE

If we are to believe that all life began in the primeval slime that eventually constituted the oceans, then we would expect similarities in all vertebrates from the most simple to the most complicated. All creatures that live in the sea's aqueous environment where the specific gravity is similar to that of their own bodies can be considered weightless. The necessity for oxygen, food, and reproduction is the same as for other vertebrates. Because of weightlessness only cartilage is needed to maintain the body form; the only muscle attachment is for the tail, enabling it to wave from side to side for locomotion. The effect of gravity on these lifeforms can only be observed in the backward slant of the vertebral appendages, which occurs because the fish, in its constant search for food, always points with its nose upstream into the prevailing current.

In fishes the pelvis is rudimentary.[3] The pelvic girdle is represented merely by a transverse bar of cartilage placed in front of the cloaca (Fig. 1-1A). This bar does not connect directly with the vertebral column except by that part of the lateral trunk musculature that extends from the tail into the body. Two strands of fibers (the caudopelvic strands), one on each side of the ventral tail musculature, are directed from behind forward to the pelvic bar. Behind the cloaca in the midline, the caudopelvic strands closely approximate each other, but as they approach the pelvic bar the fibers diverge to allow the cloaca to pass between them. This muscula-

ture forms the most conspicuous part of the body and consists of horizontally placed fibers that can be divided into two parts, dorsal and ventral, by a well-marked lateral line. In front of the pelvic bar, the lower part of the ventral musculature which encloses the body cavity is obliquely placed. This appears to arise from the longitudinal fibers that pass downward and forward to the median ventral line. The fibers which arise from the anterior border of the pelvic bar pass directly forward.

Power,[4] in 1948, after reviewing the above arrangement described by Paramore, suggested that the rudimentary pelvic floor is formed by a backward continuation of the rectus abdominis, namely the fibers which arise from the anterior border of the pelvic bar (Fig. 1-1 B). The pelvic part of the recti is attached behind to the tail (the two caudopelvic strands), while these strands attach anteriorly to the movable pelvic girdle. The cloaca passes out between these primitive representatives of the levator ani (caudopelvic strands) which can compress the cloaca simply by pulling the pelvis backward (Fig. 1-1C). This makes the pubocaudalis a caudal contin-

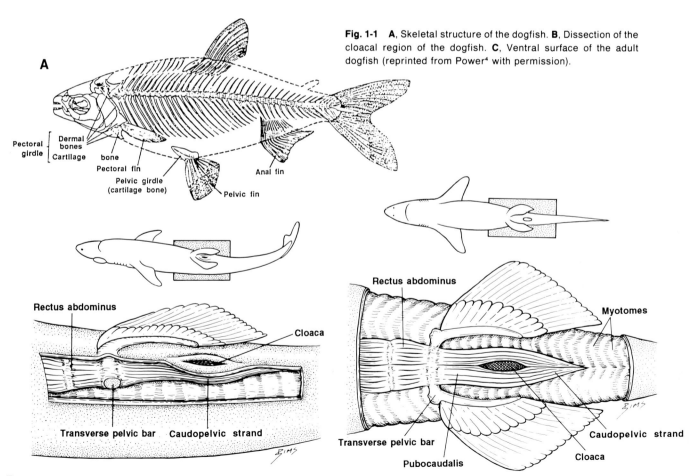

Fig. 1-1 A, Skeletal structure of the dogfish. **B**, Dissection of the cloacal region of the dogfish. **C**, Ventral surface of the adult dogfish (reprinted from Power[4] with permission).

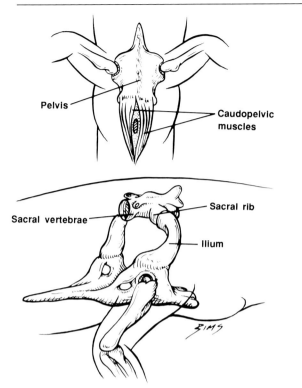

Fig. 1-2 Dissection of the salamander Maculosus showing the caudopelvic muscles.

uation of the rectus abdominus element.

Again, since fish are in a virtually gravity-free environment, the cloaca does not possess a sphincter muscle. The pressure of water on all sides of the body tends to prevent an extrusion of any part from within, such as excrement or ova. When extrusion of visceral contents becomes a necessity, the pressure from without must be overcome by an increasing pressure from within. The posterior fixation of the pelvic bar and the limitation of the size and dilatability caused by this fixation may be factors necessitating an increased visceral pressure during the passage of the usual copious amount of ova. This is accomplished by the oblique fibers in the ventral wall (corresponding to the internal oblique muscles of higher vertebrates) which by their contraction divert the increase in pressure toward the cloaca.

Nature has begun to realize the need for a bony pelvic girdle and in some fishes the ilium is already present as an outgrowth from each side of the pelvic bar.

AMPHIBIA

The necessity for a pelvic girdle arose when the first vertebrates (the amphibians) ventured onto land. These were not entirely land-based animals, as they returned to the water to lay their eggs. They breathed air by developing a rib cage and strong abdominal muscles. In the Devonian period when amphibians first appeared, the substitution of legs for fins enabled their survival. The creatures could crawl from one pool, where fish lay dying from lack of water, to another which provided an adequate supply of food. When on land they aided the intraabdominal vacuum necessary for breathing by sitting on their perineal orifices.

In some species, such as the salamander (Fig. 1-2) the ilium reaches and attaches to the rib on the single sacral vertebra by an articulation that allows to-and-fro movement of the pelvis on the spine. In the menobranchus (Fig. 1-3) the dorsal growth is incomplete, so that the pelvis is freely movable. The adult form of the salamander lives entirely on land and does not possess gills, whereas menobranchus is wholly aquatic and exhibits large external gills.

Fig. 1-3 Dissection of the menobranchus showing the caudopelvic muscles. The cloacal passage has been cut through on a plane with these muscles.

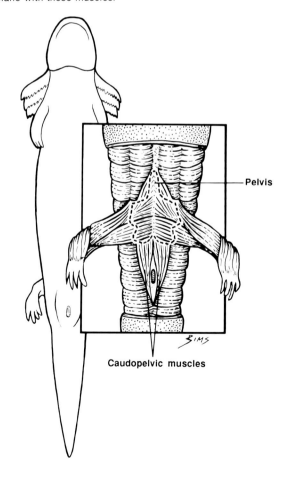

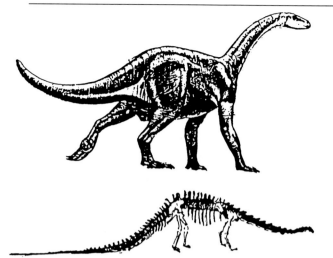

Fig. 1-4 A quadruped dinosaur and its skeletal structure.

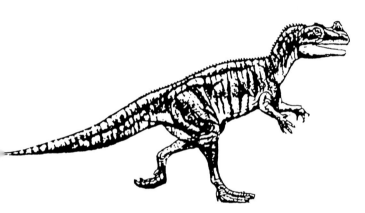

Fig. 1-5 A biped dinosaur.

In all amphibians, the caudopelvic strands form a pair of distinct and well-developed pelvic muscles separated from the lateral muscles of the trunk. These muscles proceed forward from their origin in the ventral part of the tail skeleton to insert into the posterior edge of the pelvic bar (ischia). In menobranchus, besides the recti there are three distinct layers that correspond to the external and internal oblique and transversalis muscles, whereas in the salamander an inner layer of transverse fibers corresponding to the transversalis does not exist.

The primitive recti and the puborectalis are in the same straight line separated by the caudal bar (os pubis). The rectus abdominus and external obliques are attached to the pelvis, but their contractions become efficient only by fixation of this structure. This fixation is primarily attained by the development of the caudopelvic muscles that anchor the pelvis posteriorly. These muscles are of considerable strength and pass caudally from the pelvis almost in the same straight line as the rectus abdominus, thus they are admirably adapted to resist the forward displacement of the pelvis which contraction of the recti tends to cause.

The menobranchus does not possess a cloacal sphincter because, like the fish, it is wholly aquatic. Its absence in the salamander may be explained by the well-developed caudopelvic muscles. At their insertion into the caudal bar, the inner borders of the muscles almost reach the midline, and when they contract synchronously they compress the cloaca, obviating the development of a separate sphincter.

LAND-BASED VERTEBRATES

The earliest land-based vertebrates (the reptiles) differed from the ancient amphibians in that they developed a large amnion type of egg that provided the embryo with a fluid environment on land. This released the reptiles from bondage to the marine environment. Migration to the land was an extraordinary evolutionary success and these reptiles, the dinosaurs, remained the dominant species for 150 million years.

Although there were many different types of dinosaurs, there were two main forms: one, a permanent quadruped (Fig. 1-4), was a vegetarian; the other was a bipedal flesh eater (Fig. 1-5). The quadruped was probably slower, less intelligent, and survived by synthesizing protein from plant life. The bipeds were the hunters, using their tails as lethal weapons and utilizing protein by eating their siblings as well as other species. These reptiles never stopped growing. Their size was determined by how long they lived and the availability of food to satisfy their voracious appetites. The fact that they lived for a long time and that food was plentiful is illustrated by their enormous length and weight.

But why were there two types of dinosaurs? The answer may become apparent if we digress to discuss certain similarities in the primates. The structural differences between the large gibbon or simian and the small African anthropoids or small gibbon are similar in degree and in nature to those which separate the gorilla from the chimpanzee. During the greater part of the Pleistocene epoch, mankind was also separated into two distinct types, the Neanderthal and the modern.[1] The gibbon, African anthropoids, and Pleistocene man represent three successive stages in the evolution of the highest primates. It is remarkable that there should be at each stage a process which led to a separation into two kinds, one a massive brutal form, restricted in its numbers and distribution, and the other less brutal,

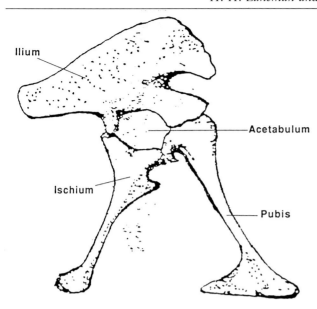

Fig. 1-6 The triradiate pelvis of the quadruped dinosaur consists of three prongs joined at the acetabulum: the ilium, ischium, and pubis.

widely distributed, and divided into numerous varieties of race. The simian, the gorilla, and the Neanderthal man are representatives of the brutal type; the gibbons, chimpanzees, and modern human types are representatives of the latter.

There is no doubt that the evolution of bipedalism affected the pelvic bones in the dinosaur. In the quadruped the vertical column formed an upward arch to help sustain the ponderous body, since there was no limitation to growth apart from the availability of food. The legs therefore were also massive and inserted into laterally placed acetabulae, and the free ends of the long bones gravitated vertically downward. The pelvis therefore had to be very strong and had three prongs: the ilium, the ischium, and the pubis fused at the acetabulum (Fig. 1-6). In the biped species the vertebral column was relatively straight and, similar to the quadruped, the legs inserted into laterally placed acetabulae. As a result of the biped state and massive weight of the abdomen, a major change had to occur in the pelvis (Fig. 1-7). The ilium and ischium maintained their relative positions but the pubis descended downward and backward to lie adjacent to the ischium. The major change was brought about by the development of a new bony process that projected forward from the pubis and was related to the narrowed and elongated ilium, resulting in a four-pronged pelvis. This development was the first indication that the pubis would be one of the pri-

mary supports of the weight of the contents of the abdominal cavity in opposition to the effects of gravity.

The dinosaurs themselves possessed the seeds of their own destruction. Perhaps they could have survived had they returned to a less cumbersome ancestral type, but one of the lessons of evolution is that unsuccessful modifications should be discarded.

The dinosaur became extinct but other reptiles survive and flourish. Two successful species that have survived to the present day are the iguana and the crocodile. They had similar requirements for survival in that they needed to vary their internal pressure and required a bony pelvis that was stronger and firmly attached to the sacrum. Because of the rise in internal pressure during active movement, greater body wall muscle contraction has evolved to impart rigidity to the trunk. Even during rest, muscle tone is maintained and applies pressure to the splanchnic venous system, which is important to the accessory circulatory mechanisms.

Thus we see that in reptiles there is a need for a fixed pelvic girdle. Paramore describes at least two sacral vertebrae present which are either ankylosed by fibrous tissue or fused together. In addition the iguana has developed so that the ends of the ribs are tightly bound together by fibrocartilage to form a broad area for the attachment of the ilium which restricts movement between them. Since the sacroiliac articulation is placed behind the acetabular joint, it may permit a certain amount of to-and-fro movement of the pelvis on the spine. In contrast, the pelvis in the crocodile may be

Fig. 1-7 Four-pronged pelvis of the biped dinosaur. Note the anterior projection of the pubis.

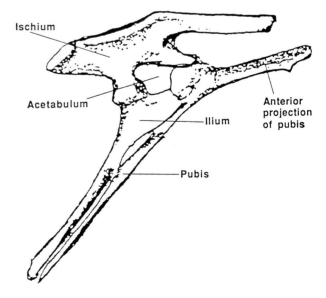

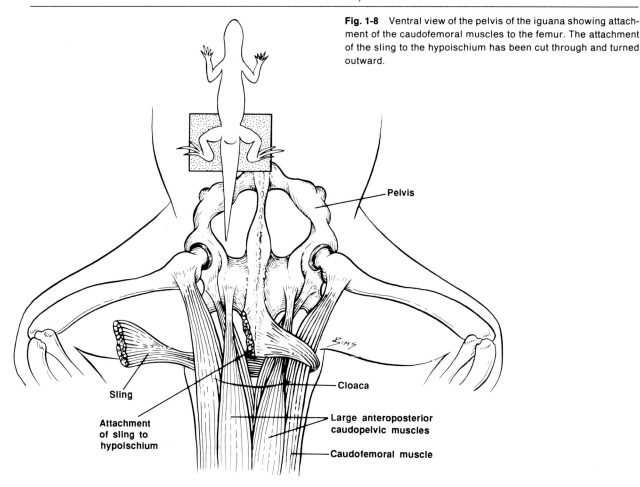

Fig. 1-8 Ventral view of the pelvis of the iguana showing attachment of the caudofemoral muscles to the femur. The attachment of the sling to the hypoischium has been cut through and turned outward.

immovably fixed to the spine. In both, the pelvic girdle is completed inferiorly by the junction of the pubic and ischial bones, and in some cases forms a single median symphysis.

In the iguana there are two well-developed caudopelvic muscles on each side, one being larger than the other (Fig. 1-8). The much larger muscles are of considerable length and serve to fix the pelvis posteriorly, and to a certain degree compress the cloaca at its sides. Traced anteriorly they rapidly diminish in size and give rise to tendons which insert into a bony protuberance on each side of the ventrolateral aspect of the pelvis. The smaller and much shorter caudopelvic muscles arise from the fascial septum in the angle between the larger caudopelvic muscles immediately behind the cloaca. These pass forward and outward, crossing the deep surface of the larger muscle to insert into the ventrolateral aspect of the pelvis behind the posterior lip of the acetabulum more laterally to the insertion of the larger muscle. Because the insertion of these muscles is lateral and not medial, they cannot exert much pressure on the

cloaca. In view of this inadequacy, the cloaca is provided with two crescent-shaped muscles, disposed transversely, one in front and the other behind, which serves as an efficient sphincter to close its orifice that opens on the surface as a transverse slit.

There is a further mechanism by which continence is maintained. The large caudofemoral muscle (Fig. 1-9A), located immediately dorsal to the belly of origin of the larger caudopelvic muscle, reaches anteriorly to the caudal limit of the pelvis where it abruptly passes outward over a sling to attach to the upper part of the femur. This sling (Fig. 1-9B) is formed by a tendon inserted between a dorsal and a ventral muscle. Paramore refers to the dorsal muscle as the lateral caudopelvic muscle which arises from the transverse processes of the anterior caudal vertebrae. It is composed of posterior and anterior fibers that form the thickest part and pass almost directly downward to end in the short flat tendon forming this sling. The ventral muscle, which keeps this tendon in place, arises from the hypoischium and passes outward and upward to insert into that

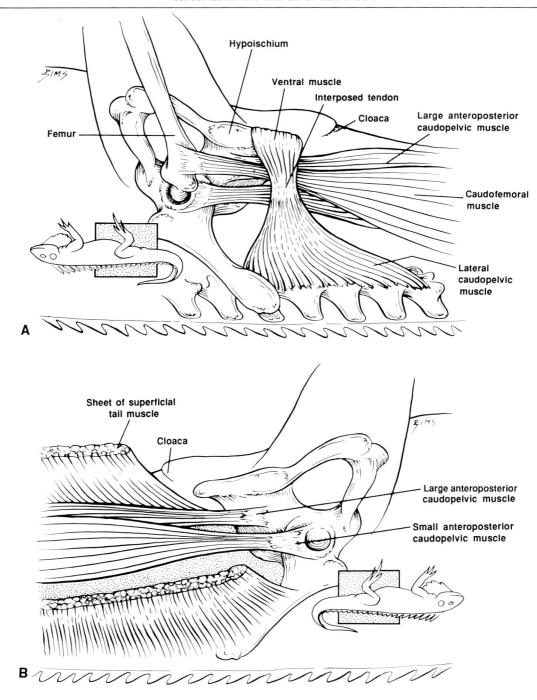

Fig. 1-9 A, Dissection of the iguana from the right side showing the caudofemoral muscle and the sling in position. The sling consists of a dorsal muscle, the lateral caudopelvic muscle, and a ventral muscle that arises from the ischium with an interposed tendon. **B,** Dissection of the iguana from the left side. The sheet of superficial tail musculature has been cut through and turned upward with the large anteroposterior caudopelvic muscle displaying the small anteroposterior caudopelvic muscle. The lateral caudopelvic muscle, the caudofemoral muscle, and the femur have been removed.

tendon. This mechanism, along with that of the other side, is capable of exerting bilateral compression upon the body cavity and the cloaca. Continence is achieved in the crocodile in essentially the same way.

In reptiles the advance in structure caused by an increase in general activity also correlates with a change in respiration. The ribs are embedded in the body wall musculature, which besides the recti consists of external and internal oblique and transversalis muscles. The ribs pass obliquely downward and backward almost as far as the pelvis; anteriorly their ventral ends are united to the sternum, while posteriorly they lie freely in the ventral part of the flank musculature. The transversalis muscle is placed between the pelvis and the anterior limit of the thorax. Its fibers cover the internal aspect of the ribs and pass transversely to the ventral midline, crossing the ribs obliquely. On the dorsal wall of the thorax, internally, a vertebrocostalis muscle is present on each side. These muscles arise from the vertebral column and pass obliquely outward and forward to insert into the ribs at their angles by slips that interdigitate with the attachment of the transversalis. During inspiration, because of the presence of ribs and the expansion of the forepart of the trunk (thorax), a much larger quantity of air enters and distends the lungs. During expiration, the function of the transversalis and vertebrocostal muscles is to increase intrathoracic pressure which, by compressing the thorax, results in the ejection of the respired air from the lungs. The abdominal wall musculature also participates in expiration. Without a rise in visceral pressure during expiration, the increase in intrathoracic pressure would as readily displace the lungs posteriorly into the abdomen as it would cause the ejection of air anteriorly, and decrease its effectiveness. Because of the greater internal pressure during expiration, the lungs are bodily compressed more and more anteriorly until they are displaced from their celomic location and become thoracic organs. In reptiles the musculature of the diaphragm separating the thorax from the abdomen is not present. The reptile's heart is shut off from the peritoneal cavity by the pericardium.

MAMMALIAN QUADRUPEDS

In the mammalian quadruped the body cavity containing the viscera is compartmentalized by interposing the thoracic diaphragm. With the two-compartment system, control over internal pressure is improved and oxygenation of the tissues better assured by the synchronous action of the abdominal wall musculature and the thoracic diaphragm.

Some anthropologists believe that the first mammals evolved parallel to the dinosaurs. These huge reptiles

kept the mammalian population suppressed; in order to survive, the bone structure was hardened and the limbs were placed directly beneath the weight-bearing centers for better running. Development of placental reproduction enabled a prolonged growth and maturation period inside of the uterus so that shortly after birth the young would be able to retreat from danger and survive. Although the evolutionary process solved the various problems by producing a closed pressure system, the pelvic floor remained a problem. Here nature had to contend with seals and counterseals to adapt to the emerging excretory, urinary, and reproductive tracts.

Smout and Jacoby[5] remind us that in the pronograde mammals the bony pelvic shelf formed by the symphysis pubis is largely responsible for sustaining the weight of the pelvic viscera, while the caudal muscles lying at right angles to the bony pelvic floor (the symphysis) guard the pelvic outlet against variations in intraabdominal pressure. The caudal muscles consist of the pubococcygeus, which arises from the iliopectineal line at the brim of the pelvis and the ischiococcygeus (homologous to the coccygeus in humans) which arises from the pelvic aspect of the ischial spine. These bilateral and symmetrically arranged striated muscles all insert into the root of the tail.

The root of the tail (coccygeal vertebrae) has a wide range of movement in the dorsoventral plane and controls the free part of the tail that extends distally from the tail root along the length of the tail. The caudal muscles are able to occlude the pelvic outlet efficiently, with or without movement of the tail. In the pronograde mammal, such as the dog, the pressure in the pelvis never becomes so great during the maintenance of normal postures to require additional support; but when the dog barks, leaps, or runs, the internal pressure in the pelvis increases, and for better control of this pressure the root of the tail is brought into apposition with the perineum. For instance, if we pick up a cat or a dog by the scruff of the neck and hold it vertically, the tail naturally takes this position. If we pull the tail away and let go, it returns immediately to the perineum. In these animals, the pelvic floor outlet is a vertical mesial slit formed by the posterior free margins of the pubococcygei that stretches from the midline of the symphysis pubis to the midline of the root of the tail (Fig. 1-10). This does not prevent the escape of visceral contents, since that is provided by the voluntary intrinsic sphincters of the rectum and the anal canal. The purpose is to maintain equal pressure to prevent visceral extrusion. Thus the caudal muscles not only perform movements of the tail, but they also increase intraabdominal pres-

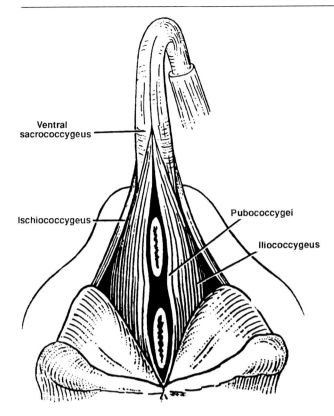

Fig. 1-10 External view of the pelvic floor of the dog showing the vertical mesial slit formed by the posterior free margins of the levator ani muscles (pubococcygei). The slit extends from the midline of the symphysis pubis to the midline of the root of the tail; the visceral canals are bilaterally compressed by muscular boundaries. The arrow indicates the position where the pubococcygei are tied together by some fibromuscular tissue passing from side to side between the vagina and the rectum.

sure and influence closure of the sphincters by their contraction.

The predatory habits of the carnivorous mammals cause marked rises of pressure in the pelvis, necessitating well-developed sphincters, pubococcygeal and iliococcygeal muscles, and a strong tail-closing apparatus. In herbivorous mammals pelvic pressure is never so great because of their relatively sedentary life. They do not tense their hindquarters in readiness to leap or use their limbs to strike down prey, and there is little need for great increases in internal pressure. Their pelvic outlets are located at the highest level of the abdominal cavity. Although the herbivore's sphincter development is adequate, the development of the pubococcygeal and iliococcygeal muscles is minimal. Thus it is lifestyle differences that explain the different closure of the pelvic outlet.

PRIMATES

As far as we know, the gibbon is the earliest known form in which the axis of the body is transformed from the pronograde to the orthograde posture. In this ancient form the remarkable changes which adapted the body to the upright posture are already evolved. All the ancient monkeys are of small size. The gibbon (Fig. 1-11), compared with those very early forms, is comparatively large; but when compared to man, the African anthropoids and the orangutan, it is small, being only a fifth to an eighth of their size (Fig. 1-12). The gibbon represents the stock from which the large-bodied anthropoids and man arose, probably some time before the beginning of the Miocene epoch. None of the existing anthropoids can be regarded as a human ancestor.

Although the human genealogic tree which we have constructed will be modified with future discoveries, the sequence of events in the evolution of the human body is becoming clear. Keith[1] suggested that "the great mass of his brain and his nude skin were evidently the latest of human acquisitions; the adaptation of the lower limbs for walking and the modification of his teeth to their present form were earlier modifications of his structure. The size of his body and structure were still older human features, while the chief structural

Fig. 1-11 Skeletal structure of the African gibbon.

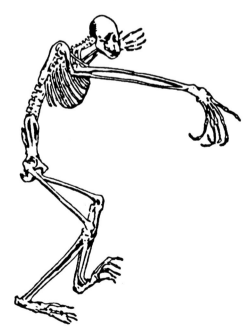

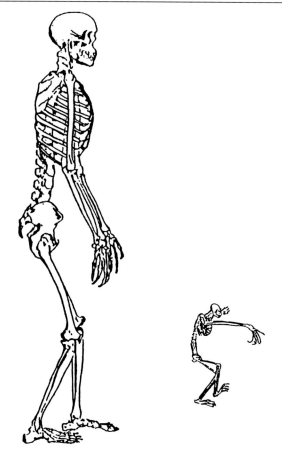

Fig. 1-12 Comparison of sizes of the skeletal structures of Australian man (left) and the African gibbon (right).

modifications to adapt the body to an upright or vertical posture, were of ancient origin."

In the assumption of the upright posture, the caudal muscles must support the pelvic viscera since the symphysis, which is largely responsible for this function in the pronograde, becomes part of the abdominal wall. As yet, the body had not completely adapted to the new way of living, and as long as the erect position was maintained the pelvic floor muscles had difficulty in meeting the greater variations in pressure produced by activity. In the early primates the internal pressures were controlled by forceful contractions of the caudal muscles that drew the root of the tail forward against the perineum and held it there. This was obviously an inefficient mechanism since the intense pressure imposed on the pelvic floor muscles must have limited the time during which they could remain in the erect posture. Further modification in the great apes and man led to the disappearance of what Paramore[3] had described

as "the perineal shutter of Sir Arthur Keith." Since the distal free part of the tail that protruded between the legs served no further purpose, it was discarded. Subsequently the coccygeal segments were flexed forward on the sacrum and incorporated into the closing mechanism of the pelvis. The caudal muscles that formerly guarded the bony outlet were now to form the pelvic floor.

Until the vertical posture had become habitual, the intense pressure imposed upon the pelvic floor muscles must have led to their fatigue from overuse. One might think that the muscles would respond by hypertrophy, but instead they degenerated. It was this degeneration that led to the regression of the muscular elements with a compensatory development of tendon and fascia. The pubococcygeus and coccygeus retained their primitive origin; the pubococcygeus mainly attached to the anococcygeal raphe, and the coccygeus muscle itself became more tendinous. The iliococcygeus lost its origin from the pelvic brim and moved to the side wall of the pelvis along the tendinous arch, which together with the pubococcygeus formed the compact levator ani muscle. All the caudal muscles retained their primitive insertion into the coccyx. Because of this regression, Fothergill[6] (1907) considered the pelvic muscles to be the vestigial remnants of the tail-moving muscles that were incapable of supporting the pelvic organs, and thus not useful in a repair operation. He had to postulate, therefore, that the cardinal ligaments are the main supports of the pelvic viscera. This regression came to a standstill as evidenced by the fact that the striated muscles of the pelvic floor remain a viable entity during the resting or static states. During activity and with the loss of the perineal shutter, the rises in pressure were great and tended to cause the escape of the viscera from the abdominopelvic cavity, as in prolapse and hernia. Further adaptations were required in the structure of the pelvic floor and the bony pelvis to support the pelvic viscera before a truly upright posture could be maintained. These adaptations are observable in the progressive changes of the pelvis from newborn to maturity.

MATURATION OF THE HUMAN FEMALE PELVIS

The Neonate

The pelvis in the newborn infant, unlike that in the adult, is somewhat funnel-shaped (Fig. 1-13). The sacrum is straight and vertical, the promontory absent,

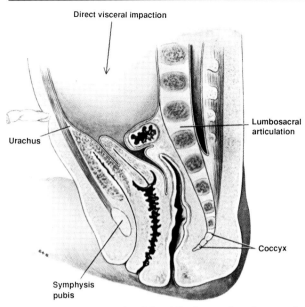

Fig. 1-13 Funnel-shaped pelvis of the human female neonate showing the direct impaction of abdominal pressure on the visceral mass directly above the pelvic floor outlet.

and the lumbosacral articulation is placed somewhat higher above the level of the pubes than in the adult. The coccyx has already become flexed. The pelvic cavity is almost parallel to the long axis of the abdominal cavity; it is long and narrow, both from front to back and from side to side, and is completely filled by the urethra, the vertically placed vagina and rectum, and by connective tissue. Because of the relatively small size of the cavity, the bladder and uterus are abdominal organs, and the cervix is high in the pelvis.

At birth, the start of respiration gives rise to a pressure in the abdominopelvic cavity that never ceases but changes with variable contractions of the thoracic diaphragm and the abdominal wall musculature. This pressure is augmented by the infant's crying, being held vertically, eating, and evacuation of stool. Because the pelvic cavity is almost in a straight line with the long axis of the abdominal cavity, the pressure produced directly compresses the visceral mass and is transmitted to the pelvic floor. Although direct impactions on the visceral mass tend to cause the organs in the abdominal cavity to enter the pelvis, they also tend to cause the escape of the viscera through the pelvic floor outlet. In the infant, we know that the pelvic floor retains the viscera in their normal positions by utilizing the same type of tissue (antagonistic muscles) against that which causes the rise in pressure. The pelvic floor muscula-

ture, like that of the abdominal wall and thoracic diaphragm, is connected with and controlled by the central nervous system. Striated muscle, of which the pelvic floor is largely composed, is capable of displaying a continuous tonus at rest and responds rapidly to the stress of excessive activity. During straining the pressure in the abdominopelvic cavity rises as an effect of the contraction of the abdominal wall and the simultaneous contraction of the pelvic floor musculature. The actions of the two are coordinated and integrated like all antagonistic groups of muscles, and by their concerted action give rise to the maintenance of a pressure equilibrium that keeps the organs in their normal location.

The Growing Child

When the growing child begins to walk, run, and play, the diaphragm becomes more muscular. The effect of a suddenly produced contraction of the diaphragm is to direct the visceral impaction somewhat forward toward the hypogastrium (Fig. 1-14A). Clinically this can be demonstrated by placing the hand on the lower abdomen and palpating its marked bulging on coughing. There is no doubt that the sudden excursions of pressure meet with the resistance of the anterior abdominal wall muscles and are reflected downward and posteriorly toward the lower sacrum, and the recurring impactions directed to the lower sacrum cause its concavity which becomes marked in the adult pelvis. This concavity is the result of two forces: (1) the visceral thrust from above, which is directed downward and backward, and (2) the forward pull of the pelvic floor musculature on the terminal part of the sacrum and on the coccyx away from its original vertical position. In this way the angulation of the vertebral column at the sacrum (lumbar lordosis) exaggerates the sacral promontory. Because of the lumbar lordosis, and thus the recession of the pelvic cavity from the abdominal wall, the pelvic and abdominal bones are no longer in the same vertical plane but become angulated at the superior strait of the pelvic inlet. Since the sacrum bears the brunt of visceral impactions, the pelvic floor musculature itself is safeguarded from the full effect of sudden visceral thrusts.

Modification of the pelvic structure occurs. The pelvic floor aperture (the genital or levator hiatus), is no longer a longitudinal slit extending throughout the length of the pelvic floor as in pronograde mammals such as the dog. It now becomes confined to the lowest level of the anterior part of the floor, so prolapse of the viscera is much less likely to occur. In the erect posture, the pelvic floor does not form a sling in the normal

Fig. 1-14 **A,** Abdominopelvic cavity in the mesial saggital plane showing the direction of visceral impactions (arrows) produced by sudden increased contraction of the diaphragm. The lower arrow indicates their deflection by the resistance of the lower abdominal wall into the curve of the sacrum posteriorly. **B,** Lateral view of the visceral canal passing through the pelvic floor aperture showing the mechanism of closure of this aperture by the puborectalis. Note that in the erect posture, **A,** the pelvic floor musculature is almost horizontal.

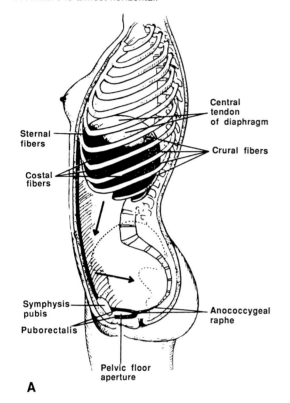

A

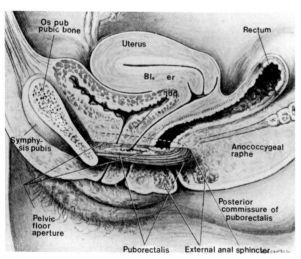

B

woman as much as it forms an almost flat plate. This floor slopes downward and forward from its attachment to the coccyx in a gentle curve toward the pubes, here becoming almost horizontal (Fig. 1-14B). The upper surface of the pubic bones and symphysis slope backward and slightly downward to meet the pelvic floor at its lowest level, and situated here medially and centrally is the aperture abutting the pubic bones.

The intrapelvic urethra, vagina, and rectum pass through this aperture to gain access to the external surface of the body. This is reached after the excretory viscera traverse the superficial tissue, in which they now diverge. Here their terminations are surrounded by the voluntary sphincter mechanisms and come into relationship with the superficial muscles.

The Adolescent

The measurements of the hiatus at rest are quite small, but at times become stretched and extremely dilated according to the volume of the visceral contents to be passed, such as during the delivery of the fetal head through the birth canal. An almost new muscle appears, the puborectalis, segmented off from the pubococcygeus. This muscle together with the pubococcygeus forms the boundaries of the hiatus, and guards the pelvic viscera from extrusion through the pelvic floor aperture. During activity the greater pressure reaches the hiatus in the levator muscles indirectly by reflection from the sacrum and diffusion through the visceral mass, thereby becoming attenuated. On reaching the aperture, the musculature guarding the hiatus contracts, thereby narrowing the hiatus and normally tends to prevent escape of the viscera. Thus it is the variable and constant thoracoabdominal and pelvic pressures which determine the change in shape of the pelvis, the evolution of its floor, and the position of its aperture by which these pressures can be successfully withstood and an equilibrium maintained.

The Adult Female

Anatomists have described the pelvic walls and floor as forming the sides of a steep funnel with a large aperture at its lowest part and the pelvic viscera situated to a considerable extent over the pelvic aperture (Fig. 1-15A). This is true in the dead. In the cadaver, the loss of muscle tone and elongation of the muscle fibers results in a considerable descent of the pelvic floor with increased obliquity of the coccyx and enlargement of the aperture. Similar conditions are found in the living in whom the pelvic floor has been damaged by child-

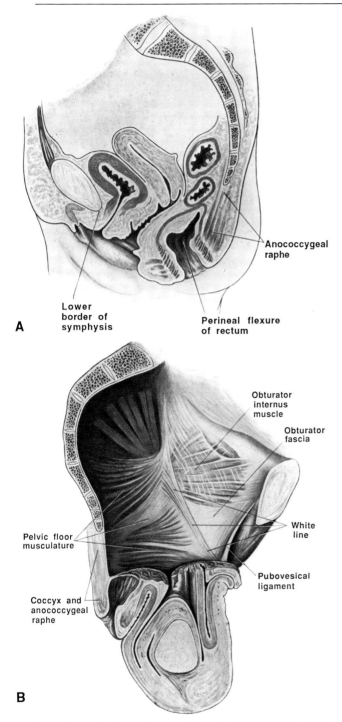

A

Lower border of symphysis

Anococcygeal raphe

Perineal flexure of rectum

Obturator internus muscle

Obturator fascia

White line

Pubovesical ligament

Pelvic floor musculature

Coccyx and anococcygeal raphe

B

Fig. 1-15 **A**, Section of the pelvis showing descent of the pelvic floor and simulation of a funnel caused by postmortem relaxation of the musculature. **B**, Section of a pelvis with advanced prolapse showing the transformation of the pelvic cavity into a funnel from pathologic causes. The coccyx is almost vertical and most of the pelvic floor musculature is atrophic. Note that the white line (insertion of levator ani) has become detached from the area of the symphysis and elongation and thickening of the pubovesical ligament has occurred.

birth or weakened by other conditions which predispose to prolapse of the viscera through the pelvic floor aperture (Fig. 1-15B). In these cases, that part of the pelvic floor musculature which attaches to the coccyx, having lost its muscle tone, causes the coccyx and the anococcygeal raphe to become more or less vertical according to the yield of the musculature inserted into it; also, the concavity of the sacrum may be reduced. Such pelves are typically funnel shaped.

The pelvic cavity in the normal living human does not present the appearance of a funnel. In these, the outline of the cavity in the median sagittal plane is curvilinear, and approaches a semicircle except for a bulge posteriorly in the region of the sacrum (Fig. 1-16). As we know, the change in shape of the sacrum, that is, its concavity, and the pelvic floor, instead of dipping downward in a funnel-like way passes from its attachment to the coccyx downward and forward in a gentle curve toward the pelvic floor aperture and by its sides to the pubes. Because of the physiologic properties of striated muscles, the pelvic floor manifests a tonic contraction that is continuous although it varies under different conditions. Thus instead of a funnel leading to the aperture, the pelvic cavity in the median plane resembles a section of a truncated cone (or parabola) the long axis of which passes approximately through the center of the pelvic inlet obliquely to its plane much more backward than downward, reaching the junction of the fourth and fifth sacral vertebrae represented by the line A–B (Fig. 1-16). This long axis, projecting in the

Fig. 1-16 The normal pelvic cavity in the anteroposterior plane resembles a section of a parabola, the long axis of which (A–B), instead of being vertical, passes more backward and downward.

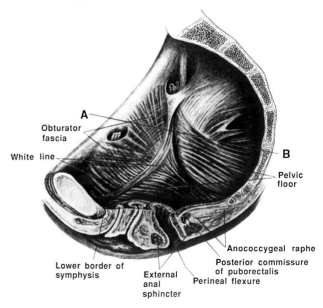

A

Obturator fascia

White line

B

Pelvic floor

Anococcygeal raphe

Posterior commissure of puborectalis

Perineal flexure

Lower border of symphysis

External anal sphincter

opposite direction, passes through the hypogastrium and strikes the lower part of the abdominal wall, which has considerable clinical significance (Halban and Tandler, 1907).[10]

The downward thrust from above plays the major role that forces the uterus and bladder, which are abdominal organs in the newborn, into the pelvis. It is a slow process that begins in infancy. Their descent correlates with the distention of the pelvic cavity itself. The distention is also an adaptation because in the infant and child the immature pelvis is not strong enough to resist the pressure. These phenomena explain the posterior bulging, the recession of the pelvis and the marked concavity of the sacrum, which are not explained by the pull of the muscles used in standing, walking and running, and the weight of the legs. They explain the enlargement of the pelvic cavity transversely, which occurs below and behind the level of the femoral thrust. With growth the pelvis bulges, but in the adult this is resisted with increased strength caused by further osseous and muscular development achieving equilibrium.

Development of the Levator Ani

It is reasonable to expect that the levator ani would be a variable feature of the pelvic floor anatomy when we reflect on its phylogeny and regression which occurred when the primates assumed the orthograde position. Thompson[7] compared the morphology of the levator ani in the tailed apes and humans and pointed out the reduction in mass and thickness of the posterior portion of the muscle after the disappearance of the tail, which is wholly converted into fibrous tissue so that only the lateral and anterior parts exist. It was claimed that the change to the orthograde posture and the dragging forward of the visceral canals to the lowest level of the pelvic floor exposed the aperture to a much greater pressure and thus to the increased tendency to visceral protrusion. In consequence, the pubococcygeus was profoundly modified so that a large number of fibers, losing their connection with the coccyx, pass around the rectum to form a sling. Holl[8] gave these fibers the name of puborectalis or sphincter ani. The anatomic dissections performed by Paramore[2] showed that the muscle surrounding the aperture in the pelvic floor is much more conspicuous than that situated laterally. The thickness of the musculature really consists of two distinct parts: the pubococcygeus which is more or less in the same plane as, and continues posteriorly with, the rest of the pelvic floor musculature (the iliococcygeus and coccygeus); and the puborectalis, situated just below this in a different plane. Both arise from the pubic

bones more or less horizontally and form the medial borders of the genital or levator hiatus. The intrapelvic urethra, the vagina, and the rectum pass through this aperture to reach the external surface of the body. This is reached after the excretory viscera traverse the superficial tissues where they now diverge. As they leave the hiatus, the viscera are provided with sphincter mechanisms which also serve to stabilize and support them in their short journey to reach the perineum. The muscles and fascia of the perineum are commonly referred to as the inferior or urogenital diaphragm. Its action and that of the superior diaphragm are well coordinated. This muscle group derives its origin from the cloacal sphincter muscle which is intimately related to the levator ani muscle, and both are ultimately derived from the third and fourth sacral myotomes. Since the cloaca gives origin to the muscle group composing the urogenital diaphragm and the external anal sphincter, the embryological development of these structures needs to be reviewed.

Embryological Development of the Pelvic Floor

By the fifteenth day after fertilization the implanted human embryo is a flat bilaminar disc consisting of two layers of cells, a columnar ectoderm forming the floor of the amniotic cavity and a layer of flattened endodermal cells comprising the roof of the yolk sac. Early in the third week of embryonic life, in the midline of the future caudal end, the embryonal cells of the primitive streak sink below the surface and spread out laterally between the ectoderm and endoderm to form the mesoderm, the middle layer of the embryonic disc. There are two remaining sites in the midline of the embryo where the mesoderm fails to separate the ectoderm from the adherent underlying endoderm. One of these bilaminar regions is found cephalad to the developing notochord and is destined to become the oropharyngeal membrane; the other lies caudal to the primitive streak and forms the cloacal membrane located in the ventral portion of the embryo caudal to the genital tubercle.

In the early embryo the allantois and the hind gut terminate in a common cavity, the cloaca. An ectodermal depression develops under the root of the tail and sinks in toward the gut until only the thin cloacal membrane remains between the gut and the outside. This ectodermal depression is called the proctoderm. The division of the cloaca is affected by the development of the urorectal fold that grows caudally toward the cloacal membrane. As the ingrowth of this fold cuts progressively deeper into the cloaca, a wedge-shaped mass of mesenchyme accompanies it and forms a dense septum (the urorectal septum) between the urogenital sinus anteriorly and the rectum posteriorly. This separation of the cloaca is completed before the cloacal membrane ruptures so that its two parts open independently.

Power[4] referred to the investigations of Eggeling (1886) and Popovsky (1889), who held the opinion that with the formation of the common cloaca, the orifice of its cavity is surrounded by a sphincter muscle. The appearance of this muscle as a distinct entity can first be seen in a two-month embryo and, although for the most part it completely surrounds the orifice of the urogenital sinus and anus, a few fibers begin to decussate between the two openings. In this way the primitive cloacal sphincter begins to divide into an external anal sphincter behind and a sphincter of the urogenital sinus in front.

The sphincter ani may be differentiated into several layers and becomes a trilaminar muscle. The urogenital sphincter also differentiates but in a more decisive manner. Slowly after the urogenital sinus opens on the surface of the embryo, the ventral end of the sphincter becomes slightly attached to the precartilaginous anlage of the pubic os. When the sinus (the ventral division of the cloaca) first opens to the outside, it differentiates into the urethra. Consequently, the ventral part of the urogenital sphincter develops into the urethral sphincter and migrates to a deeper plane. At a later date the fused end of the Müllerian ducts, which have made contact with the dorsal surface of the urogenital sinus, descend along the posterior wall of the sinus to form the vagina. The dorsal end of the urogenital sphincter surrounds the opening of the primitive vagina and becomes the vaginal sphincter (bulbocavernosus muscle) which retains a tendinous raphe in the midline and probably gives rise to the perineal superficial and deep muscles. A similar opinion is shared that the deep perineal muscles are the last of the perineal muscles to appear in the human embryo and that most of its development occurs postnatally. Because the urethral and vaginal sphincters are attached ventrally to the primitive pubis it is from there that the ischiocavernosus muscle develops.

Functional Aspects of the Urogenital Diaphragm

There is very little known of the origin of the urogenital diaphragm. Langman[9] has shown that in the human embryo the muscle mass is covered on both aspects by a primitive connective tissue and is poorly developed.

Later, in response to functional requirements and physical activities, it probably becomes the strong fascial sheets of connective tissue constituting the urogenital diaphragm. Davies[11] describes the urogenital diaphragm as a continuity of the endopelvic connective tissue. According to Power[4] "this statement does not contribute to its origin, but shows that the various fascial layers in the pelvis are continuous with each other—a very usual occurrence throughout the whole body."

The voluntary muscles of the outlet, because of their common origin, sometimes exhibit a trilaminar structure corresponding to that of the abdominal wall. This is illustrated best by the external anal sphincter. Thompson[7] describes the sphincter in its most differentiated form as trilaminar, but occasionally, particularly in women, there are two separate layers. Because of their morphogenesis, all the muscles have similar nerve supplies and exhibit comparable reflex physiologic functions. Early in development their primary function is to contain the closed contents, whereas in the adult this has been largely modified and their main function is to provide the means whereby the involuntary excretory viscera can be brought under voluntary control, namely to establish continence and voluntary defecation. The dual functions require a storage reservoir, a sphincter mechanism to control the outflow of the reservoir, a sensory mechanism so that an awareness of rectal filling reaches the conscious level and another mechanism whereby the evacuation of stool is under voluntary control. In the course of development, the terminal part of the alimentary canal is surrounded by skeletal muscular sphincters. Because of the dual origin of the anorectal mechanism (one visceral and the other somatic) this specialized region is complicated from both anatomic and physiologic points of view.

The anal canal, approximately 2.5 to 4.0 cm in length, is composed of mucosa, submucosa, an internal sphincter and longitudinal muscle; it is innervated by the autonomic nervous system and therefore not subject to voluntary control. The innervation is through branches of the pudendal nerve which not only provide a continuing resting tonus to the musculature but also come into play as antagonistic muscles in response to increases in intraabdominal pressure.

The upper half of the anal canal is lined by columnar celled, mucus-secretory endodermal epithelium. In the course of embryonic development ectoderm migrates into the lower half of the canal where it is lined by stratified squamous epithelium and is very sensitive; it is richly supplied with nerve filaments from the inferior hemorrhoidal branches of the pudendal nerve. This innervation enables the mucosa to act as a sensory component of the mechanism of continence. The slightest stimulation causes reflex contraction of the external sphincters.

The longitudinal muscle coat of the rectum is continued below into the wall of the anal canal and is inserted into the skin of the anal margin. The inner circular muscle coat of the rectum progressively thickens as it extends downward and at the pectinate line forms the powerful internal sphincter muscle that invests the anal canal. Parks[12] states that physiologically it exists in a continuously tonic state unlike circular muscle elsewhere, and is certainly responsible for part of the maintained closure of the anal canal.

The external anal sphincter makes an important contribution to the tonic closure of the anal canal. It maintains tone during waking hours, it is minimal in sleep, and the magnitude of tone corresponds with any maneuver that elevates intraabdominal pressure except for straining at defecation when the tone decreases. Both the pelvic floor and the external anal sphincter respond reflexively.

SUMMARY

The evolutionary process is a biologic continuum. Although we assume that the highest evolved form of life is homo sapiens, all historical evidence from fossils and other sources indicates that because only the fittest survive, further evolution is inevitable. Without change the species becomes extinct. The human female has evolved in such a way that she is able to overcome the stress of gravity in the erect biped posture and yet is still able to deliver babies with large brains, enabling life-long learning. Unfortunately this causes trauma to the pelvic floor during childbirth and the weakest spot in the pelvic floor, the vagina, becomes the progenitor of subsequent pelvic relaxation. In the past women with small pelves and a genetic predisposition for large babies were dealt with by nature in the same way that all

weak traits are treated—they died in labor. Thus the weakness was eliminated. The development of modern obstetrics with instrumental and operative delivery now allows such women to survive. The trauma of delivery, perhaps unnoticed at the time, damages the muscles and fascia of the pelvic floor. Most women compensate through their reproductive lives, but ultimately nature delivers the final blow by withdrawing her hormones, leading to atrophy and eventual prolapse. Since menopause is a natural condition of civilization complicated by increased life span, then prolapse also represents a response to intervention in a normal if wasteful process. Is medical intervention interfering with a process of evolution where only the fittest should survive? Review of the evolution of our species may determine where the seeds of our own possible destruction were sewn.

REFERENCES

1. Keith A. Certain phases in the evolution of man. *Br Med J.* 1912;88:788–790.
2. Paramore RH. *The Statics of the Female Pelvic Viscera.* London: H.R. Lewis Company; 1918;1:348–349.
3. Paramore RH. The evolution of the pelvic floor in nonmammalian vertebrates and pronograde mammals. *Lancet.* 1910;1:98, 1393–1399.
4. Power RMH. The embryological development of the levator ani muscle. *Am J Obstet Gynecol.* 1948;55(3):367–381.
5. Smout CVF, Jacoby F. *Gynecological and Obstetrical Anatomy and Functional Histology.* 3rd ed. Baltimore: Williams & Wilkins; 1953:76–77.
6. Fothergill WE. On the pathology and the operative treatment of the pelvic viscera. *J Obstet Gynaecol Brit Emp.* 1907;13:410–419.
7. Thompson P. *Myology of the Pelvic Floor.* Manchester, England: Victoria University Press; 1899.
8. Holl M. Die Muskeln und Fascien des Beckenausganges. In: Bardeleben H, ed. *Handbuch der Anatomie des Menchen.* Jena, Germany: Fischer; 1897;7:2.
9. Langman J. *Formation of the Mesodermal Area in Medical Embryology.* 4th ed. Baltimore: Williams & Wilkins; 1982: 47.
10. Halban J, Tandler J. *Anatomie und Etiology der Genital Prolapse Been Weibe.* Wilhelm Braumuller; Wien und Leipzig; 1907.
11. Davies, GW. Abdominal and pelvic fascia with surgical application. *Surg Gynec Obstet.* 1932;54:495.
12. Parks AG. Anorectal incontinence. *Proc Roy Soc Med.* 1975; 68:681–690.

CHAPTER 2

Anatomy of Genital Support

John O. L. DeLancey   A. Cullen Richardson

INTRODUCTION

The surgical procedures that are commonly employed to correct genital prolapse were developed during an era when antibiotics and blood transfusions were not available, and when anesthesia was often lethal. Because of the risk of abdominal exploration without these supporting services, as well as the possibility of postoperative intraabdominal sepsis, these operations were performed by the vaginal route. Surgical procedures were devised through an empiric approach to these problems and were not based on any particular anatomic observations concerning the nature of genital prolapse.

Over the past century the advent of safe anesthesia, blood transfusion, and antibiotics has provided us with the opportunity to approach the problems of pelvic organ prolapse in any one of a number of ways. The most rational approach to deciding on surgical therapy is to understand the mechanism of normal support and then to determine the ways in which it has failed. Once these two factors are understood, then a surgical approach that addresses these individual problems can be undertaken.[1] This chapter will describe the different parts of the supportive mechanism which will allow each individual part to be assessed and their specific defects appreciated.

GENERAL PRINCIPLES OF SUPPORT

Although the details of the pelvic floor will be described later, it is important to define what we mean by this somewhat general term. The top of the pelvic floor is the peritoneum that covers the pelvic viscera and walls, and the bottom of the floor is the skin of the vulva, perineum, and buttocks (Fig. 2-1A). It is composed of several structures arranged in general layers. The pelvic viscera, along with their attachments to the pelvic walls through the endopelvic fascia, form the first layer. Below this lies the levator ani muscles that form a diaphragm across the pelvic cavity with a cleft in its anterior portion through which the urethra, lower vagina, and anus exit. Next is the urogenital diaphragm (perineal membrane) that spans the anterior portion of the pelvic outlet and connects the perineal body to the ischiopubic rami (Fig. 2-1B). It also helps to affix the lower urethra to these bones. Finally, the bulbocavernosus, ischiocavernosus, and superficial transverse perineal muscles lie in the superficial area of the anterior outlet while in the posterior portion of the outlet, the anal sphincter is found. Together these structures form the floor that seals off the lower aspect of the pelvic cavity.

In order to understand the role of the pelvic floor, it is necessary to appreciate its unique position in the

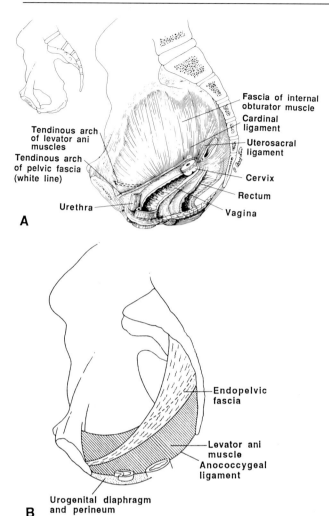

A

B

Fig. 2-1 **A**, Sagittal view of the pelvic floor. Inset shows orientation of drawing. **B** shows the layering of support.

It is evident from summarizing these layers that there are three types of tissue in the pelvic floor: striated muscle, fibromuscular tissue, and fibrous tissue. The striated muscles are under voluntary control, and are capable of rapid contraction in response to increases in load. In addition, like the external anal sphincter, they exhibit resting activity, so that they provide constant support even at rest. The various portions of the endopelvic fascia and visceral ligaments contain smooth muscle and are properly termed fibromuscular tissue. Although traditionally thought to consist of primarily fibrous tissue, only a quick inspection under the microscope is needed to realize the error of this view. Abundant quantities of smooth muscle are embedded within a fibrous matrix, and in many areas it predominates. This smooth muscle, although little studied, must modulate the activities of this complex sustentacular apparatus. There are certain areas of the pelvic connective tissue, however, where pure dense regular collagen is found. These structures are truly fibrous tissue and include the tendinous arch of the pelvic fascia and the fasciae over the obturator internus muscle.

It is a fundamental principle that all soft tissue struc-

Fig. 2-2 Sagittal view of the abdominopelvic cavity showing the position of the pelvic floor at the bottom of this space. Dashed line indicates the posterior extent of the peritoneal cavity. Details of abdominal wall layering at two different layers are shown to the left.

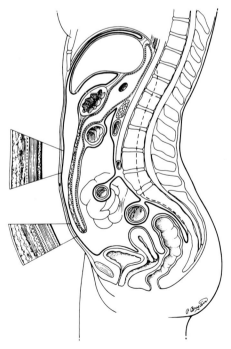

body. The abdominopelvic cavity has a cylindrical shape. Its top is formed by the respiratory diaphragm, while the vertebral column and muscles, along with the abdominal wall muscles, make up its sides. The pelvic floor forms the bottom of this cylinder and it is upon this pelvic floor that the support of the contents of the abdominopelvic cavity depend for support (Fig. 2-2). Rather than being an uninterrupted layer like the uninterrupted walls of the abdomen, the pelvic floor is traversed by the urethra, vagina (in the female) and the rectum. Therefore, it must not only support the pelvic and abdominal organs during the stress of increases in abdominal pressure, but it must also allow for opening of the pelvic floor to accommodate various excretory functions and parturition.

tures within the body depend upon their attachments to bone for support. The pelvic floor is no different than any other region in this regard. All of the support offered by the pelvic floor depends on its connection to the pelvic bones. Without this connection to the skeletal framework it would not exist. This chapter describes not only the fascial and muscular layers, but also considers how they are attached to their bony superstructure. This is important not only to an understanding of anatomy, but also to understanding where breaks in this system of support occur.

The structure of the pelvic floor and its attachments to the pelvic bones are an evolutionary solution to the need for support of the abdominal and pelvic organs that lie over the large opening of the pelvic canal. There are two forces that the pelvic floor must oppose in providing this support: gravity and increases in abdominal pressure. Of these two, the latter is by far the most important in the development of prolapse. In cases of prolapse, the organs don't fall out, but rather they are pushed out. Understanding the structure of the pelvic floor and how it resists these forces is critical to understanding the diagnosis and management of pelvic support defects. This chapter describes the structures that are responsible for these tasks.

OVERVIEW OF SUPPORT

The Mechanism of Prolapse

Before beginning a detailed description of pelvic anatomy it is helpful to take a look at the structural concepts that are involved in pelvic support. A mechanical analogy can help with an understanding of the process of genital prolapse. All forms of gynecologic prolapse involve downward protrusion of the vaginal wall through the pelvic floor. The vagina is normally in a position, relative to the abdominal cavity, similar to an in-turned finger of a surgical glove, as Bonney pointed out.[2] This "invaginated" finger can be turned outward by compressing the air within the glove driving the finger downward. This concept is illustrated in Fig. 2-3. There are three mechanical means by which this can be prevented: constriction, suspension, and a flap valve closure.

Constriction of the lower portion of the invagination occludes the opening through which prolapse would occur. Its suspension to the walls of the enclosed space attaches it in such a way that downward prolapse is impossible. The flap valve closure acts by pinning the invagination against the inner wall of the cavity. In this

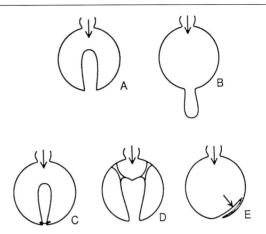

Fig. 2-3 The mechanical aspects of support. **A** is an invagination within an enclosed space. **B** shows a pressure increase, causing eversion. The following mechanisms prevent eversion: **C** Constriction of the pelvic floor; **D** Suspension of the vagina from the pelvic walls; **E** Positioning of the vagina over the pelvic wall that results in a flap valve closure.

way, increases in pressure within the cavity force the invagination against the wall, thereby trapping it in place. This is an unusually strong mechanism because the greater the increase in pressure, the greater the force pinning the invagination in place. It is evident that the flap valve closure is the by-product of suspension and the position of the pelvic floor.

The tissues of the pelvic floor act through a combination of these three mechanisms. The fibromuscular tissue of the endopelvic fascia that constitutes the cardinal and uterosacral ligaments, as well as the pubocervical fascia, acts to suspend the cervix and the vagina within the cavity of the pelvis. Constriction is provided by the levator ani muscles. The medial portion of this muscle forms a U-shaped strap that begins on the pubic bone and passes around the back of the rectum to return to the pubic bone on the other side. Contraction of this muscle constricts the lumen of the vagina by pulling it forward against the pubic bone and closing the pelvic floor.

The flap valve mechanism results from the suspension of the vagina by the cardinal and uterosacral ligaments in the posterior pelvis and by the anterior traction of the levator ani muscles. These opposing forces keep the apex of the vagina and the cervix over the levator plate, thereby keeping it in the position where flap-valve closure may occur.[3] It is probable that any one of these mechanisms can be defective and yet the others can work satisfactorily, resulting in satisfactory support. Once the synergistic nature of these different components fails, then progressive damage to the overall support mechanism leads to manifest prolapse.

Therefore, there are several different aspects to the support mechanism. These correspond to the layers of the pelvic floor mentioned earlier. In the first layer, the viscera are connected to the pelvic walls by a fibromuscular suspensory apparatus of ligaments and fasciae. Below this layer, a horizontal diaphragm of strong muscle closes off the pelvic cavity and pinches the viscera closed against the pubic bones. Finally, superficial transverse perineal, bulbocavernosus, and external anal sphincter muscles as well as the perineal membrane help maintain the viscera in place and constrict their lumens.

Anatomy of Support

In order to understand the structures that make up this floor, a brief description of the pelvic walls will assist in comprehending their lateral attachments. The ischial spines are a key structure in understanding the pelvic floor. They lie in a plane that spans the pelvic cavity and where many important parts of the pelvic floor are attached. This level is roughly diamond shaped with the spines at the lateral point (Fig. 2-4). Extending posteriorly from the spines are the sacrospinous ligaments. They form the lower border of the fixed pelvic walls and the posterior limit of the pelvic diaphragm. Extending anteriorly from the spines is a fibrous band, the tendinous arch, that attaches anteriorly to the lower portion of the pubic bone. As this band nears its anterior end, it splits into two portions: one is the tendinous arch of the pelvic fascia, from which the pubocervical fascia arises; the other is the tendinous arch of the levator ani, from which the levator ani muscles arise.

Fig. 2-4 Fascial and muscular layers of the pelvic floor.

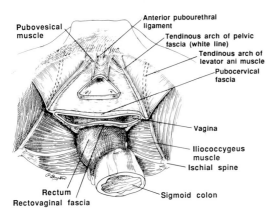

Pubovesical muscle
Anterior pubourethral ligament
Tendinous arch of pelvic fascia (white line)
Tendinous arch of levator ani muscle
Pubocervical fascia
Vagina
Iliococcygeus muscle
Ischial spine
Rectum
Rectovaginal fascia
Sigmoid colon

These fibrous bands lie on the inner surface of the obturator membrane. Above this layer are the ligaments that suspend the viscera, and below this layer are the perineal membrane and the muscles of the pelvic outlet.

Ligaments and Fasciae

The ligaments and fasciae that suspend the pelvic organs are not ligaments like those in the knee, or fasciae like the rectus sheath covering the rectus abdominus muscles. Each of these latter structures are made of dense regular collagen that is organized in parallel fibers aligned along lines of force. The ligaments of the pelvic organs are visceral ligaments and are a felt-like meshwork of fibrous tissue that contains considerable quantities of smooth muscle. Although their fibers generally lie along lines of tension, they are far less regular than the fibers of true tendons.

The endopelvic fascia is one continuous body of connective tissue. There are innumerable regional names that have been applied to various portions of this tissue, and often are more confusing than they are useful. We will restrict our comments to the functionally important aspects of this tissue.

The easiest way to understand the connections of the uterus and the vagina to the pelvic walls is to recall their embryologic derivation. The paramesonephric ducts begin as small paired tubes, similar to segments of intestine, that are attached laterally to the pelvic walls by a small mesentery. As they come to the midline, they pull their mesentery along with them until they meet in the midline and fuse. As is true with a segment of intestine, there are vessels in the mesentery, and these form the adnexal, uterine, and vaginal vessels. The fibrous sheet of the mesentery becomes the cardinal and uterosacral ligaments that attach the cervix and upper vagina to the pelvic walls. Lower in the pelvis where the vagina nears the pelvic wall, they represent the pubocervical fascia. In this way there is a sheet of fibrous tissue that attaches each side of the genital tract to the pelvic side walls.

The uppermost portion of this suspension apparatus is composed of the cardinal and uterosacral ligaments and their downward continuation to blend with the pubocervical fascia (Figs. 2-5, 2-6). These are two aspects of a single structure. As previously mentioned, they are composed of an admixture of smooth muscle and connective tissue. The cardinal ligament portion of this complex is primarily perivascular connective tissue that runs along the uterine vessels,[4] while the uterosacral ligaments are predominantly smooth muscle and fibrous tissue.[5] The cardinal ligaments arise from the

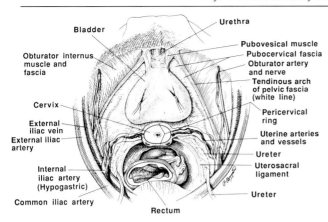

Fig. 2-5 Cardinal and uterosacral ligaments and pubocervical fascia.

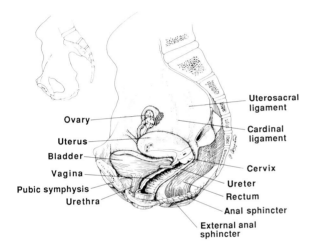

Fig. 2-6 Sagittal view of the upward suspension provided by the cardinal and uterosacral ligaments. Inset shows orientation of drawing.

area of the greater sciatic foramen, while the uterosacral ligaments extend to originate from the second through fourth sacral vertebrae. They invest the cervix, forming a pericervical ring, and extend downward to envelop and suspend the upper portion of the vagina. These ligaments suspend the cervix to the pelvic walls through their attachments to the pericervical ring.

In addition to attachments to the vagina and cervix, these suspensory ligaments have a portion which envelops the base of the bladder as the cardinal ligaments of the bladder. As the bladder is separated from the cervix and vagina, this band can be made visible, and is called the *bladder pillar*.

As previously mentioned, there is no separation between the cardinal and uterosacral ligaments. The uter-

osacral ligaments form the medial borders of the two cardinal-uterosacral ligament complexes and as such form a distinct boundary. It is this edge that appears as a sharp well-defined line when seen at laparotomy or laparoscopy, or felt on pelvic examination. The cardinal ligament extends laterally from this, and is not palpable because a finger cannot be brought to bear on its exposed surface.

As these fibrous tissues extend along the vagina their attachments gradually change from suspending the viscera upwards, as is true of the cardinal ligaments, and begin to attach the vagina laterally to the tendinous arch of the pelvic fascia (Fig. 2-5). This is the transition from the cardinal/uterosacral ligaments to the pubocervical fascia that is formed by the lateral connection of the pubocervical fascia at the tendinous arch to the pelvic side wall.

The midportion of the vagina comes into closer contact with the pelvic walls than the upper portion that is suspended by the cardinal/uterosacral complex. This portion of the vagina forms a transverse flattened oval attached at each side to the pelvic wall (Fig. 2-4). The front of this is formed by the pubocervical fascia and the back by the rectovaginal septum. The pubocervical fascia is bounded posteriorly where it blends with the cardinal ligaments. Laterally and anteriorly it attaches to the tendinous arch of the pelvic fascia. These latter structures are fibrous bands that are suspended from the lower portion of the pubic symphysis, located one centimeter from the midline and one centimeter above the pubic arch, to the ischial spine. The urethra pierces the pubocervical fascia in its anterior portion to exit the pelvis. The pubocervical fascia has abundant smooth muscle embedded within it, and varies in its development from one region to another.

Posteriorly the rectovaginal septum is a sheet of fibromuscular tissue that lies adjacent to the vagina.[6] It is found ventral to the rectovaginal space. Superiorly it blends with the cardinal/uterosacral complex that suspends its upper portions, while inferiorly it fuses with the perineal body. Laterally it attaches to the superior fascia of the pelvic diaphragm.

Muscles

The pubococcygeus and iliococcygeus are the muscles that support the pelvic viscera (Fig. 2-7) and together they are referred to as the levator ani muscles. A preferable term for the pubococcygeus would be the pubovisceral muscle[7] because it has several components that attach to the pelvic viscera, including ones properly

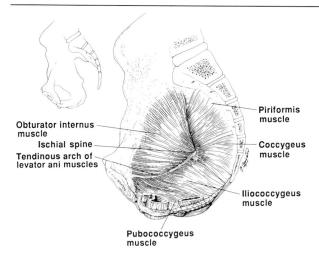

Obturator internus
muscle
Ischial spine
Tendinous arch of
levator ani muscles

Piriformis
muscle

Coccygeus
muscle

Iliococcygeus
muscle

Pubococcygeus
muscle

Fig. 2-7 Levator ani muscles (pubococcygeus and iliococcygeus). Inset shows orientation of drawing.

referred to as pubovaginalis, puborectalis, and pubococcygeus, although the latter term is used so commonly that we will not abandon it here. The important thing is to understand what it is and what the muscle does. The pubococcygeus muscles begin on the inner surface of the pubic bones, pass down into the anus between the internal and external sphincters, form a sling around the dorsal aspect of the anorectal junction, and return to the pubic bone on the other side. The medial portion of these muscles is attached to the vagina as it passes beside its lumen and the portion of the muscle between the vagina and the pubic bone is known as the pubovaginalis. There is no direct attachment of these muscles to the urethra. This is a considerable bulk of muscle that on dissection or cross section has a relatively pale color, suggesting that it is a fast twitch muscle capable of rapid contraction.

The flat iliococcygeus muscle begins from a membranous insertion to the inner surface of the obturator internus muscle at the tendinous arch of the levator ani. It is darker in color, suggesting a slow twitch high oxidative composition. The two sheets from either side are joined in a midline raphe just above the anal-coccygeal raphe. The coccygeus muscle is fixed in position by its bony origin and insertions on either side and is not mobile. It is therefore not included in the terminology of the levator ani (although it is part of the pelvic diaphragm). That portion of the pubococcygeus that attaches to the coccyx and the junction of the two iliococcygeal muscles form a shelflike portion of the pelvic floor behind the anus and in front of the coccyx. This has been referred to clinically as the levator plate

and its angle of inclination reflects the activity of both the pubococcygeus muscles as well as the iliococcygei. This is the shelf that the pelvic viscera rest on.

Physiologic studies have clearly demonstrated that the levator ani group of muscles is similar to the external anal sphincter and that it exhibits constant activity.[8] This is true even at rest, in contrast to the usual voluntary muscles that are active primarily when willfully contracted. The activity of these muscles provides a resilient and functional shelf on which the other viscera may rest.

Support of the Pelvic Outlet

Lying below the level of the levator ani muscles is the urogenital diaphragm. Previous descriptions of the urogenital diaphragm as a trilaminar structure with two layers of fascia separated by the deep transverse perineal muscle are incorrect.[9] The perineal membrane is a single layer of tissue that spans the area between the ischiopubic rami and the striated muscle that is associated with it and is represented by the compressor urethrae and urethrovaginal sphincter muscles that are part of the striated urogenital sphincter. They lie just cephalad to the perineal membrane and are continuous with the striated urethral sphincter.

Although the perineal membrane in the male is a continuous sheet from side to side on which the prostate and viscera may rest, in the female it has a large opening for the vagina. Its support, therefore, results from the attachments of this membrane to the vagina and perineal body. In this way two sheets of tissue extend from the ischiopubic ramus to the perineal body on either side. At rest these fibers are probably not stressed because of the support in this area provided by the tonic activity of the levator ani muscles. During increases in intraabdominal pressure or with relaxation of the levator ani muscle, however, this sheet would support the perineal body and introitus.

Lying below the level of the perineal membrane are a group of muscles that can be referred to as the external genital muscles. These include the ischiocavernosus, bulbocavernosus, and superficial transverse perineal muscles (Fig. 2-8). The first two of these muscles probably have little supportive role and are primarily involved in sexual function. The bulbocavernosus originates from the surface of the clitoris and covers the vestibular bulb, passing posteriorly to terminate in the area of the perineal body. The ischiocavernosus muscle has a similar origin to the bulbocavernosus, both arising over the ventral surface of the clitoral crus, from

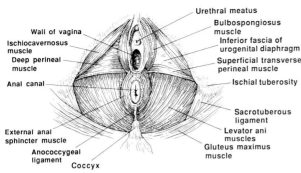

Fig. 2-8 External genital muscles and the urogenital diaphragm (perineal membrane).

which it terminates on the ischiopubic ramus. Contraction of these two muscles increases the pressure within the erectile tissues of their associated structures. The superficial transverse perineal muscles lie at a level that spans the dorsal edge of the perineal membrane. Their origin is from the inner aspect of the ischial pubic rami near the ischial tuberosity and contraction therefore helps to elevate the perineal body if it is in a plane below the level of these muscle insertions. The more superficial structures within the external genitalia such as Colle's fascia and the superficial fascia of the perineum probably have little to do with perineal support.

The external anal sphincter is a teardrop shaped muscle with its apex anchored at the coccyx. It exerts some dorsal traction on the anus that opposes the ventral traction of the pubococcygeus muscle. This attachment to the coccyx probably has some influence in supporting the perineal body in which the anterior portion of the muscle is embedded.

Mechanical Interactions

These anatomical observations indicate that the pelvic viscera are supported by a combination of muscular and fibrous tissues. In the past there was a tendency to debate which of these two elements was the one that provided support. The fact that this issue remained unresolved despite more than 100 years of argument suggests that both elements play a role. Support is provided by an interaction of the fibrous connective tissue and the muscular support.

SUMMARY

The pelvic organs are maintained in their position by a combination of connective tissue and striated muscle.

The connective tissue includes some smooth muscle and forms ligaments and fasciae that attach the organs to the pelvic walls. These include the cardinal and uterosacral ligaments as well as the pubocervical and rectovaginal fasciae. The striated muscle of the levator ani pulls the organs against the pubic bone, closing the opening in the pelvic floor and providing a relatively horizontal shelf for the organs to rest on. Interaction between these connective tissues and muscular elements is responsible for normal support, and damage to either of these elements can contribute to genital prolapse.

Previous descriptions of the pelvic floor support mechanism attempted to isolate only one factor responsible for pelvic support, but were unable to provide satisfactory explanations for the diversity of defects that are seen in patients with prolapse as well as the objective observations of pelvic floor damage following childbirth. Each individual portion of the support mechanism has a characteristic structure that has evolved in response to a structural need. Understanding the mechanism of pelvic support is similar to understanding the way in which any mechanical device works. To understand how a watch works one must understand not only the dynamics of the spring and fly wheel, but also how the escapement and gear mechanisms work. It is no more correct to say that the ligaments are responsible for normal function of the pelvic floor than it is to say that the watch spring is what makes the watch work. Without the pelvic floor musculature the ligaments would ultimately fail and without the gears and escape mechanism the watch could not keep its orderly mechanism functioning.

As we begin to understand the role that each of these individual elements play, we begin to have a better understanding of the mechanism of prolapse. This is a new and challenging era of surgical gynecology and one that should greatly improve the functional results of our operations. Although vaginal hysterectomy and anterior posterior colporrhaphy are usually effective in relieving the symptoms of genital prolapse, they have not demonstrated particularly long lasting or universally effective results and have also sometimes been the cause of dyspareunia and sexual dysfunction. Furthering our understanding of pelvic floor function will allow us to improve our treatments and thereby better serve our patients.

REFERENCES

1. Richardson AC, Lyons JB, Williams NL. A new look at pelvic relaxation. *Am J Obstet Gynecol.* 1976;126:568–573.

2. Bonney V. The principles that should underlie all operations for prolapse. *J Obstet Gynaecol Br Emp.* 1934;41:669–683.

3. Nichols DH, Milley PS, Randall CL. Significance of restoration of normal vaginal depth and axis. *Obstet Gynecol.* 1970;36:251–256.

4. Range RL, Woodburne RT. The gross and microscopic anatomy of the transverse cervical ligaments. *Am J Obstet Gynecol.* 1964;90: 460–467.

5. Campbell RM. The anatomy and histology of the sacrouterine ligaments. *Am J Obstet Gynecol.* 1950;59:1–12.

6. Nichols DH, Milley PS. Surgical significance of the rectovaginal septum. *Am J Obstet Gynecol.* 1970;108:215–220.

7. Lawson JON. Pelvic anatomy: pelvic floor muscles. *Ann R Coll Surg Engl.* 1984;54:244–252.

8. Parks AG, Porter NH, Melzak J. Experimental study of the reflex mechanism controlling muscles of the pelvic floor. *Dis Colon Rectum.* 1962;5:407–414.

9. Oelrich TM. The striated urogenital sphincter muscle in the female. *Anat Rec.* 1983;205:223–232.

CHAPTER 3

Physiology of Micturition

J. Andrew Fantl   Debra A. Miller

INTRODUCTION

The lower urinary tract, composed of the bladder and urethra, serves two functions: the storage and timely elimination of urine. During storage, the bladder acts as a reservoir and the urethra as its sphincter. During micturition, the bladder contracts to expel its contents through the urethra, now representing an active conduit. Both bladder and urethra are neurophysiologically related and should be considered as one unit. Evacuation of urine is accomplished during micturition through the coordinated actions of both bladder and urethra. Storage and efficient elimination of urine therefore results from the anatomic integrity of both structures and the coordination of function mediated by the integration of autonomic and somatic peripheral mechanisms by the central nervous system. The purpose of this chapter is to review the role of each structure as it pertains to normal lower urinary tract functioning.

STORAGE PHASE

The Bladder

During the filling of the bladder, urine enters the bladder at a rate of approximately 2 ml per minute.[1] The rate varies depending on circumstance, such as overhydration or underhydration and the use of diuret-

ics. The detrusor responds to filling with minimal changes in intravesical pressure. This requires the bladder to be distensible, and that detrusor activity be inhibited. Characteristics of bladder response to filling can be evaluated in terms of four parameters: sensation, compliance (accommodation), capacity, and stability.

Sensation

Sensation is difficult to evaluate because of its subjective nature. Criteria and methodology for its assessment are not yet well developed; however, evaluation of its normalcy or abnormality should be attempted. Sensation is usually described in terms of the volume of urine at which the individual experiences the first sensation to void, and that volume which causes an uncomfortable fullness or urge to void. This last is considered a reflection of maximum cystometric bladder capacity.

At some point during filling, usually assumed to be at the time of the first sensation to void, control of detrusor reflex contraction is required. Cerebral cortical pathways provide voluntary inhibition of micturition and also serve to mediate recurrent reflex inhibition at a local level. The detrusor is a unique smooth muscle organ because it is the only such viscera of the body under voluntary control. Abnormalities of sensation are encountered with various peripheral conditions such as diabetic neuropathy, polyneuritis, and after radical hysterectomy. Centrally occurring disease (Parkinson's disease and multiple sclerosis) can also be manifested by changes in bladder sensation.

The bladder is capable of significant distention without concomitant increase in intravesical pressure. This phenomenon is termed *accommodation*. Compliance represents a mathematical term and is defined as the change in bladder pressure for a given change in bladder volume. It is calculated by dividing the bladder volume change by the change in intravesical pressure before and after filling.[2] A normal bladder can contain 400 to 700 ml with pressure changes of less than 15 cm H_2O. As the limits of structural capacity are reached, compliance and accommodation decrease.

Compliance

Compliance is subject to passive and dynamic influences. Passive influences are inherent in the structure of the bladder wall itself. Properties inherent in smooth muscle structure enable it to lengthen without a proportional increase in tension. The amounts of elastin and collagen in the bladder wall also influence compliance. Compliance is reduced and accommodation decreases when the bladder wall is distended beyond maximum stretch. Active forces influencing detrusor compliance include the volume of fluid within the bladder, the rate of filling, that portion of intraabdominal pressure transmitted to the bladder, and the degree of detrusor activity. Conditions which increase the collagen content of the bladder wall (recurrent infection, radiation therapy) or increased detrusor activity can decrease bladder compliance and its capacity.

During filling, the normal bladder is remarkably resistant to provocative maneuvers such as heel bouncing, coughing, and rapid filling. Through central nervous system maturation and acquired behavioral education (toilet training), an individual exerts voluntary control over detrusor muscle activity. An infant voids by detrusor contraction stimulated by critical volumes. Through specific training, these autonomic responses are inhibited by cortical impulses.

Capacity

Bladder capacity ranges from 400 to 700 cc. Capacity, however, is not particularly diagnostic when evaluated separately from other parameters. It is usually assessed in light of compliance and accommodation. An abnormally large or small bladder which manifests normal compliance is not pathologic.

Capacity may also be affected by extrinsic factors. A vesicovaginal or urethrovaginal fistula may prevent a bladder from reaching maximum capacity. An incom-petent urethral sphincter mechanism may also preclude a normal bladder from filling to capacity.

Evaluation of bladder capacity, therefore, increases understanding of bladder function and/or dysfunction but must be interpreted in light of all other parameters.

Stability

Bladder stability is necessary for continence. A bladder is termed stable if it does not involuntarily contract despite provocation. An unstable bladder is one that is shown objectively to contract, spontaneously or on provocation, during the filling phase while the individual is attempting to inhibit micturition. These contractions can occur without any associated symptoms or can be related to strong sensations of urinary urgency with or without concomitant urinary incontinence.[3]

Evaluation

The storage phase of bladder (detrusor) function is urodynamically evaluated by the cystometrogram. During cystometry, bladder sensation, compliance, and detrusor stability may be assessed. Single channel cystometry monitors intravesical pressure. It does not however, take into consideration intraabdominal forces which can affect intravesical pressure measurements. Multichannel cystometry simultaneously measures intraabdominal and intravesical pressures (Fig. 3-1). Pressure increases caused by the Valsalva maneuver are then subtracted from total intravesical pressure, resulting in measurement of the pressure created by detrusor activity alone. This technique is thought to provide a more accurate assessment of true detrusor activity. In general, it is believed that multichannel cystometry (subtracted provocative cystometry) is less likely to produce false positive results when instability is diagnosed. Negative results obtained with single channel cystometry are likely to correlate better than positive results. Controversy still exists over which method provides the most reliable information. Bhatia[4] has recommended ambulatory (continuous monitoring) cystometric evaluation as the most sensitive method for detecting detrusor stability abnormalities.

Although cystometry can identify maximal bladder capacity, the observation is somewhat subjective and dependent on variables such as the laboratory setting itself, the choice of distention media (CO_2 vs water), the route and rate of bladder filling, and so on. Functional bladder capacity can be estimated by the use of a urinary diary. The patient records on paper each voided volume within a specified period of time, usually a week. This provides information on frequency as well

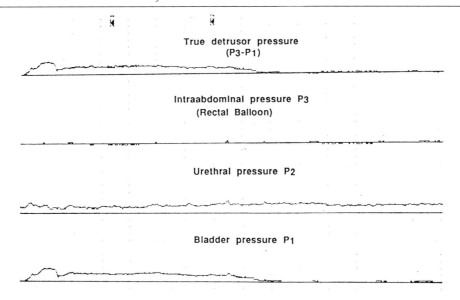

Fig. 3-1 Multichannel cystometrogram of a patient with detrusor instability. P_1 = intravesical pressure, P_2 = intraurethral pressure, P_3 = intraabdominal pressure, and $P_3 - P_1$ = the true detrusor pressure.

as the amount of urine voided. This information is considered the patient's functional capacity because it is measured under normal conditions.

The Urethra

During filling, the female urethra should be considered in its entirety as the sphincter of the bladder. Continence is maintained as long as the intravesical pressure does not exceed intraurethral resistance. The urethral resistance at rest is derived from three main sources: the periurethral striated muscles, urethral smooth musculature and elastic connective tissue, and the submucosal vascular bed. Each contributes approximately one third of total urethral resistance.[5,6] Urethral smooth muscle extends the length of the urethra and is contiguous with the detrusor. The intrinsic striated urethral muscle fibers extend from 20% to 60% of total urethral length, and the striated muscles of the perineal membrane (urogenital diaphragm) are found from 50% to 80% of the total urethral length.[7] (Fig. 3-2)

The proximal urethra is a mobile structure and is of

Fig. 3-2 Urethral landmarks (based on the work of DeLancey[7]). (Reprinted from Fantl JA, *Genuine Stress Incontinence* Philadelphia: JB Lippincott Co, with permission.)

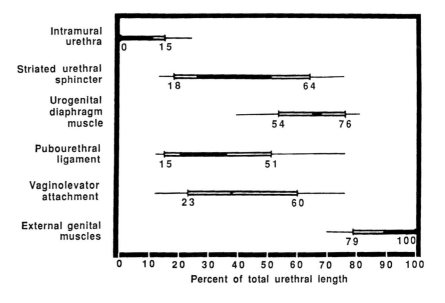

primary importance in urethral sphincteric function.[8] This requires that the structures supporting this area be anatomically supported actively by the muscles in the pelvic floor and statically by various ligamentous supports that extend from the posterior portion of the pubis to the urethra. DeLancey describes a connection between the vagina and levator muscles in an area approximately 20% to 60% of the length of the urethra in its mobile region.[7,9,10] The levator muscles indirectly provide a degree of support to the bladder neck during the storage phase of bladder function. On the other hand, opening of the bladder neck occurs at onset of micturition as these muscles relax.

Resting urethral resistance is augmented by factors such as the transmission of pressure from the abdomen to the urethra (pressure transmission). Acute increments of intraabdominal pressure are transmitted to the proximal urethra, maintaining the pressure gradient between bladder and urethra. This occurs as long as the bladder neck maintains its retropubic position and therefore depends on adequate bladder neck suspension. In continent women, sudden increases of intraabdominal pressure are transmitted to the bladder and urethra. In fact, observations show that at times the rise in urethral pressure is greater than that expected by simple transference of intraabdominal pressures. This suggests that in addition to adequate pressure transmission, other mechanisms occur during stress.[11] The striated muscles of the urogenital diaphragm as well as those intrinsic to the urethra are thought to provide voluntary and reflex contractility to the urethral sphincter during stress, Valsalva maneuver, or other motions resulting in abrupt increases in intraabdominal pressure.

Several tests of urethral sphincteric function during storage phase have been described. The choice depends on clinical vs investigatory objectives, complexity of the specific case, as well as individual preferences.

Evaluation

Direct Visualization Test

With the bladder filled to maximal cystometric capacity, the patient is requested to cough. Leakage of fluid observed through the external meatus, occurring at the acme of the cough effort indicates evidence of urethral incompetence during stress. Care must be taken to avoid overdistention of the bladder, its mechanical displacement (such as with use of a posterior vaginal blade) or inadvertent levator ani relaxation. The external meatus should be visible to the investiga-

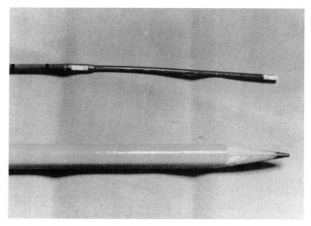

Fig. 3-2 Urethral landmarks (based on the work of DeLancey[7]). (Reprinted from Fantl JA, *Genuine Stress Incontinence* Philadelphia: JB Lippincott Co, with permission.)

tor and the spurt of fluid should occur simultaneously with the cough.

Urethral Pressure Profilometry (UPP)

Measurements of intraurethral pressure can be accomplished using different techniques. The majority of urodynamic units today utilize microtip transducers as shown in Fig. 3-3. The subtraction of the pressure measured in the urethra from that measured in the bladder is referred to as the *urethral closure pressure* (UCP). The UCP can be determined at rest (passive UPP) or during repetitive cough efforts (dynamic UPP). Passive UPP provides information on the sphincter mechanism at rest, or the intrinsic sphincteric mechanism. Severely damaged urethras such as those seen after multiple surgical interventions for urinary incontinence or radiation therapy are typical examples of clinical circumstances leading to reduced intrinsic sphincter mechanisms with very low UCP during passive testing. It should be pointed out that passive UCP does not represent a discriminator between sphincteric competence or incompetence, but rather an indicator of overall intrinsic urethral sphincteric function.

The competency of the urethra during exertion is tested during the dynamic UPP. During every cough, the urethral closure pressure and pressure transmission are monitored and individual segments of the urethra are evaluated for competence (Fig. 3-4). A zero or negative closing pressure at the peak of an exertion is considered consistent with urethral incompetence at that given urethral segment. If a zero or negative closing pressure is found across the entire functional urethral length, the

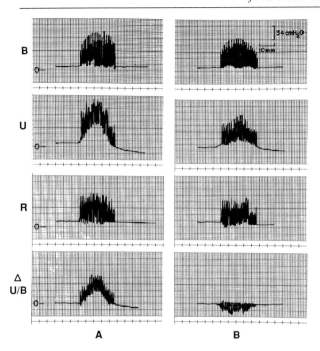

Fig. 3-4 Dynamic urethral closure pressure profiles in stress continent (**A**) and stress incontinent (**B**) women. In the lower right diagram intravesical pressure consistently exceeds urethral pressure, leading to negative closing pressure. *B* = intravesical pressure, *U* = urethral pressure, *R* = intraabdominal pressure, and Δ*U/B* = difference between intravesical and urethral pressures.

urethra is considered urodynamically incompetent. Results of direct visualization tests and dynamic profilometry in both stress continent and stress incontinent women are shown in Table 3-1.[12]

Another way to use dynamic UPP is to consider the ratio of measurements of the pressure transmission to the bladder and urethra. It has been found that pressure transmission ratios below 90% are more likely to indicate urethral sphincteric incompetence than if they are above 90%, at which values urethral sphincteric incompetence is rare.[13]

There are many other described techniques to assess sphincteric competence. These include radiologic observations during fluoroscopy, ultrasonographic visualizations, as well as other sophisticated tests such as the fluid bridge test, electrical conductance test, and others. Most of these techniques should be considered complimentary and not exclusive of each other. In addition, these should be used according to the complexity of each case. Sensitivity and specificity of most of these diagnostic tools are still not available. Clinical judgment and correlation between the patient's symptom complex and the observed test results remains a crucial part of the appropriate use and interpretation of all urodynamic observations.

THE EMPTYING PHASE

In normal women, micturition usually occurs as a result of the voluntary relaxation of the levator ani and urethral sphincter with subsequent sustained contraction of the bladder. Complete emptying of the bladder contents occurs. Fluoroscopic observation during voluntary voiding shows the bladder neck to descend and assume a funnel shape before detrusor contraction.[14] During the descent of the bladder neck, a progressive drop in intraurethral pressure has been demonstrated. This occurs approximately three seconds prior to detrusor contraction.[14] The detrusor contraction usually does not exceed 50 cm of H_2O. The tonus of the smooth

Table 3-1
Results of Direct Visualization Tests and Dynamic Urethral Profilometry in Incontinent and Continent Patients

| | Direct Visualization Test | | | | Dynamic Urethral Profilometry | | | | | |
| | Positive | | Negative | | Positive | | Equivocal | | Negative | |
Group	n	%	n	%	n	%	n	%	n	%
Incontinent (n = 84)	52	62	32	38	50	59	24	29	10	12
Continent (n = 31)	1	3	30	97	0		6	19	25	81

Incontinent patients have symptoms of stress urinary incontinence. Continent patients had sensory symptomatology but no urinary incontinence. Both groups had no other objective lower urinary tract dysfunction.
(Reproduced with permission from Fantl, JA et al.[12])

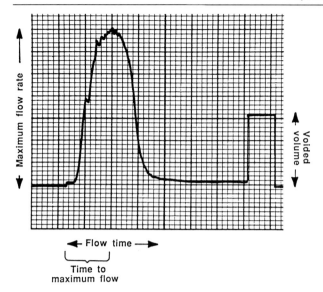

Fig. 3-5 Normal uroflow with uroflowmetric parameters diagrammed.

intermittent or interrupted flow patterns, may be more representative of emptying phase difficulties than the parameters themselves. If repetitive uroflowmetric tests indicate possible dysfunction, pressure flow studies and further assessment are indicated.

Pressure flow observations evaluate the emptying phase of lower tract function with detailed simultaneous pressure measurements of the bladder, urethra, and abdomen. Abnormal mechanisms of voiding (detrusor sphincter dyssynergia, anatomic obstruction, voiding without detrusor contraction, voiding with Valsalva maneuver) can be identified in this fashion. As it requires invasive monitoring, a significant number of patients are unable to void under these conditions. Among those who are able to void, catheter placement itself may create artifactual results. Electromyelograph study of the striated urethral muscle fibers can be used in conjunction with pressure flow studies. Its use has not become popular other than when neuropathic conditions are suspected.

and striated muscle fibers of the urethra is reduced by inhibition of their motor neurons located in the second, third, and fourth sacral spinal segments. Coordination with detrusor contractions occurs via modulation of the central nervous system.

Though initiation is most often a voluntary act, maintenance of micturition is an autonomic function. Local reflexes mediate sustained detrusor contractions. Afferent input is received from tension receptors in the bladder as well as afferents in the proximal urethra. Mahoney describes twelve reflexes involved in bladder function, five of which sustain micturition.[15]

Evaluation

The voiding phase of lower urinary tract function is assessed in several ways. Uroflowmetry is one of the most commonly used methods. Its main clinical use has been in the evaluation of men with urethral obstruction. Although rare in females, this dysfunction can occur as a result of surgery for genuine stress incontinence or in cases of severe prolapse.

Urinary flow rate is the volume of urine expelled through the urethra per unit of time. Several parameters are usually measured in a typical uroflowmetric curve (Fig. 3.5). The volume voided seems to be the one main factor affecting uroflowmetric parameters, and a wide range of normal values exist. Voiding dysfunction should be suspected when parameters are not within such variations. Characteristics of the curve, such as

---

Box 3-1
International Continence Society
Classification of Lower Urinary Tract
Dysfunction

I. Storage phase
   A. Bladder function
      1. Detrusor activity
         a. normal
         b. overactive
      2. Bladder sensation
         a. normal
         b. increased (hypersensitive)
         c. reduced (hyposensitive)
         d. absent
   B. Urethral function
      1. Normal
      2. Incompetent
II. Voiding phase
   A. Bladder function
      1. Acontractile
      2. Underactive
      3. Normal
   B. Urethral function
      1. Normal
      2. Obstructive
         a. overactivity
         b. mechanical

SUMMARY

Normal micturition involves voluntary control of a smooth muscle organ. There is central nervous system integration of local neural reflex arcs resulting in efficient storage and elimination of urine at appropriate times. Coordination of bladder and urethral function is essential to normal voiding and depends on the integrity of these peripheral and central neural pathways.

Disorders of lower urinary tract function can occur in either the storage or voiding phase and can be caused by dysfunction of bladder, urethra, or their neural control (see Box 3-1). Disturbances of cortical or behavioral abilities can lead to incontinence even though the structure and function of the lower urinary tract remains intact.

REFERENCES

1. Torrens M, Morrison J. *The Physiology of the Lower Urinary Tract.* London: Springer–Verlag; 1987:343.
2. Abrams P, Blaivas JG, Stanton SL, et al. The standardization of terminology of lower urinary tract function. *Scand J. Urol.* 1988;114:5–19.
3. Fantl JA, Hurt WG, Dunn LJ. Dysfunctional detrusor control. *Am J Obgyn.* 1977;129:299.
4. Bhatia NN, Ostergard DR. Urodynamics in women with stress urinary incontinence. *Obstet Gynecol.* 1982;60:552.
5. Rud T, Andersson KE, Asmussen A, et al. Factors maintaining the intraurethral pressure in women. *Invest Urol.* 1980;17:343.
6. Awad SA, Downie JW. Relative contributions of smooth and striated muscles to the canine urethral pressure profile. *Br J Urol.* 1976;48:347.
7. DeLancey JOL. Structural aspects of the extrinsic continence mechanism. *Obstet Gynecol.* 1988;72:296.
8. Lund CJ, Benjamin JA, Tristan TA. Cinefluorographic studies of the bladder and urethra in women: I. Urethrovesical relationships in voluntary and involuntary urination. *Am J Obstet Gynecol.* 1957;74:896.
9. DeLancey JOL. Correlative study of paraurethral anatomy. *Obstet Gynecol.* 1986;68:91.
10. DeLancey JOL, Starr RA. Histology of the connection between the vagina and levator muscles: implications for urinary tract function. *J Rep Med.* 1990;35:765.
11. Constantinou CE, Govan DE. Spatial distribution and timing of transmitted and reflexly generated urethral pressures in healthy women. *J Urol.* 1982;127:964.
12. Fantl JA, Hurt WG, Bump RC, et al. Urethral axis and sphincteric function. *Am J Obstet Gynecol.* 1986;155:554–558.
13. Bump RC, Copeland WE, Hurt WG, Fantl JA. Dynamic urethral pressure/profilometry pressure transmission ratio determinations in stress incontinent and stress continent subjects. *Am J Obstet Gynecol.* 1988;159:749.
14. Tanagho EA, Miller ER. Initiation of voiding. *Br J Urol.* 1970;42:175.
15. Mahoney DT, Laberte RO, Blais DJ. Integral storage and voiding reflexes: neurophysiologic concept of continence and micturition. *Urology.* 1977;10:95–106.

FURTHER READING

Blaivas JG. Pathophysiology of lower urinary tract dysfunction. Symposium on female urology. *Urol Clin of North Am.* May 1985;12(2):215-224.
Constantinou CE. Resting and stress urethral pressures as a clinical guide to the mechanism of continence in the female patient. Symposium on female urology. *Urol Clin of North Am.* May 1985;12(2):247-258.
Gosling J. The structure of the bladder and urethra in relation to function. *Urol Clin North Am.* 1979;6:31.
Sutherst JR, Brown MC. Comparison of single and multi-channel cystometry in diagnosing bladder instability. *Br J Med.* 1984;288:1720.
Tanagho EA, Miller ER. Initiation of voiding. *Br J Urol.* 1970;42:175.
Walters MD, Shields LE. The diagnostic value of history, physical examination and the Q-tip cotton swab test in women with urinary incontinence. *Am J Obstet Gynecol.* 1988;159:145.

CHAPTER 4

Anatomy and Physiology

4A   The Vagina

Victoria M. Maclin

INTRODUCTION

The vagina is the passageway between the vulva and uterine cervix often referred to as a potential space. In its usual resting state it is collapsed with anterior and posterior walls touching one another. However, its functions as coital organ, seminal receptacle, and passageway for menstrual effluent and natural childbirth require morphologic and physiologic versatility.

In the following pages, vaginal embryology and its associated controversy are discussed along with a review of vaginal anatomy. Recent studies in sexual physiology will be subsequently considered against the background of Masters and Johnson's classic model of sexual response. The controversies over vaginal versus clitoral orgasm are addressed and finally, the vagina's role in fertility is briefly discussed.

EMBRYOLOGY

The urethra and vagina share similar embryologic origins. The epithelium of the female urethra is entirely derived from endoderm of the urogenital sinus, while the fibromuscular layers are derived from surrounding splanchnic mesenchyme.[1,2] The vagina's epithelium is also derived from urogenital sinus endoderm. However, considerable controversy arises over whether or not its proximal portion originates from the müllerian

ducts.[2-9] The prevailing concept is described here.

The müllerian (or paramesonephric) ducts originate as longitudinal invaginations in the mesodermal epithelium of the urogenital ridges, lateral to the mesonephric ducts (Figs. 4A-1A-C).[2] The paired müllerian ducts migrate caudally, crossing anterior to the mesonephric ducts and then fuse in the midline after reaching the dorsal wall of the urogenital sinus (Fig. 4A-2A).[2,4-7] Fusion proceeds in a cranial direction forming the epithelial core of the uterovaginal canal or primordium. The caudal end of the uterovaginal primordium indents the dorsal wall of the urogenital sinus, creating a protuberance referred to as Müller's tubercle (Fig. 4-2A).[1,5-7] This is the site of the future hymen. The segment of urogenital sinus caudal to Müller's tubercle becomes the vaginal vestibule.[1]

Contact of the uterovaginal primordium with the urogenital sinus induces the formation of paired endodermal outgrowths, the sinovaginal bulbs (Fig. 4A-2A).[2,5,6] These sinovaginal bulbs proliferate and fuse to form the vaginal plate (Fig. 4A-2B). The vaginal plate elongates between the urogenital sinus and caudal uterovaginal primordium and invades the latter up to the level of the future cervix (Figs. 4A-2C-D)[3,5,7] thereby replacing the central core of mesodermal (müllerian) epithelium with sinus endoderm. The central cells of the vaginal plate subsequently degenerate and a vaginal lumen lined with epithelium of sinus endodermal origin is formed. The fibromuscular layers of the vagina are

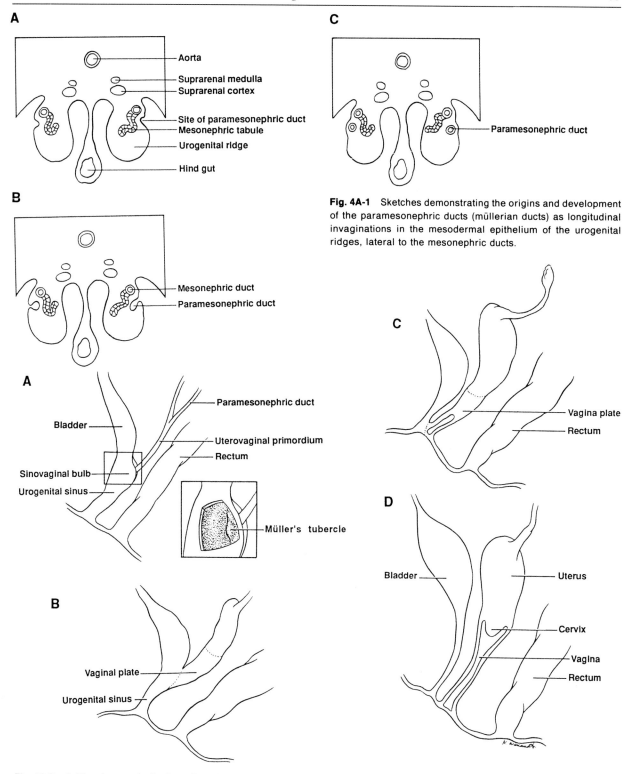

Fig. 4A-1   Sketches demonstrating the origins and development of the paramesonephric ducts (müllerian ducts) as longitudinal invaginations in the mesodermal epithelium of the urogenital ridges, lateral to the mesonephric ducts.

Fig. 4A-2   A, The uterovaginal primordium develops from fusion of the paired paramesonephric ducts. Contact of the caudal tip of the uterovaginal primordium with the urogenital sinus forms a posterior indentation, Müller's tubercle, and induces development of the sinovaginal bulbs, paired endodermal outgrowths of the urogenital sinus. **B,** The sinovaginal bulbs fuse and elongate between the urogenital sinus and the uterovaginal primordium to form the vaginal plate. **C and D,** The central cells of the vaginal plate degenerate to form a vaginal lumen.

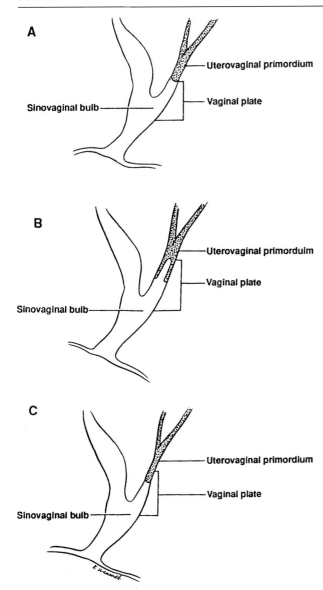

Fig. 4A-3 Sketches exemplifying three different theories of vaginal plate development. Vaginal plate develops from **A** sinovaginal bulbs only, **B** from sinovaginal bulbs and distal uterovaginal primordium joined by invasion of the former into the latter, **C** sinovaginal bulbs and uterovaginal primordium joined end to end.

derived from surrounding splanchnic mesenchyme.[2,5]

The actual area of controversy revolves around the components and dynamics of the vaginal plate (Fig. 4A-3). There seem to be three arguable concepts of vaginal plate development; the vaginal plate is formed by (1) sinovaginal bulbs alone[2] (Fig. 4A-3A), or (2) sinovaginal bulbs and distal uterovaginal primordium

joined by invasion of the former into the latter up to the level of the future cervix[3,5,7] (Fig. 4A-3B), or (3) sinovaginal bulbs and uterovaginal primordium joined end to end[9] (Fig. 4A-3C). In the first two processes, canalization of the vaginal plate would result in a vaginal epithelium derived entirely from sinus endoderm. In the third process the epithelium would have dual sinus and müllerian origins.

While some investigators believe that the vaginal epithelium consists of proximal müllerian and distal urogenital sinus components,[8,9] others subscribe to the theory of sole sinus derivation by virtue of the second previously described process. Considering some evidence that squamous epithelium derived from endoderm characteristically has a greater glycogen storage capacity than squamous epithelia otherwise derived, Ulfelder and Robboy[7] concluded that normal vaginal epithelium, which contains abundant glycogen throughout, must derive entirely from urogenital sinus endoderm. They presented a convincing argument for the latter in their comparison of the histologic characteristics of vaginal epithelium in cases of testicular feminization versus a case of distal vaginal agenesis. In the former deformity, the vagina is derived entirely from urogenital sinus and consists of stratified squamous epithelium containing large quantities of cytoplasmic glycogen. In the case of distal vaginal agenesis, the vagina is derived solely from müllerian precursors and histologically revealed adenosis (characterized by mucinous glands) and glycogen-poor metaplastic squamous epithelium. This vaginal epithelium was comparable to that found in DES-exposed women. Ulfelder and Robboy submitted that in cases of distal vaginal agenesis and DES exposure, cranial migration of sinus endoderm with replacement of müllerian epithelium fails to occur or is teratologically impaired, respectively.

ANATOMY

The vagina is a fibromuscular tubal structure bounded anteriorly by the bladder and urethra and posteriorly by the rectum (Fig. 4A-4). It extends from the vestibule to the cervix and is referred to as a potential space because while in the resting position, the anterior and posterior walls are in apposition to one another.[10]

The vagina is lined by stratified squamous epithelium which is thin in low estrogen states (prepubertal and postmenopausal) and thickens with either physiologic or exogenous estrogen stimulation. The thickened epithelium forms transverse folds or rugae. Underlying the

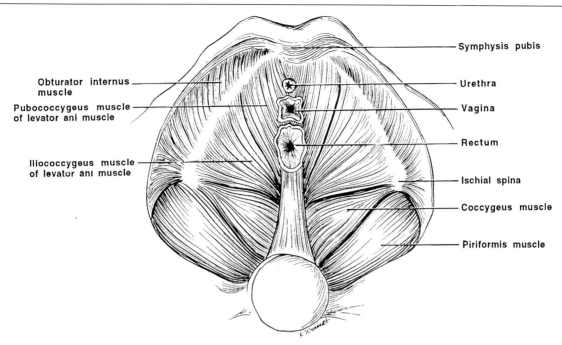

Fig. 4A-4 The pelvic diaphragm, composed of the levator ani, the coccygeus, the obturator internus, and piriformis muscles. The levator ani, consisting of the medial pubococcygeus and the lateral iliococcygeus, are divided in the midline by the interlevator cleft through which pass the urethra, vagina, and rectum.

epithelium is the lamina propria which contains a dense network of elastic fibers. Collagen fibers extend from the elastic fibers to the underlying muscular layers.[11]

The muscular layer has been described on the one hand as a bilayer of smooth muscle, with an inner circular layer and outer longitudinal layer.[10] Alternatively, Platzer and others[11] have described the arrangement of these muscular fibers as right and left turning spirals whose crossings produce obtuse angled grids supported by elastic fibers. This arrangement affords a greater capacity for stretch. Cranially, the muscle fibers merge into the myometrium. In the lower vagina, the smooth muscle is reinforced by striated muscle fibers which enclose the caudal half of the urethra and terminate in the lateral and posterior vaginal walls forming the urethrovaginal sphincter. The vagina's muscular layer is surrounded by the perivaginal portion of the endopelvic fascia.[10-12]

Masters and Johnson in their classic observations of female sexual response[13] established that the unstimulated vagina has a length from fourchette to posterior fornix of 7 to 8 cm and a transcervical width (just anterior to the resting cervix) of 2 cm. With sexual arousal, the vagina is capable of significant enlargement. There is an involuntary lengthening and distention

of the inner two thirds of the vaginal barrel such that length increases by as much as 5 cm and transcervical width increases by as much as 5.25 cm. Furthermore, this distention causes flattening of the vaginal epithelial rugal pattern. The vagina's outer third distends minimally during early sexual arousal, but eventually becomes grossly engorged due to vasocongestion, reducing the outer luminal size and forming the orgasmic platform. This and other aspects of sexual physiology are discussed later in this chapter.

Vaginal Support Mechanisms

The vaginal support mechanism is intimately related to that of the urethra, bladder, and rectum. This support is provided by the endopelvic fascia, the pelvic diaphragm, and the urogenital diaphragm.

The endopelvic fascia consists of the reflections of the superior fascia of the pelvic diaphragm on the urethra and bladder, the vagina and lower uterus, and the rectum.[12] Fibrous connections between these reflections form, anteriorly, the pubovesicocervical fascia, and posteriorly the rectovaginal septum. The pubovesicocervical fascia extends from the symphysis pubis and from the tendinous arch to insert onto the cervix at the level of the internal os, therefore running the entire length of the anterior vaginal wall. The rectovaginal septum, on the other hand, covers the middle two thirds of the posterior vaginal wall superiorly blending with the cardinal-uterosacral complex and inferiorly with the perineal body. The upper 2 to 3 cm of posterior vagina is covered on its outer surface by the peritoneum of Douglas' pouch. The lower posterior vaginal wall and rectum diverge and are separated by the muscles of the perineal body.[10]

Further support of the vagina, along with the urethra, bladder, and rectum is provided by the pelvic diaphragm and urogenital diaphragm. While the pelvic diaphragm is composed of the levator ani, the coccygeus, the obturator internus and piriformis muscles,[12] the levator ani, for the sake of this discussion, are most important (Fig. 4A-4). The levator ani consist of the medial pubococcygeus muscles and the lateral iliococcygeus. The pubococcygeus muscles are separated in the midline by the interlevator cleft through which pass the urethra, vagina, and rectum.[12] The pubococcygeus arise from the posterior surfaces of the pubic rami and pass posteromedially around the lateral walls of the vagina with fibers terminating in the fascia of the perineal body, interdigitating with the longitudinal muscle of the rectum, and with some fibers reaching the coccyx. These insertions create the inclined levator plate responsible for the vaginal axis which normally angles approximately 10 to 15° below the horizontal pelvic line. The iliococcygeus arise from the ischial spines and obturator internus fascia and insert into the coccyx with some fibers interdigitating superficially with the external anal sphincter and transverse perineal muscles.

The urogenital diaphragm lies external and inferior to the levator ani. This muscular-fascial diaphragm is composed of striated muscle and an inferior fascial layer (see Chapter 2). It extends between the ischiopubic rami and is pierced by the urethra and vagina.[10,12] Within the superficial compartment lies the superficial transverse perineal muscles, the ischiocavernosi and the bulbocavernosi. The superficial transverse perinei arise from the ischial tuberosities and insert on the perineal body posterior to the vagina. The ischiocavernosi arise from the ischial tuberosities and inferior ischial rami and insert into the crura of the clitoris and the anterior surface of the pubic symphysis. The bulbocavernosi arise from the perineal body, pass anteriorly around the vagina enveloping the vestibular bulbs, and insert into the clitoris.

Blood Supply

The arterial blood supply to the vagina derives from the uterine, vaginal, inferior vesical, medial rectal, and internal pudendal arteries.[11]

The cervicovaginal branches of the uterine artery supply the vaginal fornices and the superior third of the vagina. The vaginal artery, which originates near the cervix as a branch of the uterine artery, supplies the medial third of the vagina as well as the urethra. Branches of the inferior vesical artery supply the medial and inferior anterior vaginal wall and the pudendal artery supplies the most caudal vagina (beneath the urogenital diaphragm). The medial rectal artery sends branches to the posterior vaginal wall and the azygos artery, formed by adventitial anastomoses of all the aforementioned arteries, and supplies the upper posterior vaginal wall. All of the arteries supplying the vaginal wall contain intima pads consisting of circular and longitudinal smooth muscle which facilitate regulation of blood flow.[11]

The vagina is drained by the vaginal venous plexus. This plexus anastomoses with the venous plexus of the uterus, rectum, and bladder. In the most inferior section of the posterior vaginal wall the veins form a cavernous body which is connected to the vestibular bulbs.[11] Like the vaginal arteries, the paravaginal veins contain intima pads which may aid in tamponading venous blood flow from the vagina.

Nerve Supply

The nerves supplying the vaginal walls originate mostly in the uterovaginal plexus which derives from the pelvic plexus and is located within the cardinal ligament.[11] The pelvic plexus receives preganglionic sympathetic fibers from the inferior thoracic and superior lumbar segments via the inferior mesenteric and superior hypogastric plexuses.[11] Preganglionic parasympathetic fibers are received from the second, third, and fourth sacral segments. The nerves from the uterovaginal plexus send branches to the vaginal muscularis and lamina propria.[11]

Krantz[14] described ganglion cells in the perivaginal fascia forming aggregates typical of ganglia. These are located primarily in the lateral vaginal walls and anteriorly between the bladder and vaginal wall. He presumed these ganglia to be parasympathetic terminal neurons of the cranial segments of the vegetative nervous system. Nerve fibers passing through the ganglia without synapses were presumed to be sympathetic fibers. Krantz also noted nerve fibers supplying the vaginal muscularis and large vessels. A few fibers were noted to terminate in the tunica propria and vaginal epithelium as free nerve endings. No sensory corpuscles are contained within the muscularis, tunica propria, or epithelial layer,[14] coinciding clinically with the lack of light touch, pressure, or pain sensation within the vagina.

SEXUAL PHYSIOLOGY

Vaginal Pressure Areas

Masters and Johnson asserted that the vagina provides the "primary means of heterosexual expression of the human female."[13] Not only does the vagina undergo marked physical changes in response to psychogenic and somatogenic erotic stimuli, it can impart as well as mediate perception of intensely pleasurable erotic sensation during coitus by virtue of its pressure areas.

The outer third of the vagina constricts and generates increased pressure both voluntarily and involuntarily during arousal and orgasmic response. This constriction occurs as a result of introital and lower vaginal muscle contractions as well as vasocongestion of erectile genital tissue (cavernous bodies) in the vestibular bulbs and lower posterior vaginal wall. This vasocongestion is caused by (1) relaxation of arterial intima pads allowing increased blood flow into the cavernous bodies, (2) prevention of blood flow away from the tissues due to contraction of venous intima pads, and (3) contraction of external muscle sphincters on larger veins.[15] The muscular contribution to introital constriction is effected primarily by contraction of the previously described bulbocavernosus muscle, which encircles the introitus. This contraction also facilitates clitoral vasocongestion by compressing venous drainage.

The levator ani, particularly the medial pubococcygeus muscles, function as lower vaginal constrictors. The pubococcygeus muscles can be palpated as thick bands on either side of the vagina. Their role as facilitators or enhancers of erotic sensory perception has been an area of extensive but inconclusive study. In 1952, Kegel[16] reported that "sexual feeling within the vagina is closely related to muscle tone" and that "restoration of the function of the pubococcygeus muscle invariably brought about a degree of improvement in sensory perception of the vagina." He based his conclusions on anecdotal evidence; patients reported improved sensations during coitus after performing resistance pubococcygeal exercises. In 1979, Graber and Kline-Graber[17] supported Kegel's findings with a retrospective correlational study. They found that coitally orgasmic women had greater pubococcygeal strength than those who were clitorally (noncoitally) orgasmic or anorgasmic. Messe and Geer[18] subsequently demonstrated that pubococcygeal muscle tensing during sexual fantasy enhanced subjective and objective measures of sexual arousal. Based on the well-established premise that increased vaginal blood flow occurs with sexual arousal, they measured vaginal pulse amplitude (VPA), which is an index of vaginal blood flow, during muscle tensing alone and during erotic fantasy with and without muscle tensing. They found that fantasy with tensing provoked a greater VPA than fantasy alone. The investigators, however, did not attempt to correlate strength of muscle contraction with degrees of sexual arousal. Interestingly, Chambless and others[19] found that there was no correlation between pubococcygeal strength and pleasurability of vaginal sensations during coitus or frequency and intensity of orgasm. Freese and Levitt[20] also found no correlation between strength of voluntary muscle contractions and orgasmic function. Unfortunately, the impact of pubococcygeal strength on sexual function may never be clearly elucidated because of the difficulty of reconciling subjective perceptions with objective physiologic measurements.[21]

Phases of Sexual Response

Masters and Johnson made a major contribution to our understanding of the human sexual response. They summarized their observations within the context of a four phase model which encompassed the entire sexual response cycle. While their observations were criticized for their subjectivity and lack of objective measurement, deference to their model has endured because it simplified the complexities of sexual physiology. The four phases of this model are the excitement phase, the plateau phase, the orgasmic phase, and the resolution phase. These phases are discussed with regard to the changes effected in the vagina.

Excitation and Plateau Phases

During the excitation phase, there is arousal in response to psychogenic or somatogenic stimuli. Within the vagina, this arousal is manifested within seconds by lubrication. Masters and Johnson likened this lubrication to a "sweating" phenomenon, describing individual droplets that appeared on the vaginal walls and eventually coalesced to form a "smooth, glistening coating for the entire vaginal barrel."[13] They speculated that this fluid was likely a transudate, recognizing the lack of glandular elements in the vaginal walls. The walls also undergo a color change from purplish-red to dark purple. Excitation is further characterized by lengthening of the inner two thirds of the vagina and widening or expansion of the transcervical diameter.

During the plateau phase, there is further increase in the width and depth of the vagina. However, the most important characteristic of plateau is the development of the orgasmic platform: vasocongestion and swelling of the outer third of the vagina, including the vestibular bulbs, to the extent that the central lumen of the outer third is markedly reduced.

The change in vaginal wall color, transudation of lubricating fluid, and development of the orgasmic platform were thought by Masters and Johnson to be the result of vasocongestion of the perivaginal and vestibular vasculature, though they did not objectively measure these vascular phenomena. Since their 1966 publication, vaginal responses (such as increased blood flow and lubrication) to erotic stimuli were the subject of extensive study. Qualitative and quantitative increases in vaginal blood flow were documented using various techniques including photoplethysmography,[15,21,22] measurements of power consumption of heated electrodes,[15,23] radiotelemetric vaginal temperature monitoring,[24] and xenon clearance measurements.[15] Using the latter technique, a fivefold increase of vaginal blood flow from a baseline of 5 to 10 ml up to 30 to 50 ml/min/100 g was demonstrated. Vaginal surface oxygen tension was also shown to increase as a result of increased arterial blood flow.[15,25]

Using vaginal plethysmography and heated electrode power consumption techniques it was shown that increased blood flow occurs within seconds of clitoral stimulation.[15] This rapid physiologic response to somatogenic stimulation is thought to be mediated by a local spinal cord reflex arc. The afferent impulses are carried via the pudendal nerve, the efferent impulses through the pelvic nerve are carried via the pudendal nerve, and the efferent impulses' parasympathetic outflow are carried via sacral roots S_2 through S_4. Arousal effected by psychogenic stimuli (auditory, olfactory, gustatory, visual, or fantasy) may be mediated through arousal centers in the brain or through sympathetic outflow from T_{12} through L_3.[15] Indeed, studies in paraplegic men have shown that psychogenic erections (the corollary to vagi-

nal vasocongestion) can occur even in the presence of a transected sacral spinal cord.

Psychogenic and somatogenic stimuli work synergistically, while somatogenic stimuli alone can be temporally more provocative than psychogenic stimulation. Henson and others[22] studied labial temperature and vaginal blood volume responses to visual and tactile stimuli and demonstrated that both parameters increased more rapidly during masturbation than during erotic film visualization.

Vaginal lubrication or transudation is better understood after considering the factors affecting normal vaginal fluid dynamics. In the unstimulated state, approximately 75 % of the vaginal fluid produced during a day is reabsorbed.[26,27] This reabsorption is secondary to the active transport of sodium from the vaginal lumen into the subepithelial tissue against an electrochemical gradient. Water diffuses passively from the lumen into the subepithelial space following sodium.[26,28,29] Indeed sodium and chloride ion concentrations in vaginal fluid are considerably lower than those found in plasma.

During sexual arousal there is a fourfold increase in vaginal fluid production.[26] The sodium and chloride concentrations in this fluid also increase.[28] Vaginal pH increases significantly[30] and might have a positive correlation with the duration of erotic stimulation and arousal. Preti and others[31] reported that organic compounds produced by intravaginal microflora (in the nonstimulated state) such as C_2 to C_5 aliphatic acids, hydroxybutanone, dimethylsufone, cresol, 2-piperidine, and indole undergo dilution and decrease in concentration during arousal. Furthermore, they noted increased concentrations of lipid constituents believed to be derived from plasma. These arousal-induced changes in vaginal fluid pH, electrolyte content, and organic compound content indicate that increased vaginal fluid production during arousal resulted from transudation of fluid from plasma. Wagner postulated the mechanism underlying this transudation.[26] Increased arterial blood flow leads to an increased pressure gradient across the capillary wall, facilitating transcapillary flow of fluid into the extracellular space. This fluid transudes from the extracellular space through vaginal epithelial intracellular channels and pores, saturating the epithelium's limited reabsorptive capacity for sodium ion.[26]

Orgasmic Phase

During the orgasmic phase, the inner two thirds of the vagina remain expanded. The outer third, specifically the orgasmic platform, undergoes a series of regu-

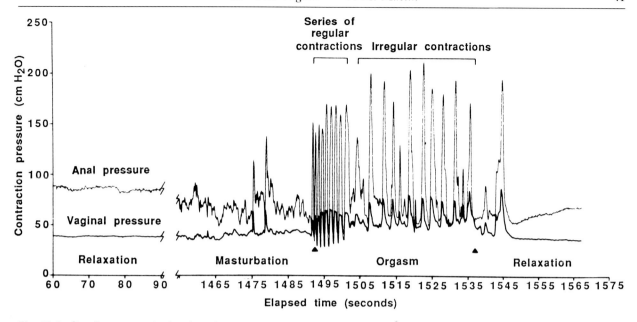

Fig. 4A-5 Simultaneous vaginal and anal pressure monitoring demonstrating that vaginal and anal orgasmic contractions occur synchronously. Closed triangles indicate perceived start and end of orgasm. (Reprinted from Bohlen, et al[35] with permission.)

lar involuntary contractions. Masters and Johnson[13,23] describe these contractions as occurring at initially 0.8 second intervals. The number of contractions range from a minimum of 3 to 5 to a maximum of 10 to 15 with a gradually increasing intercontraction interval and decreasing intensity. The authors never state specifically which muscles are involved, though another investigator using a pressure transducer in the vaginal lumen and digital palpation has suggested that orgasmic contractions include all the muscles of the urogenital diaphragm as well as the levator ani.[33]

The pattern of regular involuntary orgasmic contractions described by Masters and Johnson was also demonstrated by Gillan and Brindley using electromyographic monitoring of the lower vaginal wall.[34] However, these investigators found the initial intercontraction interval to be 0.6 seconds. Bohlen and others[35] showed that the mean intercontraction interval increased linearly at an increment of approximately 0.1 second and that the amplitude of the pressure wave form increased through the first half of the regular contractions, then decreased. Furthermore, with simultaneous vaginal and anal pressure monitoring, they demonstrated that vaginal and anal orgasmic contractions always occur synchronously with the anal contractions having greater amplitude than the vaginal contractions (Fig. 4A-5). This is not surprising considering that fibers of the iliococcygeus muscles interdigitate

with the external anal sphincter. However, this finding was contrary to that of Masters and Johnson, who stated that orgasmic rectal sphincter contractions do not always occur.[32] Considering that Bohlen's findings were based on objective measurements as opposed to subjective observation, his conclusions are probably more accurate.

Bohlen and coworkers described distinct types of female orgasm based on the pattern of contractions recorded during the perceived orgasmic period. These were designated types I, II, and IV (Fig. 4A-6). (The type III contraction pattern had only been observed in men). Type I orgasms were characterized by the regular series of 7 to 13 involuntary contractions occurring over a mean duration of 13.1 seconds with a linear increase in intercontraction interval and a uniformity of waveform. Type II orgasms were characterized by the series of regular contractions (as in type I) followed by a series of irregular contractions in which the waveforms and intervals varied irregularly. The mean orgasmic duration was 50.6 seconds. In the type IV orgasm with a mean duration of 24.4 seconds, no regular pattern of contractions was recorded. There were only nonuniform contractions with fluctuating pressures. The pressure recordings prior, during, and following perceived orgasm were indistinguishable. Interestingly, the authors noted that type IV pattern was similar to recordings of voluntary contractions, posing the question of

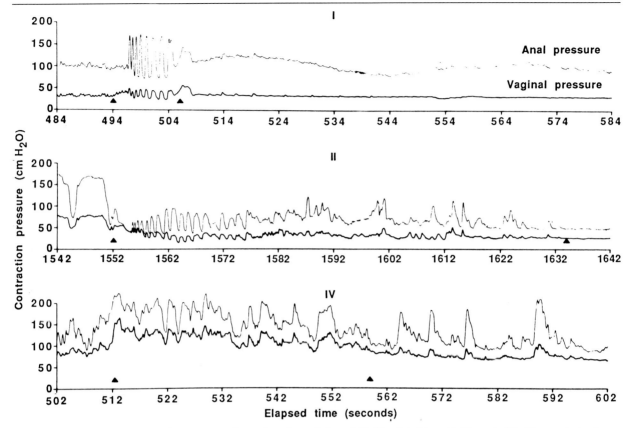

Fig. 4A-6 Orgasmic contractions representing pattern types I, II, and IV. (Reprinted from Bohlen, et al[35] with permission.)

whether or not some women were able to control their involuntary contractions during orgasm or were perceiving some less pronounced, preorgasmic change as orgasm.

This leads to the more difficult question of whether orgasm should be defined by cognitive perception or by objective physiologic criteria. The inability to reconcile these two aspects to one another presents recurring problems in sexual physiology research. Masters and Johnson encouragingly observed that "the number and intensity of orgasmic platform contractions are direct measures of subjective severity and objective duration of the particular orgasmic experience."[32] However, a relatively recent report by Levin and Wagner indicated no significant correlation between the recorded duration and the subjectively graded intensity of orgasm.[23] The graded intensity also failed to correlate with the measured increase in vaginal blood flow using heated electrode power consumption methodology. Levin and Wagner simply concluded that factors other than duration influence the subjective assessment of orgasmic pleasure. Unfortunately, psychologic components pre-

sent intangible variables which confound assessing the relative contribution of various anatomic and physiologic factors to the orgasmic experience.[21]

Resolution Phase

During the resolution phase the vasocongestion in the outer third of the vagina that forms the orgasmic platform regresses. The diameter of the outer lumen thus increases over the course of 3 to 4 minutes. The expansion of the inner two thirds also decreases. The lateral and posterior walls undergo an "irregular, zonal type of relaxation" and the cervix and anterior wall descend toward the posterior wall. The color change in the vagina undergoes a slower retrogressive process, taking as long as 10 to 15 minutes according to Masters and Johnson.[13] This was attributed to a protracted return of vaginal blood flow to baseline, substantiated by both vaginal plethysmography and heated electrode monitoring.[15,22] Similarly, vaginal surface oxygen tension also returns to baseline over a period of 10 to 30 minutes after orgasm.[15,25]

Vaginal vs Clitoral Orgasm

During the first half of this century, Freud postulated that there were two types of female orgasm, vaginal and clitoral. The vagina was considered the locus of mature female eroticism, while clitoral orgasms were deemed infantile.[36] Masters and Johnson, on the other hand, refuted this dogma and asserted that no distinction could be made between vaginal and clitoral orgasm. They contend that the clitoris is the "center of female sensual focus" and all orgasmic responses result either from direct or indirect clitoral stimulation.[37]

The relative lack of vaginal sensory innervation as demonstrated by Krantz[14] certainly mitigated in favor of Masters and Johnson's contentions. Krantz's microscopic studies of vaginal nerve supply revealed no mediators of touch (such as Meissner corpuscles, Merkel tactile discs) or pressure (pacinian corpuscles) within the vaginal walls. There was also a paucity of free nerve endings (mediators of pain) noted to terminate in the vaginal epithelium. In contrast, the clitoris contained both Meissner corpuscles and Merkel tactile discs as well as a rich supply of pacinian corpuscles and free nerve endings. Accordingly, Kinsey and coworkers[38] found that the vaginal walls were "quite insensitive" to tactile stimulation while clitoral stimulation evoked intense and immediate erotic response. Indeed, Kaplan[39] postulated that orgasm is a reflex with its sensory component being clitoral stimulation and its motor component circumvaginal contractions.

The lack of vaginal superficial tactile sensitivity seems irrelevant when considering the mediators of vaginal erotic sensitivity suggested by its various proponents.[16,17,40-48] Erotic perception was attributed to structures deep, but intimately related to, the vaginal surface.

Kegel,[16] as mentioned earlier, believed that the centers of female erotic sensory perception were located in the pubococcygeus muscles and that the more toned the pubococcygeus, the greater the likelihood of achieving orgasm. Graber and Kline-Graber[17] supported this hypothesis, reporting that orgasmic women had greater tone than anorgasmic women. Ironically, only 17% of the orgasmic women were coitally orgasmic.

Another proposed source of vaginal erotic sensitivity which sparked considerable controversy is the Grafenberg spot (G-spot), named for the investigator who first described it in 1950. This erotically sensitive area palpable through the anterior vaginal wall has been suggested to be composed of periurethral glandular tissue (Skene's glands) homologous to the male prostate. With digital or penile tactile stimulation through the anterior vaginal wall, this area, which was reported to range in diameter from 2 to 4 cm, swells and is possibly the source of an ejaculatory release from the female urethra at the time of orgasm. Addiego and others[40] extensively studied a subject who could be consistently stimulated to orgasm by specific stimulation of this spot and also ejaculated a substance that was chemically distinguished from urine. This ejaculate contained high levels of prostatic acid phosphatase and low levels of urea and creatinine as compared to urine. Belzer and colleagues[42] reported similar results from seven subjects whose specimens were not collected in the presence of an investigator. Goldberg and others[43] attempted to replicate the findings of Addiego and Belzer in their study of 11 women, six of whom claimed to be ejaculators. Two independent examiners were able to locate an area characteristic of the G-spot in only four of the eleven women, and this area was present in only two of six ejaculators. All ejaculates were chemically indistinguishable from urine, suggesting that the orgasmic urethral expulsion could be the result of urinary incontinence.

The existence of a G-spot was further repudiated by the work of Hoch[44] who, during the systematic "sexological" examination of 56 women was unable to demonstrate a G-spot. This examination in the presence of the woman's sexual partner, entailed a routine pelvic examination followed by progressive clockwise palpation of the entire vaginal wall from lower to upper vagina. With the patient's verbal feedback the areas of erotic sensitivity were identified and stimulated to the plateau level of arousal. Interestingly, 96% of women reported erotic sensitivity along the entire anterior vaginal wall and 98% reported no erotic sensitivity in the area of the pubococcygeus muscles.

Alzate and Londono[45] modified Hoch's sexological examination method by examining and stimulating their subjects up to or just short of orgasm. Two thirds of 48 volunteers had anterior wall sensitivity while one third were found to have increased posterior wall sensitivity. In none of the subjects could a G-spot be palpated. Sixteen of 48 subjects were stimulated to the point of orgasm and none of the orgasmic subjects produced an ejaculate. In a subsequent replication study,[46] Alzate demonstrated erogenous zones on both the upper anterior wall and lower posterior wall. Surprisingly, one subject with posterior wall sensitivity produced a urethral ejaculate at orgasm that was chemically indistinguishable from urine.

These latter studies cast considerable doubt on both the existence of a G-spot and the occurrence of a female ejaculate emanating from periurethral glands. Even the previous studies documenting elevated levels of prostatic acid phosphatase are suspect in view of possible contamination by an endogenous vaginal acid phosphatase.[47]

In Hoch's study[44] 100% of 56 subjects were initially coitally anorgasmic or orgasmic only with external genital stimulation. Identification of anterior vaginal wall sensitivity resulted in subsequent achievement of orgasm with continuous penile or digital stimulation of the anterior vaginal wall in 64% of subjects. Hoch attributed the anterior wall sensitivity in part to the epithelial free nerve endings and adventitial ganglia described by Krantz,[14] to unmyelinated fibers in the subepithelial region of the vaginal lamina propria forming plexuses around blood vessels, and to a network of pseudocorpuscular nerve endings, anterioles and capillaries (homologous to the corpus spongiosum penis) in the pubovesicocervical fascia. Hoch contended that the sensory input from vaginal wall stimulation should be considered a cocomponent (along with clitoral sensory input) to the sensory arm of the orgasmic reflex.[48] Further support for anterior vaginal wall erogeneity was provided by a recent study demonstrating increased anterior vaginal wall sensitivity to electric stimuli.[49]

In spite of this vaginal erotic sensitivity, the incidence of coital anorgasmia is quite high. Hoch reports that 34% of female patients reporting for sex counseling are orgasmic only with self or partner noncoital stimulation.[48] Other studies suggest that coital anorgasmia may be as high as 60% to 80%.[17,45] This problem was attributed to several factors. First, expansion and lengthening of the inner two thirds of the vaginal barrel might limit penile contact with the upper anterior vaginal wall.[50] Second, orgasm latency in the female is longer than in the male,[38] therefore male orgasm and cessation of penile thrusting may occur prior to female orgasmic release. Third, and probably most importantly, certain coital positions might limit the ability to adequately stimulate the anterior vaginal wall. Alzate emphasizes that pressure exerted at an angle to the vaginal wall is necessary to most efficiently evoke erotic response.[50] Coitus performed in the missionary position allows the penis to move parallel with the axis of the vagina, failing to adequately provide direct pressure to the anterior vaginal wall. Indeed, coitally orgasmic women have reported the most optimal coital positions to be the female superior and the rear-entry positions.

VAGINAL FUNCTION IN FERTILITY

The function of the vagina in fertility may be limited to its role as a seminal receptable and reservoir. The anatomic orientation of the vagina in the resting state as well as its alterations during arousal exemplify its excellent adaptation to this role.

The axis of the vagina angles 10 to 15° below the horizontal pelvic line. Therefore, the transcervical plane rests below the fourchette of the vaginal outlet when a woman lies in the supine position. This gravitational advantage is augmented by the changes in the vaginal canal that occur during the excitation and plateau phases of sexual arousal. As described in a previous section, during excitation there is ballooning of the inner two thirds of the vagina with the greatest effect at the transcervical plane. The uterus and cervix elevate creating a tenting effect. During the plateau phase, the development of the orgasmic platform and consequent narrowing of the outer third of the vagina augments the damming effect of the perineal body, promoting retention of the seminal plasma in the inner vaginal vault. After orgasm and during resolution, the cervicouterine elevation abates and the cervix descends into the seminal pool.[13]

Normal vaginal pH ranges between 4 and 5, a level generally considered deleterious to sperm survival. Some consideration was given to the buffering capacity of vaginal transudate, but it was shown that after arousal, pH increases by only as much as 0.5 to 0.7.[30] The amount of increase is related to the duration of erotic stimulation and the amount of transudation. Since buffering of vaginal pH to 7.0 or more is desirable for sperm viability, the buffering capacity of vaginal transudate alone is inadequate. Indeed, the seminal plasma itself plays the major role in buffering vaginal acidity. It was shown that within 8 to 9 seconds of ejaculation,[13,51] vaginal pH can rise to more than 7 with the pH subsequently declining to baseline over the course of 6 to 7 hours.[13] Progressively motile sperm were recovered from the vaginal pool for as long as 2 hours after ejaculation.[13]

Motile sperm were recovered from cervical mucus within seconds of coitus.[52] This early entry into the cervical mucus may be caused by rapid transport,[53,54] independent of flagellar movements. Studies in laboratory animals showed that transport may be secondary to vaginal or cervical muscular contractions promoted by seminal plasma factors or occurring as a reflex in response to mechanical vaginal distention.[54] These contractions may be of relatively short duration, therefore subsequent entry of sperm into cervical mucus is likely due to swimming activity.

Finally, in the past some speculation was given to the potential role of vaginal transudate in influencing early reproductive events (that is, sperm capacitation).[31] Considering that seminal plasma was shown to decapacitate previously capacitated sperm and to inhibit capacitation in vitro,[53] it seems unlikely that sperm capacitation can commence until after the sperm have left the vaginal seminal pool and have entered the cervical mucus. While sperm have been shown to capacitate in vitro after swimming through a column of cervical mucus, the primary site for completion of capacitation is thought to be the fallopian tube.[55]

SUMMARY

The vagina is an organ of controversial embryologic origin with primary functions that commence during the reproductive years. Its most repetitive and important function is as a coital instrument, though it is also a seminal receptacle and passageway for menstruation and natural childbirth. Its morphologic and physiologic changes in response to sexual arousal allow it to function efficiently during coitus to impart pleasurable sensations through its pressure areas and receive stimulation possibly to orgasm via structures within its anterior vaginal wall. The vagina's role in fertility is limited. It may facilitate rapid transport of sperm into the uterus, but it is likely only a good seminal receptacle.

REFERENCES

1. Tanagho EA. Developmental anatomy and urogenital abnormalities. In: Raz S, ed. *Female Urology*. Philadelphia: WB Saunders Co.; 1983.
2. Moore KL. The urogenital system. In: Moore KL, ed. *The Developing Human: Clinically Oriented Embryology*. Philadelphia: WB Saunders Co; 1988.
3. Gondos B. Development of reproductive organs. *Ann Clin Lab Sci*. 1985; 15:363.
4. Wilson JD. Sexual differentiation. *Ann Rev Physiol*. 1978;40:279.
5. Deppisch LM. Transverse vaginal septum, histologic and embryologic considerations. *Obstet Gynecol*. 1972;39:193.
6. Sueldo CE, Rotman CA, Cooperman NR, Rana NR. Transverse vaginal septum, a report of four cases. *J Reprod Med*. 1985;30: 127.
7. Ulfelder H, Robboy SJ. The embryologic development of the human vagina. *Obstet Gynecol*. 1976;126:769.
8. Cunha GR. The dual origin of vaginal epithelium. *Am J Anatomy*. 1975;143:387.
9. Koff AK. Development of the vagina in the human fetus. *Carnegie Contrib Embryol*. 1933;24:59.
10. Mattingly RF. Relaxed vaginal outlet, rectocele, and enterocele. In: *TeLinde's Operative Gynecology*. Philadelphia: JB Lippincott Co; 1977.
11. Platzer W, Poisel S, Hafez ESE. Functional anatomy of the human vagina. In: Hafez ESE, Evans TN, eds. *The Human Vagina*. New York: Elsevier/North Holland Biomedical Press; 1978.
12. Netter FH. Normal anatomy of the female genital tract and its functional relationships. In: Oppenheimer E, ed. *The Ciba Collection of Medical Illustrations*. New York: Ciba Pharmaceutical Co; 1970;2.
13. Masters WH, Johnson VE. The vagina. In: *Human Sexual Response*. Boston: Little, Brown and Co; 1966.
14. Krantz KE. Innervation of the human vulva and vagina, a microscopic study. *Obstet Gynecol*. 1958;12:382.
15. Levin RJ. The physiology of sexual function in women. In: Epstein M, ed. *Clinics in Obstetrics and Gynaecology*. London: WB Saunders Co; 1980;7.
16. Kegel AH. Sexual functions of the pubococcygeus muscle. *Western J Surg Obstet Gynecol*. 1952;60:521.
17. Graber B, Kline-Graber G. Female orgasm: role of pubococcygeus muscle. *J Clin Psych*. 1979;40:348.
18. Messe MR, Geer JH. Voluntary vaginal muscular contractions as an enhancer of sexual arousal. *Arch Sex Behav*. 1985;14:13.
19. Chambless DL, Stern T, Sultan FE, et al. The pubococcygeus and female orgasm: a correlational study with normal subjects. *Arch Sex Behav*. 1982;11:479.
20. Freese MP, Levitt EE. Relationships among intravaginal pressure, orgasmic function, parity factors, and urinary leakage. *Arch Sex Behav*. 1984;13:261.
21. Hoon JPW. Physiologic assessment of sexual response in women: the unfulfilled promise. *Clin Obstet Gynecol*. 1984;27:767.
22. Henson DE, Rubin HB, Henson C. Labial and vaginal blood volume responses to visual and tactile stimuli. *Arch Sex Behav*. 1982;11:23.
23. Levin RJ, Wagner G. Orgasm in women in the laboratory—quantitative studies on duration, intensity, latency, and vaginal blood flow. *Arch Sex Behav*. 1985;14:439.
24. Fugl-Meyer AR, Sjogren K, Johansson K. A vaginal temperature registration system. *Arch Sex Behav*. 1984;13:247.
25. Wagner G, Levin RJ. Oxygen tension of the vaginal surface during sexual stimulation in the human. *Fertil Steril*. 1978;30:50.
26. Wagner G. Vaginal transudation. In: Beller FK, Schumacher GFB, eds. *The Biology of the Fluids of the Female Genital Tract*. New York: Elsevier North Holland, Inc; 1979.
27. Odeblad, E. Intracavitary circulation of aqueous material in the human vagina. *Acta Obstet Gynecol Scand*. 1964;43:360.
28. Wagner G, Levin RJ. Vaginal fluid. In: Hafez ESE, Evans TN, eds. *The Human Vagina*. New York: Elsevier/North Holland Biomedical Press; 1978.
29. Duncan SLB, Levin RJ. Transuterine, transendocervical, and transvaginal potential differences in conscious women measured in situ. *J Physiol*. 1976;259:27.
30. Wagner G, Levin R. Human vaginal pH and sexual arousal. *Fertil Steril*. 1984;41:389.
31. Preti G, Huggins GR, Silverberg GD. Alterations in the organic compounds of vaginal secretion caused by sexual arousal. *Fertil Steril*. 1979;32:47.
32. Masters WH, Johnson VE. The female orgasm. In: *Human Sexual Response*. Boston: Little, Brown and Co; 1966.
33. Campbell B. Neurophysiology of the clitoris. In: Lowry TP, Lowry TS, eds. *The Clitoris*. St. Louis: Warren H. Green; 1976.
34. Gillan P, Brindley GS. Vaginal and pelvic floor responses to sexual stimulation. *Psychophysiology*. 1979;16:471.
35. Bohlen JG, Held JP, Sanderson MO, Ahlgren A. The female orgasm: pelvic contractions. *Arch Sex Behav*. 1982;11:367.
36. Freud S. *Obras Completas*. Madrid: Biblioteca Nueva, 1967;1.
37. Masters WH, Johnson V. The clitoris. In: *Human Sexual Response*. Boston: Little, Brown and Co; 1966.

38. Kinsey AC, Pomeroy WB, Martin CE, Gebhard PH. *Sexual Behavior in the Human Female*. Philadelphia: WB Saunders Co; 1953.

39. Kaplan HS. *The New Sex Therapy*. New York: Brunner/Mazel Publishers; 1974.

40. Addiego F, Belzer EG, Comolli J, Moger W, Perry JD, Whipple B. Female ejaculation: a case study. *J Sex Res*. 1981;17:13.

41. Perry JD, Whipple B. Pelvic muscle strength of female ejaculators: evidence in support of a new theory of orgasm. *J Sex Res*. 1981:17:22.

42. Belzer EG, Whipple B, Moger W. On female ejaculation. *J Sex Res*. 1984:20:403.

43. Goldberg DC, Whipple B, Fishkin RE, Waxman H, Fink PJ, Weisberg M. The Grafenberg spot and female ejaculation: a review of initial hypothesis. *J Sex Marital Ther*. 1983;9:27.

44. Hoch Z. Vaginal erotic sensitivity by sexological examination. *Acta Obstet Gynecol Scand*. 1986;65:767.

45. Alzate H., Landono ML. Vaginal erotic sensitivity. *J Sex Marital Ther*. 1984;10:49.

46. Alzate H. Vaginal eroticism: a replication study. *Arch Sex Behav*. 1985;14:529.

47. Alzate H, Hoch Z. The "G-spot" and "female ejaculation": a current appraisal. *J Sex Marital Ther*. 1986;12:211.

48. Hoch Z. The sensory arm of the female orgasmic reflex. *J Sex Ed Ther*. 1980;6:4.

49. Schultz WCMW, van de Wiel HBM, Klatter JA, Sturm BE, Nauta J. Vaginal sensitivity to electric stimuli: theoretical and practical implications. *Arch Sex Behav*. 1989;18:87.

50. Alzate H. Vaginal eroticism and female orgasm: a current appraisal. *J Sex Marital Ther*. 1985;11:271.

51. Fox CA, Meldrum SJ, Watson BW. Continuous measurement by radiotelemetry of vaginal pH during human coitus. *J Reprod Fertil*. 1973;33:69.

52. Sobrero AJ, MacLeod J. The immediate post-coital test. *Fertil Steril*. 1962;13:184.

53. Overstreet JW, Katz DF, Cross NL. Sperm transport and capacitation. In: Speroff L, Simpson JL, Sciarra JJ, eds. *Reproductive Endocrinology, Infertility, Genetics*. Philadelphia: JB Lippincott Co; 1989.

54. Overstreet JW, Katz DF. Interaction between the female reproductive tract and spermatozoa. In: Gagnon C, ed. *Controls of Sperm Motility; Biological and Clinical Aspects*. Boca Raton, FL: CRC Press, Inc; 1990.

55. Suarez SS, Pollard JW. Capacitation, the acrosome reaction, and motility in mammalian sperm. In: Gagnon C, ed. *Controls of Sperm Motility: Biological and Clinical Aspects*. Boca Raton, FL: CRC Press, Inc; 1990.

CHAPTER 4

Anatomy and Physiology

4B   The Pubococcygeus Muscle

Jerry S. Benzl

INTRODUCTION

In women with pelvic relaxation there is usually associated damage to the pubococcygeus muscle. Examination reveals that this muscle is lax, atrophied, and of poor tone. Symptoms include urinary stress incontinence, genital prolapse, sexual problems, and rectal stasis.

Pelvic relaxation syndrome is a lifelong neuromuscular disorder that can be prevented or reversed by early recognition and treatment of pathologic pubococcygeus muscle dysfunction. Vaginal manometry facilitates the proper diagnosis of this dysfunction. Details of complete pubococcygeus muscle evaluation are described.

ANATOMY AND FUNCTION OF THE PUBOCOCCYGEUS MUSCLE

Within the musculofascial diaphragms which comprise the pelvic floor the pubococcygeus muscle occupies a key position: supporting the midportion of the urethra, vagina, and rectum and providing extrinsic sphincteric functions (Fig. 4B-1). The pubococcygeus muscle, which occupies a central location, has its origin in the arch of the os pubis and its insertion not only into the tip of the coccyx but also into the intrinsic musculature of the urethra, the vagina, and the rectum (Fig. 4B-2).

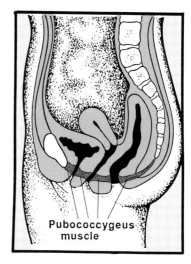

Pubococcygeus muscle

Fig. 4B-1   The pubococcygeus muscle supports and raises the floor of the pelvis. By drawing the anus, vagina, and urethra toward the pubis, these structures are constricted and their sphincteric functions are enhanced.

Histochemical analysis of pubococcygeus muscle cells have shown this muscle to consist of a heterogeneous population of large diameter, slow twitch (type I) and fast twitch (type II) muscle fibers. The predominance of the slow twitch, type I fibers suggests that the major role of the pubococcygeus muscle is to provide static visceral support. However, the significant number of fast twitch, type II muscle fibers found in the pubococ-

47

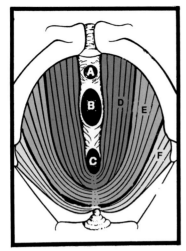

Fig. 4B-2   The pubococcygeus muscle occupies a key position within the supporting musculofascial diaphragms that comprise the pelvic floor. Its origin is from the inner surface of the superior ramus of the pubis and the spine of the ischium and also from the connecting fascia (arcus tendinous ligament) which runs along the lateral wall. Its posterior fibers insert into the coccyx; the anterior fibers insert in the midline behind and in front of the anus, vagina, and urethra. *A* = urethra; *B* = vagina; *C* = anus. *D* = pubococcygeus muscle; *E* = iliococcygeus muscle; *F* = ischiococcygeus muscle.

cygeus muscle indicate that this muscle also helps maintain urethral, vaginal, and rectal tone and assists in active closure of these structures.[1]

Pubococcygeus muscle function is normally developed during childhood and young adulthood. However, as many as 40% of adult women either lack this development or have lost the function and coordination of their pelvic muscles.[2] In patients with pelvic relaxation and genuine stress incontinence, the dynamic function of this muscle is almost always impaired, resulting in a decrease of abdominal pressure transmission to the urethra. Fortunately, pubococcygeus neuromuscular dysfunction can be prevented or reversed through muscle reeducation and exercise.[3]

ASSESSING PUBOCOCCYGEUS MUSCLE FUNCTION

The benefits of maintaining healthy pelvic muscles are so important to the health and general well-being of women that pubococcygeus muscle assessment and pelvic exercise instruction should be part of every pelvic examination.

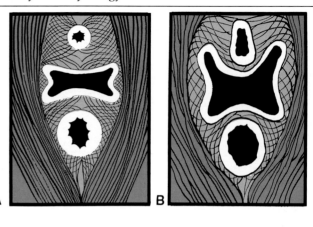

Fig. 4B-3   **A,** The well-developed pubococcygeus muscle: firm muscle and connective tissue support throughout the vagina. **B,** Atrophic pubococcygeus muscle: the atrophic muscle and vaginal connective tissue is manifest by a loose, sagging vagina.

Inspection

With the patient in the lithotomy position, observation is the first step. In women with advanced genital relaxation the perineum bulges downward, the vaginal introitus opens, exposing redundant mucosa, and the anus appears everted. In early genital relaxation the same changes are noted to a lesser degree.

A vaginal speculum examination should also be performed. The presence of cystocele, rectocele, and/or prolapse can be determined by asking the patient to bear down. To estimate how much potential supportive function the pubococcygeus muscle retains, the patient is asked to draw up instead of bearing down. If good pubococcygeus muscle function is present the perineum will be drawn up to a high position.[4]

Palpation

Vaginal palpation is performed with the index finger. A well-developed pubococcygeus muscle is manifested by firm tone throughout the entire length of the vagina (Fig. 4B-3*A*). In genital relaxation, on the other hand, the vaginal walls offer little resistance and feel thin and loose, as if detached from the surrounding structures (Fig. 4B-3*B*).

The pubococcygeus muscle, which lies in the middle third of the vagina, can be palpated on the lateral wall when the index finger is introduced to a depth of 3 to 5 cm beyond the vaginal introitus (Figs. 4B-4*A* and *B*). The muscle can be further demonstrated by asking the patient to contract it. Most patients will contract the pubococcygeus muscle when asked to pretend that they have to stop their urinary flow; other patients may

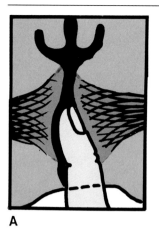
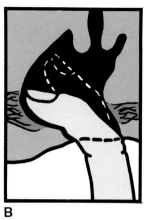

Fig. 4B-4   A, In a normal vagina, the pubococcygeus muscle is well developed and elastic tissues offer a degree of resistance in all directions. Patients can usually voluntarily contract the pubococcygeus muscle around the palpating finger. **B,** The atrophic pubococcgyeus muscle is not easily palpated and the vagina feels roomy with little lateral resistance. Many pubococcygeus muscle deficits are found to be unilateral.

produce a better contraction when asked to contract their rectal sphincter muscles. The areas in which contractions can be palpated vary with the position of the pubococcygeus and the amount of supportive function that remains. In normal patients the contractions can be felt throughout the length of the muscle, whereas in genital relaxation the pubococcygeus muscle sags and all that can be felt is slight tensing near the vaginal outlet.[5]

Approximately one third of the patients demonstrate awareness of function and good voluntary control of the pubococcygeus muscle during digital examination. By following a prescribed active pelvic muscle exercise program these patients can usually improve their pubococcygeus function with little or no additional intervention (see Chapter 13C). Other patients, however, lack awareness of pubococcygeus function and are incapable of sufficient muscle activity to promote reconstructive processes without additional instruction. These patients benefit from the biofeedback techniques of vaginal pressure manometry or electromyography.

VAGINAL PRESSURE MANOMETRY

Vaginal pressure manometry and physiotherapy of the pelvic floor muscles as treatment for urinary stress incontinence and pelvic relaxation syndrome was first popularized by Dr. Arnold Kegel in 1949.[6] Although our knowledge of pelvic floor anatomy and its dynamic function has increased considerably since that time, the basic techniques of vaginal pressure manometry remain the same.

THE PERINEOMETER

The perineometer, originally developed by Dr. Kegel, is a pneumatic device designed to help the clinician assess pubococcygeus muscle strength, help women establish awareness of pubococcygeus function, and therapeutically exercise and strengthen this muscle. It consists of a vaginal pressure sensor connected to a manometer calibrated from zero to 100 mm Hg.

When the pressure sensor is introduced into the vagina and the pelvic muscles are in a relaxed state, a static pressure reading of between 15 to 20 mm Hg indicates a normal pubococcygeus muscle resistance and normal vaginal tone. A static pressure reading of 10 mm Hg or lower usually indicates poor muscle resistance and decreased vaginal tone.

Contraction of an intact, well-developed pubococcygeus muscle can generate a pressure change of 20 mm Hg or more above the initial static pressure. Lack of awareness of function and/or pubococcygeus muscle atrophy are reflected in small or almost imperceptible increases in pressure, usually less than 5 mm Hg. Intermediate readings may be obtained in patients having awareness of function but a poorly developed or partially atrophied pubococcygeus muscle.[4,6,7]

The Perineometer as a Scientific Instrument

Several different types of perineometers are currently available and range in sophistication from simple pressure manometers to electronic instruments that assure accurate calibration (Figs. 4B-5*A* and *B*). Other perineometers utilize vaginal electromyograph sensors that measure pubococcygeus contraction electrical activity rather than the muscle contraction movements. Regardless of the type of perineometer used, one should be cautious not to focus solely on the specific pressure readings or the measured pubococcygeus muscle contraction activity. Numerous variables including the type of pressure sensor, depth of sensor placement, or patient position, size, and weight can alter the recorded values and make them pertinent only to that particular patient. The inability to standardize these variable factors limits the usefulness of the perineometer as an exact scientific instrument. Instead, the perineometer is best used clinically as a biofeedback device to focus the patient's awareness on pubococcygeus muscle function and help develop the contraction reflex.

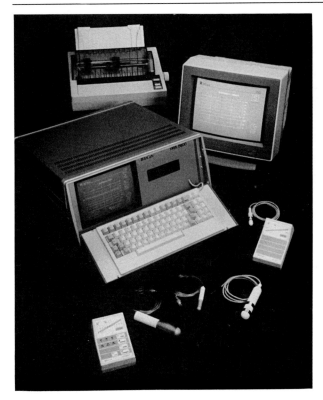

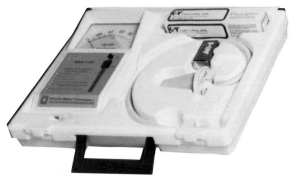

Fig. 4B-5   **A**, The PRS 8900 computerized perineometer-transvaginal electrical stimulation unit. (Manufactured by InCare Medical Products, Libertyville, Illinois.) **B**, The Gynos Perineometer vaginal pressure manometer. (Manufactured by Interactive Medical Technologies, Inc., Ventura, California.)

Clinical Applications of the Perineometer

In the office setting the perineometer provides immediate visual confirmation that the correct muscles are being exercised and greatly reduces the time required for the muscle reeducation process. The perineometer is also a useful tool for evaluating patient progress during follow-up visits. As previously mentioned, many patients have good pubococcygeus control, can easily contract this muscle, and one office training session is all that is required for them to start on a pelvic muscle exercise program.

For those patients who are unable to contract their pubococcygeus muscle, prescribing a perineometer for individual home use is of proven benefit.[8] By using the perineometer, the patient can learn by visual biofeedback when she is contracting the pubococcygeus muscle correctly, can follow a prescribed exercise program, and can monitor improvement in muscle contraction strength. In addition, the vaginal pressure sensor provides isometric resistance to the pubococcygeus muscle contractions. Isometric resistance increases the effectiveness of these exercises, particularly on the pubococcygeus muscle extensions that insert into the wall of the urethra, vagina, and rectum, thereby significantly improving their sphincteric capabilities.[9]

SUMMARY

Pubococcygeus muscle assessment and exercise training should be part of every pelvic examination. When indicated, a perineometer or similar device can be used safely for the assessment of pelvic muscle function, as a visual teaching aid, and as a home exercise device. There is ample evidence that pelvic floor muscle reeducation can in many cases alleviate the symptoms of urinary stress incontinence and pelvic relaxation syndrome. When initiated prophylactically there will probably be a decreased risk of developing lower genitourinary tract symptoms during menopause and later years.

REFERENCES

1. Koelbl H, Strassegger H, Riss PA, Gruber H. Morphologic and functional aspects of pelvic floor muscles in patients with pelvic relaxation and genuine stress incontinence. *Obstet Gynecol.* 1989; 74:789–793.
2. Kegel A, Powell TO. The physiologic treatment of urinary incontinence. *J Urol.* 1950;63:808–813.
3. Koelbl H, Hanzal E. Female stress urinary incontinence and the pelvic floor. *Int Urogynecol J.* 1990;1:150–154.
4. Kegel A. Early genital relaxation. *Obstet Gynecol.* 1956;8:545–550.
5. Kegel A. Stress incontinence and genital relaxation. *CIBA Clinical Symposium.*1952;4:35–51.
6. Kegel A. The physiologic treatment of poor tone and function of the genital muscles and of urinary stress incontinence. *Western J Surg Ob Gyn.* 1949;Nov:527–535.
7. Levitt E, Kanovsky M, Freese M, Thompson J. Intravaginal pressure assessed by the Kegel perineometer. *Arch Sex. Behav.* 1979;8: 425–430.
8. Kegel, A. Physiologic therapy for urinary stress incontinence. *JAMA.* 1951;146:915–917.
9. Jones EG, Kegel A. Treatment of urinary stress incontinence. *Surg Gynecol Obstet.* 1952;94:179–188.

CHAPTER 5

Physiology of Anal Continence and Defecation

M. M. Henry

INTRODUCTION

Generally speaking, the most important contributions to the study of structure and function of the anorectum were made by clinicians rather than by anatomists or physiologists. This anatomic region is not readily accessible for study in the cadaver and the need for scientific endeavor is more readily appreciated by the clinician in contact with patients having a functional disorder of the anal sphincter or pelvic floor (listed in Box 5-1). These disorders form an increasing component of the workload referred to a colorectal surgeon as a consequence of an aging population and a better-educated public; larger numbers of patients seek advice about their functional disabilities that have previously been regarded as untreatable.

This is a very brief account containing the anatomy and physiology relevant to an understanding of the clinical aspects of disorders of the anorectum. It is not intended that great detail be provided in a volume largely directed to gynecologic disorders.

EPITHELIUM AND VASCULATURE

The stratified squamous epithelium of the body wall skin infolds into the anal canal, where it is largely devoid of hairs and glands but is richly supplied by sensory nerve endings, particularly at the dentate line. The latter approximates to the line of fusion with the columnar epithelium continuous with the rectum. Above this level there are no recognizable sensory receptors, hence injection (that is, hemorrhoids) at this level is painless. Studies of anal canal sensation have shown that the dentate line corresponds to the most sensitive zone within the anal canal.[1] This is an important component of the sensory aspect of continence as discussed below.

The arterial supply to the rectum and anal canal is provided mainly by the superior and inferior rectal arteries. The middle rectal artery also supplies the rectum but to an extent which is probably variable. The supe-

---

Box 5-1
Functional Disorders of the Anal Sphincters and Pelvic Floor

Descending perineum syndrome
Solitary rectal ulcer syndrome
Perineal pain syndrome
Hemorrhoids
Rectal prolapse
Genital prolapse
Urinary incontinence
Anorectal incontinence
Constipation

---

rior rectal artery is the direct continuation of the inferior mesenteric artery, and its mucosal branches are said to course within the columns of Morgagni. The inferior rectal arteries are branches of the internal pudendal artery which traverse the ischiorectal fossa, divide and transmit branches through the external anal sphincter to gain access to the distal part of the anal canal. There are almost certainly extensive intramural anastomoses between the superior and inferior rectal vessels. Whatever the precise anatomic arrangement, much of the rectum and anal canal remains viable if both the superior and inferior rectal arteries are divided. Venous drainage is via veins which course with the main arterial supply. Hemorrhoids are now considered to be cushions of mucosa which carry a largely arterial supply and arteriovenous shunts[2] rather than varicosities of the anal venous circulation (hemorrhoidal bleeding is usually arterial). It is possible that these cushions of tissue which have erectile properties may play a role in normal anal continence by creation of simple surface tension effects created by apposition of moist mucosal surfaces. Hence some patients experience minor disturbances of continence following hemorrhoidectomy.

THE INTERNAL ANAL SPHINCTER

The internal anal sphincter (IAS) is a condensation of smooth muscle approximately 3 cm long and 5 mm wide which is continuous with the inner circular muscle of the rectum.[3] The sphincter is comprised of dense bundles of smooth muscle fibers which are separated by fascicles that run obliquely at the proximal and distal ends and horizontally in its middle section. At the anorectal junction the longitudinal smooth muscle of the rectum blends with caudal fibers of the pubococcygeus to form a conjoint longitudinal muscle layer that splits to pass both sides of the external anal sphincter. The muscle exists in a state of tonic partial contraction and is responsible for approximately 80% of resting anal pressure (Fig. 5-1).[4,5] The sphincter muscle is innervated by sympathetic nerves derived from the hypogastric (presacral nerves). Stimulation of the extrinsic presacral nerves gives rise to relaxation of the internal sphincter.[6] The muscle also relaxes reflexly in response to rectal distention.[7] This reflex, which is customarily referred to as the rectosphincteric inhibitory reflex, may be clinically tested by inflating a Miller-Abbott rectal balloon with 50 ml of air while recording resting anal pressure (Fig. 5-2). This reflex is shown to be facilitated exclusively by the intramural nerve plexuses since the

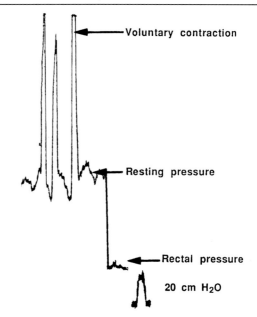

Fig. 5-1 Anal canal pressures in cm water recorded using a microballoon connected to a pressure transducer. Resting pressure is approximately 60 cm water higher than intrarectal pressure and is largely due to internal sphincter tone. During voluntary contraction (arrowed on diagram) intraanal pressure is at least doubled as a consequence of external sphincter contraction.

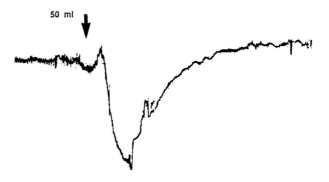

Fig. 5-2 The normal rectosphincteric inhibitory reflex. Resting anal pressure falls in response to distension of a rectal balloon with 50 ml of air.

reflex is preserved when the extrinsic neural supply to the lower gut is abolished, but the reflex cannot be obtained when the rectum is distended proximal to a myotomised segment of rectum.[6] Since the reflex is dependent on the integrity of ganglia in the muscle of the rectum, it is found absent in patients with Hirschsprung's disease, hence the diagnosis can be readily made by simple manometric methods.[8]

The IAS is responsible for generating slow waves (amplitude 5 to 25 cm water; frequency 10 to 20/min) and ultraslow waves (amplitude 30 to 100 cm water; frequency <3/min).[9] Slow waves are higher in the distal anal canal, suggesting that a vector may act to propel small quantities of rectal contents back into the rectum from the anal canal. Ultraslow waves are seen in 5% of normal subjects, but in 45% of patients with hemorrhoids and 80% of patients with anal fissures.[10,11] These observations have led to the hypothesis that these two common conditions may be caused by abnormal function within the IAS itself.

THE EXTERNAL ANAL SPHINCTER AND PELVIC FLOOR MUSCLES

These striated muscles probably derive their innervation from separate sources; the external anal sphincter (EAS) is supplied by the pudendal nerves, and the pelvic floor directly from the third and fourth motor roots that supply the muscle on its pelvic surface.[12] Both muscles display the unusual property of continuous resting electrical tone (Fig. 5-3); such activity is maintained even during sleep.[13] During such acts as coughing, voluntary contraction, sneezing, speech, or lifting there is marked recruitment of motor unit activity and a corresponding increase (interference activity) in the electromyographic response.[14] This function is mediated by a spinal reflex with afferent receptors situated within the pelvic floor muscles themselves.[15]

ANORECTAL CONTINENCE

Control of rectal contents until it is socially appropriate for them to be voided is a complex process involving many physiologic processes, the precise interrelation-

> **Box 5-2**
> **The Major Factors Considered Important in the Maintenance of Anorectal Continence**
>
> The anorectal angle
> The external anal sphincter
> The internal anal sphincter
> Sensation
>   a. of rectal distension
>   b. discrimination between flatus and feces
> Miscellaneous

ship of which remains poorly understood. A list of the factors that are currently recognized is provided in Box 5-2.

The Anorectal Angle

The angle between the lower rectum and upper anal canal (anorectal angle) is created by puborectalis contraction and is generally regarded to be crucial to the preservation of anorectal continence. The angle normally should be within the range of 60° to 105°.[16] It was observed that the anal sphincter muscles can be divided without causing gross incontinence, provided that the important puborectalis muscle remains intact.[17,18] There is considerable debate over why the angle can facilitate anal continence. Parks and colleagues believed that the angle created a flap-valve mechanism (Fig. 5-4) that raised intraabdominal pressure, causing the anterior rectal wall to close over the top of the anal canal, excluding it from rectal contents.[19] Using cine-radiologic techniques, however, Bartolo and others[20] were unable to demonstrate convincingly any flap-valve activity of the anterior rectal wall in subjects performing

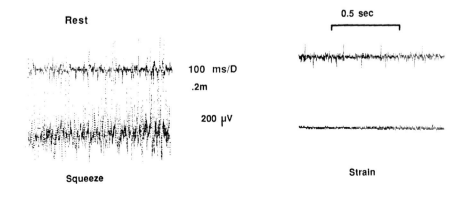

Fig. 5-3 Conventional EMG of puborectalis muscle in normal individual during resting state, during period of voluntary contraction, and during period of straining in preparation for defecation.

Rest

100 ms/D
.2m

200 µV

0.5 sec

Squeeze

Strain

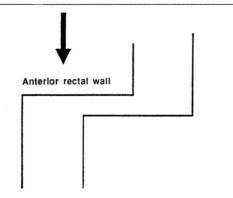

Fig. 5-4 The flap-valve. Intraabdominal pressure (arrow) is conducted onto the anterior rectal wall. When pressure increases in response to coughing, sneezing, or lifting the anterior rectal wall closes down over the top of the anal canal.

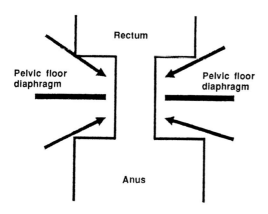

Fig. 5-5 The flutter valve. The arrows represent the lateral vector forces created by contraction of the pelvic floor muscles.

a Valsalva maneuver. Phillips and Edwards[21] demonstrated that if the anal canal was sprinkled with barium sulphate powder, a 0.5 cm segment at the anorectal angle rapidly emptied of barium when the subject moved. They surmised that this segment of rectum was subject to extraluminal forces operating in such a way that a flutter valve (Fig. 5-5) was created.

In all probability a combination of these two physical principles may well apply in addition to a simple disruption of the otherwise straight line between the rectum and anal canal. This kinking is analogous to the method by which the water supply to a hose pipe may be readily interrupted using minimum force.

The Anal Sphincters

As already stated, the anal sphincters may be divided without necessarily compromising continence. There-

fore, division of the internal sphincter (sphincterotomy) or division of the external sphincter (to treat anal fistula) usually causes only minor degrees of incontinence. It is customary to regard the internal sphincter as being responsible for a fine tuning control mechanism; that is, to provide control to flatus and to liquid stool. This concept is being challenged because some patients with IAS deficiency present with a profound functional deficit. The EAS also plays a significant part in normal anal control, although the fact that the muscle can only contract for up to 60 seconds maximum suggests that its role is limited. It may act in times of emergency, such as when the sphincters are challenged by loose stool; vigorous contraction may buy much appreciated extra time.

Sensation

As discussed above, the receptors responsible for the sensation of rectal filling probably reside in the levator muscles that lie in intimate contact with the rectum. Any pathologic process that reduces rectal distensibility (such as Crohn's disease) or interferes with contact between the rectum and pelvic floor (such as fibrosis) may lead to loss of this function and in turn lead to either incontinence or fecal impaction. The differentiation between flatus and feces is another important aspect of anal sensory function. It is almost certain that this is facilitated by the recto-sphincteric inhibitory reflex. When the rectum fills with flatus or feces, rectal distention causes reflex internal sphincter relaxation and a small sample of rectal contents enter the proximal anal canal, makes contact with the sensory receptors at the dentate line, and differentiation takes place.[22]

Miscellaneous

Other factors may play a minor role in continence. These include surface tension effects caused by hemorrhoids and vector forces acting retrogradely. In addition the valves of Houston and the rectosigmoid valve may assist continence by impeding the passage of stool.

DEFECATION

Normal defecation requires a sophisticated coordination of abdominal and pelvic muscles and rectal propulsion. The squatting position is used and intraabdominal pressure raised as a consequence of contraction of diaphragm and anterior abdominal wall muscles. Electrical activity within the pelvic floor is then reflexly inhibited, the anorectal angle straightens out such that the angle between anus and rectum approaches 180°. This, in addition to reflex internal sphincter relaxation, facilitates passage of the fecal bolus. At the termination of defecation, the internal sphincter regains its tone, closing the anal canal. Similarly, electrical tone returns to the pelvic floor and external sphincter, restoring the anorectal angle to normal.

The central mechanisms controlling defecation are not understood. Recent experiments on the cortical localization of motor cells controlling the anal sphincters suggest that there is a fast-conducting, direct pyramidal pathway to the sacral anterior horn cells supplying these muscles, thereby indicating the importance of the brain in controlling their normal function.

SUMMARY

Anal continence is influenced by a number of factors, of which sphincter contraction and in particular contraction of the pelvic floor muscles are of paramount importance. The sensation of fullness in the rectum and the special ability to discriminate between flatus and feces are necessary to alert the normal individual of the need to defecate and to identify the nature of rectal contents. Patients who lose this ability develop fecal impaction and secondary incontinence. For defecation to occur there has to be relaxation (inhibition) of tone within the pelvic floor and external anal sphincter muscles to permit passage of the fecal bolus in response to an increase in intraabdominal pressure.

REFERENCES

1. Rogers J, Henry MM, Misiewicz JJ. Combined sensory and motor deficit in fecal incontinence. *Gut.* 1988;29:5–9.
2. Thomson WH. The nature of hemorrhoids. *Br J Surg.* 1975;62: 542–552.
3. Wilde FR. The anal intermuscular septum. *Br J Surg.* 1949;36: 279–285.
4. Bennett DL, Duthie HL. The functional importance of the internal anal sphincter. *Br J Surg.* 1964;51:355–357.
5. Duthie HL, Watts JM. Contribution of the external anal sphincter to the pressure zone in the anal canal. *Gut.* 1965;6:64–68.
6. Lubowski DZ, Nicholls RJ, Swash M, Jordan MJ. Neural control of internal anal sphincter function. *Br J Surg.* 1987;74:668–670.
7. Gowers WR. The automatic action of the sphincter ani. *Proc R Soc Med.* 1877;26:77–84.
8. Callaghan RP, Nixon HH. Megarectum: physiological observations. *Arch Dis Childh.* 1964;39:153–157.
9. Hancock BD, Smith K. The internal sphincter and Lord's procedure for hemorrhoids. *Br J Surg.* 1975;62:833–866.
10. Hancock BD. Measurement of anal pressure and motility. *Gut.* 1976;17:645–651.
11. Hancock BD. The internal sphincter and anal fissure. *Br J Surg.* 1977;64:92–95.
12. Snooks SJ, Swash M. The innervation of the muscles of continence. *Ann R Coll Surg Eng.* 1986;68:45–49.
13. Floyd EW, Walls EW. Electromyography of the sphincter ani externus in man. *J Physiol.* 1953;122:500–609.
14. Taverner D, Smiddy FG. An electromyographic study of the normal function of the external anal sphincter and pelvic diaphragm. *Dis Col Rec.* 1959;2:153–160.
15. Melzack J, Porter NH. Studies on the reflex activity of the external sphincter ani in spinal man. *Paraplegia.* 1964;1:277–296.
16. Hardcastle JD, Parks AG. A study of anal incontinence and some principles of surgical treatment. *Proc R Soc Med.* 1970;63 (suppl):116–118.
17. Milligan ETC, Morgan CN. Surgical anatomy of the anal canal with special reference to anal fistulae. *Lancet.* 1934;ii:1150–1156.
18. Varma KK, Stephens D. Neuromuscular reflexes of anal continence. *Aus and NZ J Surg.* 1982;41:263–272.
19. Parks AG, Porter NH, Hardcastle JD. The syndrome of the descending perineum. *Proc R Soc Med.* 1966;59:477–482.
20. Bartolo DCC, Roe AM, Locke-Edmunds JC, Virjee J, Mortensen NJM. Flap-valve theory of anorectal continence. *Br J Surg.* 1986; 73:1012–1014.
21. Phillips SF, Edwards DAW. Some aspects of anal continence and defecation. *Gut.* 1965;6:396–405.
22. Read MG, Read NW. Role of anorectal sensation in preserving continence. *Gut.* 1982;23:345–347.

CHAPTER 6

Clinical Evaluation

Andrew M. Agosta

INTRODUCTION

The clinical evaluation of the pelvic floor is the stepping stone for all diagnostic and therapeutic decisions to be made. In order to achieve the best therapeutic success, the pelvic floor surgeon needs a knowledge and understanding of the entire pelvic floor. This chapter reviews a general philosophy concerning evaluation, some important components of the history and physical examination, as well as basic office tests to help evaluate the pelvic floor.

GENERAL PHILOSOPHY

The evaluation of pelvic floor disorders was hindered in the past by some fundamental errors. The first was the use of a compartmental approach, treated by different specialties without regard to complete pelvic floor function. One specialty dealt with the anterior compartment (lower urinary tract disorders), one with the posterior compartment (anal/rectal disorders), and another with the vaginal compartment (uterovaginal disorders). This often was done without understanding the importance of the effect on each other's compartments. An example of this compartmental approach includes patients who underwent cystourethropexy without regard to existing posterior vaginal wall defects. This not uncommonly has resulted in extension of

an enterocele postoperatively. The above demonstrates therapy of the anterior pelvic floor compartment without regard to its effect on the posterior compartment. It is well known that anterior vaginal wall elevation that occurs with a cystourethropexy may significantly alter anatomic relationships, allowing intraabdominal forces to reach the cul-de-sac directly. This leads to a relatively high incidence of enteroceles after urethropexy.[1] Leaving even a small posterior vaginal wall abnormality without correction places the patient at risk of the deficit enlarging and becoming symptomatic. Because of this, special attention at the initial office evaluation should be given to the posterior vaginal wall in all potential urethropexy patients.

Another example of poor outcome associated with compartmentalized care of the pelvic floor are cases of surgical correction of uterovaginal prolapse (treatment of the vaginal compartment) without regard to the anterior compartment. This often has resulted in a new symptom—stress urinary incontinence—requiring further surgery in the future. In cases of anterior vaginal wall prolapse (pelvic relaxation of the support structures of the anterior vaginal wall), often there is associated loss of urethrovesical junction support as well, and therefore coexisting genuine stress urinary incontinence. The symptoms of stress urinary incontinence, however, may be masked because of urethral obstruction from the prolapse. Surgical correction without regard to this possibility often will lead to the onset of a new symptom—stress incontinence—and therefore extreme patient dissatisfaction.

A second error in the handling of pelvic floor disorders involves the concept of extirpating surgery. Most training programs emphasize extirpating surgery such as hysterectomy or adnexectomy. The clinical examination therefore is done with the idea in mind of how to most easily remove a structure. In looking at standard extirpating management, there are many common scenarios that lead to important questions. Why do some women with uterine prolapse treated by total vaginal hysterectomy present later with vaginal vault prolapse? Why is anterior colporrhaphy associated with an alarmingly high failure rate, estimated to be up to 33%?[2,3] In addressing these undesirable outcomes many practitioners have put blame on patients' tissues, claiming they were atrophic and/or had poor elasticity. In other cases technical difficulty secondary to patient obesity or poor tissue planes due to scar tissue from previous surgical repairs were held responsible. While these conditions certainly can contribute to operative failure, another risk for failure must be considered—that the surgeon's choice of operation is in error. Surgical failure may accompany operations that do not restore the pelvic floor to correct anatomic position. Pelvic surgeons have placed too little emphasis on restoration of proper anatomy and likewise too little emphasis on the clinical evaluation. Obviously, if uterine prolapse is not caused by the uterus itself, but instead results from weakness in uterine as well as vaginal support structures, then removal of the uterus alone without attention to repair of the support defects will not prevent prolapse of the vaginal vault. Likewise, cases of traditional anterior colporrhaphy are inappropriate when the true defect lies laterally or superiorly instead of in the midline. By identifying all of the defects present in a given patient, the correct combination of techniques necessary for individualized treatment can be established. Therefore, it is important to first diagnose the defects by a good clinical evaluation prior to deciding on the repair technique. Instead of extirpating pelvic surgeries, the surgeon should concentrate on restorative surgery. To do this the clinical evaluation encompassing a thorough history, physical examination, and diagnostic tests must embody this concept. The examination should locate specific defects in support structures. It is logical to assume that correcting these defects, thereby restoring anatomic conditions, will give the best chance for long-term success. Knowledge of correct pelvic anatomy is paramount and must be appreciated before defects can be noted and their severity estimated. The occurrence of multiple defects at various vaginal sites is common, with each requiring its own specific reparative technique. Therefore, the blending of several restorative techniques is often necessary to achieve optimal cure. Patients should not be "fitted for the same procedure," but procedures should be tailored to the patients' specific defects. By identifying each anatomic abnormality individualized treatment can be accomplished. All abnormal support areas can be found preoperatively by a carefully performed clinical evaluation.

In summary, as in all of clinical medicine the history and physical examination are the first and most important steps in evaluation of a woman with pelvic floor disorders. Combined with a thorough knowledge of anatomy and pathophysiology of genital, urinary tract, and colorectal disorders, the properly performed clinical evaluation can guide the practitioner into appropriate use of diagnostic tests as well as management. There is a need for the pelvic surgeon to fully understand and study the entire pelvic floor so that complete restoration of normal anatomy can be accomplished.

HISTORY

It is just as important to obtain a thorough history when evaluating a female with lower urinary tract and pelvic floor disorders as in any other branch of medicine. Early in the physician–patient interview, one should obtain a description of the patient's main complaint, its frequency, duration, and a clear understanding of its magnitude or disability. Although the information obtained from history is mostly nondiagnostic, it often helps point the examiner in the right direction, thereby assisting in the selection of appropriate diagnostic tests. Patient interviews remain the most important method of obtaining the appropriate information and allow an essential physician–patient relationship to be developed. Computerized forms or questionnaires in lay terms certainly can be useful to allow more rapid patient assessment, but these clearly cannot be substituted for the quality of information gathered from a personal interview. The importance of developing a good rapport with a patient cannot be stressed enough when treating pelvic floor dysfunction.

From a practical viewpoint the examiner wants to know whether the symptoms prompting the visit are suggestive of four broad categories: symptomatic pelvic relaxation, urinary incontinence, bladder irritability, or anal/rectal disorders.

Pelvic Relaxation

Symptoms of pelvic relaxation are varied. Often more than one vaginal compartment is involved and more than one symptom is noted. On the other hand, there are many patients with pelvic relaxation disorders who are asymptomatic. Whether the relaxation is relevant or not depends on the size and extent of the disorder along with the magnitude of the patient's symptoms. Pelvic relaxation in general often causes feelings of "something falling, vaginal heaviness, pressure, or irritation." Cystoceles, in particular, may cause minimal symptoms until the anterior vaginal wall descends to a point where it approaches or protrudes through the introitus. Patients may feel or actually see the protrusion at this point. Also they may have voiding disturbances and need digital maneuvers to push the prolapse out of the way in order to void. Even without the need for digital maneuvers, the patient may have increased residual urine with subsequent complications, such as repeated urinary tract infections. Uterine and vaginal vault prolapse, along with enterocele, cause vague symptoms of pelvic pressure. These symptoms may be more pronounced in a standing position and relieved by resting supine. Rectoceles tend to cause symptoms of defecation disorders, including excessive bearing down and fecal tenesmus. They may actually require digital maneuvers (splinting) or frequent enemas to enable defecation.

Urinary Incontinence

Given a history of urinary incontinence, it is important to ascertain the duration of the problem, whether the patient uses pads, and how long absorbent protection has been necessary. It often is useful to ask which type of absorbent protection is used, such as mini-pads or an absorbent garment, in order to get an idea of the amount of urinary leakage present. A history of previous surgery on the bladder, urethra, or anterior vaginal wall is important because these may be associated with scarring, fibrosis, and denervation of the urethra. If intrinsic urethral damage is present this condition may require special surgical procedures, as opposed to a standard retropubic urethropexy to enable a good prognosis for cure.[4,5]

The bladder presents many symptoms that are nonspecific and overlapping. However, the diagnosis of stress incontinence (genuine stress urinary incontinence) most commonly is associated with leakage during coughing, sneezing, exercising, or any movement which increases intraabdominal pressure. The leakage usually occurs in small spurts at the time of the stressful event. The symptom of stress incontinence is common since 85% to 100% of patients with genuine stress urinary incontinence complain of stress incontinent symptoms.[1,6-10] However, it is a nonspecific symptom in that more than half of patients with other urologic disorders also complain of stress incontinence.[11] It has relatively poor predictive value, with a positive predictive value of 59% to 85% and a negative predictive value of 18% to 69%, indicating that this symptom does not reliably predict the diagnosis.[10,12,13] Women who have stress incontinence as their only complaint have a 60% to 90% (mean 73%) chance of having genuine stress incontinence on diagnostic testing. Of these women, 10% to 40% have detrusor instability (alone or coexistent with genuine stress incontinence).[6,8-10,12,14-20] This underscores the need for further testing prior to any surgical consideration.

Bladder Irritability

Symptoms of frequency, urgency, and urge incontinence are characteristically suggestive of an unstable bladder. These symptoms may be elicited by asking the patient if she has the strong desire to urinate even when her bladder is not very full, if she has the urge to urinate before she leaks, or if she often leaks on the way to the bathroom. Other symptoms suggestive of an unstable bladder include leakage associated with the sound, site, or feel of running water, leakage when standing up from a sitting or supine position associated with urge, urinary frequency, and nocturia. Frequency is present when the patient has more than seven daytime voids in 24 hours. Nocturia is abnormal when there are two or more times during the night that wake the patient from sleep in order to urinate. Also, enuresis or a history of previous enuresis which persisted into late childhood may increase the likelihood of an unstable bladder.[21] The symptoms of urgency or urge incontinence are very sensitive in the diagnosis of detrusor instability with 70% to 95% of patients with detrusor instability complaining of urgency.[6-10,19,20,22-25] However, these symptoms are nonspecific in that many patients with genuine stress incontinence also complain of urgency. They do have a high negative predictive value (82%) indicating that if a patient does not complain of urgency, there is less than a 20% chance of that patient having detrusor instability.[10,13] The symptoms of frequency, nocturia, and enuresis are not very sensitive or specific individually, but the chance of detrusor instability increases as the number of abnormal urologic symptoms increases.[24,26] Also these may indicate certain medical illnesses that increase urine output (e.g., diabetes mellitus, diabetes insipidus, congestive heart failure, or psychogenic water intoxication).

The symptom of continual leakage, causing the patient to complain of being constantly wet, may be associated with a bypass mechanism such as an ectopic ureter, vesicovaginal fistula, or urethral vaginal fistula. Symptoms of pain in the area of the bladder may suggest interstitial cystitis. All patients should be asked questions regarding voiding disturbances, including any difficulty in starting the urinary stream, interruption of flow, slow flow, or prolonged urination, and questions regarding urinary tenesmus.

In addition to taking a history of urinary symptoms, it is often helpful to ask the patient to fill out and return a urinary diary (Fig. 6-1). The diary consists of two 24-hour time periods in which the patient records the time she voids and the amount voided. She also records pertinent data such as the number of pads used per day, times of urinary accidents, or any associated factors. From this urinary diary a number of important facts may be obtained, such as the actual frequency of urination and episodes of nocturia. The largest voided amount suggests the patient's maximal bladder capacity, whereas the 24-hour urine output gives an idea of excessive outflow states such as diabetes mellitus or

Fig. 6-1 Twenty-four-hour urinary diary (Urolog).

UROLOG

Please keep track of your urine output for two full 24 hours. These do not have to be consecutive days. Please include a.m. and p.m. when documenting the time of day you urinate, and please measure the amount you urinate in ounces or cc's. Please indicate any time you accidentally leaked urine and any cause for the accident (example: coughing, lifting, urgency).

Example:	Time	Amount
	8 a.m.	8 oz's
	10 a.m.	less than 1 oz
	11:30 a.m.	leaked urine-couldn't measure

DAY 1		DAY 2	
TIME	AMOUNT	TIME	AMOUNT

diabetes incipidus. In general these should be considered if urine output is greater than 4 L/day.

Given a history of recurrent urinary tract infections (UTIs), it is important to elicit exactly what symptoms are associated with the patient's UTIs. Classic symptoms are increased urgency and frequency, along with dysuria and possibly hematuria. The patient should be asked how frequently the urinary tract infections occur and if urine cultures were performed. If given antibiotics in the past, it is helpful to ask the patient the interval between the start of antibiotics and improvement or resolution in her symptoms. True urinary tract infections usually have prompt improvement and resolution of symptoms with antibiotics. A history of urinary tract infections as a child may indicate congenital abnormalities. Patients should be asked whether there is an association between urinary tract infections and intercourse. The type of contraception used is important in that certain barrier methods, such as the diaphragm, may increase the incidence of urinary tract infections.[27] Also, frequent vaginal infections or sexually transmitted diseases should be considered as possible causes for the irritative symptoms. Again, voiding disturbances with increased residual urine may predispose to UTIs. Therefore questions should be asked regarding whether the patient's urine stream is forceful and whether there is tenesmus. Also ascertain whether there are any associated conditions that may lead to bladder neuropathy and voiding disturbances, such as lumbar disc disease or diabetes with peripheral neuropathy. If the patient has experienced hematuria, document whether the hematuria was resolved after antibiotics. If not, a bladder neoplasm should be ruled out along with the possibility of renal lithiasis.

Anal/Rectal Disorders

Rectal symptoms should be specifically questioned, because patients seldom voluntarily offer this type of information. Again it is important to have the patient describe in her own words the nature of her bowel problem, its frequency and duration, and how it affects her lifestyle. It is important to ask specific questions regarding fecal incontinence and whether this incontinence is related to solids, liquids, or gas. The patient should be asked whether there is sensation to defecate prior to an incontinent episode or fecal urgency, and the percentage of bowel movements controlled versus uncontrolled. The loss of sensation is frequently seen in females with impaction as a cause for their incontinence by way of a normal internal anal sphincter reflex.[28] Fecal urgency may relate to disorders such as Crohn's disease or colitis. Other important questions include those concerning constipation, which can be defined as bowel movements two or less times per week or greater than 25% straining.[29] Excessive bearing down often accompanies a history of fecal tenesmus. The type of medications used to control the bowels should be obtained and include laxatives, bulk agents, enemas, and suppositories. These will influence a patient's bowel habits along with daily intake of foods high in fiber. Again, neurologic disease can influence bowel function and therefore it is important to list a history of any surgery or injury to the spine. Also, the patient should be asked questions concerning hematochezia, melena, hemorrhoids, change in bowel habits, or change in the size of stool. It is important to know if any known bowel disorders exist, such as ulcerative colitis, Crohn's disease, diverticulosis, rectal polyps, bowel cancer, or irritable bowel syndrome. Also it may be useful to know if any bowel studies were performed, such as barium enema, sigmoidoscopy, colonoscopy, or defecography.

Following the gynecologic and urologic history, a thorough medical, surgical, and obstetric history is obtained, along with a complete list of the patients' medications that might influence bladder and bowel symptoms.

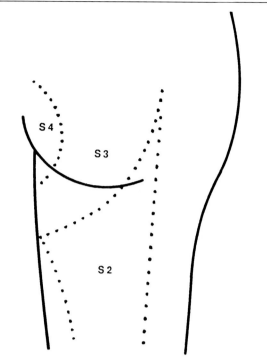

Fig. 6-2 S2, 3, 4 Sensory Dermatomes. Patient's right buttock and posterior thigh viewed.

CLINICAL EXAMINATION

Neurologic Examination

In patients with bladder symptoms the physical examination should begin with a neurologic evaluation of the S2 to S4 lower micturition center.[30] The evaluation includes lower deep tendon reflexes, Babinski (plantar) reflex, and sensation over the inner thigh, vulvar, and perirectal areas (sensory dermatones representing S2 to S4, Fig. 6-2). Also the bulbocavernosis reflex should be elicited by tapping the clitoris and noting a reflex contraction of the perirectal muscles. This represents the motor component of S2 to S4. It should be noted, however, that the absence of this reflex may not imply neurologic disease, because approximately 10% of normal adults do not have a bulbocavernosis reflex strong enough to be elicited.[31] Twenty percent to 30% of patients with muscular sclerosis,[32] Parkinson's disease,[33] or other CNS disease have primary complaints of urinary incontinence, emphasizing the need for good neurologic screening exams.

Urethral Axis

The urethral axis or Q-Tip test was introduced in 1972 by Crystle and coworkers[34] to measure urethral vesical junction mobility. The test is performed with the patient in the supine lithotomy position. A sterile lubricated cotton swab is inserted through the urethra into the bladder. It is then withdrawn to the level of the urethral vesical junction, indicated by an increased resistance to pulling.[35] Using an orthopedic goniometer with an attached level to indicate the horizontal position, the patient is asked to strain and the maximum straining angle (from horizontal) is measured (Fig. 6-3). A straining angle greater than 30° from horizontal indicates urethral hypermobility.[36,37] Although most studies have concentrated on the diagnostic value of the Q-Tip test without substantiation of its accuracy in measuring urethral mobility, at least based on limited data, it appears that the Q-Tip test accurately quantitates urethral mobility. The accuracy of the Q-Tip test seems best when the Q-Tip is placed at the level of the urethral vesical junction or proximal urethra, rather than within the bladder, midurethra, or distal urethra. Bladder fullness does not alter the test result significantly. It is an easy and inexpensive method of quantifying mobility of the bladder neck and proximal urethra, provided the tip of the Q-Tip is properly placed.[35]

Recently the Q-Tip test was criticized as being unable to diagnose or predict urethral incompetence.[36] This test alone is not useful in diagnosing stress incontinence or detrusor instability. Instead, it simply gives information on urethral mobility.[35] The urethral axis may be clinically useful, however, as long as the examiner understands its function and limitations. First, the test is very sensitive, with 90% to 100% of patients with unrepaired genuine stress incontinence having a straining Q-Tip angle greater than 30°. However, it is nonspecific in that more than half of continent females and patients with other urologic disorders also have a Q-Tip test result greater than 30°. One benefit is its negative predictive value, in that if a patient has a straining Q-Tip angle less than 30° with no previous surgery, it is somewhat unlikely that she has genuine stress urinary incontinence.[11] Of course further testing would need to be performed to confirm this.

Fig. 6-3 Sterile Q-Tip applicator and orthopedic goniometer used in assessing urethral axis (Q-Tip test). **A** shows resting axis, **B** shows straining axis upon Valsalva maneuver.

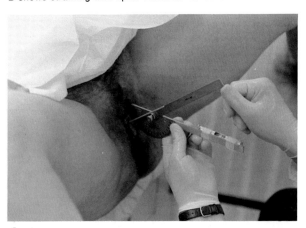

A

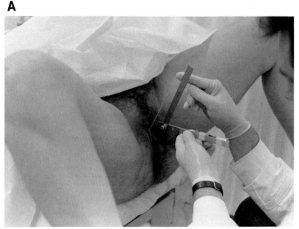

B

Furthermore, based on limited data there is some indication that in patients with intrinsic urethral damage as the cause of stress incontinence (low pressure urethra or Type III incontinence), a normal Q-Tip test may be a poor prognostic indicator of operative success with a suburethral sling. In a recent article by Summitt and coworkers,[38] females with low urethral closing pressure, defined as $\leq$ 20 cm/H_2O in the sitting position with a full bladder, 93% (27 of 29 patients) with a positive Q-Tip test were objectively cured of their incontinence. Only 20% (1 of 5 patients) with a negative Q-Tip test were cured with a suburethral sling. This suggests that the urethral axis during straining may influence the type of surgical procedure chosen. Perhaps this subgroup of patients would be better served with management such as an artificial urinary sphincter or periurethral collagen injections. Because of the small number of patients with a negative preoperative Q-Tip test, the statistical power of the above study is questioned, and a larger sample is needed to confirm results.

Cystometrogram

Simple cystometrics (eyeball cystometrics) can be accomplished in the office setting without the use of electronic equipment. A Foley catheter is placed in the bladder after the patient voids. A postvoid residual urine sample is collected and recorded. This urine sample is also used for analysis and culture. A 50 cc syringe without its piston is attached to the end of the Foley catheter to use as a funnel for filling the bladder. The syringe is held approximately 15 cm above the symphysis pubis. Sterile water is poured into the syringe in 50 cc increments (Fig. 6-4). The patient's sensation to filling is evaluated by asking for her first sensation (100–150 cc), sensation to fullness (comfortable desire to urinate—200–250 cc), sensation to marked fullness (strong desire to urinate—300–350 cc) and maximal capacity ("I can't hold any more"—400–600 cc). If at some point in the examination the meniscus rises instead of its normal slow descent into the catheter, the examiner should place a hand on the patient's abdomen. In the absence of any palpable abdominal muscle contraction, this then implies detrusor instability.[39]

Standing Stress Test

In patients who complain of urinary incontinence, a standing stress test should be performed. This is accomplished with the patient in the upright position with a comfortably full bladder. The patient is asked to cough

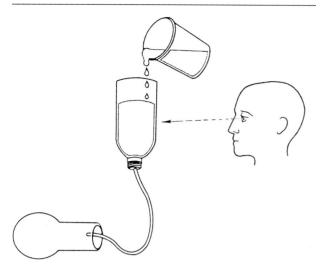

Fig. 6-4 Simple office or "eyeball" cystometrogram.

vaginal apex in patients after hysterectomy (Fig. 6-5B). The prolapse should be raised with an attempt to mimic the anatomic result that would be achieved by surgical correction of the prolapse, being very careful to avoid overcorrection. This placement prevents descent of the uterus or vaginal apex and displacement of the anterior vaginal wall during stress. The stress test now is performed in the usual manner. The patient is asked to cough and perform the Valsalva maneuver with the examiner looking for urinary leakage from the urethra.[41]

Fig. 6-5 Anterior vaginal wall relaxation *(A)* before and *(B)* after prolapse reduction with lower half of Sim's speculum. Reprinted with permission from The American College of Obstetricians and Gynecologists (*Obstet Gynecol* 1988;72(3):292).

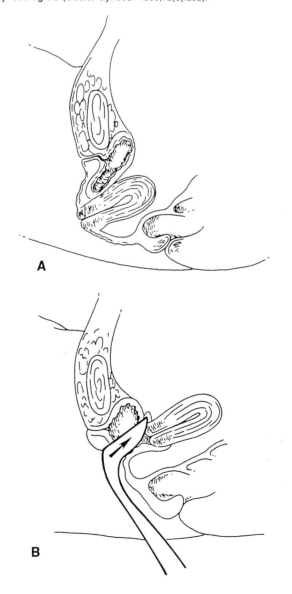

and perform the Valsalva maneuver while the examiner observes for any urinary leakage from the urethral meatus. Direct observation of urine leakage with spurts at the same time as a cough or Valsalva maneuver may be suggestive of urethral sphincteric incompetence. Delayed loss, prolonged loss of urine, or no urinary loss on provocation may suggest other causes for incontinence, most notably detrusor instability, and further testing should be pursued. A positive standing stress test has the highest predictive values (both positive and negative values 89%) for the diagnosis of genuine stress urinary incontinence of all the office tests.[12]

One exception that requires special note is the patient who has severe uterovaginal prolapse with anterior vaginal wall relaxation protruding to the level of or beyond the vaginal introitus during straining. Often such relaxation has coexisting loss of urethrovesical junction support, but the patient remains paradoxically continent. A stress test should be performed on these individuals with or without symptoms of urinary leakage. This may help identify patients with genuine stress incontinence who will manifest the symptoms of their incontinence only after prolapse reduction surgery. The basis of their paradoxical continence is related to mechanical urethral obstruction that may be caused by physical kinking of the urethra as the prolapse is accentuated with stress.[40] The stress test should be performed in this setting with careful reduction of the uterovaginal prolapse with the lower half of a Sim's speculum (Fig. 6-5A). The speculum should be positioned so that its leading edge is in the anterior fornix just in front of the anterior lip of the cervix or with the leading edge at the

Perineal Descent

Perineal descent syndrome involves a number of symptoms relating to abnormal descent of the perineum during straining. It was first recognized by Parks in 1966.[47] It may be initiated by abnormal bowel habits with straining[42,43] or by nerve damage caused during childbirth.[44] The most prominent clinical feature is pronounced difficulty of defecation with excessive straining and a sense of incomplete emptying. Perineal descent encourages anterior rectal wall prolapse into the lumin of the anal canal, causing obstruction from the free passage of stool during defecation. Also this places the anterior mucosa in contact with the epithelium below the dentate line, which is rich in sensory fibers, giving the sensation of continued fullness in the rectum (fecal tenesmus). There may be symptoms of rectal discharge, bleeding, and perineal pain, along with a change in the caliber of the stool becoming "pencil-like."[45] There is concern that continued perineal descent may cause increasing stretch nerve injury to the pudendal nerve, eventually leading to loss of anal sphincter function and subsequent fecal incontinence.[46-50]

Clinically abnormal descent can be recognized by the observation that the perineum "balloons" below the bony outlet of the pelvis during a straining effort.[48] The extent of perineal descent can be measured in relationship to the plane of the ischial tuberosities using a perineometer. The perineometer is an instrument with a movable pillar that rests on the anal verge while two fixed legs rest on the ischial tuberosities[45,51] (Fig. 6-6). The amount of descent should not be greater than two centimeters.[51,52] Although compared to radiologic measurements this technique may underestimate the amount of perineal descent,[53] the clinical measurement with the perineometer is reproducible, easily accomplished as part of the office examination, and does not involve radiation exposure.

PELVIC RELAXATION

Anterior Vaginal Segment

Evaluation of pelvic relaxation is best accomplished with the patient in the somewhat upright position since the true extent of relaxation cannot always be appreciated in the supine lithotomy position. This can be accomplished by way of a rotating birthing chair, reverse Trendelenberg position on some examination tables, or positioning the patient with additional cushions on a standard examination table. To evaluate the ante-

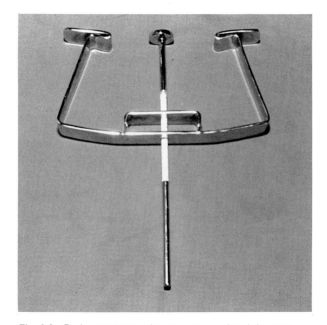

Fig. 6-6 Perineometer used to measure perineal descent.

rior vaginal wall, the lower half of a Sim's speculum is inserted into the vagina and downward traction is applied. The patient is then asked to perform the Valsalva maneuver and any displacement is visualized. A cystocele is present when there is a descent of the anterior vaginal wall. This may be secondary to damage and relaxation of the vaginal mucosa itself or of its supporting tissues. It is important for the physician to assess both the amount of displacement and also attempt to locate the sites involved in loss of support. To understand where a specific defect is causing a cystocele, it is important to understand the anatomy of the anterior vaginal wall. The support of the anterior vaginal wall occurs at its lateral sulci by way of its lateral attachments to the arcus tendineus from the pubic symphysis to the level of the ischial spines. Superior to the ischial spines the attachment also is at its lateral sulci to the cardinal ligaments and corresponding perivascular connective tissue at the apex of the vagina.[54,55] With this in mind it is easily seen that cystoceles can be secondary to loss of support in one or a combination of three areas: central defects (distention or pulsion cystocele), lateral defects (displacement or traction cystocele), or vaginal apex defects (cystoceles secondary to uterovaginal descensus). Distention cystoceles are secondary to overstretching of the vaginal wall and/or atrophic changes of aging causing weakness of the intrinsic structural components. As a result, rugal folds are diminished or may disappear. Lateral sulci are intact. Displacement cystoceles are secondary to loss of the lateral attachment and support of the vagina. Usually there are relatively well-preserved rugal folds and disappearance of the lateral sulci.

The examiner can use two other additional clues to help diagnose lateral wall defects. First, the index finger is placed along the area of the lateral sulci and the patient asked to hold her urine or squeeze her vagina or rectum. When there is good lateral wall support the patient's anterior vaginal wall is pulled upward and laterally. With a defect in this area, however, there is a reduction in the upward displacement of the anterior vaginal wall. A uterine packing forcep can also be used as an adjunct to the clinical evaluation. The forcep is spread and the ends of the forcep placed simultaneously in each anterior vaginal lateral wall, elevating and supporting the vagina to its lateral sidewalls. In a lateral wall defect this will elevate and support the vagina to a normal anatomic position. The degree of uterovaginal descensus contributing to a cystocele can be judged by placing the leading edge of a Sim's speculum at the vaginal apex or anterior fornix just in front of the anterior lip of the cervix and elevating that superiorly to its normal position. The patient is then asked to strain once more while maintaining support to the vaginal vault and the degree of cystocele is reevaluated. An anterior cystocele (urethrocele) occurs when there is rotational descent of the bladder neck during straining. As with all other types of anterior vaginal wall relaxation, this may occur in conjunction with other defects or as an independent defect.

Posterior Vaginal Segment

To evaluate the posterior vaginal wall the Sim's speculum is removed, rotated, then reinserted into the vagina and upward traction is applied. Again the patient is asked to perform the Valsalva maneuver. Similarly, a rectocele is present when there is descent of the posterior vaginal wall. Damage may be secondary to distention or disruption of the rectovaginal septum (Denonvilliers' fascia). Rectoceles may be termed as low, mid, or high position, depending on the area for the structural or supporting weakness. Also it is important to visualize and palpate the perineum for evidence of loss of perineal support. With the speculum still in place it is helpful to perform a rectal examination to verify the presence or absence of any abnormal caliber of the rectum or irregular distensability of the anterior rectal wall. At the time of the rectal examination palpation for any irregularity or mass should be performed, including fecal impaction. Impaction may predispose a patient to

fecal incontinence by way of reflex relaxation of the internal anal sphincter.[28] Also an estimation of the basal rectal tone and maximum squeeze rectal tone should be attempted. A bidigital rectal vaginal examination should then be performed to examine for any palpable mass ballottable between the examiner's fingers upon straining, indicative of an enterocele.

Superior Vaginal Segment

To evaluate the superior vaginal compartment, first a thorough bimanual examination should be performed in the usual manner to feel for any pelvic masses. During the examination particular attention should be placed on the vaginal axis. The normal vaginal axis is in a horizontal position when the patient is upright. Therefore in lithotomy position with insertion of one or two fingers the axis of the vagina should be found to move posteriorly toward the sacrum. By downward traction of the examiner's fingers the levator ani muscles (levator plate) can be palpated. The anterior vaginal wall lies on the posterior vaginal wall, which in turn lies on the levator plate. With a horizontal levator plate this helps prevent uterovaginal prolapse as well as cystocele formation. In patients with a vertical vaginal axis and poor levator plate on palpation, the forces causing uterovaginal and anterior vaginal wall pelvic relaxation are more active. These patients then are subject to the risk for uterovaginal prolapse. Again this demonstrates the importance of considering the status of the entire pelvic floor as opposed to evaluating one specific compartment. Uterovaginal descensus is evaluated using the examiner's index finger placed very gently on the cervix or vaginal cuff. The cuff can usually be palpated by the previous surgical scar along with dimpling in its lateral edges. The patient in the upright position is asked to strain and the examiner's finger follows the descent of the apex. It is often helpful to document the amount of descent down the length of the vagina.

Grading Pelvic Relaxation

Standardization for the classification of pelvic relaxation and relaxation severity (grading) enhances the sharing of accurate and complete information to facilitate treatment. Too often relaxation disorders are vaguely defined and there is a need for standardization of terms in order to compare data between patients and to better communicate with physicians.

The following grading system (referenced from Baden and Walker's writings)[56,57] is an easily remembered and useful system, although it is not the only grading system proposed.[58] Until a universally accepted grading system is available it will be necessary to also narratively describe the defect.

In grading urethroceles, cystoceles, prolapse, and rectoceles, the following system can be used[56,57]: Grade 0 corresponds to normal. Grade 1 is descent of the component to one-half distance toward the vaginal introitus with a Valsalva maneuver. Grade 2 is from one-half to the level of the introitus. Grade 3 is progression through the hymenal ring. Grade 4 is maximal descent through the hymenal ring with straining or descent through the introitus at rest.

Enterocele Grade 0 is considered normal when there is no more than two centimeters of cul-de-sac peritoneum between posterior cervix and rectum. Grade 1 is a herniation of the peritoneal pouch between the rectal and vaginal walls down to one-fourth distance toward the hymenal ring. Grade 2 is herniation from one-fourth to one-half the distance toward the hymenal ring. Grade 3 is herniation from one-half to three-fourths the distance and Grade 4 is a herniation to the hymenal ring.

SUMMARY

This chapter reviewed the techniques of performing a thorough history, complete physical examination, and simple diagnostic office testing in the evaluation of lower urinary tract, anorectal, and pelvic relaxation disorders. All of the above disorders are intimately related and often found in conjunction with one another. Also, the management of one specific disorder has direct influence on the presentation of symptoms from another. Because of this interrelationship between specific components of the pelvic floor, the philosophy of a complete evaluation including investigation of all pelvic floor components on each patient was stressed. Keeping this concept in mind and using the tools for evaluation outlined in this chapter, a great deal of information regarding the pelvic floor function can be gathered during one simple office visit. Specific additional diagnostic testing or direct management decisions are then tailored to each patient.

REFERENCES

1. Cardozo LD, Stanton SL. Genuine stress incontinence and detrusor instability—a review of 200 patients. *Br J Obstet Gynecol.* 1980;87:184.
2. Schram M. Cystocele etiology. *NY State J Med.* March 1976: 370–372.
3. Schram M, Schram D. Cystocele repair—a modified technique. *Obstet Gynecol.* 1967;29:447
4. Sand PK, Bowen LW, et al. The low-pressure urethra as a factor in failed retropubic urethropexy. *Obstet Gynecol.* 1987;69:399–402.
5. Horbach NS, Blanco JS, et al. A suburethral sling procedure with polytetrafluoroethylene for the treatment of genuine stress incontinence in patients with low urethral closure pressure. *Obstet Gynecol.* 1988;71:648–652.
6. Drutz HP, Mandel F. Urodynamic analysis of urinary incontinence symptoms in women. *Am J Obstet Gynecol.* 1979;134:789.
7. Glezerman M, et al. Evaluation of reliability of history in women complaining of urinary stress incontinence. *Eur J Obstet Gynecol Reprod Biol.* 1986;21:159.
8. Jarvis GJ, Hall S, et al. An assessment of urodynamic examination in incontinent women. *Br J Obstet Gynecol.* 1980;87:893.
9. Sand PK, Hill RC, Ostergard DR. Incontinence history as a predictor of detrusor stability. *Obstet Gynecol.* 1988;71:257.
10. Walters MD, Shields LE. The Diagnostic value of history, physical examination, and the Q-tip cotton swab test in women with urinary incontinence. *Am J Obstet Gynecol.* 1988;159:145.
11. Walters MD. The history and physical examination in women with urinary incontinence. In: *American Uro-Gynecologic Society Quarterly Report,* January 1989;7(1).
12. Fischer-Rasmussen W, Hansen RI, Stage P. Predictive values of diagnostic tests in the evaluation of female urinary stress incontinence. *Acta Obstet Gynecol Scand.* 1986;65:291.
13. Quigley GJ, Harper AC. The epidemiology of urethral-vesical dysfunction in the female patient. *Am J Obstet Gynecol.* 1985; 151:220.
14. Abrams P, Feneley R, Torrens M. The clinical contribution of urodynamics. In: Chism DG, ed. *Urodynamics.* New York: Springer–Verlag; 1983:144.
15. Byrne DJ, Hamilton Stewart PA, Gray BK. The role of urodynamics in female urinary stress incontinence. *Br J Urol.* 1987;59:228.
16. Kadar N. The value of bladder filling in the clinical detection of urine loss and selection of patients for urodynamic testing. *Br J Obstet Gynecol.* 1988;95:698.
17. Korda A, Krieger M, et al. The value of clinical symptoms in the diagnosis of urinary incontinence in the female. *Aust NZ J Obstet Gynecol.* 1987;27:149.
18. Kuzmarov IW. Urodynamic assessment and chain cystogram in women with stress urinary incontinence. *Urology.* 1984;24:236.
19. Moolgaoker AS, Ardran GM, et al. The diagnosis and management of urinary incontinence in the female. *J Obstet Gynecol Br Commonwealth.* 1972;79:481.
20. Webster GD, Sihelnik SA, Stone AR. Female urinary incontinence: the incidence, identification, and characteristics of detrusor instability. *Neurourol Urodyn.* 1984;3:235.
21. Whiteside CG, Arnold EP. Persistent primary eneuresis: a urodynamic assessment. *Br Med J.* 1975;A:364.
22. Arnold EP, et al. Urodynamics of female incontinence: factors influencing the results of surgery. *Am J Obstet Gynecol.* 1973; 117:805.
23. Awad SA, McGinnis RH. Factors that influence the incidence of detrusor instability in women. *J Urol.* 1983;130:114.
24. Cantor TJ, Bates CP. Comparative study of symptoms and objective urodynamic findings in 214 incontinent women. *Br J Obstet Gynecol.* 1980;87:889.
25. Farrar DJ, Whiteside CG, et al. A urodynamic analysis of micturition symptoms in the female. *Surg Gynecol Obstet.* 1975;144:875.
26. Kajansuu E, Kauppila A. Scored urological history and urethrocystometry in the differential diagnosis of female urinary incontinence. *Ann Chir Gynecol.* 1982;71:197.
27. Fihn SD, Latham RH, Roberts P. Association between diaphragm use and urinary tract infection. *JAMA.* 1985;254:240–245.
28. Henry MM, Swash M. Faecal incontinence, B: pathogenesis and clinical features. In: Henry MM, Swash M, eds. *Coloproctology and the Pelvic Floor.* London: Butterworths; 1985:223.

29. Drossman DA, Sandler RS, et al. Bowel patterns among subjects not seeking healthcare. *Gastroenterology.* 1982;83:529–534.

30. Bradley WE. Urologic oriented neurologic examination. In: Ostergard DR, ed. *Gynecologic Urology and Urodynamics.* Baltimore: Williams & Wilkins Co; 1985:63.

31. Bruskewitz R. Female incontinence: signs and symptoms. In: Raz S, ed. *Female Urology.* Philadelphia: WB Saunders; 1983:45–50.

32. Beck PR, Warren KG, Whitman P. Urodynamic studies in female patients with multiple sclerosis. *Am J Obstet Gynecol.* 1981;139: 273.

33. Galloway NTM. Urethral sphincter abnormalities in Parkinsonism. *Br J Urol.* 1983;55:691.

34. Crystel D, Charme L, Copeland W. Q-tip test in stress urinary incontinence. *Obstet Gynecol.* 1972;38:313.

35. Karram MM, Bhatia NN. The Q-tip test: standardization of the technique and its interpretation in women with urinary incontinence. *Obstet Gynecol.* 1988;71:807.

36. Montz FJ, Stanton SL. Q-tip test in female urinary incontinence. *Obstet Gynecol.* 1986;67:258.

37. Sand PK, Bowen LW, Ostergard DR, et al. Hysterectomy and prior incontinence surgery as risk factors for failed retropubic cystourethropexy. *J Reprod Med.* 1988;33:171.

38. Summitt RL Jr, Bent AE, Ostergard DR, Harris, TA. Stress incontinence and low urethral closure pressure. Correlation of preoperative urethral hypermobility with successful suburethral sling procedures. *J Reprod Med.* 1990;35(9):877–880.

39. Ouslander JG, Leach GE, Staskin DR. Simplified tests of lower urinary tract function in the evaluation of geriatric urinary incontinence. *JAGS.* 1989;37:706.

40. Richardson DA, Bent AE, Ostergard DR. The effect of uterovaginal prolapse on urethrovesical pressure dynamics. *Am J Obstet Gynecol.* 1983;146:901–905.

41. Bump RC, Fantl JA, Hurt WG. The mechanism of urinary continence in women with severe uterovaginal prolapse: results of barrier studies. *Obstet Gynecol.* 1988;72:291.

42. Kiff ES, Barnes PRH, Swash M. Evidence of pudendal neuropathy in patients with perineal descent and chronic straining at stool. *Gut.* 1984;25:1279–1282.

43. Snooks SJ, Nicholls RJ, et al. Electrophysiological and manometric assessment of the pelvic floor in solitary rectal ulcer syndrome. *Br J Surg.* 1985;72:131–133.

44. Snooks SJ, Swash M, et al. Injury to innervation of pelvic floor sphincter musculature in childbirth. *Lancet.* 1984;2:546–550.

45. Henry MM. Descending perineum syndrome. In: Henry MM, Swash M, eds. *Coloproctology and the Pelvic Floor.* London: Butterworths; 1985:299–302.

46. Jones PN, Lubowski, DZ, et al. Relation between perineal descent and pudendal nerve damage in idiopathic faecal incontinence. *Int J Colorect Dis.* 1987;2:93–95.

47. Parks AG. Anorectal incontinence. *Proc R Soc Med.* 1975;68:681–690.

48. Parks AG, Porter NH, Hardcastle JD. The syndrome of the descending perineum. *Proc R Soc Med.* 1966;59:477–482.

49. Henry MM, Parks AG, Swash M. The anal reflex in idiopathic faecal incontinence: an electrophysiological study. *Br J Surg.* 1980;67:781–783.

50. Parks AG, Swash M, Urich H. Sphincter denervation and anorectal incontinence and rectal prolapse. *Gut.* 1977;18:656–665.

51. Henry MM, Parks AG, Swash M. The pelvic floor musculature in the descending perineum syndrome. *Br J Surg.* 1982;69:470–472.

52. Mahieu P, Pringot J, Bodart, P. Defecography: I. description of a new procedure and results in normal patients. *Gastrointest Radiol.* 1984;9:247–251.

53. Oettle GJ, Roe AM, et al. What is the best way of measuring perineal descent? A comparison of radiographic and clinical methods. *Br J Surg.* 1985;72:999–1001.

54. DeLancey JOL. Anatomy and physiology of urinary continence. *Clin Obstet Gynecol.* 1990;33:298.

55. Edmonds PB, Richardson AC. Clinical evaluation of pelvic support defects (videotape). Danbury, Conn: Davis-Geck; 1987.

56. Baden WF, Walker TA. Physical diagnosis in the evaluation of vaginal relaxation. *Clin Obstet Gynecol.* 1972;15:1055.

57. Baden WF, Walker TA, et al. Preoperative evaluation of vaginal relaxation. *Group Prac.* 1970;19:28.

58. Beecham, CT. Classification of vaginal relaxation. *Am J Obstet Gynecol.* 1980;136:957.

CHAPTER 7

Anatomic Investigation

7A   Radiologic Investigation

7A1   The Anorectum and Vagina

Frederick M. Kelvin   Giles W. Stevenson

INTRODUCTION

A variety of static and functional imaging techniques are used in the investigation of anorectal disorders (Table 7A1-1). In patients with disorders related to defecation, the rectum frequently has a normal configuration at rest. Studies which provide only static anatomic information, such as barium enema and computed tomography, are therefore of limited value. Evacuation proctography (defecography) is a radiologic method of observing the act of defecation and recording the information on videotape, by cineradiography or on digital film. Defecography is frequently the only method that allows recognition of functional abnormalities related to defecation. Balloon proctography is a relatively simple technique that provides predominantly morphologic information about the anorectal region that has been largely superseded by evacuation proctography.

Colonic transit studies are often used in patients with chronic constipation in order to attempt to distinguish between normal colonic transit, delayed colonic transit caused by colonic inertia, and delayed colonic transit resulting from rectal outlet obstruction.

Anal endosonography yields highly detailed images of the internal and external anal sphincters. Early experience with this relatively new technique suggests that it will play a valuable role in investigating disorders involving the anal canal and its sphincters. Pelvic floor ultrasonography (see Chapter 7B) provides a method

Table 7A1-1

Radiologic Techniques for Investigating Anorectal Dysfunction

Major Role	Minor Role
Evacuation proctography	* Magnetic resonance imaging
Colonic transit studies	Barium enema
Anal endosonography	Computed tomography
	Balloon proctography
	Pelvic floor ultrasonography

*Potential major role

for assessing the anorectal angle and puborectalis movement without the use of ionizing radiation; clinical experience with this technique is still limited.

Radiologic evaluation of the vagina alone is rarely necessary, as most disorders affecting the vagina are readily accessible to clinical assessment. The anatomic relationship of the vagina to the rectum at rest and during defecation is demonstrated by opacifying the vagina at the time of evacuation proctography.

This chapter provides a description of those radiologic procedures that are helpful for investigating defecatory disorders. Evacuation proctography, colonic transit studies, and anal endosonography will be stressed, as these currently represent the most clinically useful radiologic studies. Magnetic resonance imaging has considerable potential for the overall assessment of pelvic prolapse.

BARIUM ENEMA

Several films of the rectum, including lateral and anteroposterior views, are routinely obtained during the course of a barium enema examination. The anal canal is usually not visualized, however, and only those rectal disorders which alter the normal appearances at rest, such as proctitis or rectal neoplasia, can be readily diagnosed. The main role of the barium enema examination in patients being investigated for pelvic floor disorders is to exclude underlying neoplasm or other colorectal abnormalities. Disorders of the pelvic floor generally do not produce abnormal findings on barium enema examination. The solitary rectal ulcer syndrome constitutes a relative exception; suggestive findings of rectal mucosal irregularity or mass effect are sometimes revealed with barium enema, although evacuation proctography remains the essential radiologic investigation. In addition, lateral diverticula of the rectum have been demonstrated on barium enema[1]; they probably represent an extreme example of mucosal herniation through the levator ani and may also be seen during evacuation proctography in patients with prolonged constipation and straining.

MAGNETIC RESONANCE IMAGING AND COMPUTED TOMOGRAPHY

Both magnetic resonance imaging and computed tomography graphically display pelvic viscera and their interrelationships. Magnetic resonance imaging has proved particularly useful because of its ability to depict the pelvis in multiple planes. Both techniques are able to demonstrate the levator anus muscle, at least in part (Fig. 7A1-1).

Magnetic resonance (MR) imaging has recently been used to assess both the normal anorectum[2] and pelvic prolapse.[3] Fast scans are obtained predominantly in the sagittal plane with the pelvic floor in a relaxed state, with the pelvic floor contracted, and during straining down. Limited experience suggests that dynamic MR imaging may provide a more precise method of determining measurements related to anorectal function than is achieved with evacuation proctography.[2] Dynamic MR imaging can evaluate prolapse involving both the anterior and middle compartments of the pelvis, as well as rectoceles and enteroceles; and based on initial data, MR provides important additional information that influences the surgical repair that is performed.[3] Much further experience is needed to define the evolving role of MR imaging in pelvic floor disorders.

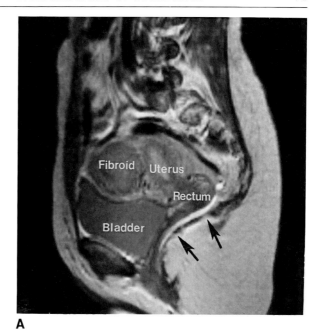

A

B

Fig. 7A1-1 Magnetic resonance image of pelvis: normal levator anus muscle. **A**, Sagittal image (TR = 2400 msec, TE = 25 msec) shows levator anus (arrows) as curvilinear structure located behind rectum. **B**, Coronal image (TR = 2200 msec, TE = 25 msec) demonstrates levator anus (arrows), below which are the ischiorectal fossae.

BALLOON PROCTOGRAPHY

In this technique, a balloon is inserted into the patient's rectum, the balloon filled with a dilute barium suspension, and the patient is then seated in the upright position on a specially constructed commode placed sideways to the radiographic table. Two lateral views of the pelvis are taken; one at rest and the other during straining as the patient attempts to evacuate the balloon. The sitting position facilitates recognition of pelvic floor weakness. This weakness is usually not demonstrable in other positions, such as those utilized during a barium enema, as the pelvic floor muscles are insufficiently stressed.

Various observations can be made from this study, including measurement of the anorectal angle, the degree of pelvic floor descent, and the patient's ability to expel the balloon.[4] While this technique does provide some physiologic information, it suffers from several disadvantages. The balloon does not accurately reflect the rectal contour so that rectal infoldings, including intussusception, may be missed. The degree of insertion of the rectal balloon may alter the anorectal angle, thereby confusing its measurement (Fig. 7A1-2). The act of defecation is not observed, and the liquid nature of the barium suspension does not approximate the consistency of fecal material. The Lahr balloon, which also attempts to measure anal sphincter pressures, provides a similar type of examination but is used in the recumbent rather than sitting position and is therefore less physiologically accurate.

The failure of balloon proctography to reliably reflect changes occurring during defecation has, in general, led to replacement of this technique by evacuation proctography. As a nonimaging method, however, the

Fig. 7A1-2 Variability of anorectal angle as determined by Lahr balloon. **A**, With patient at rest and Lahr balloon distended within rectum and anal canal, the anorectal angle *(a)* measures approximately 140 degrees. **B**, When Lahr balloon is introduced further into rectum, the axes of the rectum and anal canal are altered and the anorectal angle *(b)* is markedly reduced. It now measures approximately 95 degrees.

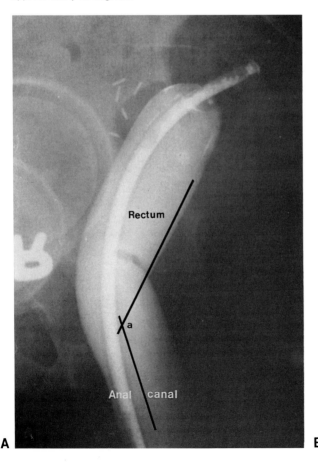
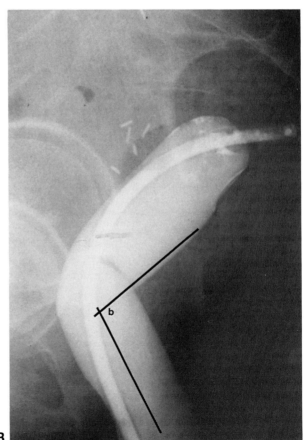

A   B

inability to expel a balloon catheter is used as a method of assessing clinically significant rectal outlet obstruction caused by nonrelaxation of the puborectalis or anal sphincter.

EVACUATION PROCTOGRAPHY (DEFECOGRAPHY)

Evacuation proctography provides a dynamic assessment of the act of defecation by recording the rectal expulsion of a thick barium paste that approximates the consistency of feces. A more liquid barium suspension is usually unsuitable as it can be evacuated with relatively little muscular force. In addition, many individuals instinctively contract the pelvic floor tightly when there is liquid in the rectum in order to prevent leakage, and this may result in misleading values for the rest, squeeze, and strain measurements during proctography. Because evacuation proctography is currently the most heavily used radiologic technique for investigating pelvic floor disorders, its method of performance and normal appearances will be discussed in some detail prior to a consideration of abnormal findings.

Technique

There is considerable variation in the method of performing evacuation proctography. Many investigators, however, have adopted a method similar to that of Mahieu and coworkers, who developed the first simplified technique applicable to routine clinical practice.[5] The examination is usually completed within 15 minutes.

No bowel preparation is required, as the rectum is usually empty. A thick barium paste is used. This is available commercially (Anatrast, E-Z-EM Co., Westbury, NY 11590) or, alternatively, a more viscous barium suspension can be prepared from barium powder and potato starch. Prior to rectal filling, the vagina is opacified. A variety of methods are used for opacifying the vagina, including insertion of a contrast-soaked tampon,[6] and a piece of gauze soaked in barium.[5] The latter approach enables movement of the rectovaginal septum to be studied. We have recently observed a patient in whom anterior rectal wall invagination and intussusception were demonstrated during proctography without a vaginal tampon, but these were not seen when a vaginal tampon was in place. A tampon may act as a splint, and either barium-soaked gauze or barium alone appear to be preferable for assessment of the rectovaginal septum.

The barium paste is then introduced into the rectum via a rectal tube by means of a caulking gun. An orthopedic cement gun designed for hip replacement work is ideal, although expensive. This high quality instrument lasts indefinitely and is easier to use than caulking guns from hardware stores. Initial introduction of 30 ml to 50 ml of liquid barium appears to improve coating of the rectal mucosa and aid visualization of abnormalities such as intussusception. The barium paste is then injected until the patient experiences discomfort due to rectal distention or until about 250 ml have been instilled. As the tube is withdrawn, a small amount of contrast is injected to delineate the anal canal. Finally, a small amount of barium is smeared on the patient's skin just behind the anal orifice. This enables the length of the anal canal to be measured.

The patient then sits on a specially constructed commode[7] in the lateral position in relation to the adjacent upright fluoroscopic table. A radiopaque ruler or spring within the commode enables corrected measurements of distances in the sagittal plane to be made. Usually three lateral spot films of the rectum and anal canal are then obtained: the first at rest, the second on squeezing the anal sphincter tightly closed, and the third on straining down without evacuation. Finally, the patient is asked to evacuate the rectum and this process is recorded on videotape. Unless evacuation is rapid, one or two spot films can usually be obtained during rectal emptying. Patients with difficulty in emptying the rectum should be asked if they normally use additional maneuvers to aid evacuation; if so, they should be encouraged to perform these maneuvers in order to assess the effect on defecation.

Certain technical modifications may be invoked.[8] In patients with a history of marked difficulty in evacuation, a liquid barium suspension may be substituted for the barium paste, and a second examination using the paste is performed only if the liquid is satisfactorily expelled. If an enterocele or sigmoidocele is suspected, the small bowel or sigmoid colon can be first opacified with barium.[5,6] Anteroposterior and oblique views may be helpful in patients with unusual or confusing radiographic findings obtained in the lateral projection.

Normal Appearances

As experience with evacuation proctography has accumulated, it has become clear that the normal range of appearances is considerably wider than was initially appreciated.[9–11] Much of the data that follows represents the findings of Shorvon and colleagues,[9] who performed evacuation proctography on 23 nulliparous

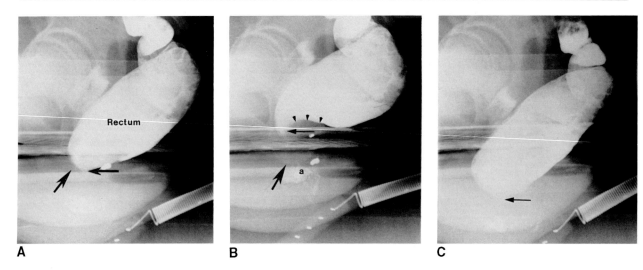

A   B   C

Fig. 7A1-3 Normal evacuation proctogram. **A,** With subject sitting at rest, the anorectal junction (thin arrow) lies very close to the level of the inferior margin of the ischial tuberosity (broad arrow), and the anal canal is closed. Note spring with 1 cm markers to allow accurate measurement of midline structures. **B,** When the anal sphincter is squeezed tightly closed, the anorectal junction (thin arrow) rises above the level of the ischial tuberosity (broad arrow). Note elevation of the posterior wall of the distal rectum (arrowheads) caused by contraction of the pelvic floor muscles. The position of the anal orifice is identified by an oval collection of barium *(a).* **C,** On straining, the anorectal junction (arrow) has descended but the anal canal remains closed.

women who were under 35 years of age, all of whom had no anorectal symptomatology. Fig. 7A1-3 illustrates a normal evacuation proctogram and the various parameters which can be assessed from the examination. These parameters include a number of features that can be measured, such as the anorectal angle (ARA), the position of the anorectal junction, the length of the anal canal, and the rectosacral gap. Changes in these measurements can be assessed both on maneuvers such as squeezing and straining, as well as during defecation. Morphologic changes such as rectocele and intussusception can be observed, and the speed and completeness of rectal emptying can be recorded.

At rest, the anal canal is usually closed, although in one series of normal volunteers it was noted to be open in 3 of 23 women.[9] The ARA is most commonly measured between the axis of the anal canal and a line drawn along the posterior border of the distal rectum (Fig. 7A1-4). The latter line is often difficult to define because of the curvature of the posterior rectal wall. An alternative method is to draw the rectal line through the central axis of the rectal lumen. There is considerable variation in measurement of the ARA, regardless of whether the posterior rectal wall or the central axis of the rectum is used.[12] Thus, skepticism is warranted when comparing ARA measurements made by different individuals.

The normal resting ARA has a range of 70° to 135°[9]; in most normal subjects, however, this

angle does not exceed 120°. The importance of the ARA derives from the fact that the angle is produced by the puborectalis sling, which is generally rec-

Fig. 7A1-4 Anorectal angle: methods of measurement. The anorectal angle as measured between the axis of the anal canal and the posterior wall of the rectum (white lines) is less than the anorectal angle when a line drawn through the central axis of the rectum (black lines) is substituted for that along the posterior rectal wall.

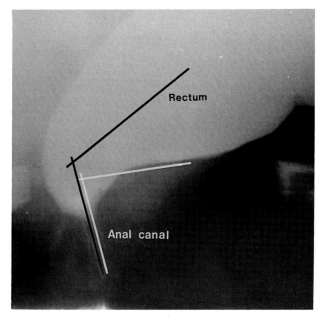

ognized to play a major role in maintaining continence. However, both because of the inexactness of its measurement and its wide range of normal values, caution should be exercised when assessing its significance.

The mean position of the anorectal junction at rest (Fig. 7A1-3*A*) in women is 4 mm above the inferior margin of the ischial tuberosity, with one standard deviation of 13 mm.[9] The rectosacral gap at the level of the third sacral segment usually does not exceed 10 mm.[9] The mean length of the anal canal at rest in women, as measured at proctography, is 1.6 cm.[9] This is less than the manometrically derived measurement, which averages 3.7 cm.[13] The radiographic anal canal is measured from the external anal orifice inferiorly to the point where the parallel walls of the anal canal meet the cone-shaped walls of the distal rectum. Pressure readings at manometry may be obtained from this cone-shaped area, suggesting that it is actually part of the anal canal. This would explain the discrepancy between anal canal lengths as determined manometrically and at proctography.

On squeezing, the anorectal junction rises (Fig. 7A1-3*B*) and the ARA becomes more acute as a result of contraction of the puborectalis and the levator ani muscles, the latter of which may produce a more generalized elevation of the posterior rectal wall. Lengthening of the anal canal occurs in two thirds of young women[9]; this increase in length could be due at least in part to closure of the funnel-shaped cone of the radiographic distal rectum.

On straining, the puborectalis and levator ani muscles should relax, leading to both an increase in the ARA and descent of the anorectal junction (Fig. 7A1-3*C*). The latter is associated with shortening of the anal canal (mean change 2 mm) in most women.[9] However, there may be a paradoxical decrease in the ARA on straining, which probably results from contraction of the pelvic floor muscles because of the fear of incontinence. The straining film before defecation is, therefore, the least useful of the static images. It is our impression that straining after defecation provides more information and we now usually defer this maneuver to the end of the examination.

Defecation is initiated by opening of the anal canal, which assumes a funnel-like shape starting at its proximal end. In normal subjects, the maximal width of the anal canal does not exceed 2 cm.[10,11] Using a relatively thin barium suspension, Bartram and coworkers[10] found that the average time for the anal canal to open fully was 4.5 seconds, and rectal emptying was completed within 30 seconds, with an average of 11 seconds. Complete emptying of the rectum is seen in only half the normal population.[4,11]

Pelvic floor descent on defecation is estimated by the degree of descent of the anorectal junction, which is most easily measured in relation to the inferior margin of the ischial tuberosity (Fig. 7A1-3). Alternatively, the tip of the coccyx can be used as a bony landmark. Usually, the anorectal junction does not descend more than 3.5 cm in young females, and descent is less than 4.5 cm in 95%.[9] In older females, the position of the pelvic floor at rest is significantly lower, but there is decreased pelvic floor descent on straining.[14] Pelvic floor descent as measured at proctography is considerably greater than clinical assessment of perineal descent which is measured with the patient lying down and only straining. The discrepancy is exaggerated by the further shortening of the radiographic anal canal that occurs on defecation. Therefore, the terms "perineal descent" and "pelvic floor descent" should not be used interchangeably.

Deformities of the rectal wall such as rectocele and intussusception may be observed during normal and abnormal defecation. These are discussed further below.

Abnormal Findings

Many findings may be demonstrated on evacuation proctography (Table 7A1-2), several of which frequently coexist in the same patient. Some caution is necessary when assessing the clinical relevance of proctographic findings. For example, a small rectocele is a frequent finding in normal young women. Intrarectal intussusception of minor degree is also a normal finding.[9] Emotional factors, particularly embarrassment when asked to defecate, must be considered when evaluating possible obstructed defecation.

Rectocele

A rectocele is visualized on proctography as an outpouching of the anterior rectal wall, which usually is obvious only during defecation (Fig. 7A1-5). Its formation reflects relative weakness of the rectovaginal septum. A rectocele appears to act as a diverticulum by retaining contrast during straining and defecation, thereby leading to a sensation of incomplete rectal emptying. The patient may, therefore, strain down repeatedly in an attempt to empty the rectocele and achieve complete evacuation. In severe cases, digital pressure on the perineum in front of the anus or on the posterior vaginal wall may alleviate this problem; the success of this maneuver can be assessed during the proctogram.

Rectoceles are common in asymptomatic females. In one series, rectoceles were found on proctography in 81% of healthy young women[9]; all but one of these

Table 7A1-2
Main Findings on Evacuation Proctography

Observations	Measurements
Rectal intussusception	Low anorectal junction at rest
Rectocele	Excessive pelvic floor
Enterocele	descent
Sigmoidocele	Inability to elevate pelvic
Persistent puborectalis	floor
impression (spastic pelvic	Increased separation of
floor syndrome)	vagina from rectum
Nonrelaxing anal sphincter	
Anal incontinence	

rectoceles was less than 2 cm in depth. Small rectoceles that do not retain contrast, and which are not associated with obstructive defecation, should therefore be accepted as normal.

While most rectoceles are detected on clinical examination, they are often accompanied by other findings at proctography, such as enterocele or rectal intussusception[15] (see Figs. 7A1-7, 8, 11, and 12). Lack of recognition of these coexistent disorders may explain why treatment limited to surgical repair of the rectocele often fails. Utilization of proctography prior to rectocele repair in patients with disordered defecation is

Fig. 7A1-5 Rectocele. Film obtained during evacuation shows a large rectocele that is indenting the posterior wall of the vagina. Note the collapsed normal rectum.

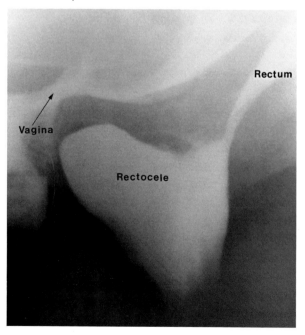

therefore prudent. Transrectal rather than transvaginal repair, or rectal imbrication via the transvaginal route, may be indicated if incomplete emptying of the rectocele is present.

In some patients repair of the rectocele may be unnecessary. For example, Kodner has found that patients treated surgically for rectal intussusception who have had refractory rectoceles have not needed additional surgery to correct the rectocele.[8] This raises the possibility that at least some rectoceles are the result of repeated straining secondary to a preexisting defecation disorder, such as rectal intussusception, rather than the primary cause of the patient's obstructive symptoms.

Intussusception

Rectal intussusception is a relatively frequent finding at evacuation proctography. It is important to recognize, as it is generally accepted to be the initiating mechanism in rectal prolapse. The intussusception almost always starts about 6 cm to 8 cm inside the rectum.[16] The infolding originates on the anterior wall in 62% of cases, is annular in 32%, and arises posteriorly in the remainder.[15] When the infolding measures 3 mm or less, it is likely to represent only mucosal prolapse and not a full-thickness intussusception.[8] Thus, minor rectal infoldings may merely reflect pleating of redundant mucosa as the rectum collapses and are a normal finding.

Intussusception confined to the rectum may not be of immediate consequence. Downward extension of the intussusception into the anal canal (rectoanal intussusception) is, however, usually regarded as abnormal (Fig. 7A1-6). This often produces a sensation of incomplete evacuation or blockage, which the patient sometimes learns to relieve by placing a finger in the anal canal to "push back the plug." The blockage may lead to further straining and intussusception, thereby creating a vicious circle of events. When the rectal wall descends further and protrudes through the anal orifice, that is, when complete rectal prolapse occurs, the diagnosis is usually clinically obvious.

Internal intussusception in which the intussusception stops short of the anal orifice is frequently difficult to detect clinically (occult rectal prolapse). In this situation evacuation proctography is necessary for its recognition. It is important for patients to attempt complete rectal evacuation during proctography, because in some cases the intussusception only develops at the end of defecation. Other findings may be seen on proctography

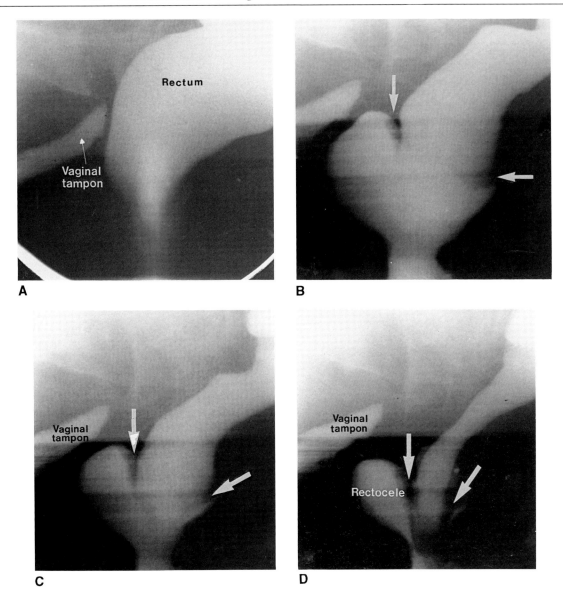

Fig. 7A1-6   Rectoanal intussusception. **A**, At rest, the configuration of the rectum is normal. **B**, As evacuation is initiated, an infolding develops on both the anterior wall (vertical arrow) and the posterior wall (horizontal arrow) of the rectum. This represents the beginning of the intussusception. **C** and **D**, The infoldings (arrows) become progressively deeper as evacuation continues. In **D**, the intussusception has extended into the anal canal, thereby forming a rectoanal intussusception. A rectocele is also present. (Courtesy of D. Mezwa, Royal Oak, Michigan.)

in rectal prolapse, including abnormal separation of the rectum from the sacrum and a redundant sigmoid colon; these may be the result rather than the cause of the prolapse.

Complete rectal prolapse can be mistaken clinically for prolapsing hemorrhoids; in this situation hemorrhoidectomy will fail to improve symptoms and may result in incontinence.[8] It is therefore wise to perform proctography in any patient with hemorrhoids who has symptoms of rectal outlet obstruction in order to exclude intussusception or obstructed defecation of other etiology.

Proctography may also be useful following rectopexy; persistent intussusception may be found in those who fail to improve, whereas the intussusception is no longer seen in patients who become symptomfree.[16]

Enterocele

An enterocele is a prolapse of the small bowel or its mesentery into an abnormally deep pouch of Douglas. At proctography, it is suspected when increased separation of the opacified vagina from the upper rectum is seen on straining or defecation. Rectovaginal separation greater than 2 cm should always be considered suspicious for an enterocele. This finding may be associated with indentation of the anterior rectal wall. If abnormal separation of the vagina from the rectum is observed, the proctogram is repeated after first opacifying the entire small bowel with orally administered barium. Loops of small bowel are then seen to fill the gap between the vagina and upper rectum (Fig. 7A1-7). Sometimes the enterocele is only identified at the end of defecation, after repeated straining on the part of the patient. Some investigators routinely opacify the small bowel prior to proctography in order to maximize detection of enteroceles.

Enteroceles are difficult to detect on physical examination; in our experience and that of others, proctography is a much more sensitive method of diagnosis.[17,18] In some patients differentiation between an enterocele and a rectocele cannot be made with conviction on physical examination. Proctography distinguishes between these two entities and demonstrates when they coexist.

The search for an enterocele at surgery can be difficult and time consuming. Many enteroceles probably go unrecognized at the time of surgery because the patient is recumbent and relaxed rather than upright and straining down. Failure to recognize and prophylactically repair an enterocele at the time of surgery frequently leads to subsequent enlargement of the enterocele and progressive symptomatology, thereby necessitating a repeat operation.[19] The risk of an enterocele is particularly high when the cul-de-sac has been exposed by a surgical procedure that pulls the vagina forward, for example, Burch urethropexy or following hysterectomy. Such patients, in particular, should be evaluated by evacuation proctography prior to undergoing surgery for pelvic prolapse.

Fig. 7A1-7 Enterocele. **A,** Toward the end of evacuation, the collapsed rectum becomes markedly separated from the opacified vagina. There is also a large rectocele. **B,** Following oral ingestion of barium to opacify the small bowel, the proctogram was repeated. Film obtained toward end of defecation shows that the vaginal separation from the rectum is caused by prolapsed small bowel, indicating the presence of an enterocele. Note the collapsed rectum.

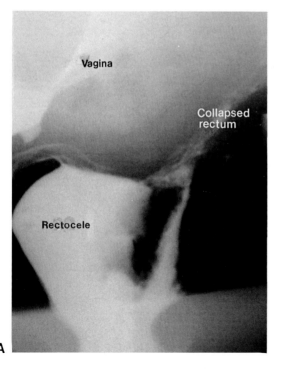
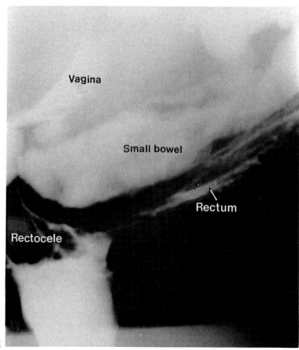

A

B

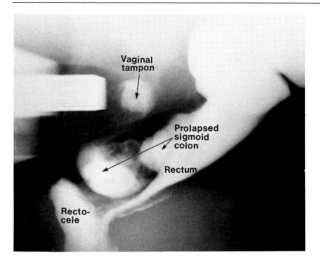

Fig. 7A1-8 Sigmoidocele. In this patient, the separation of the vaginal tampon from the rectum is caused by prolapsed sigmoid colon, i.e. a sigmoidocele. Note that there is a coexistent rectocele.

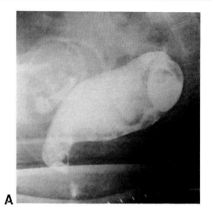
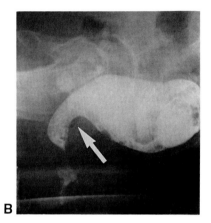
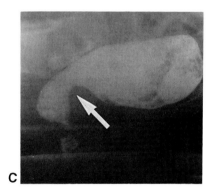
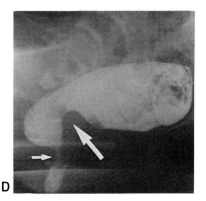

Sigmoidocele

Abnormal separation of the vagina from the upper rectum may also be due to a prolapsed uterus or a sigmoidocele. A sigmoidocele, which is a prolapse of redundant sigmoid colon into a deep pouch of Douglas, is less common than an enterocele. It is also readily overlooked on physical examination. Radiographic detection (Fig. 7A1-8) sometimes requires opacifying the sigmoid colon by limited barium enema and then repeating the proctogram.

Persistent Puborectalis Impression (Spastic Pelvic Floor Syndrome)

The anorectal angle normally increases on straining as a result of relaxation of the puborectalis muscle. The extent of this increase is usually considerable, ranging from 20° to 40°.[4,11] In a subgroup of patients with impaired evacuation, proctography demonstrates either an unaltered or a decreased anorectal angle on straining or defecation; these findings are frequently the result of a persistent or paradoxical increase of the puborectalis

Fig. 7A1-9 Persistent puborectalis impression of a patient with history of difficulty initiating defecation. **A**, At rest, the appearances are unremarkable. **B**, On squeezing down, a very prominent puborectalis impression (arrow) is seen. **C**, During straining, the puborectalis fails to relax and its impression (arrow) is essentially unchanged. **D**, On attempted evacuation, the puborectalis (large arrow) remains contracted and there is virtually no relaxation of the anal sphincter (small arrow).

impression (Fig. 7A1-9). This appearance is often relatively persistent, with the result that evacuation may only be achieved after multiple attempts at straining and defecation.

Electromyography of the puborectalis and external sphincter muscles in these patients during straining has shown that instead of the normal reduction in activity, activity in these muscles is increased. The patient therefore appears to attempt to defecate against a contracting pelvic floor. This entity, which frequently results in longstanding and often painful defecation, has been referred to by a variety of names, including the spastic pelvic floor syndrome,[20] anismus, and paradoxical contraction of the puborectalis.

The syndrome appears to be fairly common. Persistent contraction of the puborectalis may be a contributing factor in the development of other pelvic floor disorders, including the solitary rectal ulcer syndrome, the descending perineum syndrome, and rectal intussusception.

Some patients may contract their pelvic floor muscles during proctography because of embarrassment at the thought of defecating without total privacy. Because it is difficult to exclude this contributing factor to the proctographic findings, electromyography is usually performed for confirmation of the diagnosis, prior to commencing biofeedback or other treatment.

Nonrelaxing Anal Sphincter

In some patients with obstructed defecation, the puborectalis relaxes and the pelvic floor descends but the anal canal fails to open, presumably due to nonrelaxation of the internal and/or external anal sphincter. We have observed this in patients with painful hemorrhoids, anal fissure, and tumors of the spinal cord. In some patients with these findings, no underlying cause can be ascertained. Occasionally, posterior or posterolateral pouches are seen arising from the rectum (Fig. 7A1-10); these pouches probably represent herniations of rectal mucosa through the levator ani caused by chronic straining, irrespective of the etiology of the outlet obstruction.

Solitary Rectal Ulcer Syndrome

The solitary rectal ulcer syndrome (SRUS) is a chronic benign condition affecting predominantly young patients characterized by ulcerative or other inflammatory changes in the rectum that are related to chronic straining during defecation. Patients typically have a history of passage of blood or mucus from the rectum, together with persistent straining. However, only about one half of the patients with SRUS report this typical history.

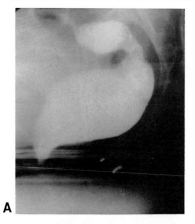

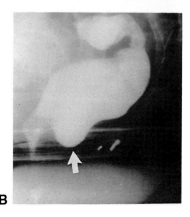

Fig. 7A1-10 Posterolateral pouch in outlet obstruction. **A,** The appearance of the proctogram at rest is normal in this patient with a history of chronic straining and constipation. **B,** On attempted defecation, the anal sphincter does not relax and a posterior rectal bulge (arrow) appears that is due to posterolateral herniation of the rectal wall through the levator ani.

Definitive diagnosis requires rectal biopsy that shows the characteristic finding of smooth muscle fibers extending into the epithelial layer. Suggestive changes may be present on proctoscopy or double contrast barium enema examination. Evacuation proctography is very helpful for showing the underlying defecatory disturbance. The name of the syndrome is misleading, as the ulcer is not the most obvious feature.

Barium enema most commonly shows thickening of the rectal folds and/or rectal spasm. Nodularity of the rectal mucosa, anteriorly or laterally, and rarely posteriorly, may be mild or gross enough to produce an irregular rectal mass. Ulceration may be detectable in the nodular area. Less often, there is fine surface granularity or stricture. Regardless of reported history, these findings should prompt proctoscopy and biopsy,

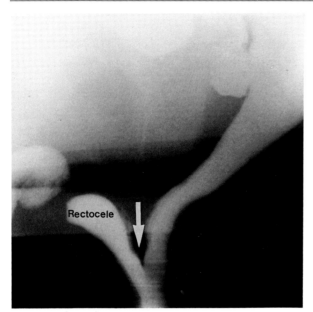

Fig. 7A1-11   Solitary rectal ulcer syndrome. Evacuation proctography in a patient with this syndrome demonstrates a deep rectal intussusception (arrow), together with a rectocele. (Courtesy of D. Mezwa, Royal Oak, Michigan.)

as well as evacuation proctography. The latter examination is almost always abnormal. In the majority of cases, rectal intussusception is present (Fig. 7A1-11); this frequently is either rectoanal or complete.[21] A persistent puborectalis impression is demonstrated less often.

The close relationship between rectal intussusception and SRUS is important both pathogenetically and from the viewpoint of treatment. It is believed that chronic straining leads to mucosal prolapse or intussusception, which ultimately causes pressure necrosis and ulceration of the rectal wall due to ischemia or mechanical trauma. The observation that intussusception originates in the anterior rectal wall in approximately two thirds of cases, and that this location is the main site of abnormality in SRUS, supports this contention.[21] Many patients with SRUS are helped by rectopexy, presumably because of the frequent association with intussusception. It appears that evacuation proctography may be useful in predicting the outcome of rectopexy in SRUS. Those with delayed rectal emptying (> 30 seconds) and abnormal perineal descent are likely to have a poor outcome from this operation.[22]

Descending Perineum Syndrome

The descending perineum syndrome, in which patients have pronounced difficulty with defecation result-ing in long periods of straining, was defined originally by radiologically measuring the descent of the anorectal junction on straining. Subsequently, the syndrome has been considered present if, using a simple clinical device (the perineometer), the plane of the perineum balloons below that of the ischial tuberosities during straining.[23] As discussed earlier, perineal descent is normally less than the descent of the pelvic floor. A comparison of the perineometer to proctographic assessment of pelvic floor descent has shown the unreliability of the former method.[24]

The syndrome is an important component of many disorders involving obstructed defecation and may ultimately lead to anal incontinence as a result of stretch injury to the pudendal nerve. Even single episodes of straining can damage the pudendal nerve, albeit temporarily, as evidenced by increased pudendal nerve terminal motor latency measurements.[25] Abnormal pelvic floor descent associated with straining is thought to be a major factor in causing stretch-induced nerve injury, thereby weakening the pelvic floor muscles that are responsible for maintaining continence. Lesaffer[26] had early success in treating pelvic floor descent with a perineal support device that minimizes pathologic descent and nerve stretch.

Proctography is valuable both to assess abnormal descent of the anorectal junction and to demonstrate associated abnormalities that cannot be shown clinically, particularly internal intussusception (Fig. 7A1-12).

Anal Incontinence

Radiologic evidence of major anal incontinence at proctography is unusual unless both puborectalis and anal sphincter tone are affected. Loss of puborectalis function is suggested by an exaggerated anorectal angle at rest (> 120° to 135°) and failure of the anorectal angle to decrease on squeezing (Fig. 7A1-13). This is usually associated with a failure of elevation of the posterior rectal wall. Loss of external sphincter function is suggested by inability, on squeezing down, to close an anal sphincter that was open at rest. In this situation, the anal canal frequently exceeds 2 cm in diameter. In Shorvon and colleague's study,[9] the finding of an open anal canal at rest in 3 of 23 normal volunteers is hard to explain. It suggests caution in trying to interpret a proctographic finding in isolation from consideration of the clinical problem.

Incontinent patients may be classified as those with sphincteric trauma, those with idiopathic (neurogenic) incontinence, and those with associated prolapse, or

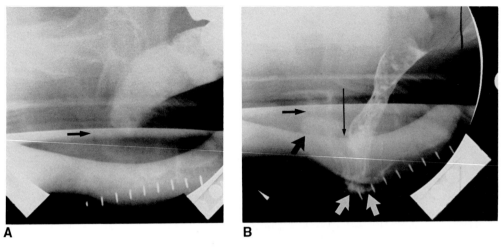

Fig. 7A1-12   Descending perineum syndrome with prolapse. **A,** At rest, the appearances are normal. The anorectal junction is at the level of the ischial tuberosity (arrow). **B,** At the end of evacuation, major intussusception occurs with abnormal descent of the anorectal junction and external prolapse (white arrows). Note the rectocele (large black arrow), intussusception (vertical arrow), and level of the ischial tuberosity (horizontal arrow).

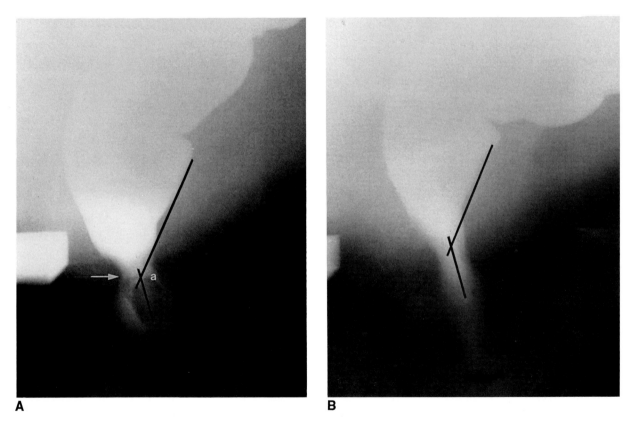

Fig. 7A1-13   Anal incontinence. **A,** There is gross anal incontinence at rest, with a patulous anal canal (arrow). The anorectal angle *(a)* is abnormally wide, measuring approximately 150 degrees. **B,** On squeezing down, the anal canal remains open and there is essentially no change in the anorectal angle, although there is some elevation of the posterior rectal wall.

combinations of each of the three. Radiologic visualization of an atonic anal sphincter is usually superfluous.

It was long believed that a widened anorectal angle caused by a weak puborectalis sling could be restored to normality by postanal repair.[4] More recent evaluation using current proctographic techniques has shown no significant change in the anorectal angle following post-anal repair.[27] In this study, those who were improved by the operation had a significantly longer anal canal (both at rest and during defecation) and less pelvic floor descent preoperatively than those who did not benefit by the postanal repair.

Patients with rectal prolapse are frequently incontinent, partly because the intussusception dilates the internal sphincter. Defecography is important in the incontinent patient in order to detect rectal prolapse; in such patients, a rectopexy may be performed initially, with postanal repair being reserved for those patients with persistent incontinence.[28] Other manifestations of chronic straining, such as a low pelvic floor, abnormal pelvic floor descent, or an enterocele, may be seen at proctography.

In many so-called idiopathic cases, it is likely that chronic straining leads to progressive weakness of the pelvic floor, and ultimately to incontinence as a result of neurogenic damage. In this way, it may be speculated that obstructed defecation and anal incontinence may merely represent different stages in the evolution of a single disease process. We found that patients with constipation as well as patients with anal incontinence had an anorectal junction position that was lower than normal controls. The constipated group showed the same amount of pelvic floor elevation as the controls, whereas the incontinent group had almost no ability to elevate the pelvic floor. Thus both clinical groups had evidence of a ballooned pelvic floor, but the constipated group still had an intact neuromuscular response, while the incontinent group had become unable to respond. These findings support the hypothesis that the straining associated with constipation can lead to incontinence.

Conclusions

Evacuation proctography provides considerable information about functional disorders of defecation, particularly those related to obstructed defecation and chronic constipation or straining. It is also useful in patients with anal incontinence to provide an overview of the disorder, to record the status of the puborectalis and sphincters, and to demonstrate any associated prolapse. Evacuation proctography permits measurement of the anorectal junction level at rest, and demonstrates whether pelvic floor movement is preserved. It is also useful for follow-up to show improvement in these parameters in response to treatment.

Clinical decisions should not be formulated on the basis of proctographic findings alone. These require careful integration with the patient's clinical findings, as well as with other investigatory techniques including electromyography, manometry, and colonic transit studies. Because of the overlap of normal and abnormal appearances at proctography, it is especially important to take into account the nature and severity of clinical symptoms before making management decisions.

COLONIC TRANSIT STUDIES

Patients with constipation may have impaired colonic function (colonic inertia) or obstructed defecation, or a combination of both. Colonic transit studies are often used in an attempt to separate these underlying etiologic disturbances.

Some authors recommend stopping all medications and putting the patient on a fiber-supplemented diet while performing the study. Others perform one transit study with the patient taking their usual diet and medication and then perform a second transit study with the patient on laxatives. This has the advantage of recording the patient's normal state and also demonstrates whether the loaded colon can be cleared by laxatives.

In its most simple form, the patient ingests, at a specific time on day 1, 20 small radiopaque markers that are contained within a single capsule (Sitzmarks, Lafayette Pharmacal, Fort Worth, TX 76109). A single plain abdominal radiograph is then taken on day 5 to determine the location and extent of elimination of the markers. Normal individuals usually excrete at least 80% of the markers within 5 days.[29] Patients who retain more than 20% of the markers should have plain abdominal radiographs taken at 2- to 3-day intervals until all the markers have been passed (Fig. 7A1-14). Retained markers can be assigned to the right colon, left colon, or rectosigmoid by dividing the abdomen into three areas (Fig. 7A1-14A).

This technique can be refined to assess segmental delays in colonic transit by obtaining plain abdominal radiographs at daily intervals until all the markers are passed. Mean transit through each of the three colonic segments is approximately 12 to 15 hours, resulting in a total colonic mean transit of approximately 36 to 45 hours. Colonic transit may be slower in the elderly. An alternate method of assessing segmental transit involves the ingestion of different-shaped markers on each of 3 successive days, followed by a plain abdominal radiograph on day 4 and, if necessary, at 2- to 3-day intervals until all markers are passed.[30] This technique of assessing segmental transit reduces the number of films re-

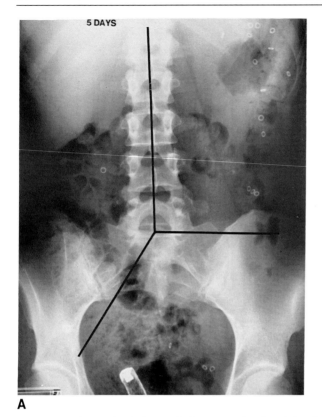
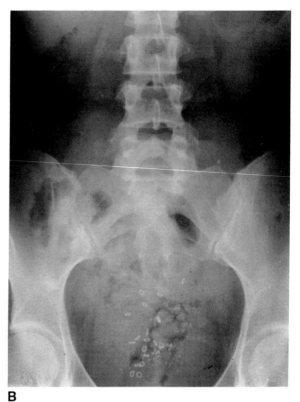

Fig. 7A1-14 Delayed colonic transit due to rectal outlet obstruction. **A,** Plain abdominal film obtained 5 days after ingestion of 20 radiopaque markers. Virtually all the ringlike markers have been retained within the colon. The abdomen can be divided into 3 areas (black lines) in order to roughly assess segmental localization of the retained markers within the large bowel. **B,** A further plain abdominal radiograph taken 2 days later shows aggregation of the markers with the rectum and rectosigmoid colon, thereby suggesting rectal outlet obstruction. Subsequent evacuation proctography demonstrated a large rectocele. The patient's sense of incomplete evacuation was greatly improved following repair of the rectocele.

quired with no loss of accuracy, and is therefore preferred because of reduced radiation dose. However, further films may be required if clearance is not complete by the fourth day.

A daily, single capsule technique wherein 20 markers are ingested every day for five days with a single radiograph on the morning of day 6 may also be used. Further films are never required. Most young adults have less than 40 markers remaining; those with mild delay, or the elderly, may have up to 60 markers, and those with severe delay have more than 60 markers still present in the abdomen. Colonic transit scintigraphy is a more sophisticated technique that provides detailed information about segmental transit.[31]

Based on segmental colonic transit studies, Wald[32] divided patients with severe idiopathic constipation into three groups: those with normal transit, those with generalized colonic inertia, and those with left-sided or rectosigmoid slowing. Generalized colonic inertia is suggested by abnormal retention of markers throughout the colon, whereas the aggregation of the markers in the rectum or rectosigmoid suggests obstructed defecation (Fig. 7A1-14). The interest in distinguishing between these two disorders is in part related to therapeutic considerations; patients with generalized colonic inertia may benefit from colectomy, whereas those with delayed rectosigmoid transit require full investigation of the pelvic floor followed by appropriate local therapy. Unfortunately, these therapeutic distinctions may not always hold true. For example, there is some evidence that patients with an evacuation abnormality, when treated by colectomy, have as good an outcome as those without such an abnormality.[33] Interestingly, the degree of defecatory impairment as assessed at evacuation proctography does not appear to correlate with measurements of colonic transit, suggesting that both colonic inertia and an evacuation abnormality may have a role in the etiology of constipation.[34]

ANAL ENDOSONOGRAPHY

Anal endosonography is a recently developed technique that provides high-resolution images of the anal canal, including the internal anal sphincter (IAS) and external anal sphincter (EAS). The technique was developed in England at St. Mark's Hospital. Initial experience suggests that anal endosonography will play a major role in the assessment of disorders affecting the anal canal and its sphincters.

A Bruel and Kjaer ultrasound scanner with a 7-MHz rotating endoprobe is used. A specially designed hard plastic cone filled with degassed water is screwed onto the end of the probe to protect it and to provide effective acoustic coupling within the anal canal.[35] The lubricated cone is introduced with the patient in the left lateral position, and a series of radial images are obtained as the probe is slowly withdrawn down the anal canal. The examination takes 5 to 10 minutes to perform, and causes no more discomfort than routine digital examination.

The normal appearances of the anal canal are illustrated in Fig. 7A1-15. Five distinct layers can usually be identified: the mucosa, submucosa, IAS, intersphincteric plane, and EAS. The smooth muscle of the IAS is clearly visualized as a homogeneous, hypoechoic circular band measuring 2 mm to 3 mm in width. The stria-

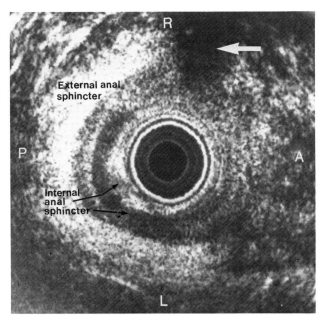

Fig. 7A1-16 Defects in external and internal anal sphincters secondary to obstetric trauma. Patient who developed incontinence following childbirth requiring episiotomy and forceps delivery. The internal anal sphincter is intact posteriorly and on the left, but no hypoechoic band is identified anteriorly and toward the right, indicating deficiency. A large V-shaped notch (white arrow) is seen anterolaterally on the right within the external anal sphincter, consistent with a traumatic defect following episiotomy in this area. *P* = posterior, *A* = anterior, *R* = right, *L* = left. (Courtesy of C. Bartram, London, England.)

Fig. 7A1-15 Normal anal endosonography. Radial image with probe in anal canal. The different layers of the normal wall are shown.

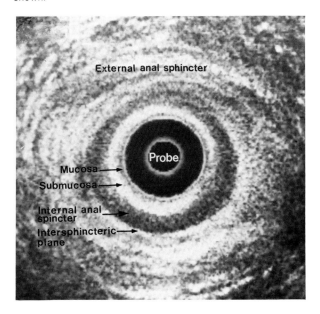

ted muscle of the EAS has different acoustic properties, with variable echogenicity and a linear pattern, resulting in a streaky appearance. Between the two sphincters, a narrow echogenic band is present. This represents the intersphincteric plane. In some subjects, a thin hypoechoic complete or partial ring of longitudinal muscle is identified within the intersphincteric plane. Immediately adjacent to the water-filled plastic cone, the anal mucosa and submucosa are visualized. Frequently, the hypoechoic mucosa can be differentiated from the more echogenic submucosa.

Anal endosonography has already been shown to be of value in the investigation of fecal incontinence. Incontinence caused by obstetric or surgical trauma to the anal sphincters is traditionally assessed by digital examination, manometry, and electromyographic mapping of the EAS. Traumatic defects in the IAS and EAS can readily be demonstrated by anal endosonography (Fig. 7A1-16). The technique provides an alternative to electromyography for mapping the defects in the EAS. In this respect, a high degree of correlation between the two techniques has been demonstrated.[36] Anal endosonography has the benefit, however, of being essentially painless and much less time-consuming; and for these reasons it has now replaced electromyographic mapping of the EAS at St. Mark's Hospital.

Endosonography also provides an accurate picture of the IAS, for which routine electromyography is not available. The thickness, length, and symmetry of the IAS can be demonstrated, in addition to any focal defect.[37] The IAS contributes about 80% of the resting pressure in patients with an intact EAS. There may well be a correlation between the thickness of the IAS and the resting pressure.[37] With increasing age, the IAS thickens and becomes more echogenic.[38]

Further applications of anal endosonography include the evaluation of perianal sepsis and anal fistulae.[39] The location of a fistulous track or abscess can be determined, as well as its relationship to the intersphincteric plane and sphincters. This is particularly important in anal fistulae; sepsis localized to the intersphincteric space can be laid open in its entirety, whereas transsphincteric spread may require cutting part of the EAS, with the associated risk of incontinence. Fig. 7A1-17

illustrates a transsphincteric abscess. Anal endosonography may also be useful in patients with unexplained chronic anal pain, as it may detect a small, clinically unsuspected abscess or fistula.[37]

RADIOLOGIC EVALUATION OF THE VAGINA

The vagina is readily identified by computed tomography, ultrasonography, and magnetic resonance imaging. Anatomy texts frequently depict the vagina as having an almost vertical axis. This appears to be a consequence of rectal distention, which is often present at autopsy. Particularly when the vagina is lax, it tends to have an oblique or horizontal axis. If evacuation proctography is carried out in such a patient, the vagina is then seen to assume a vertical orientation secondary to the rectal distention.

Vaginography is occasionally required for demonstration of the source of a vaginal fistula. The examination is performed by injecting water-soluble contrast into the vagina after introduction of a Foley balloon catheter and gently inflating its balloon to seal the intro-

Fig. 7A1-17 Transsphincteric abscess. A large hypoechoic area representing an abscess extends posteriorly from the internal anal sphincter, which is deficient in the area of the abscess. The abscess extends into and through the external anal sphincter, indicating its transsphincteric nature. *P* = posterior, *A* = anterior, *R* = right, *L* = left. (Courtesy of C. Bartram, London, England)

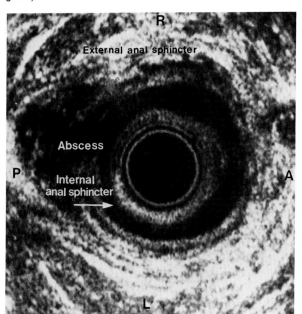

Fig. 7A1-18 Rectovaginal fistula. Single contrast barium enema shows a fistulous tract (arrow) connecting the lower rectum to the vagina that is extensively opacified via the fistula.

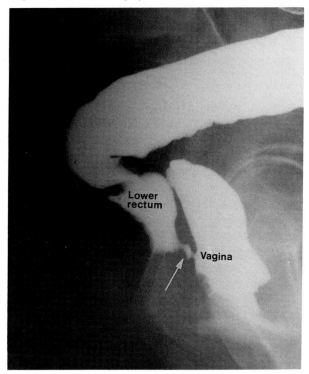

itus. Rectovaginal fistulae, however, are more usually demonstrated by barium enema examination (Fig. 7A1-18).

The important relationship of the vagina to the rectum, and movement of the rectovaginal septum, is demonstrated during evacuation proctography, as already discussed. Rectovaginal separation during defecation or straining is crucial for the detection of enteroceles and sigmoidoceles.

SUMMARY

Rational therapy for disorders of defecation requires objective documentation of the underlying problem. Evacuation proctography often demonstrates the multifactorial nature of the functional disturbance. It is especially useful in evaluating the patient with chronic constipation or straining who may have a treatable cause of rectal outlet obstruction. Repair of pelvic prolapse requires identification of all its components in order to reduce the risk of surgical failure. Evacuation proctography contributes to surgical planning by identifying clinically unsuspected enteroceles and sigmoidoceles, as well as coexistent disorders of rectal evacuation.

Colonic transit studies can suggest the presence of generalized colonic inertia as a cause of chronic constipation. Anal endosonography is particularly useful for mapping the extent of traumatic damage to the external anal sphincter. Dynamic magnetic resonance imaging will almost certainly play an increasing role in the assessment of pelvic floor disorders, because it can show all pelvic structures on a single image without the need for initially opacifying either the vagina or rectum.

REFERENCES

1. Halpert RD, Crnovich FM, Schreiber MH. Rectal diverticulosis: a case report and review of the literature. *Gastrointest Radiol.* 1989;14:274–276.
2. Kruyt RH, Delemarre JBVM, Doornbos J, Vogel HJ. Normal anorectum: dynamic MR imaging anatomy. *Radiology.* 1991; 179:159–163.
3. Yang A, Mostwin JL, Rosensheim NB, Zerhouni EA. Pelvic floor descent in women: dynamic evaluation with fast MR imaging and cinematic display. *Radiology.* 1991;179:25–33.
4. Preston DM, Lennard-Jones JE, Thomas BM. The balloon proctogram. *Br J Surg.* 1984;71:29–32.
5. Mahieu P, Pringot J, Bodart P. Defecography: 1. Description of a new procedure and results in normal patients. *Gastrointest Radiol.* 1984;9:247–251.
6. Shorvon PJ, Stevenson GW. Defaecography: setting up a service. *Br J Hosp Med.* 1989;41:460–466.
7. Bernier P, Stevenson GW, Shorvon P. Defecography commode. *Radiology.* 1988;166:891–892.
8. Finlay IG (moderator). Proctography: symposium. *Int J Colorect Dis.* 1988;3:67–89.
9. Shorvon PJ, McHugh S, Somers S, Stevenson GW. Defaecography findings in normal volunteers: results and implications. *Gut.* 1989;30:1737–1749.
10. Bartram CI, Turnbull GK, Lennard-Jones JE. Evacuation proctography: an investigation of rectal expulsion in 20 subjects without defecatory disturbance. *Gastrointest Radiol.* 1988;13:72–80.
11. Goei R, van Engelshoven J, Schouten H, Baeten C, Stassen C. Anorectal function: defecographic measurement in asymptomatic subjects. *Radiology.* 1989;173:137–141.
12. Penninckx F, Debruyne C, Lestar B, Kerremans R. Observer variation in the radiological measurement of the anorectal angle. *Int J Colorect Dis.* 1990;5:94–97.
13. McHugh SM, Diamant NE. Anal canal pressure profile: a reappraisal as determined by rapid pull-through technique. *Gut.* 1987;28:1234–1242.
14. Pinho M, Yoshioka K, Ortiz J, Oya M, Keighley MRB. The effect of age on pelvic floor dynamics. *Int J Colorect Dis.* 1990;5:207–208.
15. Mahieu P, Pringot J, Bodart P. Defecography: II. contribution to the diagnosis of defecation disorders. *Gastrointest Radiol.* 1984; 9:253–261.
16. Goei R, Baeten C. Rectal intussusception and rectal prolapse: detection and postoperative evaluation with defecography. *Radiology.* 1990;174:124–126.
17. Kelvin FM, Maglinte DDT, Hornback JA, Benson JT. Pelvic prolapse: assessment with evacuation proctography (defecography). *Radiology.* In press.
18. Brubaker L, Retzky S, Smith C, Saclarides T. The role of dynamic proctograms in the evaluation of women with genital prolapse. Presented at 12th Annual Meeting of the American Uro-gynecologic Society; October 25, 1991; Newport Beach, Calif.
19. Nichols DH. Enterocele. In: Nichols DH, Randall CL, eds. *Vaginal Surgery.* Baltimore: Williams & Wilkins; 1989:313–327.
20. Kuijpers HC, Bleijenberg G. The spastic pelvic floor syndrome: a cause of constipation. *Dis Col Rect.* 1985;28:669–672.
21. Goei R, Baeten C, Arends JW. Solitary rectal ulcer syndrome: findings at barium enema study and defecography. *Radiology.* 1988;168:303–306.
22. Finlay IG, Bartram CI, Nicholls RJ. Can videoproctography and anorectal physiology predict outcome after rectopexy for the solitary rectal ulcer syndrome? *Gut.* 1987;28:A1361.
23. Henry MM, Parks AG, Swash M. The pelvic floor musculature in the descending perineum syndrome. *Br J Surg.* 1982;69:470–472.
24. Oettle GJ, Roe AM, Bartolo DCC, McC Mortensen NJ. What is the best way of measuring perineal descent? A comparison of radiographic and clinical methods. *Br J Surg.* 1985;72:999–1001.
25. Lubowski DZ, Swash M, Nicholls RJ, Henry MM. Increase in pudendal nerve terminal motor latency with defaecation straining. *Br J Surg.* 1988;75:1095–1097.
26. Lesaffer LPA. Perineal support device. In: Smith LE, ed. *Practical Guide to Anorectal Testing.* New York: Igaku Shoin; 1990:205–208.
27. Yoshioka K, Hyland G, Keighley MRB. Physiological changes after postanal repair and parameters predicting outcome. *Br J Surg.* 1988;75:1220–1224.
28. Penninckx FM (moderator). Faecal incontinence: symposium. *Int J Colorect D.* 1987;2:173–186.
29. Hinton JM, Lennard-Jones JE, Young AC. A new method for studying gut transit times using radioopaque markers. *Gut.* 1969; 10:842–847.
30. Metcalf AM, Phillips SF, Zinsmeister AR, MacCarty RL, Beart RW, Wolff BG. Simplified assessment of segmental colonic transit. *Gastroenterol.* 1987;92:40–47.

31. Krevsky B, Maurer AH, Fisher RS. Patterns of colonic transit in chronic idiopathic constipation. *AM J Gastroenterol.* 1989;84: 127–132.

32. Wald A. Colonic transit and anorectal manometry in chronic idiopathic constipation. *Arch Int Med.* 1986;146:1713–1716.

33. Kamm MA, Hawley PR, Lennard-Jones JE. Is colectomy for severe idiopathic constipation a success? *Gut.* 1987;28:A1343.

34. Turnbull GK, Bartram CI, Lennard-Jones JE. Radiologic studies of rectal evacuation in adults with idiopathic constipation. *Dis Col Rect.* 1988;31:190–197.

35. Law PJ, Bartram CI. Anal endosonography: technique and normal anatomy. *Gastrointest Radiol.* 1989;14:349–353.

36. Law PJ, Kamm MA, Bartram CI. A comparison between electromyography and anal endosonography in mapping external anal sphincter defects. *Dis Col Rect.* 1990;33:370–373.

37. Bartram CI, Law PJ. Anal endosonography. Technique and applications. In: Herlinger H, Megibow A, eds. *Advances in Gastrointestinal Radiology.* St. Louis: Mosby Year Book; 1991;101–115.

38. Burnett SJD, Bartram CI. Endosonographic variations in the normal internal anal sphincter. *Int J Colorect Dis.* 1991;6:2–4.

39. Law PJ, Talbot RW, Bartram CI, Northover JMA. Anal endosonography in the evaluation of perianal sepsis and fistula in ano. *Br J Surg.* 1989;76:752–755.

C H A P T E R   7

Anatomic Investigation

7A   Radiologic Investigation

7A2   Plain Films of the Abdomen and Pelvis

G. Byington Pratt

INTRODUCTION

Despite the development of new technology, a number of abnormalities can be detected simply with either plain films of the pelvis or abdomen or traditional contrast studies of the urinary tract. The typical plain film may be obtained for other reasons, but it can give a great deal of information regarding the lower urinary tract and pelvic floor. Similarly the conventional contrast examinations—intravenous pyelogram (IVP) and voiding cystourethrogram—are still the first radiographic studies performed. The information gained from these can be expanded by ultrasound and computed tomography (CT). The role of magnetic resonance (MR) imaging is not fully established.

PLAIN FILMS

Conventional plain films of the abdomen, pelvis, and spine may reveal bone abnormalities that are of significance in regard to bladder floor abnormalities. These include fractures involving the innominate bones, particularly the obturator rings or symphysis pubis. Fractures of the lumbar spine or sacrum could cause neurologic abnormalities.

Partial and complete agenesis of the sacrum has high correlation with congenital abnormalities of the urinary tract when three or more segments of the spine are involved. Spina bifida can be a manifestation of diastematomyelia and tethering of the filum terminale. These may be associated with neurologic deficit and neurogenic bladder. However, at least 10% of the population has nonfusion of the spinous processes of a vertebra without other findings.

Degenerative changes of the spine, including disk space narrowing, degenerative osteophyte formation, and spondylolithesis, may also result in neurologic changes in bladder function. Either benign or malignant tumors or metastatic involvement of the lumbosacral spine can be identified on plain film studies. Similarly, tumors with their origin within or adjacent to the spine, such as neurogenic tumors, might be detected by their mass, destruction of vertebrae, or by erosion of the vertebral pedicle. Defects of the sacrum from either primary or secondary tumors or anterior myelomeningocele are encountered.

The soft tissue shadows may reveal a distended bladder, vascular calcification, or old injection sites of heavy metal. The latter was a treatment for tabes dorsalis that can cause loss of bladder sensation. Today, such injection sites are seldom seen in patients younger than 70 years old.[1]

Evidence of infection either in soft tissues or in bone might also be detected by a mass or mottling of the soft tissue shadow. Osteomyelitis could be detected by destruction of the cortex or trabecula of the bone and periosteal reaction.

CONTRAST STUDIES OF THE URINARY TRACT

Contrast studies of the urinary tract may be performed to evaluate outflow obstruction, to identify a fistula, and to evaluate voiding dysfunction. The voiding cystourethrogram can show whether the obstruction is in the bladder neck or in the distal urethra.[2] In the 1960s there was a great deal of interest in bladder neck obstruction in young children as a cause of urinary infection.[3] But later studies showed that the presumed obstruction was not as significant a contributor to infections as previously thought.[4] Still, the cystogram has the value of showing the bladder capacity, trabeculation, or diverticula. Reflux into the ureters and upper urinary tract can also be detected. The voiding phase shows the bladder neck and urethra and also displays the extent of bladder floor descent during voiding. The voiding cystogram delineates the length of the urethra and gives an estimate of relative meatal stenosis. A fistula to or from the bladder may be the result of infection, surgery, tumor, or granulomatous colitis. A urethrogram utilizing a catheter with double balloons to occlude the urethra both proximally and distally can detect extravasation of the urethra and diverticula of the urethra.

The chain cystourethrogram was introduced in the 1950s and articles discussing its role are still in the current literature.[5] Some authors still feel that the posterior urethral vesical angle is important. An angle equal to or greater than 115° was considered a diminished posterior angle, with some correlation to stress urinary incontinence.[6]

More recently, an article states that the chain cystogram is obsolete and the urodynamic technique is the standard for evaluating voiding difficulties.[7] That author contends that the videourodynamic (VUD) examination is most useful in studying cases of stress incontinence and detrusor instability.

The intravenous pyelogram reveals evidence of chronic changes in the kidney either from infection with hydronephrosis and loss of parenchyma, ureteral pelvic junction narrowing, or congenital abnormalities of the kidneys such as duplication. Duplication may be associated with an ectopic ureter, which infrequently enters the urethra as an ectopic ureterocele distal to the trigone of the bladder. But incontinence will occur only if the ectopic ureter enters the urethra distal to the bladder neck or in the vagina.

A recent study of patients with stress incontinence and control patients emphasized the use of the cystourethrogram.[8] The authors found no differences in the radiographic findings between patients with pelvic relaxation with or without stress urinary incontinence. They went on to say that the findings of change in the posterior urethral angle and of urethrovesical junction at the most dependent point of the bladder may simply reflect pelvic relaxation. They concluded that the cystourethrogram should not be relied on for the work-up of urinary incontinence. However, this test may still be useful for detection of other abnormalities of the urinary tract.

MAGNETIC RESONANCE IMAGING

Magnetic resonance (MR) imaging is a blossoming area of investigation. Although the cost of these studies is high, the absence of radiation makes it attractive. In addition, views of the pelvis can be produced in planes of section not available on computed tomography (CT).

A recent article proposes the use of MR imaging for evaluation of the urethra.[9] Another uses it to study various forms of pelvic floor descent.[10] In it the authors give MR criteria for diagnosing abnormal descent of the three pelvic compartments. These are based on measurement of organ position during straining related to the pubococcygeal line.

SUMMARY

A number of abnormalities which may involve the urinary tract and pelvic floor can be detected with either simple plain film studies of the pelvis and spine, magnetic resonance imaging, or contrast studies including IVP, cystourethrograms, and urodynamics.

Radiographic visualization of the lower urinary tract during bladder filling and voiding (voiding cystourethrography) is considered by some to be an important part of the urodynamic evaluation of patients, especially those with neurologic disorders.[11] The National Institutes of Health's Urinary Incontinence Consensus Statement[2] concluded that "video urodynamic evaluation requires special expertise. Its role is limited to the more elusive incontinence problems."

The debate over different methodology obviously includes the expense involved in utilizing technology as well as radiation exposure. More widespread applicability of ultrasound videourodynamic evaluation may come about as technology improves, including the development of liquid contrast material that can be visualized by ultrasound. Research on such technology is currently being conducted.

REFERENCES

1. Stanton S. *Clinical Gynecologic Urology.* St. Louis: CV Mosby Co; 1984.
2. Blaivas JG. Techniques of evaluation. In: Yalla SV, McGuire EJ, Elbadawi A, Blaivas JG, eds. *Neurourology and Urodynamics: Principles and Practice.* New York: MacMillan Publishing Co; 1988:155–198.
3. Davis LA, Lich R, Howerton L, Joule W. The lower urinary tract in infants and children. *Radiology.* 1961;77:445.
4. Shopfner CE. Roentgenological evaluation of bladder neck obstruction. *AJR.* 1967;100:162.
5. Yoshioka S, Ochi K, Takeuch M. Simple method for chain cystography. *Urology.* 1986;28:527.
6. Hodgkinson CD. Relationship of female urethra and bladder in urinary stress incontinence. *Am J Obstet Gynecol.* 1953;65:560.
7. Saxton HM. Urodynamics: the appropriate modality for the investigation of frequency, urgency, incontinence and voiding difficulties. *Radiology.* 1990;175:307–316.
8. Bergman A, McKenzie C, Ballard CA, Richmond J. Role of cystourethrography in the preoperative evaluation of stress urinary incontinence in women. *J Reprod Med.* 1988;33:372–376.
9. Hricak H, Secaf E, Buckley DW, Brown JJ, Tanagho EA, McAninch JW. Female urethra: MR imaging. *Radiology.* 1991;178:527–535.
10. Yang A, Mostwin JL, Rosenshein NB, Zerhouni EA. Pelvic floor descent in women: dynamic evaluation with fast MR imaging and cinematic display. *Radiology.* 1991;179:25–33.
11. Amis ES, Blaivas JG. The role of the radiologist in evaluating voiding dysfunction. *Radiology.* 1990;175:317–318.

CHAPTER 7

Anatomic Investigation

7B   Ultrasound Investigation

Vincent Lucente

INTRODUCTION

Since ultrasound evaluation of the pelvis was first described in 1958, the development of real-time imaging and, more recently, various endoprobe transducers, has dramatically affected our understanding of the functional female pelvic floor anatomy and lower urinary tract. Improving technology promises routine use of ultrasound during office evaluation of pelvic floor disorders involving both urinary and fecal incontinence. This chapter will review some of the basic principles of ultrasound and discuss its role as a diagnostic tool for a variety of disorders often associated with dysfunction of the female pelvic floor.

BASIC PRINCIPLES OF ULTRASOUND

Ultrasound refers to sound energy with a frequency above 20,000 Hz. The sound waves are produced and received by piezoelectric crystals. The sound beam is propagated as a longitudinal wave through human soft tissue at a speed of 1.54 km/sec.

Penetration of tissue depends on the frequency of the sound waves. The higher the frequency, the shorter the wavelength and less penetration. The lower the frequency, the longer the wavelength and deeper the tissue penetration.

Since frequency selection involves a compromise be-

tween better image resolution (high frequency) and deeper tissue penetration (low frequency), the decision must be based on the position of the organ(s) to be examined. For example, a 3.5 or 5.0 MHz transducer is often used to scan an intraabdominal organ such as the bladder.

A sound wave becomes attenuated as it travels through soft tissue. This phenomenon is a result of absorption, scattering, and reflection of sound waves.

Reflection occurs at different tissue interfaces because of the change in tissue density. Reflection is complete at tissue and air boundaries and necessitates the use of a coupling medium (a low density gel) to allow sound waves to enter through the skin.

Shadowing is the reduction of echo amplitude from acoustic interfaces that lie behind highly reflective or attenuating structures. This phenomenon occurs often when attempting to scan the bladder neck region transabdominally as a result of the intervening symphysis. Angulating the transducer to avoid this is limited by the abdominal panniculus, especially in an upright position during strain maneuvers.

There are various types of ultrasound transducers currently being used, each with an advantage in certain applications. A rotating crystal contained within the transducer of the sector scanner emits bursts of sound energy that travel in different directions from the transducer face, thereby producing a recognizable "pie-shaped" image. The advantages of sector scanners include easy handling of the transducer head and a very small contact site. Mechanical sector transducers may be subject to slight image distortions at the edges of the field (side lobe artifact) due to hysteresis (stopping and starting) that occurs with an oscillating transducer.

Linear-array scanners have a large number of crystals arranged in a linear fashion. The energy beams pass straight out from each crystal, generating a rectangular image as wide as the transducer itself. Recently, curved linear-array transducers have been developed. These offer the improved handling of sector scanners without the limitations of narrow proximal field widths encountered with vaginal or rectal endoprobes. At Methodist Hospital of Indiana we use a 3.5 MHz curved linear-array transducer placed at the vaginal introitus.

EVALUATION OF THE LOWER URINARY TRACT

Assessment of Bladder Neck Mobility

Over the years numerous theories have been proposed to explain the pathophysiology of genuine stress urinary incontinence (GSUI). GSUI is a condition in which the involuntary loss of urine occurs when the intravesical pressure exceeds the maximal urethral pressure in the absence of a detrusor contraction.[1] Various etiologic processes can affect the urethral sphincteric mechanism, resulting in GSUI. Hypermobility of the urethrovesical junction, with rotational descent of the proximal urethra below the region of an abdominal "pressure zone," has been associated with impairment of abdominal pressure transmission. This inefficient pressure transmission to the urethra during stress jeopardizes the urethral sphincteric mechanism and may overcome various protective factors, such as resting urethral tone and urethral length, and can lead to failed urethral competence. This excess mobility has been attributed to disruption of the anatomic supports of the region, primarily the fibromuscular vagino-levator attachments to the arcus tendinous fasciae pelvis.[2]

A variety of procedures, including the Q-Tip test, lateral chain cystourethrogram, and dynamic urethroscopy have been advocated to evaluate the functional anatomy of paravesical and paraurethral support tissues.

The Q-Tip test, although simple and well tolerated, is nonspecific for the diagnosis of GSUI. Nearly half of continent women or those with other urologic disorders have a positive Q-Tip test.[3] It is a measure of urethral

mobility but provides no associated anatomic information.

Radiographic techniques such as a lateral chain cystogram or videocystourethrography do provide anatomic information. However, these techniques require technical expertise and costly equipment while subjecting the patient to radiation and a higher complication rate.

Dynamic urethroscopy, using a 0-degree telescope, has also been recommended to assess mobility of the urethra. The scope is placed within the mid-urethra and the response of the urethrovesical junction is evaluated during Valsalva and cough maneuvers. Unfortunately, the presence of the scope itself induces mechanical artifact, and interpretation is completely subjective.

Ultrasound assessment of the bladder itself was first described by Holmes, who focused primarily on adynamic features such as residual urine, distortion of the bladder by pelvic pathology, and detection of bladder tumors.[4] Since that time, numerous studies have demonstrated real-time ultrasonography to be useful in evaluating the anatomic relationship of the bladder, urethrovesical junction (UVJ), and proximal urethra. Various techniques regarding type and placement of the transducer, mode of scanning, and positioning of patients have been advocated.

One of the first reports in the English literature of real-time ultrasonography in the evaluation of urinary stress incontinence documented the use of a linear-array transducer placed on the patient's abdomen.[5] A pediatric feeding tube was used to demonstrate the urethra. With the patient in both supine and standing positions the inclination of the urethra and the distance between the UVJ and the pubic symphysis was measured at rest and during the Valsalva maneuver. Although the authors did not definitively quantify their measurements, they did find that among continent patients little change occurred in the relative anatomic positions of the UVJ during the Valsalva maneuver compared to the altered urethrovesical relationships in incontinent patients. Their technique of placing the transducer above the pubic symphysis, angled caudally to visualize the area of interest, unfortunately provided a reduced image quality. This was, and still is the result of significant intervening tissue affecting sound wave penetration (attenuation) and acoustic shading from the symphysis itself.

Placing a linear-array transducer within the rectum to improve imaging of the bladder base and neck was described by Nishizawa and coworkers.[6] The authors described how the technique may be used to replace X-ray cystography during urodynamic imaging. Shappeero, Friedland, and Perkash used the same technique to visualize the bladder base and proximal urethra in males suspected of having neuromuscular dysfunction of the bladder.[7] They performed radiographic and sonographic voiding cystourethrograms on all patients, and concluded that the sonographic examination is as good as, and occasionally better than, the radiographic method.

The technique of using a transrectal probe for the investigation of women with urinary incontinence was introduced by Brown and coworkers.[8] However, questions arose regarding endoprobe movement during straining maneuvers, thereby creating artifact, attendant discomfort, and possible inhibition of bladder neck movement. Bergman and colleagues[9] established that insertion of the rectal probe did not alter urethrovesical junction mobility as evaluated by the Q-Tip angle change. In this study, urethrovesical junction mobility (anteroposterior) in the supine position was measured. The drop in the urethrovesical junction on straining was measured in centimeters on the ultrasound screen using internal electronic calipers. Of 44 patients with the diagnosis of GSUI, 38 had a drop in the UVJ of greater than or equal to 1 cm during straining. All patients with bladder instability, as well as 22 of the 24 patients in the control group, had a UVJ drop of less than 1 cm during straining. With this parameter the results of the series found transrectal ultrasound in the evaluation of women with GSUI to have a sensitivity of 86% and a specificity of 92%. However, the potential problems of probe or patient movement during straining were also noted by the authors.

Ultrasound cystourethrography by perineal scanning for evaluation of female stress urinary incontinence was suggested by Kohorn and others.[10] For perineal scanning, the patient is placed in a supine position with legs slightly abducted to allow access of the transducer to the perineum. A linear-array transducer in a sagittal orientation is positioned to visualize the bladder, bladder base, urethrovesical junction, and the pubis. Using this technique, Gordon and coworkers[11] compared ultrasound to lateral chain urethrocystography for the evaluation of bladder neck descent. Descent (in millimeters) was measured among 21 patients who complained of GSUI. In this study, a coefficient of determination was calculated as a measurement of the reliability of the ultrasound method compared with lateral chain urethrocystogram. The ultrasound method with a catheter compared to the cystogram was found to have a coefficient of determination of 0.73. However, 99% confidence limit ranged from as low as 0.565 to as high as

0.954. Variation between patient position (ultrasound scanning performed supine versus erect for the chain cystogram) may have contributed to less than optimal correlation. Kölbl and others[12] compared perineal ultrasound scanning performed with the patient standing to urethrocystography findings among patients with GSUI. Based on the recommendations of Green,[13] the posterior urethrovesical angle (Beta) and the angle of inclination (Alpha) with the patient in an upright position at rest and during strain were analyzed. Comparable results for both these angle measurements were found in all patients with GSUI, regardless of the diagnostic procedure.

A combined approach using a vaginal sector scanner and a linear-array transducer placed on the perineum was reported by Benson and Sumners.[14] The location of urethral egress in relation to the most dependent portion of the bladder and the displaced distance of the bladder neck during the Valsalva maneuver was assessed with the vaginal transducer. The direction of this displacement, horizontal versus vertical, was determined using the perineal transducer stabilized to the inferior aspect of the pubis and coccyx. Six of the seven patients found on urodynamic evaluation to have GSUI demonstrated the urethral egress arising from the most dependent portion of the bladder. Hodgkinson[15] emphasized that location of the internal urethral egress at the bladder's most dependent portion compromised the urethral sphincteric mechanism (Fig. 7B-1).

The magnitude of urethral vesical junction descent ranged from 6 mm to 15 mm with a mean of 10 mm. A tendency for predominantly horizontal displacement was also noted.

Transvaginal endosonography for evaluating the anatomy of the lower urinary tract in urinary stress incontinence was described by Quinn and others[16] in a series of 100 women with a range of urinary symptoms. The patients were scanned in the recumbent position. The inferior border of the symphysis was used as a "key landmark." A level mounted on the endoprobe ensured

Fig. 7B-1 The location of urethral egress in relation to the bladder's most dependent area. **A** shows its location prior to surgery. **B** shows its location after successful urethropexy surgery; note the urethral egress becomes more anterior.

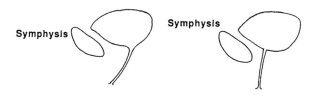

the maintenance of a horizontal position during scanning. Distortion of the anatomy by the endoprobe was reported to be easily noted during scanning and avoided by reorientation of the endoprobe. In 19 of the 23 females with primary stress incontinence the urethrovesical junction was inferior to the level of the mid-symphysis at rest, and in 18 there was opening and descent of the bladder neck during a cough. Similar findings were seen in 12 of 14 patients with recurrent stress incontinence. The authors found the technique to produce consistent views of the anatomy and to be well received by the patients.

Kölbl and Bernaschek [17] recognized regional distortion as a disadvantage in using vaginal or rectal endoprobes and developed a new method termed "introital sonography." The technique involves placing a vaginal sector scanner adjacent to the vulva just underneath the external urethral orifice, visualizing the bladder, urethrovesical junction, urethra, and symphysis. The length of the urethra, the angle of micturition, and the retrovesical angle could be measured easily. Fifteen of 20 women with incontinence symptoms were found to have GSUI, established by simultaneous combined pressure-flow and sonographic studies. Although sonographic parameters were not compared to normal controls, the method was reported to display a marked descent of the urethrovesical junction and an increase of the retrovesical angle during coughing in patients with GSUI. In five patients with detrusor instability, sonographic findings revealed a marked opening of the bladder neck during filling cystometry.

The authors outline several advantages of simultaneous introital sonographic urethrocystography and pressure-flow measurements. First, and perhaps most important, compared to endosonographic techniques, introital sonography is devoid of any potential artifact as a result of urethral or bladder neck distortion. Similarly, with the transducer placed at the introitus there is no irritation by rectal or transurethral catheters during simultaneous urodynamic measurements. Like the radiographic cystourethrogram, the sonographic findings complement the urodynamic studies. The exact location of microtip pressure transducers can easily be determined while visualizing the bladder neck and urethra during filling. This helps to exclude tonometric artifacts. The voiding phase can also be evaluated without the use of catheters. Visualization of micturition and, specifically, the patient's ability to stop voiding, which demonstrates the voluntary musculature and the urethral "milking-back" mechanism, can be evaluated (Fig. 7B-2).

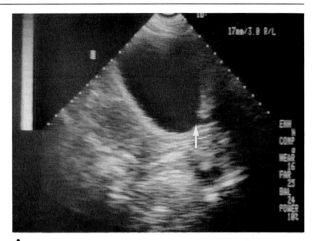

A

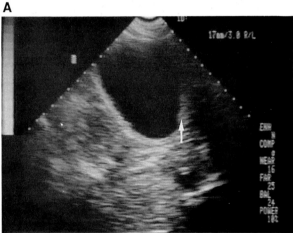

B

Fig. 7B-2   A, Ultrasound view of patient voiding. Arrow indicates open proximal urethra. **B**, Arrow indicates closed urethra during effort to stop voiding. Urethra emptied by the milking-back mechanism of striated muscle.

The technique we have developed in our urodynamic laboratory employs a curved linear-array transducer placed at the vaginal introitus. A 3.5 MHz scanner is enclosed with a condom and positioned just under the external urethral orifice to visualize the bladder, urethrovesical junction, urethra, and symphysis (Fig. 7B-3). A 10 cc balloon, 16 French Foley catheter is placed prior to scanning. The balloon is inflated with 5 cc of air and 5 cc of "hand soap" diluted with water. This creates an air/soap-bubble interface that can be clearly visualized during scanning, providing a constant horizontal reference. It enables us to easily establish X and Y coordinates as well as precise and consistent identification of the urethrovesical junction.

All patients are scanned in standing position with a

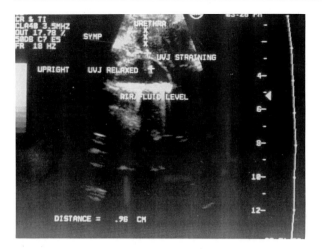

Fig. 7B-3 Vaginal introital ultrasonography (inverted orientation, feet up, head down). Horizontal air/fluid levels noted in Foley balloon. Urethrovesical junction *(UVJ)* marked at rest (relaxed) and straining. *SYMP*=symphysis. Distance, the amount of movement of the UVJ = .98 cm. (Direction of movement calculated from horizontal.)

comfortably full bladder. The examiner is positioned in front of the patient. The posterior, inferior border of the symphysis is identified and outlined or traced using electronic calipers. This outline remains on screen during all subsequent scanning and measurement recordings are determined by a second set of electronic calipers. After or during any stress maneuver, such as coughing or the Valsalva maneuver, care is taken to properly reposition the transducer to guarantee alignment of the border of the symphysis with the previously obtained outline. This ensures correction of any transducer displacement which could create artifact during dynamic testing. We have also found that the curved linear-array transducer provides a broader proximal field of view compared to a sector scanner. This enables continued visualization of the symphysis, bladder, urethrovesical junction, and proximal urethra, despite the significant mobility of these soft tissues. The parameters that are routinely noted during scanning are listed in Box 7B-1. In addition to these parameters, ureteral "spray" can also be visualized to confirm ureter patency preoperatively.

At the time of this writing, the data on these sonographic findings among patients with GSUI and normal volunteers are still being compiled. However, we have found the technique to be reproducible, well tolerated, and free of distortion or movement artifact which can affect the accuracy of all measurements.

Determination of Residual Urine Volume

Residual urine volume can also be calculated using the formula for an ellipsoid body. Measurement of bladder dimensions can be obtained from transverse and longitudinal images determining the height, breadth, and length, respectively:

$$\text{Volume} = \tfrac{4}{3} \times \text{II} \times r1 \times r2 \times r3$$
$$r1 = \text{Breadth}/2 \quad r2 = \text{Height}/2 \quad r3 = \text{Length}/2$$

The correlation between the calculated volume and catheterized residual urine has been reported to be 98%.[18] Although single catheterization may seem relatively atraumatic, avoiding this invasive procedure is appreciated, especially in pediatric patients.

Evaluation of Neuromuscular Bladder Dysfunction

Ultrasound has also proven valuable in the evaluation of the urinary tract in neuromuscular bladder dysfunction. Brandt and colleagues,[19] in a study of 36 spinal cord injury (SCI) patients, found that ultrasound evaluation of the bladder yielded significantly more diagnostic information than radiography in 27% of the patients.

Some of the disadvantages of a transrectal endoprobe in the neurologically intact patient do not apply to SCI

Box 7B-1
Sonographic Parameters in the Evaluation of Stress Incontinence

1. Location at rest of the urethrovesical junction in relationship to posterior-superior aspect of the symphysis.
2. Mobility of urethrovesical junction during Valsalva maneuver.
   a. Absolute distance
   b. X and Y displacement
3. Location of urethral egress compared to most dependent aspect of bladder.
4. Ability to elevate urethrovesical junction on "squeeze" maneuver.
5. Presence of proximal urethral opening on Valsalva maneuver in absence of detrusor contraction ("funneling").

patients. Many of them are accustomed to voiding in a supine position and most have lost sensation from the anus and rectum, making them unaware of the rectal probe.[20] Brandt and colleagues[19] demonstrated bladder trabeculation as well as dilated ureters in neuromuscular dysfunction using transabdominal sonography. Urethrovesical reflex in pediatric patients has also been demonstrated using transabdominal sonography.[21] Using all of the sonographic techniques available may entirely eliminate the indications for radiographic voiding cystourethrography in the evaluation of neuromuscular dysfunction of the bladder.

Evaluation of Urethral Diverticulum

We have found ultrasound to be valuable in evaluating urethral diverticulum (Fig. 7B-4). The often complex three-dimensional aspects of diverticula are difficult to appreciate during urethroscopy, yet are easily readable during introital or vaginal scanning. The occasional bladder stone that may form on a poorly placed suspension suture during a needle urethropexy can also be easily diagnosed sonographically.

EVALUATION OF ANAL INCONTINENCE

Interest in anorectal and pelvic floor dysfunction as a cause of bowel related symptoms is increasing, especially among urogynecologists dedicated to approaching the female pelvis as a complete entity including anorectal disorders. However, the pathophysiologic mechanisms involved in these disorders, including fecal incontinence, are still only partially understood. Current knowledge is largely based on investigational studies such as defecography, anal manometry, and anal electromyography. These techniques provide information about anosphincteric, puborectalis, levator ani muscle, and rectal wall function; all of these contribute to normal bowel storage and emptying.[22]

The physiologic mechanisms of fecal continence are complex. However, two basic muscular mechanisms have been described which are important in maintaining continence. The external anal sphincter squeezes the anal canal, lengthening it and increasing its resistance. The puborectalis draws the distal rectum forward, creating a flap-valve effect preventing the transmission of intraabdominal pressure directly into the anal canal.[1] Although controversy exists regarding the relative importance of these two functions, both are routinely measured during evaluation of fecal incontinence, providing insight into the pathophysiology of this condition.

Anal sphincteric function is commonly measured by anal manometry, whereas puborectalis function is indirectly assessed by measuring the anorectal angle during defecography. Although the clinical relevance of anorectal angle measurement continues to be debated, the discrepancies in the literature may be a result of lack of standardization of the technique and evaluation.[23] As such, the true predictive value of the anorectal angle measurement remains to be determined, yet its present interpretation of representing puborectalis, and perhaps the remaining levator ani musculature, appears a valid contribution to fecal continence studies.

Both anal sphincteric function and determination of the anorectal angle can be readily performed with the use of ultrasound and a Lahr balloon. Sonographic sphincterography is performed using a transducer, either a vaginal endoprobe or a curved linear-array transducer, specifically placed on the perineum to visualize a cylindrical balloon within the anal canal and rectum. The deflated balloon connected by a hose to a fluid reservoir is placed into the anal canal and inflated by raising the fluid reservoir in increments. The investigator can see whether the balloon is expanded or collapsed at any given pressure as calculated by the height of the fluid bag above the level of the patient's anal canal. The highest pressure at which the patient's sphincter muscle, upon instruction, can collapse the balloon is the maximum squeeze pressure attributed to predominantly external sphincteric function. The low-

Fig. 7B-4 Ultrasound view (upright orientation) of filled urethral diverticulum posterior to mid-urethra.

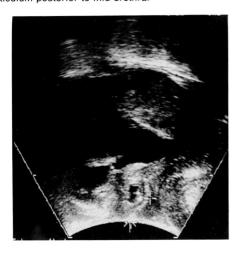

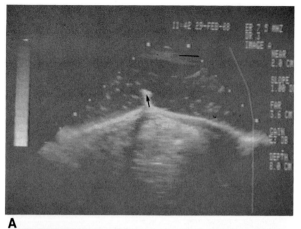

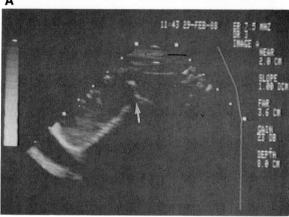

Fig. 7B-5 Anorectal ultrasound. **A** "Resting angle" with balloon in anal canal and rectum, and **B** "squeezing angle" of anorectum can be determined. Arrow indicates level of puborectalis sling.

(mean rest angle = 151.3 + 20.7, squeeze angle = 124.2 + 11.0). This information is helpful when contemplating performing a retrorectal levatoplasty (posterior anal repair) to restore the anorectal angle in incontinent patients. Also, since ultrasound does not expose the patient to radiation, rest and contract angle measurements can be repeated until the examiner is satisfied the results are truly representative. This "in-office" technique allows an objective assessment and continued evaluation without the cost, inconvenience, and radiation exposure of radiographic studies.

SUMMARY

Since the introduction of ultrasound as a diagnostic tool for stress incontinence nearly 10 years ago, technologic progress has resulted in continued improvements in resolution as well as in transducers capable of various scanning angles that are easier to handle. These developments allow improved definition of the pelvic soft tissue details.

Sonographic evaluation, as always, offers several advantages over conventional radiographic studies, including avoiding radiation, lower cost, and minimal (if any) discomfort. Not only has ultrasound proven useful as an adjunctive diagnostic tool, but it provides a method for objective postsurgery evaluation that can be performed in the office with equipment that is commonplace in obstetrics and gynecology. Perhaps most importantly, because of its safety, ultrasound studies are dynamic and can be repeated until the examiner has confidence in the accuracy of his technique and that the images produced are free of artifact and truly represent the functional anatomy.

At present, ultrasound evaluation of the female pelvic floor does not appear to provide conclusive and discriminatory diagnostic information, but does supply complementary data to be used in conjunction with other well-established tests. Given ultrasound's rapid evolution to date, along with continued refinements in laboratory technique and advancing technology, ultrasound holds even greater promise for the future. Ultrasound is a safe, reliable, convenient, and economical tool for diagnostic evaluation of the lower urinary tract and various pelvic floor disorders.

est balloon pressure at which the balloon expands within the resting anal canal is the basal or opening pressure. The contour of the flexible balloon within the anal canal and rectum can be visualized and a sonographically measured anorectal angle can be determined. The anorectal angle can be observed during relaxation "resting angle" (Fig. 7B-5A) and during voluntary contraction "squeeze angle" (Fig. 7B-5B). In several studies an increased anorectal angle was found in patients with fecal incontinence.[24,25] Similar findings were reported using ultrasound to evaluate anorectal angles and puborectalis function. Using this sonographic technique, Pittman and Benson[26] compared 10 asymptomatic women to six women with complete incontinence to solid stools. The asymptomatic women were found to have a significantly more acute anorectal angle at rest (mean rest angle = 113.5 + 10.6) and during voluntary contraction (squeeze angle = 94.5 + 11.7) than did women with incontinence to solid feces

REFERENCES

1. Abrams P, Blaivas JG, Stanton SL, et al. The standardization of terminology of lower urinary tract function. *Scand J Urol Nephrol.* 1988;114(suppl):5.

2. DeLancey JOL. Structural aspects of the extrinsic continence mechanism. *Obstet Gynecol.* 1988;72:296.

3. Walters MD, Shields LE. The diagnostic value of history, physical examination, and the Q-tip cotton swab test in women with urinary incontinence. *Am J Obstet Gynecol.* 1988;159:145.

4. Holmes JH, Hinman F Jr, eds. *Ultrasonic Studies of Bladder Filling and Contour in Hydrodynamics of Micturition.* Springfield, Ill: Charles C Thomas: 1971;303.

5. White RD, McQuown D, McCarthy TA, Ostegard, DR. Real time ultrasonography in evaluation of urinary stress incontinence. *Am J Obstet Gynecol.* 1980;138:235.

6. Nishizawa O, Harada T, Takada H, et al. A new synchronous video urodynamics. *Tohuku J Med.* 1982;136:349.

7. Shappeero L, Friedland G, Perkash I. Transrectal sonographic voiding cystourethrography: studies in neuromuscular bladder dysfunction. *AJR.* 1983;141:83–90.

8. Brown MC, Sutherest JR, Murray A, et al. Potential use of ultrasound in place of x-ray fluoroscopy in urodynamics. *Br J Urol.* 1985;57:88.

9. Bergman A, Ballard CA, Platt LD. Ultrasonic evaluation of urethrovesical junction in women with stress urinary incontinence. *Obstet Gynecol.* 1986;68:269.

10. Kohorn E, Scioscia A, Gentry P, Habbins J. Ultrasound cystourethrography by perineal scanning for assessment of female stress urinary incontinence. *Obstet Gynecol.* 1986;68:269.

11. Gordon D, Pearce M, Norton P, Stanton S. Comparison of ultrasound and lateral chain urethrocystography in the determination of bladder neck descent. *Am J Obstet Gynecol.* 1989;160:182.

12. Kölbl H, Bernaschek G, Wolf G. A comparative study of perineal ultrasound scanning and urethrocystography in patients with genuine stress incontinence. *Arch Gynecol Obstet.* 1988;244:39.

13. Green TH. Development of a plan for diagnosis and treatment of urinary stress incontinence. *Am J Obstet Gynecol.* 1962;83:632.

14. Benson JT, Sumners J. Ultrasound evaluation of female urinary incontinence. *Inter Urogyn J.* 1990;1:7–11.

15. Hodgkinson CP. Stress urinary incontinence. *Am J Obstet Gynecol.* 1970;108:1141.

16. Quinn, MJ, Beynon J, McMortensen NUJ, Smith PJB. Transvaginal endosonograph: a new method to study the anatomy of the lower urinary tract in urinary stress incontinence. *Br J Urol.* 1988;62:414.

17. Koelbl H, Bernaschek G. A new method for sonographic urethrocystography and simultaneous press-flow measurements. *Am J Obstet Gynecol.* 1989;74:417.

18. Roehrborn CG, Peters PC. Can transabdominal ultrasound estimation of post-voiding residual (PVR) replace catheterization? *Urology.* 1988;31:445.

19. Brandt TD, Harrey N, Calenoff L, Greenberg M, Kaplan P, Nanninga J. Ultrasound evaluation of the urinary system in spinalchord injury patients. *Radiology.* 1981;141:473.

20. Fellow GJ. Dynamic ultrasonography for voiding dysfunction. *Urol Clin North Am.* 1989;16:809.

21. Kessler RM, Altman DH. Real-time sonographic detection of vesicoureteral reflex in children. *AJR.* 1982;141:473.

22. Felt-Bersman RF, Luth WJ, Janssen JJWM, Meuwissen SM. Defecography in patients with anorectal disorders: which findings are clinically relevant? *Dis Colon Rectum.* 1990;33:277.

23. Shorvon PJ, McHugh S, Diamant NE, Somers S, Stevenson GW. Defecography in normal volunteers; results and implications. *Gut.* 1989;30:1737.

24. Kuypers HC, Strijk SP. Diagnosis of disturbances of continence and defecation. *Dis Colon Rectum.* 1984;27:658.

25. Skomorovski E, Henrichsen S, Christiansen J, Hegedus V. Video-defecography combined with measurement of the anorectal angle and of perineal descent. *Acta Radiol.* 1987;28:559.

26. Pittman S, Benson JT. Physiologic evaluation of the anorectum, a new ultrasound technique. *Dis Colon Rectum.* 1990;33:676.

CHAPTER 8

Manometric Investigation

8A   Urodynamics

Mickey M. Karram

INTRODUCTION

Urodynamic studies have become an integral part of the evaluation of female patients with lower urinary tract dysfunction. Unfortunately a flurry of new equipment, diagnostic procedures, and complicated testing have bewildered the clinician.[1] It has become exceedingly difficult to decide what tests are necessary to adequately evaluate patients and plan various treatment options. This is further complicated by the lack of standardized technique and terminology. The purpose of this chapter is to define certain urodynamic modalities used in the evaluation of the storage and evacuation of urine, so that there is a clear understanding of the rationale, technique, utility, and limitations of each test.

HISTORY

Urodynamic techniques date back to 1872 when Schatz accidentally discovered a crude technique for measuring bladder pressure while trying to record intra-abdominal pressure. Shortly thereafter, Dubois[2] studied the effects of changes in position on intravesical and intrarectal pressure and observed that the desire to void was associated with contraction of the detrusor. The currently popular water cystometer was designed by Lewis in 1939.[3] The advent of air cystometry[4] and car-

bon dioxide cystometry[5] simplified the procedure even further.

Drake[6] is credited with describing one of the first clinically useful urinary flow meters in 1948. Drake's work was important because he clearly demonstrated the relationship between urinary flow rate and voided volume. Von Garretts,[7] in 1956, was the first to record instantaneous flow on a photokymograph as a function of time.

In 1923, Bonney[8] devised a crude method for determining urethral pressure by measuring the minimum pressure needed to force liquid into the urethra through a catheter. The current technique for measuring urethral pressure is derived from observations made by Lapides and coworkers[9] in 1960. One year later, Enhorning[10] recorded pressure at consecutive points along the urethra using a fluid filled balloon catheter, thus obtaining a urethral pressure profile. Refinements by numerous investigators,[11,12] most notably Brown and Wickham,[13] have led to the current use of very sophisticated microtip transducers.

DEFINITIONS, CLASSIFICATION, AND RECOMMENDATIONS

In 1973, the International Continence Society (ICS) established a committee for the standardization of terminology of lower urinary tract function.[14] This report has since been revised numerous times.[15–18] The most recent recommendations[19] of this committee state that although a complete urodynamic evaluation is not necessary in all patients, some clinical or urodynamic evaluation of the filling and voiding phases should be performed.

Detrusor activity is defined as normal or overactive. An overactive detrusor is termed an unstable bladder in the absence of a known neurologic abnormality and is termed detrusor hyperreflexia if an obvious neurologic lesion is present. Urge incontinence is the involuntary loss of urine associated with a strong desire to void (urgency). Motor urgency is secondary to an overactive detrusor, whereas sensory urgency is caused by hypersensitivity.

The urethral closure mechanism may be normal or incompetent. An incompetent urethral closure mechanism is defined as one that allows leakage of urine in the absence of a detrusor contraction. Leakage may occur when intravesical pressure exceeds intraurethral pressure (genuine stress incontinence) or when there is an involuntary fall in urethral pressure (unstable urethra).

Reflex incontinence is the loss of urine due to detrusor hyperreflexia and/or involuntary urethral relaxation in the absence of the sensation usually associated with the desire to micturate. This condition is only seen in patients with neuropathic bladder and urethral disorders. Overflow incontinence is any involuntary loss of urine associated with overdistention of the bladder.

During micturition the detrusor may be normal, acontractive, or underactive. Normal voiding is achieved by a voluntary initiated detrusor contraction that is sustained and can usually be suppressed voluntarily. The acontractile detrusor is one that cannot be demonstrated to contract during urodynamic studies. Detrusor areflexia is defined as acontractility caused by an abnormality of nervous control and denotes the complete absence of a centrally coordinated contraction. Detrusor underactivity is defined as a detrusor contraction of inadequate magnitude and/or duration to effect bladder emptying within a normal time span. Some patients may have detrusor underactivity during voiding and detrusor overactivity during filling. The use of terms such as atonic, hypotonic, autonomic, and flaccid should be avoided.

CYSTOMETRY

Cystometry is the main method used for investigation of bladder storage function. It is a urodynamic test in which the pressure and volume relationship of the blad-

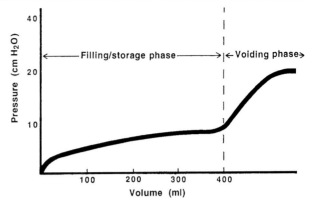

Fig. 8A-1   Normal cystometrogram showing filling and voiding phases.

der is measured (Fig. 8A-1). Cystometry is used to assess detrusor activity, sensation, capacity, and compliance. The evaluation of each factor has different implications and before any definitive conclusions can be reached, findings must be examined in the light of associated manifestations and clinical findings. A normal bladder has the power of accommodation; it can maintain an almost constant intravesical pressure throughout its filling phase regardless of volume.

The basic principle of cystometry is the simple coupling of a manometer to the inside of the bladder. A filling media is instilled into the bladder and as it fills, intravesical pressure is plotted against volume. The testing apparatus can range from simple single channel methods which can be accomplished manually or electronically, to complex methods combining electronic measurements of bladder, abdominal, and urethral pressure along with electromyography and fluoroscopy (Fig. 8A-2).

Fig. 8A-2   Sophisticated urodynamic laboratory required for multichannel studies.

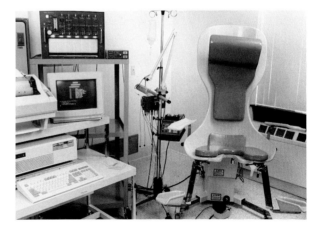

A normal cystometrogram shows an initial rise in pressure to achieve resting bladder pressure which is usually between 2 to 8 cm/H_2O. The normal adult female will experience an urge to void at 200 to 300 ml with a maximum capacity at 400 to 700 ml. Within this capacity, bladder pressure should not rise above 15 cm/H_2O, with a mean rise being 6 cm/H_2O (Fig. 8A-1).

Technique of Cystometry

Despite the widespread use of cystometry, the optimal technique for performing this test is controversial. Questions remain regarding the position of the patient, antegrade versus retrograde filling of the bladder, optimal distention medium, the temperature of the medium, the rate of filling, as well as indications for electronically subtracted cystometry.[20–24]

The commonly used infusion media for cystometry include water, carbon dioxide, and radiographic contrast material. Although the numeric values of cystometric parameters between carbon dioxide and water differ, there has not been shown to be a qualitative difference with regards to the information obtained.[20] Carbon dioxide offers the advantage of speed, convenience, and simplicity because it can be instilled at rates up to 300 ml/min.[25,26] However, there are several drawbacks to using carbon dioxide. Since it is an odorless, colorless gas, it can very easily leak through the tubing of the urethra resulting in artifactual data. Further, inaccuracies may result from the inherent compressibility of the gas and the fact that it is often irritating to the bladder mucosa. These factors combine to cause cystometric parameters to occur at smaller volumes when carbon dioxide is used. Water offers the advantage of being more physiologic than carbon dioxide. Leakage from the urethra can be easily visualized and the cystometric evaluation can be followed by a voiding study.[27]

The rate of filling of the infusion media must also be taken into consideration. The ICS has attempted to standardize filling rates by describing 3 ranges. Slow fill is less than 10 ml per minute, medium fill is 10 ml to 100 ml per minute, and fast fill is greater than 100 ml per minute. Patients with normal lower urinary tract function can tolerate most fast fill rates. The effect of filling rate on an unstable bladder is still poorly understood but fast fill methods appear to be more effective in provoking detrusor overactivity.[28] Despite this, most investigators fill the bladder at medium fill rates.

Currently it appears that the most sensitive testing position is standing.[29,30] Most urodynamic labs fill the bladder with the patient in the sitting position and then if an abnormality is strongly suspected and has not been demonstrated on sitting, the patient is asked to stand and perform various provocative maneuvers. Provocative or detrusor activating features should be used to enhance the sensitivity of cystometrics. These maneuvers are designed to reproduce the usual symptoms that the patient experiences and include coughing, straining, heel bouncing, and hearing or feeling running water. Supine cystometry is the least sensitive of all methods and may miss up to 50% of women with detrusor instability or hyperreflexia.[29,30]

A variety of catheters are used for these studies. Simple or manual cystometry can be performed with a urethral Foley catheter while electronically monitored studies require more sophisticated balloon or microtip catheters. Water filled balloon catheters or water perfusion catheters have been used with moderate success. These catheters are inexpensive, disposable, and relatively easy to use. More sophisticated laboratories, however, use sensitive microtip catheters.[31] These are available with one to six microtransducers on the catheter. They are somewhat expensive and require replacement after approximately 100 studies even with careful maintenance. The advantages of these catheters are that they are small in size, flexible, and can accurately measure rapid changes in pressure variations seen during repetitive coughing or Valsalva maneuver. They are limited by fragility and rotational artifacts (Fig. 8A-3).

Fig. 8A-3 Two microtip catheters. Note one catheter has a single microtransducer and is used for estimating abdominal pressure, while the other catheter has two microtransducers approximately 6 cm apart used to measure intravesical and intraurethral pressure. This catheter also contains a distal filling port.

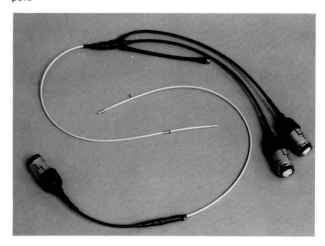

Although antegrade filling of the bladder has been used, most laboratories use retrograde filling with the distention medium at room temperature.

Single vs Multichannel Cystometry

"Eyeball" or "poor man's" urodynamics is a type of manual single channel cystometry that can be performed without any special equipment or expertise. With the patient in a dorsal lithotomy position, a Foley catheter is placed. A 50 ml syringe without its piston or bulb is attached to the catheter and held above the bladder. The patient is then asked to stand and the bladder is filled by gravity by pouring 60 ml aliquots of sterile water into the syringe (Fig. 8A-4). The patient's first sensation, urge to void, and maximum capacity is noted. The water level in the syringe should be closely observed during filling as any rise in the column of water can be secondary to a detrusor contraction. Unintended increases in intraabdominal pressure should be avoided. The catheter is then removed and a stress test is performed in which the patient is asked to cough in a standing position. If visual loss of a small amount of urine occurs simultaneous with the cough, this is very suggestive of genuine stress incontinence. If a gush of urine occurs a few seconds after the cough, this is more suggestive of an unstable bladder. Interpretation of single-channel cystometry can, at times, be difficult because of artifact introduced by rises in intraabdominal pressure caused by straining or patient movement. Borderline or negative tests should be repeated to maximize their negative predictive value.

While single-channel electronic cystometers are commercially available,[1] in the author's opinion, they offer no distinct advantage over a carefully performed "eyeball" cystometrogram. The only real advantage of electronically measuring pressure devices is their ability to simultaneously measure and record pressures from various anatomic sites, thus obtaining subtracted pressures of importance.

Multichannel or subtracted cystometry relies on the measurement of abdominal as well as intravesical pressure, making one able to distinguish events that are secondary to rises in intraabdominal pressure versus those secondary to true changes in intravesical pressure.[32–34] Abdominal pressure can be measured either via transrectal or transvaginal catheters.[35,36] We prefer vaginally placed catheters as they are easier to clean and maintain and measurements are not cluttered by rectal peristalsis. Subtraction of intraabdominal pressure from intravesical pressure allows for the calculation of

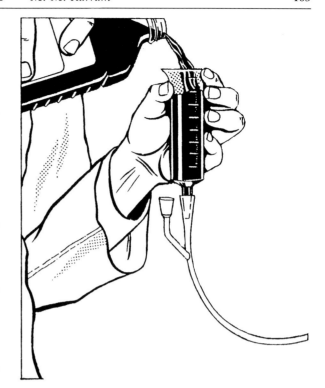

Fig. 8A-4 "Eyeball" or "poor man's" cystometry.

true detrusor pressure. Subtracted cystometry may be enhanced further by additional measurement of urethral pressure. This allows for the calculation of the urethral closure pressure, which is the difference between the urethral and bladder pressure (Fig. 8A-5). When this is performed, the urodynamicist may gain further insight into bladder and urethral function during both the storing and voiding phases.

These studies are usually performed with the patient in a sitting position on a birthing chair (Fig. 8A-2). The catheters are placed such that abdominal, vesical, and maximum urethral pressure (midurethra) are simultaneously measured. Before starting to fill, residual urine should be measured. The bladder is then mechanically filled at a constant rate. The first sensation of filling as well as the volume at first desire to void are recorded. Maximum cystometric capacity is the volume at which the patient has a strong desire to void. Effective cystometric capacity is the maximum cystometric capacity minus the residual urine.

If no detrusor instability is demonstrated during passive bladder filling, the previously mentioned detrusor provoking maneuvers should be employed (Fig. 8A-6). If, despite these maneuvers, the patient continues to

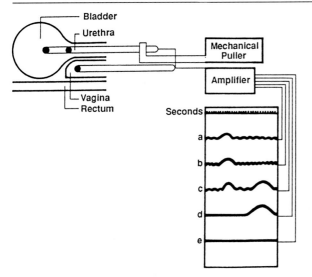

Fig. 8A-5 Simultaneous measure of intravesical, intraurethral, and intraabdominal pressures with mechanical calculation of true detrusor and urethral closure pressure. *a* = intraabdominal pressure; *b* = intravesical pressure; *c* = intraurethral pressure; *d* = urethral closure pressure; *e* = true detrusor pressure.

Fig. 8A-6 Urodynamic tracing showing cough-provoked bladder instability.

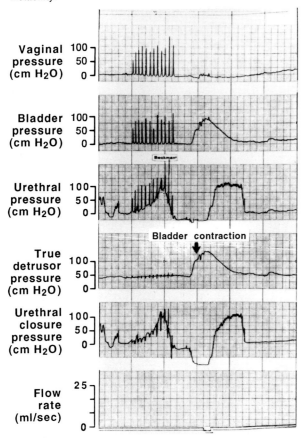

Continent   Stress incontinence

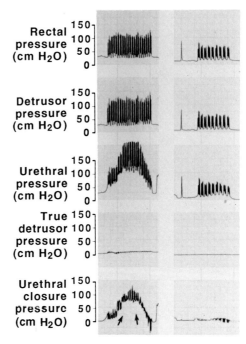

Fig. 8A-7 Dynamic urethral pressure profile in a continent female and in a patient with genuine stress incontinence. Note the differences in the pressure transmission ratio. Arrows indicate positive pressure transmission.

demonstrate bladder stability, yet is strongly suspected of having an unstable bladder, the patient can be restudied with erect cystometry and provocative maneuvers 15 to 30 minutes following the subcutaneous injection of 2.5 mg of bethanechol. This should not significantly alter the activity of the normal detrusor, but it may unmask an occult unstable one.[37-39]

If the patient demonstrates visual loss of urine simultaneous with coughing or straining in the absence of a detrusor contraction and no detrusor or urethral instability is demonstrated during the rest of the test, the patient has the urodynamic condition of genuine stress incontinence (Fig. 8A-7). If she has urine loss due to a nonsuppressible detrusor contraction in the absence of stress incontinence, then she has pure detrusor instability. If urodynamic criteria for both conditions are met, the patient has mixed incontinence (Fig. 8A-8). Up to 30% of patients with genuine stress incontinence will have coexistent detrusor instability.[40-43]

The evaluation of bladder sensation has been described by Bradley, Timm, and Scott.[43] The bladder is

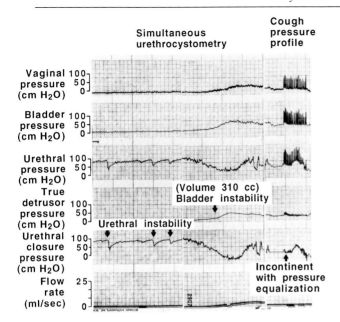

Vaginal pressure (cm H$_2$O)
Bladder pressure (cm H$_2$O)
Urethral pressure (cm H$_2$O)
True detrusor pressure (cm H$_2$O)
Urethral closure pressure (cm H$_2$O)
Flow rate (ml/sec)

Simultaneous urethrocystometry · Cough pressure profile

(Volume 310 cc) Bladder instability

Urethral instability

Incontinent with pressure equalization

Fig. 8A-8 Urethrocystometry and dynamic urethral cough pressure profile (CPP) in a patient with a combination of urethral and bladder instability as well as genuine stress incontinence.

Box 8A-1
Disorders Resulting in Abnormal Bladder Capacity

Increased bladder capacity
  Sensory neuropathy
  Chronic obstruction
  Lower motor neuron lesion

Reduced bladder capacity
  Urinary tract infection
  Bladder instability
  Upper motor neuron lesion
  Genuine stress incontinence
  Bladder contraction due to fibrosis
    (interstitial cystitis, tuberculosis)
  Enuresis

---

capable of exteroception (touch, pain, temperature) and proprioception (stretch). Bladder sensation may be decreased or increased. Decreased sensation is usually regarded as neuropathic (e.g., diabetes, tabes dorsalis, cauda equina lesions); however, extremes of increased and decreased sensation are more common in clinical practice. Hypersensitive bladders that are not associated with a rise in detrusor pressure are common in females, and many cannot be explained by infection or an infiltrative process (sensory urgency). With cystometry these patients can be divided into two groups: those who can be distracted from their symptoms and tolerate a normal bladder capacity, and those who cannot. The former group may respond to psychosomatic therapy; the latter do not.[44]

There are various neurologic and nonneurologic conditions that result in abnormalities in bladder capacity with or without significant changes in detrusor pressure. These conditions are listed in Box 8A-1.

Indications for single channel or "eyeball" cystometry versus subtracted or multichannel cystometry have been debated extensively[45]; however, very few comparisons exist in the literature. One study by Ouslander and coworkers[46] reported a sensitivity of 75% in patients undergoing supine simple cystometry when compared

to multichannel testing in a geriatric population. Sutherst and Brown[45] compared single channel and multichannel urodynamics in a blind cross-over study of 100 incontinent women. They noted single-channel cystometry to be 100% sensitive and 89% specific compared to multichannel studies. Multichannel cystometry has a higher sensitivity for picking up low pressure detrusor contractions, sometimes termed subthreshold instability. This has been defined as a rise in detrusor pressure less than 15 cm/H$_2$O which results in either symptoms or urinary leakage.[47] Multichannel techniques definitely improve the specificity of cystometry by avoiding false positives created by increases in abdominal pressure. Whether the cost of multichannel testing is justified depends on therapeutic options and risks to the population studied. Box 8A-2 lists the author's indications for multichannel testing.

Most urodynamicists view multichannel cystourethrometry as the gold standard by which the accuracy of other tests are compared, but it is not a perfect test. Ambulatory monitoring studies have shown that the pick-up rate of diagnosis of an unstable or hyperreflexic bladder can be further increased when patients are placed on continuous outpatient monitoring.[48,49] In one study the diagnosis, based on multichannel urodynamics, was significantly revised in 60% of patients after continuous monitoring was performed.[49]

URINARY FLOW RATE

Since urinary flow rate is the product of detrusor action against outlet resistance, a variation from the

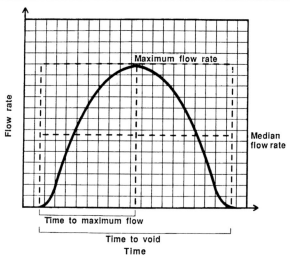

Fig. 8A-10 Graphic representation of normal uroflow curve.

Box 8A-2
Indications for Multichannel Urodynamics

1. Complicated history.
2. Single channel studies are inconclusive.
3. Recurrent urinary loss after previous surgery for stress incontinence.
4. Voiding dysfunction in the absence of significant pelvic relaxation.
5. Urgency/frequency in the absence of cystitis.
6. Lower urinary tract dysfunction following pelvic radiation or radical pelvic surgery.
7. Nocturnal enuresis.
8. Urge incontinence not responsive to therapy.
9. Neurologic disorders.
10. Continuous leakage.

---

normal flow rate may reflect dysfunction of either. Flow rate is defined as the volume of fluid expelled via the urethra per unit time and is expressed in milliliters per second.

Simple uroflowmetry is performed by asking the patient to void into a special commode; urine is funneled into a flow meter which records volume versus time (Fig. 8A-9). Every effort should be made to allow

Fig. 8A-9 Instrumentation for spontaneous uroflowmetry.

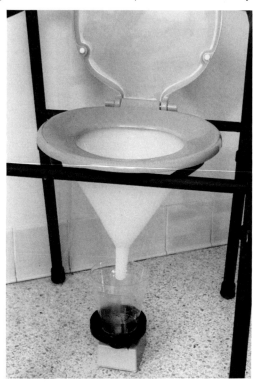

the patient to void in private to diminish the possibility of a psychological inhibition so common in a laboratory setting. The following parameters can be obtained during a uroflowmetric evaluation:

1. The flow rate, that is, the volume of urine passed in ml/sec.
2. Maximum flow rate.
3. Total flow time.
4. Total volume voided.
5. Average flow rate.
6. Post-void residual.

Normal values include a maximum flow of approximately 25 mm/sec recorded in about 5 seconds, normally appearing on a graph as a single, smooth curve over 15 to 20 seconds (Fig. 8A-10). In normal micturition the flow curve should rise steeply and the length of time to maximum flow should be less than one third of the total voiding time. Maximum flow depends on age, voided volume, and position. It has been empirically stated that maximum flow rates of less than 15 mm/sec for voided volumes greater than 200 ml are indicative of an abnormally reduced flow. However, since flow rate is determined by the relationship between detrusor force and urethral resistance, and since these may vary considerably and still produce adequate bladder emptying, there can be no precise definition of a normal or a low flow rate. What is clinically relevant is that borderline flow rates require further urodynamic assessment.[50-52]

Curve patterns refer to the configuration of the uroflowmetric curve. Continuous flow is usually consid-

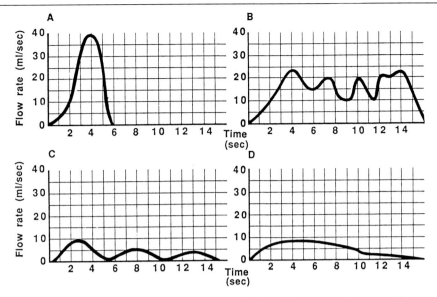

Fig. 8A-11 Graphic representation of various uroflow patterns. **A,** Superflow commonly seen with poor urethral resistance. **B,** Interrupted pattern due to intermittent sphincter activity. **C,** Interrupted stream during straining to void. **D,** Abnormal flow rate characteristic of detrusor outlet obstruction.

ered the normal pattern. The curve is considered intermittent when the flow rate drops and subsequently increases. Multiple peak pattern is used to describe a downward deflection of the flow rate that does not reach 2 ml/sec or less[51] (Fig. 8A-11).

Abnormal uroflowmetric curves can be seen anytime there are factors present that could potentially affect detrusor contractility and/or urethral resistance. Detrusor contractility can be potentially affected by neuropathic lesions, pharmacologic manipulation, intrinsic muscle dysfunction, or psychogenic inhibition. Urethral resistance can be impaired by tissue trophic changes producing atrophy or fibrosis, drug effects such as alpha-adrenergic stimulation, striated muscle contraction secondary to pain or fear, or urethral axis distortion secondary to pelvic relaxation. Detrusor external sphincter dyssynergia is a condition in which there is lack of synergism between the detrusor muscle and the external striated sphincter and can lead to an obstructive syndrome.[53,54]

Residual urine is the volume of urine remaining in the bladder immediately after the completion of micturition. This can be measured by catheterization, ultrasound, or radioisotope methods. What constitutes a significant residual is not universally established, but its absence does indicate efficient voiding.

Uroflowmetry is a simple screening technique to objectively document voiding dysfunction. A normal flow rate in females does not necessarily indicate a normal

voiding mechanism. For example, some women may have normal flow rates in the absence of any detrusor contraction if sphincteric relaxation is assisted by an increase in intraabdominal pressure from straining. To define voiding mechanisms and objectively establish the basis of a patient's voiding dysfunction, more complex pressure flow studies must be performed.[32,33,52,55] These involve the monitoring of abdominal, intravesical, and detrusor pressures synchronously with the flow rate (Fig. 8A-12). The specific parameters and ICS-

Fig. 8A-12 Technique for performing pressure/flow studies. The patient must be able to void around catheters.

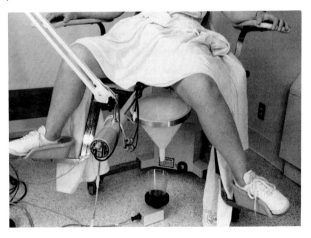

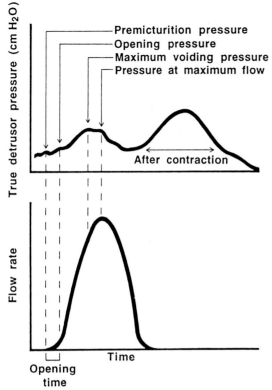

Fig. 8A-13 International Continence Society terminology and specific parameters for pressure/flow studies.

recommended terms are shown in Fig. 8A-13. Urethral pressure can also be monitored to assure there is complete urethral relaxation during the voiding mechanism. Several attempts have been made to integrate the parameters of pressure-flow studies into a single factor. However, these factors are based on models which do not take into account the urethral shape, distensibility, and voided volume.

Depending on age, menopausal status, voided volume, and presence or absence of lower urinary tract dysfunction, females can void by any combination of detrusor contraction, abdominal straining, and urethral relaxation[52] (Table 8A-1) (Fig. 8A-14). In females who void in the absence of a detrusor contraction, it is im-

Table 8A-1

Potential Voiding Mechanisms on
Pressure/Flow Studies

Urethral Relaxation	Bladder Contraction	Abdominal Straining
1. Present	Absent	Absent
2. Present	Present	Absent
3. Present	Absent	Present
4. Present	Present	Present

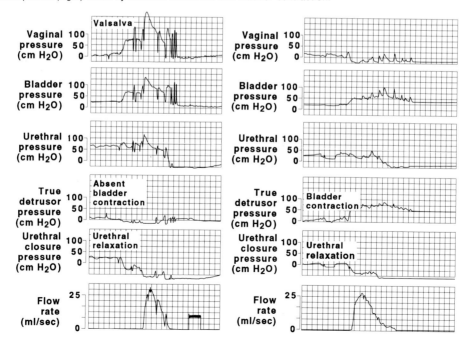

Fig. 8A-14 Voiding mechanisms in two patients. Note the first patient *(left)* voids by urethral relaxation and Valsalva maneuver whereas the second patient *(right)* voids by urethral relaxation and bladder contraction.

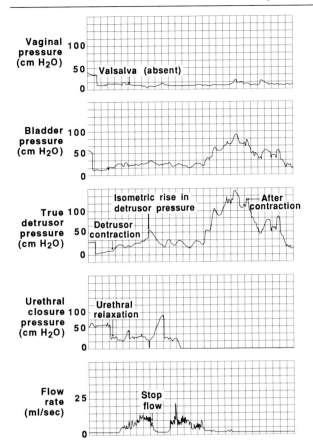

Fig. 8A-15   Pressure/flow study with "stop test." Note isometric rise in detrusor pressure simultaneous with stoppage of flow.

portant to perform a "stop test,"[56] as this is the only method of diagnosing an acontractile detrusor. To perform this test, urine flow must be suddenly interrupted on command by closing the urethra. Some women are only able to achieve cessation of flow by inhibition of the detrusor, which takes several seconds. When the urethra can be closed voluntarily, the detrusor contraction becomes isovolumetric and increases to a maximum (Fig. 8A-15). If the patient cannot interrupt her own stream, it may be necessary to physically occlude the urethra via a catheter or elevation of anterior vaginal wall.

The main clinical use of pressure flow studies is to document the mechanism of abnormal voiding. If the patient has symptoms and signs of abnormal voiding with low flow rates and voids with a high detrusor pressure, she is probably voiding against an obstruction. On the other hand, if a patient has low flow rates and voids with minimal or no rise in detrusor pressure, then her voiding dysfunction is probably secondary to an acontractile or underactive detrusor. Also, patients with absent or small detrusor contractions are at higher risk for retention problems following antiincontinence surgery.[50,57]

Video-Pressure Flow Studies

The combination of the previously described individual tests with radiographic techniques has made it possible to study both the filling and voiding functions of the bladder and urethra under direct fluoroscopic vision. This method of evaluation has been employed much more frequently in Europe than in the United States.[58]

These tests are performed by infusing radiographic contrast material for cystometry. Urodynamic parameters are transduced and displayed on a storage oscilloscope. A television camera scans the oscilloscope screen and the resulting image is displayed on a television monitor. The fluoroscope image of the bladder and urethra is electronically mixed with that of the urodynamic data and displayed on the same monitor.

Commonly cited advantages of video studies include the consolidation of multiple evaluation modalities into one examination, providing information regarding anatomy and function of the lower urinary tract under various provocative conditions. Descent of the bladder neck, milk back of urine from the urethra to the bladder, and bladder neck funnelling all may be visualized during the simultaneous recording of bladder, urethra, and abdominal pressure. Asymptomatic abnormalities such as urethral or bladder diverticulum also may be noted.[32,58] The major disadvantages of this modality are the radiation exposure (approximately 800 millirads), cost, technical expertise, and support necessary for its use.

URETHRAL PRESSURE STUDIES

The urethral pressure profile is a graphic recording of the pressure within the urethra at each point along its length. Contributing to normal urethral compliance and pressure are smooth and striated muscle activity, the fibroelastic component of the urethral wall, vascular tension due to the rich, spongy network around the urethra, and an extrinsic compression component secondary to the pelvic floor muscles.

These studies can be performed using balloon catheters in which one or more small balloons are mounted on the same catheter and transmit pressure by fluid filled lines to the transducer. With frequent and careful calibration to compensate for membrane characteristics, they are accurate and have a rapid response time. More recently microtip catheters have been used. These eliminate zero errors and facilitate measurement in different postures and under dynamic situations such as coughing. Other variables besides catheter types can include different infusions, perfusion rates, catheter sizes, catheter withdrawal rates, and tubing lengths. All of these must be taken into consideration during the interpretation of these studies.[59-61]

To perform a passive urethral pressure profile, the catheter is placed as previously described for urethrocystometry, except that the urethral transducer moves through the urethra rather than remaining stationary in the zone of maximum urethral pressure (Fig. 8A-5). The profile is recorded by withdrawing the urethral transducer with the microtip directed laterally[62] through the urethra at a constant speed, usually via a mechanical withdrawal device; however, this can also be performed manually. The pressure recorded by this transducer is charted on graph paper that is moving at the same speed as the catheter. If bladder pressure is recorded simultaneously, the urethral closure pressure can be calculated.

Recommended nomenclature for urethral pressure profiles was proposed by the ICS.[14-19] The most frequently measured parameters are: 1) the maximum urethral pressure which is the maximum pressure of the profile, 2) the maximum urethral closure pressure which is the difference between the maximum urethral pressure and the bladder pressure, and 3) the functional urethral length which is the length of the urethra along which the pressure exceeds the bladder pressure. Other parameters such as anatomic or total length and area underneath the profile can also be calculated (Fig. 8A-16).

Normal values will vary slightly between different techniques, tending to be higher with microtip transducers. It has been documented by Rud[63,64] that the mean urethral closure pressure shows a downward trend with age. His studies noted a mean urethral closure pressure of 90 cm/H_2O in females less than 25 and a mean pressure of 65 cm/H_2O in females greater than 64 years of age. The average functional urethral length is approximately 2.4 to 2.8 cm/H_2O and tends to increase up to 50 years of age with a decline thereafter. The menopause appeared to be a significant factor. There is no variation in any parameter during the menstrual cycle.

A normal urethral pressure profile is usually symmetric but it is not uncommon to see vascular pulsations, as

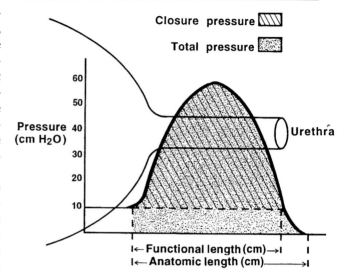

Fig. 8A-16 Graphic representation of urethral pressure profile.

blood pressure accounts for approximately one third of the urethral closure pressure. Rarely, a twin peak profile can be seen and this may be associated with previous bladder neck surgery or urethral diverticulum.[65]

The diagnostic value of static urethral pressure profilometry is limited because it is a study that is carried out during rest. Although certain trends are noted in patients with lower urinary tract dysfunction, there is so much overlap with normal patients that these trends cannot be used as reliable diagnostic indicators.[66] One potential benefit of measuring maximum urethral closure pressure in stress incontinent patients may be in the diagnosis of what has been termed the "low pressure urethra."[67,68] This is further discussed under stress incontinence.

The diagnostic yield of profilometry can be increased by the addition of dynamic factors such as Valsalva maneuvers, voluntary squeeze, and most commonly, coughing. These studies are performed by asking the patient to cough with maximum effort as the catheter is withdrawn through the urethra. Profiles may be performed by continuous or incremental withdrawl with maximum coughs at regular intervals throughout the functional length of the urethra. It is also important that the recorder be set so that the entire amplitude of each cough spike in the bladder and urethra is captured on the recording paper. These studies are best performed with microtip catheters rather than balloon catheters.[69,70]

In normal continent women, the proximal portion of

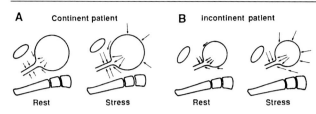

Fig. 8A-17 **A,** Graphic representation of pressure transmission to bladder and urethra in a continent female, and **B,** a female with genuine stress incontinence.

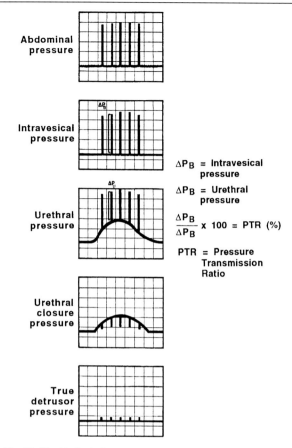

ΔP_B = Intravesical pressure

ΔP_B = Urethral pressure

$\dfrac{\Delta P_B}{\Delta P_B}$ x 100 = PTR (%)

PTR = Pressure Transmission Ratio

Fig. 8A-18 Method of calculation of pressure transmission ratio during cough pressure profile.

the urethra is located above the level of the urogenital diaphragm. This means that the bladder and the major portion of the sphincteric mechanism are above the lower anatomic limit of the abdominal cavity. In this location the bladder and proximal urethra are subject to equal transmission of rapid increases in intraabdominal pressure (Fig. 8A-17). Thus the urethral closure pressure is unchanged and urine remains in the bladder.

The pressure transmission ratio from an individual cough is calculated by dividing the amplitude of the urethral pressure spike by the amplitude of the corresponding bladder pressure spike and multiplying the quotient by 100 (Fig. 8A-18). By definition which follows from Enhorning's principle, genuine stress incontinence occurs when the pressure in the bladder exceeds the maximum pressure in the urethra, thus producing a pressure transmission ratio of less than 100%.[71] In young, continent females with well-supported bladder necks, coughing or other provoking factors to increase intraabdominal pressure results in a sphincteric response of accentuation of urethral closure pressure. The ability of this sphincter to generate additional pressure occurs probably secondary to reflex mechanisms that become operative during increased intraabdominal pressure.[72,73]

Thus stress or dynamic urethral pressure profiles can be used to objectively demonstrate pressure equalization between the bladder and the urethra in the absence of a detrusor contraction, which then meets all the terms of the ICS definition of genuine stress incontinence (Fig. 8A-7). Also one can actually calculate the pressure transmission ratio, thus expressing the deficit in transmission between the urethra and the bladder in quantitative terms[73,74] (Fig. 8A-18). The clinical use of dynamic profiles remains controversial, as it has been shown by numerous investigators that much crossover exists between normal symptomatic females and those suffering from lower urinary tract dysfunction.[72–74]

OTHER TESTS COMMONLY PERFORMED IN CONJUNCTION WITH URODYNAMICS

Measurement of Bladder Neck Mobility

Most females with primary genuine stress incontinence respond favorably to surgeries aimed at elevating and stabilizing the proximal urethra in a high retropubic position. For this reason it is felt by many that the measurement of bladder neck descent during stress is important in the evaluation of the incontinent female.[75–78] Bladder neck descent can be measured by radiologic techniques, ultrasound techniques, or by the simple placement of a lubricated Q-tip to the level of the bladder neck and measuring the angle of deflection during straining using an orthopedic goniometer.[78] Although numerous investigators have stated that a straining angle of greater than 30 degrees indicates a "positive test,"[77] it is our opinion that these results are best reported by actually stating the maximum straining angle.[78] It must be continually reemphasized that measurement of bladder neck mobility is not diagnostic of lower urinary tract dysfunction. Its only purpose is to document this mobility prior to undertaking surgical procedures that are aimed at elevating and stabilizing the bladder neck.

Cystourethroscopy

Endoscopy is commonly performed in the evaluation of female patients with lower urinary tract dysfunction. An endoscopic evaluation of the lower urinary tract should be undertaken to either facilitate the diagnosis of certain conditions, to rule out coexistent potential diagnoses, or to help in choosing appropriate management. There is very little data currently available to either support or refute the routine use of cystourethroscopy in females with lower urinary tract dysfunction. Karram and Angel[79] recently completed a retrospective review of more than 120 patients with various problems in the storage and evacuation of urine. The conclusions of this review note that endoscopic evaluation was of very little use in patients with primary stress incontinence, detrusor instability or a combination of both. It was, however, useful in patients with recurrent incontinence, patients with painful bladder syndromes, such as urethral syndrome or interstitial cystitis, and patients with voiding dysfunction that was not secondary to pelvic relaxation. Very poor correlation between findings on dynamic urethroscopy and eventual urodynamic diagnosis in incontinent females was also noted.

COMMON URODYNAMIC FINDINGS OF VARIOUS CONDITIONS

Stress Incontinence

Stress urinary incontinence is a generic term and can be used to describe a symptom, a sign, or a condition. The symptom of stress incontinence is present when patients state that they have involuntary urinary loss, whereas the sign is the objective demonstration of urinary loss, and the condition is the urodynamic demonstration of urinary loss, which requires the measurement of intravesical, intraabdominal, and intraurethral pressure with mechanical calculations of true detrusor and urethral closure pressure (Fig. 8A-7). Whether all patients who present with the symptom of stress incon-

tinence require detailed urodynamic testing is controversial. In the author's opinion the minimum work-up of these patients should include history, physical exam, urine culture, residual urine, assessment of urethrovesical junction mobility, a stress test to objectively demonstrate urine loss, and simple cystometry to confirm normal detrusor function.

The measurement of maximum urethral closure pressure, although controversial, may be of assistance in choosing appropriate surgical therapy in these patients. The low pressure urethra has been empirically defined as a maximum urethral closure pressure of less than 20 cm/H_2O and is considered by some to be an indication of poor urethral function. The clinical applicability of this, although very controversial, may be that these patients are at higher risk for unsuccessful conventional bladder neck surgery and may require more obstructive procedures to cure their incontinence.

In patients who will undergo bladder neck surgery for stress incontinence, the preoperative performance of voiding studies may help predict which patients will require prolonged bladder drainage. Bhatia and Bergman[57] noted that patients who void without a detrusor contraction had a much higher incidence of prolonged catheterization than those who void with a detrusor contraction.

In patients with complicated histories, prior surgical failures, or in whom these simple tests are inconclusive, more detailed urodynamic testing should be undertaken (see Box 8A-2).

Detrusor Instability

In the normal female, the detrusor muscle should be under voluntary control. The diagnosis of detrusor instability is made when there is a rise in detrusor pressure that is considered not to be caused by bladder compliance as defined by the ICS. These abnormalities may produce urgency and urge incontinence or may be asymptomatic.

Uninhibited detrusor contractions on cystometry may appear in different ways. The first is multiple detrusor contractions with pressure normalization after each contraction. A second pattern is detrusor contractions appearing one after another with continuous pressure accumulation. A third type of pattern has been described in which a rise in bladder pressure is steady. This pattern may not represent involuntary detrusor activity since it can occur in patients with fibrosis or inflammatory changes and is more properly termed a poor or low compliance bladder (Fig. 8A-19).[80]

If urethrocystometry is performed in patients with

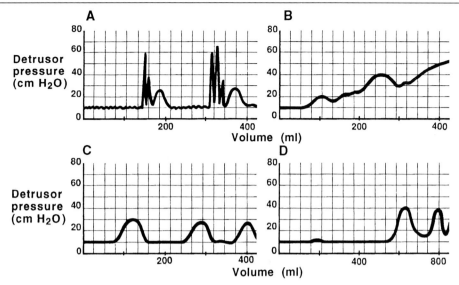

Fig. 8A-19 Various cystometric patterns. **A**, Cough- or stress-provoked detrusor instability. **B**, Consistent rise in intravesical pressure which is better termed a low compliance bladder. **C**, Detrusor instability with phasic contractions in which pressure returns to baseline after every contraction. **D**, Subthreshold instability with normal terminal contraction.

detrusor instability, one notes that detrusor contractions are almost always preceded by a drop in urethral pressure. A recent study by Bergman and coworkers[81] looked at the urethral pattern in women with detrusor instability in order to learn whether urethral pressure changes may be the cause rather than the effect of the bladder contraction. They evaluated 72 women with detrusor instability and noted patients to have one of two patterns with regards to urethral pressure change. The first pattern demonstrated uninhibited bladder contractions that preceded any change in urethral pressure while the second pattern noted a urethral pressure drop of greater than or equal to 20 cm H_2O 2 to 5 seconds prior to the detrusor contraction. They also noted that the patients who had urethral relaxation prior to the detrusor contraction responded better to alpha sympathomimetic drugs, while those patients without urethral pressure changes responded more favorably to anticholinergic drugs.[82,83]

Resnick and others recently identified another subset of detrusor instability in elderly institutionalized females. Their study noted that some incontinent females had detrusor contractions that produced incontinence but did not effectively empty the bladder. Detailed testing revealed that impaired contractility was the reason for impaired emptying, thus the condition was termed detrusor hyperactivity with impaired contractility. It may represent the last stage of detrusor instability in which there is a deterioration of detrusor function.

Urethral Instability

The unstable urethra was first described by McGuire in 1978[84] and is currently a very controversial condition. The ICS states that an involuntary fall in urethral pressure may cause urinary incontinence; however, terms such as "unstable urethra" await further data and precise definition.[19] Variations in maximum urethral closure pressure of insignificant magnitude to produce a negative closure pressure are frequently observed in normal asymptomatic females and the clinical significance of such pressure variations is unclear. These pressure variations have been labeled urethral instability by certain investigators although they do not fit criteria to meet the current definition laid down by the ICS. It is probably preferable to term these patients as having unstable urethral pressure,[85] as it makes a useful distinction between pressure variations which lead directly to incontinence and those which are potentially contributory (Fig. 8A-20). Such variations in urethral pressure have been identified in approximately 10% to 20% of females[86] with lower urinary tract symptoms and several studies have more specifically related these changes to sensory urge than to either motor urge or stress

A

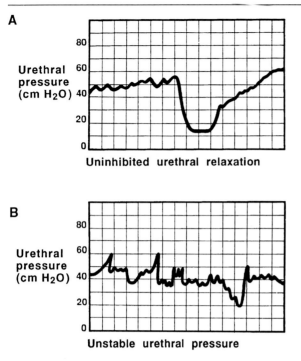

Fig. 8A-20 Graphic representation to show the difference between **A**, uninhibited urethral relaxation and **B**, unstable urethral pressure.

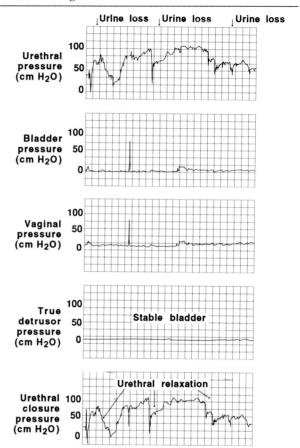

Fig. 8A-21 Urodynamic tracing in a patient with uninhibited urethral relaxation. Note the bladder remains stable.

incontinence. Different amplitudes of variations have been employed in various studies as criteria for the diagnosis of unstable urethral pressure. Some studies have used a cutoff of 15 cm/H_2O[87-89] while others have arbitrarily used a discrimination point of 20 cm/H_2O. Cordoza and Versi[90] advocated a value of 25 cm/H_2O, having found the distribution of variation of maximum urethral closure pressure was least skewed in postmenopausal women when this cutoff was employed.

Sand and colleagues[89] recently identified a rare cause of urinary incontinence in which there is a drop in maximum urethral closure pressure associated with involuntary loss of urine without a rise in detrusor pressure. This condition is best termed uninhibited urethral relaxation (Fig. 8A-21).

Neurologic Disease

Urodynamic findings in patients with neurologic dysfunction depend on the severity and location of the lesion.[91,92] Lower motor neuron lesions of the sacral segments present with retention problems secondary to

detrusor areflexia if the bladder neck is intact. If the bladder neck is incompetent either from sympathetic denervation or from another cause, the patient may give a history of both incontinence and difficulty voiding. If the neurologic insult is above the sacral outflow tracts, patients will usually have involuntary detrusor contractions (detrusor hyperreflexia). If the lesion spares the neural connections between the pontine micturition center and the sacral micturition center, voiding occurs in a coordinated fashion (urethral relaxation and detrusor contraction). If, however, this pathway is impaired, detrusor external sphincter dyssynergia results. In this condition the patient is unable to void because of simultaneous contraction of the detrusor muscle and the external striated urethral sphincter (Fig. 8A-22).[93,94] In patients with multiple sclerosis the lesions are commonly multifocal and urodynamic findings are unpredictable.[95] Also since these patients are subject to ex-

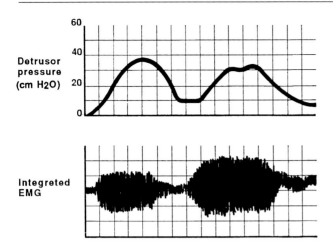

Fig. 8A-22 Graphic representation of a patient with detrusor external sphincter dyssynergia. Note the simultaneous contraction of the detrusor muscle and the urethral sphincter.

acerbations and bouts of remission, it is important to test the patient when she is symptomatic. [95,96]

Severe Pelvic Relaxation

Evaluation of patients with severe pelvic prolapse should include an assessment of the lower urinary tract. These women may have underlying incontinence and/or voiding dysfunction. Severe pelvic relaxation may cause a stress incontinent patient to become continent from the downward descent of the viscera posterior and superior to the urethra producing kinking and obstruction. When the prolapsed contents are reduced and visceral descent is limited, it has been shown that 36% to 80% of patients have underlying genuine stress incontinence exposed. [97–99] This potential stress incontinence can be elicited by performing a stress test after gentle reduction of the prolapsed contents with either a pessary or a Sim's speculum. One group of investigators found it helpful to perform pressure transmission ratios on these patients, as they noted that if pressure transmission was greater than 100% with pessary reduction, then patients needed only conventional anterior vaginal repair. Whereas if transmission ratios were less than 100%, a bladder neck suspension was necessary in conjunction with anterior repair. [99]

Uroflowmetry and determinations of residual urine should also be performed in these patients to objectively define any underlying voiding dysfunction. More complicated pressure/flow studies may be needed in some patients to evaluate detrusor function.

URODYNAMICS IN PERSPECTIVE

The purpose of urodynamic testing is to identify and quantitate the etiologic factors that contribute to lower urinary tract dysfunction. Since the bladder is a notoriously poor witness and responds to a variety of pathologies with the same symptoms, the need for urodynamics testing becomes very important before directing therapy. Although an accurate history is very important, numerous studies have documented poor correlation between patients' symptoms and urodynamic findings. [100,101] On the other hand, the validity of any diagnosis based on urodynamic data is linked to the patient's symptoms and the reproduction of those symptoms during the testing session. It is therefore important for the urodynamicist to correlate the urodynamic data with all other clinically relevant information. This is possible only if the urodynamicist is the physician who takes the history, performs the physical exam, interprets other tests, explains the diagnosis, and plans a reasonable management plan.

Another important but rarely discussed aspect of urodynamic testing is the cost-effectiveness of these studies. There is growing belief that too many expensive instruments have been purchased by too many gynecologists and urologists who do not have the time or expertise either to learn basic urodynamics or to perform the tests in a reproducible manner. In 1979 McGuire[102] published the results of a poll to survey the cost of urodynamic investigations. This study concluded that major urodynamic testing is largely confined to university laboratories where part of the initial and continuing costs of equipment can be defrayed from sources other than patient charges. Practical urodynamic testing at the office level was confined to flow rates and simple cystometry. A more recent retrospective study by Miller and colleagues[103] concluded that the expense and effort of running a urodynamic unit are justified when more than 200 patients are studied per year. One important issue which has not been addressed yet is how often urodynamic testing prevents inappropriate surgery.

SUMMARY

Urodynamic studies are an integral part of the evaluation of lower urinary tract dysfunction in females. However, these tests are still evolving and there is a need for more controlled studies to clarify controversies regarding indications, techniques, and interpretation.

REFERENCES

1. Blavias JG. Machines for measuring urodynamics. *Contemp Obstet Gynecol.* 1990(Suppl:Technology):99–110.
2. Dubois P. Uber den Druck in der Harnblase. *Arch Klin Med.* 1876;17:148.
3. Lewis LG. A new clinical recording cystometer. *J Urol.* 1939;41:638.
4. Merrill DC, Bradley WE, Markland C. Air cystometry: 1. Technique and definition of terms. *J Urol.* 1971;106:678.
5. Bradley WE, Timm GW, Scott FB. Cystometry: III. Cystometers. *Urol.* 1975a;5:843.
6. Drake WM. The uroflowmeter: An aid to the study of lower urinary tract. *J Urol.* 1948;59:650.
7. Von Garretts B. Analysis of micturition: A new method of recording the voiding of the bladder. *Acta Chir Scand.* 1956;112:326.
8. Bonney V. On diurnal incontinence of urine in women. *J Obstet Gynecol.* Br Commonw. 1923;30:358.
9. Lapides J, Ajemian EP, Stewart BH, Breskey BA, Lichtwart JR. Further observations on the kinetics of the urethrovesical sphincter. *J Urol.* 1960;84:86.
10. Enhorning G. Simultaneous recording of intravesical and intraurethral pressure. *Acta Chir Scand.* 1961;276(suppl):1.
11. Tanagho EA, Miller ER, Myers EH, Corbett RK. Observations on the dynamics of the bladder neck. *Br J Urol.* 1966;38:72.
12. Tanagho EA, Myers EH, Smith DR. Urethral resistance, its components and implications: I. Smooth muscle components. *Invest Urol.* 1969;7:136.
13. Brown M, Wickham JEA. The urethral pressure profile. *Br J Urol.* 1969;41:211.
14. Bates P, Bradley WE, Glen, et al. First report on the standardization of terminology of the lower urinary tract function. Urinary incontinence. Procedures related to the evaluation of urine storage: cystometry, urethral closure pressure profile, units of measurement. *Br J Urol.* 1976;48:39; *Eur Urol.* 1976;2:274; *Scand J Urol Nephrol.* 1976;11:193; *Urol Int.* 1976;32:81.
15. Bates P, Glen E, Griffiths D, et al. Second report on the standardization of terminology of lower urinary tract function. Procedures related to the evaluation of micturition: flow rate, pressure measurement, symbols. *Acta Urol Jpn.* 1977;27:1563; *Br J Urol.* 1977;49:207; *Scand J Urol Nephrol.* 1977;11:1977.
16. Bates P, Bradley WE, Glen E, et al. Third report on the standardization of terminology of lower urinary tract function. Procedures related to the evaluation of micturition: pressure flow relationships, residual urine. *Br J Urol.* 1980;52:348; *Eur Urol.* 1980;6:170; *Acta Urol Jpn.* 1980;27:1566; *Scand J Urol Nephrol.* 1980;12:191.
17. Bates P, Bradley WE, Glen E, et al. Fourth report on the standardization of terminology of lower urinary tract function. Terminology related to neuromuscular dysfunction of lower urinary tract. *Br J Urol.* 1981;52:333; *Urology* 1981;17:618; *Scand J Urol Nephrol.* 1981;15:169; *Acta Urol Jpn.* 1981;27:1568.
18. Abrams P, Blaivas JG, Stanton SL, et al. Sixth report on the standardization of terminology of lower urinary tract function. Procedures related to neurophysiological investigations: electromyography, nerve conduction studies, reflex latencies, evoked potentials and sensory testing. *World J Urol.* 1986;4:2; *Scand J Urol Nephrol.* 1986;20:161.
19. Abrams P, Blaivas JG, Stanton SL, et al. The standardization of terminology of lower urinary tract function. *Scand J Urol Nephrol.* 1988;114(suppl):5.
20. Gleason DM, Bottaccini MR, Reilly RJ. Comparison of cystometrograms and urethral profiles with gas and water media. *Urology.* 1977;9:155.
21. Colstrup H, Andersen JT, Walter S. Detrusor reflex instability in the male. Fact or artifact? A randomized crossover study of the influence using a balloon catheter during rapid fill CO_2 cystometry. *Neurourol Urodynam.* 1982;1:183.
22. Arnold EP, Webster JR, Loose H, et al. Urodynamics of female incontinence: factors influencing the results of surgery. *Am J Obstet Gynecol.* 1973;117:805.
23. Brown ADG. The urodynamic management of female urinary incontinence. MD Thesis. Edinburgh. Cited by Turner-Warwick R, Brown ADG. *Urol Clin North Am.* 1974;6:203.
24. Cass AS, Ward BD, Markland C. Comparison of slow and rapid fill cystometry using liquid and air. *J Urol.* 1970;104:104.
25. Merrill DC, Rotta JA. A clinical evaluation of detrusor denervation supersensitivity using air cystometry. *J Urol.* 1974;111:27.
26. Merrill DC, Bradley WE, Markland C. Air cystometry. II. A clinical evaluation of normal adults. *J Urol.* 1972;108:85.
27. Jorgensen L, Lose G, Andersen JT. Cystometry: H_2O or CO_2 as filling medium? A literature survey of the influence of the filling medium on the qualitative and the quantitative cystometric parameters. *Neurourol Urodynam.* 1988;7:343.
28. Klevmark B. Motility of the urinary bladder in cats during filling at physiologic rates: I. Intravesical pressure patterns studies by a new method of cystometry. *Acta Physiol Scand.* 1974;90:565.
29. Sand PK, Hill RC, Ostergard DR. Supine urethroscopic and standing cystometry as screening methods for the detection of detrusor instability. *Obstet Gynecol.* 1987;70:57.
30. Arnold EP. Cystometry-postural effects in incontinence effects in incontinent women. *Urol Int.* 1974;29:185.
31. Bruskewitz R, Raz S. Urethral pressure profile using microtip catheters in females. *Urology.* 1979;16:303.
32. Blaivas JG. Multichannel urodynamic studies. *Urology.* 1984;23:421.
33. Massey A, Abrams P. Urodynamics of the female lower urinary tract. *Urol Clin North Am.* 1985;12:231.
34. Penders L, De Leval J. Simultaneous urethrocystometry and hyperactive bladders: a manometric differential diagnosis. *Neurourol Urodynam.* 1985;4:89.
35. McCarthy TA. Validity of rectal pressure measurements as indication of intraabdominal pressure changes during urodynamic evaluation. *Urology.* 1982;20:657.
36. Al-Taher H, Sutherst JR, Richmond DH, Brown MC. Vaginal pressure as an index of intraabdominal pressure during urodynamic evaluation. *Br J Urol.* 1987;59:529.
37. Lapides J, Friend CR, Ajemian EP. Denervation supersensitivity as a test for neurogenic bladder. *Surg Gynecol Obstet.* 1962;114:141.
38. Merrill DC, Rotta J. A clinical evaluation of detrusor denervation supersensitivity during air cystometry. *J Urol.* 1974;3:27.
39. Melzer M. The Urecholine test. *J Urol.* 1972;108:729.
40. Karram MM, Bhatia NN. Management of coexistent stress and urge urinary incontinence. *Obstet Gynecol.* 1989;73:4.
41. McGuire EJ, Savastano JA. Stress incontinence and detrusor instability/urge incontinence. *Neurourol Urodyn.* 1985;4:313.
42. Lockhart JL, Vorskman B, Pohtano VA. Anti-incontinence surgery in females with detrusor instability. *Neurourol Urodyn.* 1984;3:201.
43. Bradley WE, Timm GW, Scott FB. Cystometry: V. Bladder sensation. *Urology.* 1975;6:654.
44. Torrens M, Abrams P. Cystometry: symposium on clinical urodynamics. *Urologic Clinics of North Am.* 1979;6:71.
45. Sutherst JR, Brown MC. Comparison of single and multichannel cystometry in diagnosing bladder instability. *Br Med J.* 1984;288:1720.
46. Ouslander JG, Staskin D, et al. Clinical versus urodynamic diagnosis in an incontinent geriatric female population. *J Urol.* 1987;137:68.
47. Coolsaet BLRA, Blok C, Van Venrooij GEPM, et al. Subthreshold detrusor instability. *Neurourol Urodynam.* 1985;4:309.
48. Bhatia NN, Bradley WE, Haldeman S. Urodynamics: Continuous Monitoring. *J Urol.* 1982;128:963.

49. Bhatia NN, Bradley WE, Haldeman S, Johnson BK. Continuous ambulatory urodynamic monitoring. *Br J Urol.* 1982;54:357.

50. Abrams P, Torrens M. Urine flow studies. *Urol Clin North Am.* 1979;6:71.

51. Fantl A J. Clinical Uroflowmetry. In: Ostergard DR, ed. *Gynecologic Urology and Urodynamics.* 2nd ed. Baltimore: Williams & Wilkins Co; 1985;125–132.

52. Tanagho EA. Urodynamics: Uroflowmetry and female voiding patterns. In: Ostergard DR, ed. *Gynecologic Urology and Urodynamics.* 2nd ed. Baltimore: Williams & Wilkins Co; 1985;117–124.

53. Bradley WE. Urologically oriented neurological examination. In: Ostergard DR, ed. *Gynecologic Urology and Urodynamics.* 2nd ed. Baltimore: Williams & Wilkins Co; 1985;63–68.

54. Bradley WE. Urodynamics: integration of electromyography with cystometry and urethral pressure profiles. In: Ostergard DR, ed. *Gynecologic Urology and Urodynamics.* 2nd ed. Baltimore: Williams & Wilkins Co; 1985;101–116.

55. Tanagho EA, McCurrcy E. Pressure and flow rate as related to lumen caliber and entrance configuration. *J Urol.* 1971;105:583.

56. Susset JG, Brissot RB, Regnier CH. The stop-flow technique: a way to measure detrusor strength. *J Urol.* 1982;127:489.

57. Bhatia NN, Bergman A. Urodynamic predictability of voiding following incontinence surgery. *Obstet Gynecol.* 1984;63:85.

58. Barnick CG, Cardozo LD, Benness C. Use of routine videocystourethrography in the evaluation of female lower urinary tract dysfunction. *Neurourol Urodynam.* 1989;8:447.

59. Abrams PH. Perfusion urethral profilometry. *Urol Clin North Am.* 1979;6:103.

60. Abrams PH, Martin S, Griffiths D J. The measurement and interpretation of urethral pressures obtained by the method of Brown and Wickham. *Br J Urol.* 1978;50:33.

61. Tanagho EA. Membrane and microtransducer catheters: their effectiveness for profilometry of the lower urinary tract. *Urol Clin North Am.* 1979;6:110.

62. Anderson RS, Shepherd AM, Feneley RCL. Microtransducer urethral profile methodology: variations caused by transducer orientation. *J Urol.* 1983;119:727.

63. Rud T. The urethral pressure profile in continent women from childhood to old age. *Acta Obstetricia et Gynecologica Scandinarica.* 1980;54:331.

64. Rud T, Andersson KE, Asmussen M, Hunting A, Ulmsten U. Factors maintaining the intraurethral pressure in women. *Invest. Urol.* 1980;17:343.

65. Bhatia NN, McCarthy TA, Ostergard DR. UPPs in women with urethral diverticula. Proceedings of the Xth annual meeting of the International Continence Society. Los Angeles; 1980:25–28.

66. Versi E. Discriminant analysis of urethral pressure profilometry data for the diagnosis of genuine stress incontinence. *Br J Obstet Gynecol.* 1990;97:251.

67. McGuire EJ. Urodynamic findings in patients after failure of stress incontinence operations. *Prog Clin Biol Res.* 1981;78:351.

68. Sand PK, Bowen LW, Panganiban R, et al. The low pressure urethra as a factor in failed retropubic urethropexy. *Obstet Gynecol.* 1987;69:399.

69. Rowan D, James ED, Kramer AEJL, et al. Urodynamic equipment: technical aspects. Produced by the International Continence Society Working Party on Urodynamic Equipment. *J Med Eng Technol.* 1987;1:57.

70. Bump RC. The urodynamic laboratory. *Obstet Gynecol Clin North Am.* 1989;16:795.

71. Enhorning G. Simultaneous recording of the intravesical and intraurethral pressure. *Act Chir Scand.* 1961;276S:1.

72. Richardson DA. Value of the cough pressure profile in the evaluation of patients with stress incontinence. *Am J Obstet Gynecol.* 1986;155:808.

73. Bump RC, Copeland WE Jr, Hurt WG, Fantl JA. Dynamic urethral pressure profilometry pressure transmission ratio determinations in stress-incontinent and stress-continent subjects. *Am J Obstet Gynecol.* 1988;159:749.

74. Hilton P, Stanton SL. Urethral pressure measurement by microtransducers: the results in symptomfree women and in those with genuine stress incontinence. *Br J Obstet Gynaecol.* 1983;90:919.

75. Crystle CD, Charme LS, Copeland WE. Q-tip test in stress urinary incontinence. *Obstet Gynecol.* 1971;38:313.

76. Walters MD, Diaz K. Q-tip test: a study of continent and incontinent women. *Obstet Gynecol.* 1987;70:208.

77. Bergman A, McCarthy TA, Ballard CA, et al. Role of the Q-tip test in evaluating stress urinary incontinence. *J Reprod Med.* 1987;32:273.

78. Karram MM, Bhatia NN. The Q-tip test: standardization of the technique and its interpretation in women with urinary incontinence. *Obstet Gynecol.* 1988;71:8078.

79. Karram MM, Angel OH. Indications for cystourethroscopy in females with lower urinary tract dysfunction. Proceedings of the 11th Annual AUGS Meeting, October 31–November 3, 1990; Tarpon Springs, Fla.

80. Webster GD. *The Unstable Bladder in Female Urology,* Raz S, ed. Philadelphia: WB Saunders; 1983:139–161.

81. Bergman A, Koonings PP, Ballard CA. Detrusor instability. Is the bladder the cause or the effect? *J Reprod Med.* 1989;34:834.

82. Resnick NM, Yalla SV, Laurino E. The pathophysiology of urinary incontinence among institutionalized elderly persons. *N Engl J Med.* 1989;320:1.

83. Resnick NM, Yalla SV. Detrusor hyperactivity with impaired contractile function. *JAMA.* 1987;257:3076.

84. McGuire EJ. Reflex urethral instability. *Br J Urol.* 1978;50:200.

85. Hilton P. Unstable urethral pressure: toward a more relevant definition. *Neurourol Urodyn.* 1988;6:411.

86. Kulseng-Hanssen S. Prevalence and pattern of unstable urethral pressure in one hundred seventy-four gynecologic patients referred for urodynamic investigation. *Am J Obstet Gynecol.* 1983;146:895.

87. Fossberg E, Beisland HO, Sauder S. Sensory urgency in females. Treatment with phenylpropanolamine. *Eur Urol.* 1981;7:157.

88. Ulmsten U, Henriksson L, Iosif S. The unstable female urethra. *Am J Obstet Gynecol.* 1982;144:93.

89. Sand PK, Bowen LW, Ostergard DR. Uninhibited urethral relaxation: an unusual cause of incontinence. *Obstet Gynecol.* 1986;68:645.

90. Cardozo L, Versi E. Urethral instability in normal postmenopausal patients. Proceedings of the XVth annual meeting of the International Continence Society. London; 1985:115–116.

91. Bradley WE, Rockswold GC, Timm GW, et al. Neurology of micturition. *J Urol.* 1976;115:481.

92. Bradley WE, Timm GW, Scott FB. Innervation of the detrusor muscle and urethra. *Urol Clin North Am.* 1974;1:3.

93. Blaivas JG, Sinnha HP, Zayed AAH, Labib KB. Detrusor-external sphincter-dyssynergia. *J Urol.* 1981;125:542.

94. Blaivas JG, Sinnha HP, Zayed AAH, Labib KB. Detrusor-external sphincter-dyssynergia: a detailed EMG study. *J Urol.* 1981;125:545.

95. Blaivas JG, Bhimam G, Labib KB. Vesicourethral dysfunction in multiple sclerosis. *J Urol.* 1979;122:342.

96. Blaivas JG. Management of bladder dysfunction in multiple sclerosis. *Neurology.* 1980;30:12.

97. Bump RC, Fantl JA, Hurt WG. The mechanism of urinary continence in women with severe uterovaginal prolapse: results of barrier studies. *Obstet Gynecol.* 1988;72:291.

98. Richardson DA, Bent AE, Ostergard DR. The effect of uterovaginal prolapse on urethrovesical pressure dynamics. *Am J Obstet Gynecol.* 1983;146:901.

99. Bergman A, Koonings PP, Ballard CA. Predicting postoperative urinary incontinence development in women undergoing operation for genitourinary prolapse. *Am J Obstet Gynecol.* 1988;158:1171.

100. Farrar DJ, Osborne JL, Stephenson TP, et al. A urodynamic view of bladder outflow obstruction in the female: factors influencing the results of treatment. *Br J Urol.* 1976;47:815.

101. Powell PH, Shepard AM, Lewis P, et al. The accuracy of clinical diagnosis assessed urodynamically. In: Zinner NR, Sterling AM, eds. *Female Incontinence.* New York: Alan R. Liss, Inc; 1981: 201.

102. McGuire EJ. Patient costs for urodynamic testing. *Urology* 1979;16:426.

103. Miller RA, Barod RK, Chapman J, Fergus JN. The clinical value and cost of a district hospital urodynamic unit. *Br J Urol.* 1982; 54:635.

Manometric Investigation

8B   Anorectal Manometry

N. W. Read   W. M. Sun

INTRODUCTION

Disorders of anorectal function are more common in women than men. Eight times as many women than men suffer from fecal incontinence. This is due to the very high incidence of obstetric trauma and postpartum weakness of the pelvic floor, leading to neuropathy of the pudendal nerve. The irritable bowel syndrome is at least twice as common in women than men. Severe constipation in young to middle-aged adults is almost entirely a disease of women; it fluctuates during the menstrual cycle, is often more severe during pregnancy, and may present for the first time after hysterectomy. A functional test that can identify the abnormalities in these conditions would certainly help surgeons or physicians.

Why Do Manometric Recordings?

The anorectum is a complicated mechanism that is involved in two major functions: control of defecation and the preservation of continence. It consists of a rectal reservoir, two concentric sphincters, one composed of smooth muscle, the other of striated muscle, and sensors in the pelvic floor and rectum that modulate the contractile activity of both the sphincter and the distal colon. Disorders of defecation, either constipation or incontinence, may result from defects in several different components of the anorectal mechanism.

When combined with measurements of rectal sensation and sphincter electromyography, anorectal manometry can assess the function of the different components of the anorectal mechanism under physiological conditions. Thus, these tests provide a direct assessment of what the surgeon or physician wants to know. That is, how well does the anorectum preserve continence or facilitate defecation, and what component of the mechanism is faulty? Manometric measurements of sphincter function are operative; they provide insights into pathophysiologic mechanisms. More complex neurophysiologic tests may be required to indicate the etiology.

Anorectal function tests complement neurophysiologic tests in the investigation of anorectal disorders. For example, if sphincter function tests show a profound weakness of the external sphincter that is not associated with an obvious anatomic defect or perineal descent, or if external sphincter responses to rectal distention or increases in intraabdominal pressure are absent, then neurophysiologic (and possibly neuroanatomic) tests should be considered to identify the site of the lesion.

METHODOLOGY FOR MEASUREMENT OF ANORECTAL PRESSURES

The pressures measured in the anorectum depend on the technique used to measure them. Pressures in the anal canal can be measured by perfused catheters, sleeve catheters, water-filled balloons, and force transducers. Each technique studies a somewhat different aspect of contractile activity and has particular advantages and disadvantages. Since the muscular components of the anorectum are so close to each other, measurement of pressures from multiple closely spaced sites discriminates between the function of each component.

Perfused Side Holes

In modern perfusion systems, a narrow multilumen anal probe constructed from low compliance tubing, and equipped with side-opening ports is connected via external pressure transducers to a perfusion apparatus (pressurized bottles containing distilled [degassed] water connected to the transducers via capillary tubing). The pressures measured by perfused side holes depend on the compliance of the catheter system and the rate of perfusion. Systems employing low compliance catheters respond rapidly to changes in pressure, and if the catheter bore is sufficiently small, they utilize very low flow rates (0.2 ml/min^{-1}) thus avoiding excessive accumulation of fluid in the rectum.

The pressure recorded in each catheter is an index of the resistance to flow of fluid out of the catheter. In the anal sphincter, where the muscular wall is closely apposed to the side opening of the catheter, fluid is initially trapped in a relatively small space, and pressures may increase until fluid escapes. The point at which this occurs has been termed the yield pressure[1,2,3] and is influenced by the surface tension between adjacent walls of the canal as well as by the muscular tone. For comparative results, it is important that fluid is perfused into the canal until the yield pressure is attained. In modern systems, this point is reached rapidly.

A side-opening port localizes a contraction in the anal canal better than an end-opening where the wall is not apposed to the outflow from the catheter. Perfused side holes are less useful for recording pressures in a large hollow organ, such as the rectum, where a contraction anywhere within the space may cause a rise in pressure.

Sleeve Sensors

A sleeve sensor can be used in conjunction with perfused side holes to record the maximum pressure in the anal sphincter. Fluid is perfused through a sleeve or tunnel formed by a flexible silastic membrane glued over a smooth silastic base.[4] When the probe is in the anus, the sleeve spans the sphincter so that a contraction anywhere along its length will cause an increased resistance to the flow of fluid and is measured as an increase in pressure in the catheter. The sleeve sensor measures the net resistance of the whole sphincter to the flow of fluid, but it does not localize the site of resistance and it cannot distinguish between contraction of the internal anal sphincter (IAS) and the external anal sphincter (EAS).

Balloons

Fluid or air-filled balloons are connected by a catheter to pressure transducers. Because balloons distend the anal canal and rectum, the pressures measured may provide a more sensitive index of the resistance to distention than perfused side holes. Duthie and Watts[5] were unable to demonstrate any effect of anesthesia and muscle relaxants on anal tone when they used open-tipped perfused catheters, but recorded a 40% decrease in pressure using a balloon.

The pressures that are recorded depend on the size of the balloon; resistance to distention will increase as the diameter of the balloon is increased. Pressures within the anal canal are often measured by microballoons of fixed diameter (0.5 to 1.0 cm).[6,7] Microballoons avoid problems of radial pressure asymmetry (see later discussion), but by distending the anal canal, they may induce anal contraction. It is difficult to record from more than one anal site using microballoons.

The "Schuster" probe[8] consists of a rigid metal cylinder that is clamped in the anal canal by inflating two balloons so that the external balloon records the EAS contractions, while the internal balloon records predominantly the activity of the IAS. This ingenious device provides a simple and convenient means of recording external and internal sphincter components independently, although the overlap of the two sphincters limits the interpretation of the data. Another possible drawback is that large balloons that stretch the sphincter may alter anorectal contractility to a greater extent than small balloons or perfused catheters.

Rectal tone and compliance can be measured using large, floppy, thin-walled balloons inflated with increasing volumes of air and water; a condom is ideal, although smaller balloons are used to measure the contractility of the rectal ampulla.[9] The pressures recorded depend in part on the viscoelastic properties of the balloon. The latter can be determined by inflation outside the body, and the pressures so obtained are subtracted from the measurements recorded when the balloon is in situ to obtain an index of the viscoelastic properties of the rectum. Substitution of a large thin-walled plastic bag for a balloon avoids subtraction of ex vivo pressures. Large rectal balloons or bags measure the integrated pressure inside the rectal cavity; smaller balloons may be used to localize rectal contractions. The presence of fecal material, the occurrence of a high degree of contractile activity at one site and the presence of extrarectal masses may reduce rectal capacity and alter the pressure volume relationships in a rectal balloon. If a subject is lying in the left lateral position, the pressures recorded from a balloon filled with water are identical to those with an air-filled balloon.[10]

Another way of studying the properties of the rectal wall is to measure rectal volume in response to changes in pressure using a large capacity plastic bag, which is inserted into the rectum filled with water and connected to a large external fluid reservoir. The values so obtained provide a more direct index of rectal compliance. This barostat system maintains the rectal pressure constant at a low physiologic level while measuring changes in rectal volume.[11] The barostat system is, of course, ideal for studying changes in the tone of a closed viscus such as the stomach or the urinary bladder. It is less useful for studying a muscular tube such as the rectum, which is obstructed to a variable degree at its proximal end by feces or muscular contraction.

Microtransducers

Strain gauge transducers are now made sufficiently small to fit in the anal canal.[6,12–15] Microtransducers do not require perfusion of fluid and do not distend the anus, therefore they may avoid some potential sources of inaccuracy associated with balloons or perfused catheters.[6,11] The disadvantages of transducers are that they are expensive and not always very robust. They impart a rigidity to the catheter which can distort the anal pressure profiles by accentuating radial differences (see below), and they do not permit simultaneous recording from multiple anal ports. Perhaps future microtransducers will be smaller and more affordable.

THE INTERPRETATION OF ANORECTAL PRESSURES

Index of Contractile Resistance

Anal pressure is often used as an index of the resistance of the sphincter to the passage of fecal material

from the rectum. In support of this, two studies have shown that sphincter pressure is significantly correlated with the force required to pull a spherical ball through the anal canal.[16,17] Other factors, however, contribute to the resistance of the anal canal. For example, if the anorectal angle is sufficiently acute, only very low anal pressures are needed to keep the mass in the rectum.[18] The presence of hemorrhoids may add an important component to anal resistance.[19]

Whether pressures can be used to provide a useful index of resistance of the anal canal also depends on the size of the probe. Anal pressures increase when larger probes are used to measure them.[19] Pressures recorded with narrow probes may give an erroneous index of anal canal resistance to the passage of large, solid stool. Normally, the anal canal is fairly elastic and can relax to accommodate large probes,[19,20] but when the canal is infiltrated with fibrous tissue, higher pressures than normal may be recorded with large-diameter probes, but not necessarily with small-diameter probes.

Radial and Longitudinal Differences

Variations in pressures exist at different sites within the anal canal. The highest pressures are usually recorded in the lower canal, corresponding with the anatomic position of the bulk of the EAS. Radial pressures, measured by a rigid probe, are lower anteriorly than posteriorly in the upper canal, both at rest and during voluntary contraction,[21,22] approximately equal in the mid-canal, but lower posteriorly than anteriorly in the lower canal. Thus, the manometric records are consistent with the existence of a forwardly directed top loop (puborectalis sling) and a backwardly directed loop below it,[23] but they do not confirm Shafik's forward directed base loop. In recent years, sophisticated computerized systems were employed to construct three-dimensional models of the sphincter pressure profile.

The authors do not believe that radial pressure differences provide useful information. An infinitely flexible recording port will come to rest within the anal canal when opposing pressures are balanced. Thus, radial differences must be artifacts caused by the leverage of the rigid probe within the anal canal as it negotiates the anorectal angle. Radial differences are much smaller when soft flexible probes are used.[19]

Stationary versus Pull-through Measurements

Movement of the probe within the anal canal may reflexly increase anorectal pressure.[24] Thus, higher pressures may be recorded if the probe is continuously pulled through the canal than if the probe is left at one site to allow the pressure to fall to steady levels before being moved (station pull-through). We have recently shown after insertion of a 4 mm diameter probe, that the resting anal pressures gradually decline over 15 minutes before they reach a steady state.[25]

Ambulatory Recordings

Techniques are now available for recording pressures and electrical activity in the anal sphincter while the subject is carrying out his or her normal activities.[12,15] Signals from as many as six recording sites can be digitized and stored on magnetic tape using a data-logger. The tapes can be played back in the laboratory for analysis and yield a permanent record. Ambulatory techniques allow the events surrounding episodes of incontinence to be identified, and provide important documentation of the changes in anorectal pressure that occur during sleeping, walking, and eating. A major limitation of the present system is the difficulty of maintaining a sensor within the anal canal for long periods of time, and the difficulty in deciding whether a drop in

anal pressure is caused by a shift of the sensor back into the rectum or a true decline in pressure. Ambulatory recordings from the rectum avoid problems of probe movement, but interpretation of increases in pressure may be difficult unless careful records are kept of movement, talking, and coughing, which may cause changes in rectal pressure by altering intraabdominal pressure.

NORMAL RECORDS

Resting Pressures

Resting pressure in the anal canal undergoes regular fluctuations. These consist of slow waves (amplitude 5 to 25 cm/H_2O; frequency between 6/min and 20/min) and much larger and ultraslow waves (amplitude 30 to 100 cm/H_2O; frequency <3/min).[18,26,27] It seems likely that slow and ultraslow waves are generated by the IAS, because electrical recordings from the IAS show fluctuations occurring at the same frequencies,[25,28] and rectal distention reduces the tone of the IAS and abolishes both electrical and pressure fluctuations (Fig. 8B-1). Brindley[29] has suggested that electrical recordings from

Fig. 8B-1 Recordings of anorectal pressure and electrical activity of the EAS and IAS in normal subject before and during contraction of the EAS, during rectal balloon with 60 and 100 ml of air and during increased intraabdominal pressure. Channels 1 to 6 represent ports situated 0.5, 1.0, 1.5, 2.0, 2.5, and 4.5 cm, respectively, from the anal verge. Note that EAS contraction increased EAS electrical activity and anal pressures; rectal distention induced relaxation in sphincter pressure associated with abolition of the electrical oscillations, produced by IAS activity, and an increase in the electrical activity of the EAS, whereas deflation produces a rebound increase in pressure which is associated with marked increase in the slow wave oscillations; straining to blow up a balloon was associated with increases in rectal pressure, anal pressure, and EAS electrical activity. The bar (⎽⎽) indicates when subject experienced rectal sensations. *DD* = desire to defecate.

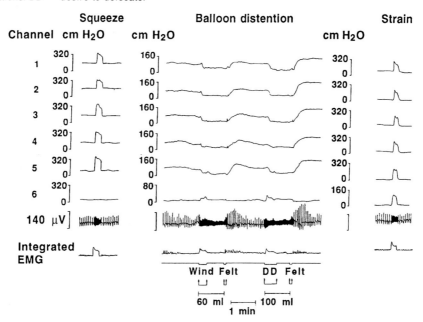

the IAS in vivo may be movement artifacts related to IAS contraction.

The frequency of the IAS slow wave is higher in the lower canal than in the upper canal.[18,30,31] These investigators wondered whether an inwardly directed contraction gradient could encourage small amounts of material in the anal canal to move back into the rectum.

Ultraslow waves are associated with particularly high resting pressures. Haynes and Read found them in about 40% of normal subjects, but only when the resting pressure was above 140 cm/H_2O.[26] Other workers have reported ultraslow waves in only 5% of normal subjects, but in 30% to 45% of patients with hemorrhoids[27,32,33] and 67% to 80% of patients with anal fissures.[34,35] Resting sphincter pressures are often very high in both of these conditions.

Tonic contraction of both the internal and external sphincters contribute to the resting pressure, though the relative contribution of each varies according to the conditions of measurement. Studies in which the EAS component was blocked by anesthesia of the pudendal nerve showed that about 15% of the resting pressure, measured by a 7 mm anal balloon, came from the EAS.[36] Sphincter pressures measured with a 3 mm microtransducer in patients before and after curarization suggest 30% of resting pressure from the EAS.[37] Bannister and others[38] compared the residual pressure after rectal distention with the resting sphincter pressure in normal subjects and estimated that the external anal sphincter could provide up to 50% of the tone of the sphincter under these conditions, but this is probably an overestimate, because rectal distention is known to increase the activity of the EAS. Finally, Bennett and Duthie[39] showed that IAS myotomy for fissures produced a 50% drop in sphincter pressure measured with narrow open-ended polyethylene tubes.

Resting anal pressure is reduced in patients with meningocele, spinal shock,[40] spinal anesthesia,[41] and in patients who have had a sacral resection with ablation of sacral nerves on one or both sides.[42] Resting anal pressure is not, however, lowered in chronic paraplegics.[40,43–45]

The activity of the IAS is modulated by the sympathetic nervous system. Stimulation of the distal end of the hypogastric nerves induces sphincter contraction.[46–50] Blockade of the sympathetic outflow with high spinal anesthesia[41] reduced resting anal pressure more than with low spinal anesthesia or with pudendal block. Finally, the tone of the IAS in vitro is reduced by about 50% after administration of a selective alpha-adrenoceptor blocker, phentolamine.[51] Lestar and colleagues[37] compared basal sphincter pressure before and

after abdominoperineal excision for cancer and concluded that the neurogenic component amounted to 53% of IAS tone. These results are contradicted by recent reports that high frequency stimulation of the presacral nerves reduced anal pressure.[52] However, it seems likely that the presacral outflow contains functionally mixed nerves rather than just adrenergic fibers,[51,53] and high frequency electrical stimulation might selectively excite the inhibitory nerves.[54]

Anal pressure is increased in the upright posture and is associated with an increased electrical activity in the external sphincter.[18] Coughing or increases in intraabdominal pressure also increase the external sphincter activity,[18,55,56] possibly by stimulation of tension receptors in the pelvic floor. Parting the buttocks in normal adults causes a brief increase in EAS activity followed by a fall in pressure.[24] Resting pressures are lower in elderly subjects compared with younger subjects.[17,22,57]

Pressures During Voluntary Contraction

Phasic contraction of the EAS is under voluntary control and is usually associated with contraction of the puborectalis sling. Voluntary contraction elevates the pressure throughout the anal canal, but the pressure rise is maximal in the lower canal where the EAS is situated.[38] Pressures induced by voluntary contraction are reduced as subjects get older.[17,57] If subjects are asked to sustain a voluntary contraction, the pressure declines to basal values over a period of up to 3 minutes.[56,58] Both the amplitude and duration of the voluntary squeeze pressure are reduced by anesthesia of the anal mucosa.[58]

Length of the Anal Canal

The length of the high pressure zone, determined by the pull-through technique, is 2.5 to 5 cm.[59] It is shorter when assessed by multiport stationary recordings (2.5 cm in males and 2 cm in females),[25] probably because pull-through excites contraction of the puborectalis, the EAS, and perhaps the IAS. The functional sphincter length is increased during conscious contraction of the sphincter[25] and reduced when the rectum is distended.[38,39]

Rectal Pressures

The rectum is often quiescent and basal pressures measured in the rectum are about 5 cm/H_2O. Rectal contractions may be induced by infusion of air or water and distention with a balloon.[60,61] Scharli and Keisewetter described three major types of rectal contractile activity: runs of simple nonpropagated contractions, occurring at a frequency of 5 to 10 min^{-1}; slower static contractions, occurring at a frequency of about 3 min^{-1} and attaining amplitudes of up to 100 cm/H$_2$O; and slow propagated contractions usually associated with anal relaxation.[61] Similar findings have been reported by other workers.[62]

Two groups have compared the runs of rectal contractions to the migrating motor complex of the small intestine.[15,63] This "rectal motor complex," however, does not migrate and occurs only at one site in the rectum. The period between consecutive runs varies from as little as 10 minutes to as much as 260 minutes, and there is no temporal relationship with the phases of the migrating motor complex of the small intestine.[64] The authors regard the phenomenon as too inconsistent to deserve the appellation "rectal motor complex."

Ingestion of a meal causes an increase in rectal motor activity that is usually associated with a desire to defecate.[62–69] The response to the ingestion of food is related to the number of calories in the meal as well as the quantity of ingested lipid.[70] Recently, Brown and others[71] showed that a drink of either caffeinated or decaffeinated coffee increases rectal motility within 4 minutes of ingestion; approximately 30% of normal university students report that coffee induces a desire to defecate.

ANORECTAL RESPONSES TO RECTAL DISTENTION

These vary according to the rate and pattern of distention.[10]

Rapid Intermittent Distention

Rapid intermittent inflation of a balloon with increasing volumes of air or liquid, mimicking rapid dumping of fecal material in the rectum, induces rectal contraction, IAS relaxation, and EAS contraction.

Rectal Pressures

The initial increase in rectal pressure that occurs when a balloon is inflated rapidly in the rectum is often followed by a secondary transient increase in pressure, probably caused by rectal contraction. The pressure then gradually subsides to a steady baseline as the rectum accommodates to the new volume. As the distending volume increases, the phasic rectal pressure response increases in amplitude and duration and the steady state pressures increase. Eventually the rectum

fails to accommodate the new volume and a large increase in steady-state pressure is observed when the balloon is distended.[10,72] This increase in pressure is often associated with pain.

The slope of the relationship between steady-state pressure and volume has been used to calculate values for rectal compliance (dV/dP). Values for the tension of the rectal wall have also been calculated from the pressure data by the Laplace law.[72] This calculation relies on the assumption that the radius of a balloon in the rectum is the same as it is outside the body.

There are major problems in comparing values for rectal compliance from different groups of patients and different centers. First, values depend on the shape and size of the balloon, its distention characteristics, and its position in the rectum. Second, values obtained during intermittent distention are very different from values obtained during ramp inflation.[10] Third, the relationship between rectal pressure and volume is sigmoid in shape (Fig. 8B-2). Thus, values for compliance calculated from one section of the profile are very different from values obtained at other regions. More recently, there has been a tendency to calculate compliance from the changes in volume and pressure induced by a single maximal or submaximal volume. This may be grossly misleading because the pressure rises steeply at these volumes and the number obtained may not be representative of the viscoelastic properties of the rectum. We recently found that values for compliance were three times higher when calculated from dV/dP at 100

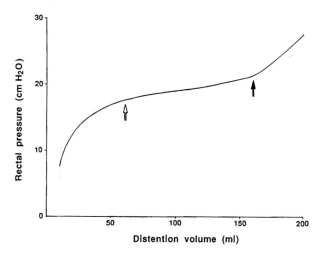

Fig. 8B-2 Diagram of the rectal pressure-volume relationship during balloon inflation of the rectum at the rate of 50 ml/min. The open arrow indicates the sensation of wind (gas), the closed arrow a desire to defecate.

ml than when compliance at each volume (10, 20, 40, 60, and 100) were averaged.[10]

Despite these limitations, rectal compliance appears to be reduced in normal elderly subjects.[73] Glick and colleagues[74] reported that the tone and compliance of the distal colon is reduced in patients with high spinal lesions; Sun, Read, and Donnelly observed similar results in the rectum.[75] White and colleagues[76] reported that rectal tone was reduced and compliance was increased in patients with low spinal lesions, but the authors were unable to confirm this finding in patients with incomplete spinal lesions.[75] The differences in results can almost certainly be explained by the methodological factors listed above.

The phasic contractile response to rectal distention is reduced or absent in patients with lesions involving the low spinal cord,[43,76] suggesting that it is mediated by a spinal reflex. It is exaggerated and induced at lower distending volumes in patients with complete supraconal lesions, indicating modulation by descending inhibitory pathways.[45]

Sensation

Normal subjects perceive rectal distention at 10 to 20 ml. The sensation, especially at low volumes, is transient but becomes prolonged and changes in quality as volume increases. Low volumes induce a sensation of gas in the rectum ("wind"). As the volume increases, the subjects experience a desire to defecate, a more urgent desire to defecate, and finally pain. Rectal sensitivity is increased in old age.[73]

Sphincter Response

Intermittent distention of the rectal balloon induces a transient increase in anal pressure that is associated with an increase in the electrical activity of the EAS[38] (Fig. 8B-1). This is followed by a decline in anal pressure and is associated with suppression of the IAS electrical oscillations.[32,40] As the rectal balloon is distended with larger volumes, the amplitude and duration of relaxation increases.[8,32,38,40,77]

On deflating the balloon, anal pressures often exceed the values observed immediately before inflation. The rebound increases in pressure are always associated with increases in the amplitude of the IAS slow wave, but only transient increases in the activity of the EAS.[32] The rebound response is absent in patients with high spinal cord lesions,[45,75] suggesting it may be mediated by activity in the sympathetic nerves.

The relaxation of the IAS in response to rectal distention is mediated by an intramural reflex; it is not abolished by spinal anesthesia in man,[41] but disappears in experimental animals after rectal application of cocaine, and after low rectal transection.[52,78,79] Schuster and coworkers[80] and Naudy and others[81] have shown that distention of the more proximal regions of the colon may cause IAS relaxation. IAS relaxation is probably modulated by activity in the spinal cord since there is no relationship between the degree of distention and the amplitude of relaxation in either patients with meningocoele,[40] patients with high spinal anesthesia,[41] or patients with high spinal lesions.[75] Patients with complete supraconal lesions still show a graded response to rectal distention, but the relaxation is exaggerated and induced at lower volumes.[45]

After an initial burst of activity, the electrical activity of the EAS reduces to a steady state which increases in amplitude and duration as the rectal volume increases. Very high levels of rectal distention are associated with an abolition of EAS activity causing a profound reduction in anal pressure.[82] This is rare in normal subjects with rectal volumes of up to 200 ml.

In patients with complete spinal transection, balloon distention of the rectum induces a brief increase in EAS activity[45,82–84] which indicates that the response is a spinal reflex.[56] The EAS response is absent during sleep.[85] Moreover, both the onset and duration of the electrical activity of the EAS are strongly linked with rectal sensation.[86] Thus the EAS response to rectal distention is heavily modulated by conscious mechanisms in normal subjects. Both sensation and EAS response are also correlated with the duration of the phasic rectal activity,[86] suggesting the possibility that both are induced by stimulation of rapidly adapting rectal mechanoreceptors.[87]

Ramp Inflation

Rectal Pressures and Sensation

Responses to rectal sensation are different if the rectum is distended by ramp inflation.[10] Normal subjects feel the typical rectal sensations in the same sequence as they do during intermittent distention: perception of the balloon, sensation of wind, desire to defecate, and finally discomfort or pain. Each sensation, however, is perceived at lower volumes during ramp inflation, and is sustained until superseded by the next sensation. The start of each sensation appears to be associated with specific points on the rectal pressure/volume profile. Sensation is first perceived during the initial rapid rise in pressure. A feeling of wind occurs near the beginning of the plateau phase when the rectum is relaxing to accommodate the increasing volume. A desire to defecate is associated with the onset of phasic rectal contractions and occurs when the rectum has reached its limit of accommodation and pressure again begins to rise steeply (Fig. 8B-2). Each sensation occurs at a sequentially lower volume when the infusion rate is slowed from 100 ml/min through 50 and 20 to 10 ml/min, and this is associated with shallower pressure volume curves, indicating greater receptive relaxation or rectal accommodation.[10] These results are incompatible with a simple volume or pressure receptor; instead they suggest the triggering of a slowly adapting tension receptor lying parallel with the circular muscle of the rectal wall.[88] Such a receptor would be subjected to a greater degree of stimulation when the rectum relaxes; and relaxation appears to take place earlier and at lower volumes when the infusion rate is lowest.

IAS Response

The internal anal sphincter may not relax at all at the slowest distention rates, even when very large volumes are infused into the rectum. IAS relaxation is not associated with rectal sensation and EAS activity during ramp inflation.[10] These results suggest that an important role of the IAS is to maintain continence when the rectum slowly fills with feces or gas.

EAS Response

The electrical activity of the EAS remains at basal levels as long as rectal distention is not perceived. The perception of the balloon increases the electrical activity of the EAS, and this increase is maintained or escalated as the infusion volumes rise. The onset of each new sensation is associated with a burst of EAS electrical activity.[10]

DYNAMIC STUDIES OF ANORECTAL FUNCTION

More information on the relationship between anorectal responses and continence may be gained by recording anorectal pressures when the rectum is distended with fluid.[26,89] This mimics the situation that occurs when the sphincter is trying to retain a large volume of liquid feces in the rectum. In the authors' studies,[26,89] saline was infused into the rectum at a rate of 60 ml/min for 25 minutes. A few minutes after the start of the infusion, a regular series of anal relaxations developed (Fig. 8B-3). After a few more minutes these were accompanied by contractions of the rectum and the EAS. The frequency of these oscillations was approximately 1/min (similar to that of the ultraslow wave) and increased as more fluid was infused.

In normal subjects, continence appeared to be maintained during rectal infusion of saline by the residual tone of the sphincter; as such, the results resemble those from ramp distention. Inhibition of sphincter tone was less than that which could be elicited by balloon distention of the rectum, and the peak rectal pressures were always lower than the lowest anal sphincter pressures. Phasic contraction of the EAS appeared to play little part in the maintenance of continence in normal sub-

Fig. 8B-3 Typical record of anal and rectal pressure fluctuation and external sphincter electromyogram (EMG) during rectal infusion of saline in a normal subject. Note that regular increases in rectal pressure occur at the same time as anal relaxations and external sphincter contractions (seen on the anal pressure and EMG channels). (Reprinted from Henry MM, Swash M, eds, *Coloproctology and the Pelvic Floor—Pathophysiology and Management*, London: Butterworths; 1983:77, with permission.)

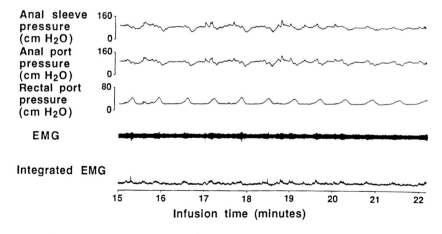

jects, since contraction was only transient and occurred before the deepest relaxation of the IAS.[26] No subject exhibited sustained forcible contraction of the EAS in an attempt to retain fluid in the rectum.[26,86] Incorporation of only very small amounts of bile acid in the infusion solution increased the rectal contractile activity and the depth of anal relaxations and caused leakage at a much earlier stage.[90]

RESPONSES TO INCREASES IN INTRAABDOMINAL PRESSURE

Increases in intraabdominal pressure caused by subjects blowing up a balloon are associated with a compensatory increase in the activity of the external anal sphincter, causing the sphincter pressure to increase above the rectal pressure and maintain continence.[25] This response is graded according to the intraabdominal pressure[91] and is thought to be triggered by receptors in the pelvic floor acting through a spinal reflex.[92] If subjects are asked to strain as if to defecate, many of them can prevent the compensatory increase in EAS activity. As a result, the sphincter pressure is lowered and defecation is facilitated. Patients with complete supraconal spinal lesions are unable to facilitate defecation by suppressing the spinal reflex.

Gender Differences in Anorectal Function

There are large differences in anorectal function between men and women.[25] Anal pressures under resting conditions and during a maximum contraction of the sphincter are lower in women than in men, particularly if they have had several children. The anal canal is also shorter in women.[93] The rectum is more sensitive to distention in women and anorectal motor responses are induced at lower volumes. Rectal compliance is lower in women than men. The only major difference in the anal response to rectal distention between men and women is that lower volumes are required to induce 50% of maximum relaxation in women.

THE USE OF ANORECTAL MANOMETRY TO IDENTIFY THE CAUSE OF FECAL INCONTINENCE

Normal Maintenance of Continence

Under resting conditions and during gradual distention of the rectum (approximately 10 ml/min) with gas or fluid, continence to rectal mucus and feces appears to be maintained by the tonic contraction of the IAS, with some assistance from tonic activity of the external anal sphincter.[10] Circularly oriented muscle fibers are unable to shorten sufficiently to seal off the anal canal unless they contract around an anal lining that is sufficiently bulky to plug the orifice. The bulk of the anal lining is increased by infolding when the sphincter is contracted, and also by the presence of expansile vascular cushions that act to seal the sphincter while stretching the muscle so that the circular muscle fibers can contract with a greater mechanical advantage.[94,95] This explains why a radical hemorrhoidectomy is associated with a high incidence of anal seepage.[96]

The sphincter is unable to maintain continence when threatened by rectal contraction, rapid rectal distention, and increases in intraabdominal pressure. This is because rapid rectal distention and contraction cause a reflex relaxation of the IAS, mediated by intrinsic nerves, whereas rises in intraabdominal pressure may be of sufficient magnitude to overwhelm the resting sphincter pressure. Continence can only be maintained under these conditions by a compensatory contraction of the EAS. The EAS response to rectal distention is heavily modulated by conscious mechanisms and is very closely linked with rectal sensation.[86]

Contraction of the EAS during relaxation of the IAS increases the resistance of the sphincter, particularly in its outermost aspect, while allowing the composition of the rectal contents to be sampled by the sensitive anal lining.[97] The sampling of the rectal contents by the anal sensors has been proposed as the mechanism whereby people can discriminate between solid stool, liquid feces, and flatus. It is possible, however, that solid and fluid (gas or liquid) rectal contents may be identified by their ability to stimulate rapidly adapting rectal stretch receptors in the rectal wall. When asked, most people report that they can perceive gaseous distention as a rectal sensation, and many normal people find it difficult to distinguish between gas and liquid when they have diarrhea.

Simultaneous contraction of the puborectalis muscle assists the EAS in maintaining continence by making the anorectal angle more acute. It is easy to see how a more acute anorectal angle impedes the entry of a solid cylindrical stool into the anal canal, but it would not aid continence to liquids unless the upper anal canal was compressed against a relatively fixed object such as the cervix uteri or the prostate gland.

The EAS and IAS contract in a reciprocal manner during attempts to maintain continence. For example, rectal distention and contraction cause relaxation of the

IAS, but a compensatory contraction of the EAS. In contrast, Salducci and coworkers[98] reported that micturition is associated with relaxation of the EAS and contraction of the IAS. This reciprocal activity may partly explain why patients who have weakness of both IAS and EAS tend to be more incontinent than those who have EAS weakness alone.

Investigation of Patients with Fecal Incontinence

Fecal incontinence can result from impairment of any of several components of the continence mechanisms. Clinical assessment of anorectal function must do the following:

1. Provide dynamic information about the integrated function of each component.
2. Mimic situations where continence is threatened.
3. Discriminate between different treatment options.
4. Be reasonably comfortable for the patient.
5. Not interfere unduly with normal physiologic function of the anorectum.

In the authors' laboratory a multichannel recording technique is used to measure pressures at multiple sites in the anus and the rectum and the electrical activity of the external and internal anal sphincters (Fig. 8B-4) under resting conditions, during conscious contraction of the external sphincter, and during threats to continence induced by rapid rectal distention and increases in intraabdominal pressure (Fig. 8B-1). Rectal sensations during rectal distention are recorded on the chart and any leakage of perfusion fluid is noted.

The recording of anorectal pressures from multiple closely spaced sites facilitates the identification of abnormalities of internal or external sphincter function. The two muscles often exhibit reciprocal activity; therefore the EAS contraction that occurs, for example, during rectal distention, can mask IAS relaxation in the outermost anal channels, but not in the inner channels. Interpretation of the manometric profiles is greatly facilitated by simultaneous recording of the electrical activities of the EAS and the IAS, allowing changes in pressure caused by the activity of those muscles to be identified. Some have questioned the use of a wire electrode to record internal sphincter electromyography (EMG) in vivo, saying that the regular oscillations may be artifacts induced by muscle movement and contraction.[29] Even if that is true, the recordings still provide a useful functional index of IAS activity, representing the regular oscillations in the activity of that muscle

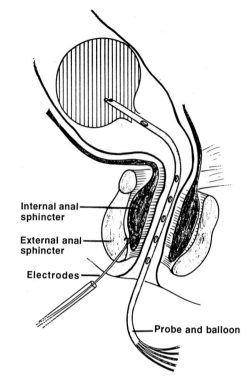

Fig. 8B-4 Diagram of the anal canal showing the different muscle components and probes used to measure pressure in multiple sites in the anal canal, and the electrical activity of IAS and EAS.

which are abolished when the muscle relaxes during rectal distention, and increase in amplitude during rebound contraction.

The authors' experience is that combined anorectal manometry and electrophysiology revealed abnormalities in all except three out of a total of 302 patients referred with fecal incontinence over a period of two consecutive years.[99] The majority of patients had several abnormalities. The test can be used with other clinical information to identify different causes of fecal incontinence, each of which logically would require a different treatment (Table 8B-1).

WEAKNESS OF THE EXTERNAL ANAL SPHINCTER

Most but not all patients (92.2%) had squeeze pressures that were below the normal range. External sphincter responses to rectal distention and increases in intraabdominal pressure were also impaired, and nearly all of these patients leaked the perfusion fluid during these maneuvers.

Table 8B-1
Causes of Fecal Incontinence That Can Be Identified by Physiological Testing

Causes	Features	Possible Treatment
Pudendal neuropathy	Perineal descent Weak conscious and reflex EAS contractions Normal electrical responses	Postanal repair
Obstetric trauma	Weak sphincter Circumferential electrical gap	Sphincter repair
Impaired rectal sensation	1. IAS relaxes at volumes that fail to induce sensation and EAS response 2. Delayed sensation and EAS response	Retraining
Low spinal lesion	Impaired rectal sensation. Reduced rectal tone. Absent EAS responses to rectal distention and increases in intraabdominal pressure	Training
High spinal lesion	Absent rectal sensation Little conscious control of EAS Enhanced reflex activity of EAS	Training
Irritable bowel syndrome	Enhanced rectal sensitivity Reduced rectal compliance Increased rectal contraction, and anal relaxation in response to rectal distention	Drugs Diet Psychotherapy
Spontaneous relaxation IAS	Inappropriate IAS relaxations under resting conditions and after squeeze and strain	? Drugs
Impaired IAS tone	Very low pressures No IAS relaxation on rectal distention	? Sympathomimetic drugs

Weakness of the EAS can result from several different mechanisms: pudendal neuropathy, trauma to the sphincter, or lesions in either the cauda equina, brain, or spinal cord. These diagnoses can be differentiated by a combination of physiologic and clinical criteria.

Pudendal Neuropathy

Pudendal neuropathy is the most common cause of fecal incontinence. More than half of our patients with weak external sphincters also exhibited abnormal perineal descent in that their pelvic floor descended more than 2 cm when they strained. Nearly all of these patients were women and most had multiple vaginal deliveries. In this group, 52% also had clinical evidence of either rectal prolapse, anterior mucosal prolapse, or solitary rectal ulcer.

Weakness of the EAS is thought to occur when the distal segment of the pudendal nerve becomes stretched and compressed against the ischial spine. This situation may arise from weakness of the pelvic floor caused by childbirth or by prolonged straining at stool. This would account for the abnormal degree of pelvic floor descent. The diagnosis can be proven by neurophysiologic tests. Single fiber or concentric needle electromyography[100] shows the prolonged motor unit po-

tentials that indicate reinnervation, whereas pre-rectal stimulation of the pudendal nerve demonstrates a prolonged pudendal nerve terminal motor latency.[101] For the vast majority of patients, however, such tests are unnecessary; the combination of perineal descent and sphincter weakness is sufficient support for the diagnosis. The only indication for neurophysiologic tests is when sphincter weakness due to a lesion in the spinal cord or cauda equina is suspected. A postanal repair is often successful, providing the pelvic floor and sphincter are not too weak.

Obstetric Trauma

It is not uncommon for patients to be referred many years after their last delivery for investigation of fecal incontinence due to anal tears. In our study,[99] 7% of women with weak external sphincters had a defect in their external sphincter ring on examination and a history of a perineal tear during childbirth. The average time from their last childbirth to the first time they sought medical help for fecal incontinence was 14 years (range 2 to 40 years). All of these patients reported that although they were aware of the threat of incontinence, they were unable to prevent it.

The sphincter defect usually results from inadequate suture of the torn sphincter. The manometric features of a mechanically weak sphincter with normal electromyographic responses cannot usually be distinguished from pudendal neuropathy, expect when a reduction in anal pressure during a conscious contraction indicates the gaping of a divided sphincter. The diagnosis requires a careful obstetric history and physical examination. Careful palpation of the anovaginal region with the index finger in the vagina and the thumb in the anus usually establishes the diagnosis. Mapping out the site of the defect by recording EAS activity around the circumference of the sphincter or by endoanal ultrasonography can facilitate diagnosis and guide the surgeon.[102]

When obstetric trauma is the only factor responsible for sphincter weakness, direct repair of the defect has a good prognosis. In many cases, obstetric trauma is associated with weakness of the pelvic floor and pudendal neuropathy. Sphincter repair is unsuccessful in patients with no EAS electrical activity.

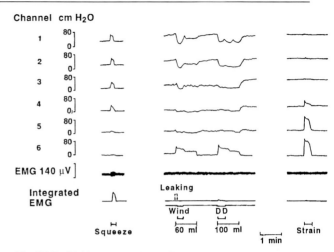

Fig. 8B-5 Multiport recordings of anal pressure and the electrical activity of the EAS during maximum contraction of the external anal sphincter, during rectal distention, and during straining (as if to defecate) in a patient with low spinal lesion. Channels 1 to 6 represent ports situated 0.5, 1.0, 2.0, 2.5, and 4.5 cm from the anal verge and in the balloon 5 to 11 cm from the anal margin. Note that there is appropriate contraction of the sphincter, but no increase in activity generated by rectal distention and increase in intraabdominal pressure.

Spinal Lesions

More than 40 patients referred to our unit with fecal incontinence over 2 years had evidence of spinal injury or disease on anorectal function testing, although injury or disease were not evident on history or physical examination. Unlike other causes of external sphincter weakness, equal numbers of men and women had evidence of spinal lesions. These patients are important to recognize because anorectal symptoms may be an early finding in progressive neurologic disease.

Occult spinal injury or disease is an important cause of incontinence associated with weakness of the EAS. The diagnosis is suspected if impaired or absent conscious contraction of the EAS is associated with blunted rectal sensitivity. The identification of low spinal cord or cauda equina lesions as opposed to high spinal lesions depends on whether EAS responses to rectal distention or increases in intraabdominal pressure are absent or enhanced.[75]

Patients with low spinal or cauda equina lesions have absent external sphincter electrical and mechanical responses to rectal distention and increases in intraabdominal pressure (Fig. 8B-5). Lesions in the cauda equina may abolish spinal reflexes by desynchronizing the volley of impulses traveling along the afferent nerves to the cord.[75]

Patients with high spinal lesions show enhanced, but transient sphincter activity during rectal distention or increases in intraabdominal pressure caused by inflating a party balloon (Fig. 8B-6). EAS activity will also be enhanced when they move their legs or cough. This keeps the anal pressures above rectal pressures so that leakage is rare. None of these patients could contract their sphincters consciously.

If a cerebrospinal cause for fecal incontinence is suspected, then neurophysiologic tests are indicated to confirm the site of the lesion, followed by neurologic consultation and sophisticated imaging techniques.

In most cases, there is no specific treatment for the neurologic condition, and patients with incontinence related to spinal lesions do not respond to anal surgery or drugs. Some success, however, may be achieved by retraining techniques, though patients who are profoundly disabled may require a colostomy.

Weakness of Internal Anal Sphincter

Weakness of the internal anal sphincter is found in a surprisingly high percentage of patients.[103] Of our patients,[99] 32% showed very low basal pressures and no IAS relaxation when the rectum was distended (Fig.

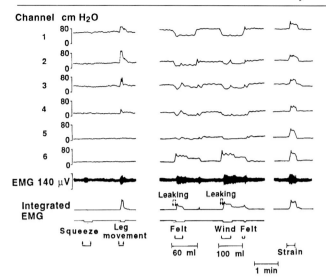

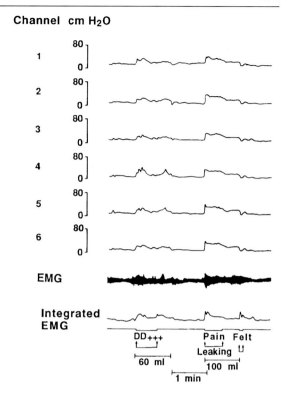

Fig. 8B-6 Recording of anorectal pressures at ports situated 0.5, 1.0, 2.0, 2.5, and 4.5 cm from the anal margin and in the balloon 5 to 11 cm from anal verge (channels 1 to 6) and the electrical activity of sphincter complex in a patient with a high spinal lesion during attempts at sphincter contraction, during rectal balloon distention with 60 and 100 ml of air, and during increases in intraabdominal pressure (strain). There is no conscious contraction of the sphincter but reflex response to rectal distention and increase in intraabdominal pressure are much increased. The pressure and EAS activity were greatly increased during leg movement.

Fig. 8B-7 Recordings of anorectal pressure and the electrical activity of the sphincter in a female patient with impaired IAS function before, during, and after inflation of a rectal balloon with 60 and 100 ml of air. Channels 1 to 6 represent ports situated 0.5, 1.0, 1.5, 2.0, 2.5, and 4.5 cm, respectively, from the anal verge. Note the absence of IAS electrical activity and the abnormally low basal anal pressures, and the absence of anal relaxation during rectal distention. This increase is associated with an increase in the electrical activity of the EAS. No rebound pressures were observed on deflating the rectal balloon. The bars (⊔) indicate when the subject experienced rectal sensation. DD = desire to defecate and + + + indicates the severity of the sensation. (Reprinted from *Gastroenterology.* 1989;97:133, with permission.)

8B-7). The latter indicated that the IAS tone was already so low that it could not relax further. The electrical record showed attenuated or absent IAS electrical oscillations. The abnormally low anal pressures rule out Hirschsprung's disease.[104–106] The absent or delayed IAS relaxation in these patients is not associated with an insensitive and hypercompliant rectum.[107,108]

Nearly all of the patients with IAS weakness also had an abnormally weak external sphincter.[103] Maximum squeeze pressures and the EAS pressure responses to rectal distention and to increase in intraabdominal pressure were lower in patients with IAS dysfunction than in any other group of incontinent patients we studied, and these patients were more severely incontinent than patients who just had weakness of the EAS. Most of these patients also had an abnormal degree of pelvic floor descent. Perhaps the extremely weak striated muscle exposes the IAS to traction by the tissues of the pelvic floor. Alternatively, the abnormal descent of the pelvic floor may damage the delicate sympathetic nerves that are thought to enhance the tone of the IAS.[28,48,51,109]

Christensen and Rich[110] suggested that excitatory nerves supplying the IAS may also travel in the pudendal nerve. If that is so, then the IAS weakness may also be due to pudendal neuropathy.

Unfortunately, our experience suggests that patients with combined EAS and IAS weakness do not do well after postanal repair. The use of pharmacologic agents to increase IAS tone needs to be explored.

Spontaneous Transient Anal Relaxation

More than a quarter of patients referred to our unit for investigation of fecal incontinence showed episodes of spontaneous IAS relaxation at rest lasting at least 15

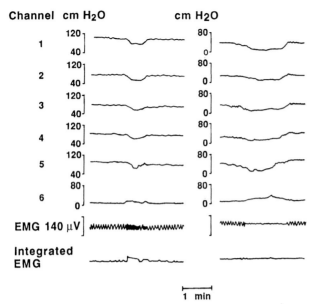

Channel cm H₂O

Fig. 8B-8 Multiport recordings of anal pressure and the electrical activities of the EAS and IAS during and after an episode of spontaneous anal relaxation in a normal subject *(left)* and an incontinent patient *(right)*. Channels 1 to 6 represent ports situated 0.5, 1.0, 1.5, 2.0, 2.5, and 4.5 cm, respectively, from the anal verge. The relaxation lasted longer in the patient and was not associated with a compensatory increase in external sphincter activity.

Transient IAS relaxations are also more common in these patients immediately after a conscious contraction or increase in intraabdominal pressure. Postsqueeze or poststrain relaxations are rare in normal subjects.

Of patients with transient anal relaxations, 75% had abnormal rectal sensitivity, typical of a subset of patients with irritable bowel syndrome. Perhaps the exquisite rectal sensitivity in these patients causes the IAS to relax in response to the slightest provocation.

Surgery is not indicated in patients with transient IAS relaxations unless there is another cause for incontinence, but perhaps the use of drugs to stabilize IAS contractions needs to be explored.

Transient relaxations of the sphincter may be important in the nocturnal incontinence observed in patients with diabetic autonomic neuropathy. Normally the colon is quiescent during sleep and does not exhibit the strong propagated contractions that are frequently seen after getting up in the morning.[114,115] Neuropathy involving the sympathetic control of the gut could conceivably result in colonic secretion and more frequent propulsive contractions. If these contractions propelled material into the rectum while subjects were asleep, they would cause a relaxation of the IAS. Because the patient is unconscious and rectal sensation diminished in this condition, the anal relaxation would not be accompanied by a compensatory contraction of the EAS,[85] and the patient would be incontinent.

seconds and reducing the pressure in the outermost anal channels by at least 20 cm/H²O[111] (Figure 8B-8). The same phenomenon is seen in a similar percentage of normal subjects, but they are able to simultaneously contract the EAS, thus maintaining the anal pressure barrier and guarding against incontinence. However, in incontinent patients, the relaxations are of a longer duration and the anal pressure falls to lower values. Few of the incontinent patients with transient IAS relaxation showed compensatory increases in EAS activity. Transient relaxations have also been observed in prolonged ambulatory recordings from the anal sphincter.

IAS relaxations are normally evoked by rectal distention, such as might be caused by the entry of flatus or feces into the rectum, or by rectal contraction.[43,112,113] Most episodes of transient IAS relaxation recorded in patients studied, however, appeared to be due either to autonomous losses of internal sphincter tone or to reductions in tone provoked by events that did not increase pressure in the rectum.[40] In this regard, Naudy and others[81] have shown that distention of more proximal regions of the colon can cause sphincter relaxation.

Impaired Rectal Sensation

The ability of the patient to perceive the distention of the rectum caused by, for example, the arrival of feces, appears to be necessary for the prompt and appropriate contractile response of the EAS.[86] EAS responses occur as soon as a rectal sensation is perceived and occur for the same period of time. Conscious perception of rectal distention is not necessary for relaxation of the IAS. Thus patients with impaired rectal sensation are incontinent because they fail to contract the EAS to compensate for a relaxation of the IAS, induced by rectal distention or contraction. Leakage of perfusion fluid is common but ceases as soon as the patient perceives the distention or leakage and contracts the EAS.[86]

Two abnormalities can be seen during manometric and electrophysiologic tests. In the first, the rectal volume that induces IAS relaxation is lower than that which induces rectal sensation and an increase in EAS activity[86,116] (Fig. 8B-9). This abnormality probably accounts for the incontinence in patients with megarec-

Channel cm H₂O

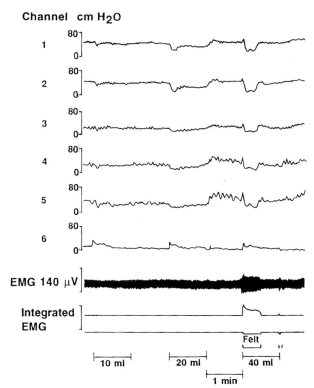

Fig. 8B-9 Recordings of anal pressures at ports situated 0.5, 1.0, 1.5, 2.0, 2.5, and 4.5 cm from the anal margin (channels 1 to 6) and the electrical activity of the EAS, during distention of a rectal balloon with 10, 20, and 40 ml of air in a patient. Note that the rectal distention of 10 and 20 ml induced IAS relaxation and increased rectal pressure but did not elicit rectal sensation, hence no electrical activity of EAS. Distention with 40 ml caused rectal sensation which induced increased electrical activity of EAS.

Channel cm H₂O

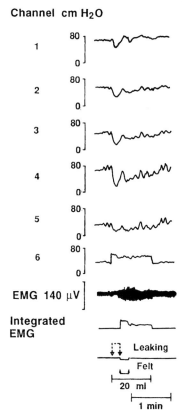

Fig. 8B-10 Recordings of anorectal pressures at ports situated 0.5, 1.0, 1.5, 2.0, 2.5, and 4.5 cm from the anal margin (channels 1 to 6) and the electrical activity of the external sphincter during distention of a rectal balloon with 20 ml of air in a patient with delayed sensation and EAS activity. Note that the rectal distention elicits a phasic rectal contraction and IAS relaxation. The rectal pressure is higher than the residual anal pressure at the beginning of the distention and leakage occurs. This ceases once the subject feels the rectal sensation, which triggers the EAS activity, increasing the anal pressure to a value higher than the rectal pressure.

tum and fecal impaction.[117] In the second, the EAS response is present but delayed[86,118] (Fig. 8B-10).

Surgery and drugs are ineffective in these patients, but success can be achieved by techniques of sensory and anal coordination retraining.

The Irritable Rectum

The condition known as irritable bowel syndrome (IBS) is probably not a single condition. We have argued that one important subset can be characterized by increased rectal sensitivity.[119] A large cohort of patients with irritable bowel syndrome have rectums that are much more sensitive to distention than normal subjects.[62,119–121] Patients feel a desire to defecate, urgent desire to defecate, and then pain at much lower rectal volumes than normal subjects. Rectal compliance is abnormally low in these patients[119] and sustained relaxa-

tion of the IAS and repetitive rectal contractions are induced at abnormally low rectal volumes (Fig. 8B-11).

Although these physiologic features are typical of the irritable bowel syndrome, they can also be found in inflammatory conditions such as ulcerative colitis[122] and solitary rectal ulcer syndrome.[123] Presumably the inflammatory changes sensitize the rectum. Patients with ulcerative colitis and solitary rectal ulcer syndrome also complain of typical IBS symptoms. The physiologic features of the irritable bowel syndrome can also be induced in normal volunteers by rectal infusion of low concentrations (1 mm) of bile acid.[90]

Of our incontinent patients, 45% had the sympto-

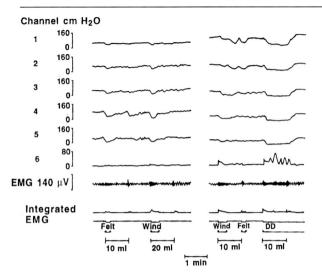

Channel cm H₂O

Fig. 8B-11 Anorectal pressure recorded during rectal distention in normal subject *(left)* and in typical IBS patient *(right)*. Channels 1 to 6 represent ports situated 0.5, 1.0, 1.5, 2.0, 2.5, and 4.5 cm from the anal verge. Note that rectal distention induces repetitive rectal contractions, sustained IAS relaxations, and a desire to defecate at lower volumes in the IBS patient compared with the normal subject.

matic and physiologic features of IBS. These patients represent about 25% of patients with IBS.[124] Rectal hyperreactivity does not usually cause incontinence if the sphincter mechanism is normal, but all of the patients with IBS and fecal incontinence had weak external sphincters and most (65%) had an abnormal degree of perineal descent. Incontinence occurs when the high rectal pressure peaks in these patients exceed the low sphincter pressure. The combination of large rectal contractions, precipitous IAS relaxation, rectal mucus, and a weak EAS makes incontinence in these patients particularly difficult to treat.

Patients with rectal prolapse and the solitary rectal ulcer syndrome also exhibit hypersensitive and hyperreactive rectums associated with extremely weak external sphincters.[123] It is not surprising that incontinence is so common in these patients.

Large Rectal Waves

There were a few patients in our series[99] who showed abnormally large rectal pressure waves ($\geq$ 20 cm/H²O, lasting $\geq$ 5 sec) during rectal distention, but did not exhibit the hypersensitivity of the irritable rectum. External sphincter responses to rectal distention were often impaired in these patients. These findings were

also quite common in patients with diabetic neuropathy (Read and Sun, unpublished observations) and it is possible they indicate damage to the autonomic nerves supplying the colon.

INVESTIGATION OF OBSTRUCTED DEFECATION

Normal Defecation

Defecation is a stereotyped sequence of actions, usually initiated by a conscious mechanism and involving a number of pelvic reflexes, that are probably coordinated by a center in the conus medullaris and controlled by a center in the pons.

Feces are propelled into the rectum by propagated colonic contractions. If the stool is large enough, rectal distention (and probably also the weight of the stool on the pelvic floor) may induce a desire to defecate. Rectal distention also induces a relaxation of the IAS and a rectal contraction that may serve to tamp the stool down into the proximal anal canal, increasing the defecatory urge. The subject sits or squats, contracts the diaphragm, contracts the abdominal muscles and levator muscles,[125,126] while relaxing the external sphincter and possibly also the puborectalis muscle, and feces are extruded. Once started, defecation continues with no conscious effort; presumably this is a result of a strong propagated colorectal contraction. Patients with complete supraconal transection of the spinal cord have automatic defecation and demonstrate exaggerated contraction of the rectum and relaxation of the sphincter in response to relatively minimal fecal amounts,[127] but when they strain to defecate they produce a paradoxical contraction of the EAS and no relaxation. This combination of defects makes it impossible for these patients to have control over defecation.

Defecation may be impaired by reduced colonic propulsion, failure of the internal anal sphincter to relax, inappropriate contraction of the external anal sphincter and puborectalis muscle, failure of the levators to lift the pelvic floor and open the anorectal angle,[125] and luminal obstruction by hemorrhoids and partial prolapse of the rectum into the anal canal. The causes of obstructed defecation can be determined and differentiated by combined anorectal manometry, electromyography, and tests of rectal sensation (Table 8B-2), but measurement of colonic transit is necessary to identify abnormal or impaired colonic propulsion. Although helpful in some patients, the arbitrary subdivision of

Table 8B-2

Causes of Obstructed Defecation That Can Be Identified by Physiological Testing

Causes	Features	Possible Treatment
Anismus	Paradoxical EAS contraction during defecation	? Retraining
Short segment Hirschsprung's disease	High anal pressures. Failure of IAS to relax on rectal distention	Sphincterotomy
Megarectum	Increased rectal compliance and capacity Reduced rectal sensation	Defecation retraining
Low spinal lesion	Impaired rectal sensation. Reduced rectal tone Absent EAS response to rectal distention and increases in intraabdominal pressure	Training
Irritable bowel syndrome	Enhanced rectal sensitivity Reduced rectal compliance Increased rectal contractility, and anal relaxation in response to rectal distention	Drugs Diet Psychotherapy
Nonprolapsing hemorrhoids	Ultra-slow waves High resting pressures Failure of outermost anal canal to relax during rectal distention	Banding Electrocoagulation Hemorrhoidectomy
Partial rectal prolapse	Very low resting pressures Failure of anal pressure to increase above rectal pressure during increases in intraabdominal pressure	Banding ? Postanal repair

patients into those with obstructed defecation and those with colonic inertia based on the evacuation of ingested radiopaque transit markers can be misleading. It now seems probable that some of the more seriously constipated patients have a central control disorder that may result in a combined impairment in colonic propulsion and sphincter relaxation.

Mechanisms of Obstructed Defecation That May Be Discriminated by Anorectal Function Tests

Anismus

Failure of the external anal sphincter to relax during defecation can be detected by asking the patient to evacuate either porridge or a solid object placed in the rectum to stimulate feces, during simultaneous recording of the electrical activity of the EMG (Fig. 8B-12). Patients with anismus fail to evacuate the object, and this is accompanied by a paradoxical increase in EAS electrical activity and a rise in sphincter pressure as the patient strains to defecate.[128–130]

Fig. 8B-12 A, Recordings of anal pressure and electrical activity of the EAS in a normal subject, and **B,** a constipated patient during attempted defecation. Note that the pressure in the anal canal and the EAS electrical activity increase during straining in the constipated patient. (Reprinted from Preston DM, Lennard-Jones JE[128] with permission.)

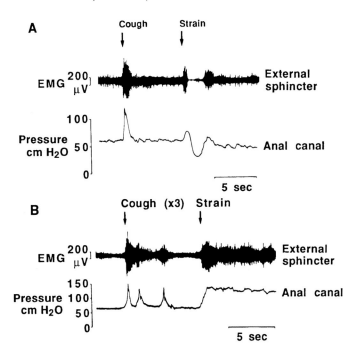

The specificity of anismus has been questioned by some investigators. It is characteristic of patients with high spinal lesions.[45] A paradoxical increase in EAS activity may also be observed in some normal subjects, possibly caused by the embarrassment of defecating while being watched.

Failure of expulsion is often not the only abnormality patients with anismus exhibit; if it were, then feces would probably collect in the rectum as impacted masses. The rectum of these patients usually is empty and many of them show abnormalities of colonic propulsion. Some patients with anismus also have a selective disturbance in rectal sensation in that the threshold rectal volume required to induce a desire to defecate is abnormally high whereas the threshold required to induce other sensations are often normal.[130] This combination of abnormalities suggests perhaps a disorder in the central nervous control of defecation.

The independent role of anismus is also questioned by the disappointing results of therapy to reduce external sphincter activity. Anal myotomy,[131,132] paralysis of the sphincter with botulinus toxin, and even colostomy have not had the anticipated levels of success in patients with anismus. Some investigators found that biofeedback training to relax the external sphincter can induce normal defecation in female patients with anismus,[133] but only after several weeks of intensive therapy. Others have had less success. It is possible that the patients are receiving more benefit from the long periods of psychologic support that accompanies the physiologic retraining. Devroede[134] has written on the important relationship between constipation and psychologic disturbance in patients with severe constipation.

Failure of the Internal Sphincter to Relax During Rectal Distention

Failure of the internal sphincter to relax during rectal distention is, in our experience, a fairly common finding during the manometric investigation of patients with constipation. Only a few of these patients have Hirschsprung's disease.

Diagnostic confusion can arise unless pressures are measured at multiple sites and combined with electromyography. For example, IAS relaxation in the outermost anal channels can be obscured by compensatory EAS contraction. Patients with nonprolapsing hemorrhoids may fail to relax the outermost part of the sphincter, possibly because the high pressure in the vascular tissue buffers the decline in anal tone.[33] Some constipated patients have abnormally low basal pressures. These patients probably do not demonstrate anal

relaxation because the sphincter has no tone and is already relaxed.[103] Finally, patients with megarectum may require abnormally large distending volumes to stimulate the rectal tension receptors that mediate anal relaxation. Since we have used combined electromyography and multiport manometry, we have only diagnosed three cases of short segment Hirschsprung's disease in the last five years. Perhaps its importance as a cause of adult constipation has been overestimated.

Most patients with severe constipation but whose sphincter is capable of relaxing have a sphincter that relaxes at an abnormally high distention threshold. In most cases this is not associated with an abnormally large rectal capacity, which requires larger volumes to stimulate tension receptors. Only very few of our younger patients had a megarectum. Furthermore, the distention threshold required to induce anal relaxation in elderly patients with megarectum is normal.[117]

A few patients have an abnormally hypertonic, hypertrophic internal sphincter[104-106] that relaxes, but often incompletely and after high degrees of distention. Kamm and colleagues[135] have recently reported a family with constipation and hypertrophy of the IAS diagnosed at ultrasound.

Hemorrhoids

It is our experience that patients with nonprolapsing or first degree hemorrhoids commonly complain of obstructed defecation; often the stools are small, require much effort to expel, and can get stuck in the anal canal behind the ballooning anal cushions.[33] Manometric studies in patients with nonprolapsing piles show abnormally high pressures and ultraslow waves.[30,33] When the rectum is distended with a balloon, pressures in the outer aspect of the anal canal remain elevated even though the internal sphincter is relaxed and the activity of the external sphincter is not increased (Fig. 8B-13). Recent observations from our laboratory suggest that high residual pressure is probably caused by the elevated pressure within the vascular spaces.[33]

Solitary Rectal Ulcer Syndrome

Patients with partial prolapse of the anterior rectal wall into the anal canal complain of a frequent urge to defecate but an inability to expel any stool despite long periods of straining. Passage of stool does not usually abolish the urge to defecate. Prolonged straining may cause the rectal wall to emerge as a red berry at the anus, and this feature may be confused with hemorrhoids. The manometric findings, however, are quite distinct. Unlike hemorrhoids, basal and squeeze pressures often are very low, the internal sphincter tone may be absent[123] (Fig. 8B-13), and the anal pressure fails to exceed rises in intraabominal pressure. These patients appear to be attempting to herniate their rectum through an extremely weak sphincter. Other patients may have normal sphincter tone, but when they increase their intraabdominal pressure the sphincter relaxes so that the rectal wall can enter the anal canal (Read and Sun, unpublished observations).

Impaired Rectal Sensitivity

Blunted rectal sensitivity is a common feature of patients with constipation. It is not usually an isolated defect. In elderly patients and children, it is commonly associated with a megarectum, increased rectal compliance, and fecal impaction; in patients with spinal disease, it is associated with weakness of the external sphincter and impairment of EAS responses to rectal distention; in young to middle-aged adults, it is often associated with reduced rectal compliance. We have recently observed that both rectal compliance and sensitivity are reduced when the rectum of normal volun-

teers is distended at a rapid instead of a slow rate.[10] It is possible that the increased tonic contraction of the rectal smooth muscle may shield in-parallel tension receptors from stimulation.

Megarectum

Megarectum is a common finding in elderly people or children with constipation. The major pathophysiologic features are an increase in rectal capacity and a profound reduction in rectal sensitivity, such that much larger volumes are required to induce a desire to defecate.[136] Thus, patients with megarectum probably become fecally impacted because they are unable to detect the presence of a fecal mass in the rectum until it is too large to be expelled. After the fecal mass is removed from the rectum, elderly patients with fecal impaction are quite able to evacuate simulated stools, if they are told that something is there.[117]

Is the reduction in rectal sensation a primary neuropathy or can it occur as a result of conscious retention of stool? The successful outcome of retraining techniques in children with fecal impaction suggest that the latter is possible. However, children with fecal impaction often have anismus. They can be successfully trained to

Fig. 8B-13 Recordings of anorectal pressure and the electrical activity of EAS and IAS in patients with solitary rectal ulcer syndrome *(left)*, nonprolapsing hemorrhoids *(right)*, during rectal balloon distention with 60 and 100 ml of air. Channels 1 to 6 represent ports situated at 0.5, 1.0, 1.5, 2.0, 2.5, and 4.5 cm from the anal verge. Note there are no anal relaxations in the outermost channels, although the inner channels showing normal relaxation and the IAS electrical activity is abolished in hemorrhoid patients. Patients with solitary rectal ulcer syndrome showed lower basal pressure, rectal distention induced increases in anal pressure, and repetitive rectal contraction.

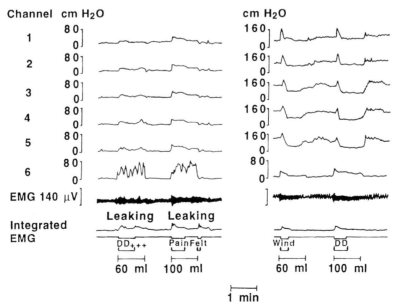

defecate, but results to retraining are poor if rectal sensation is impaired.[13] The concomitant blunting of anal and perianal sensation that is found in the elderly patient suggests a defect in nervous control[117] and response to defecation training is often disappointing.

Irritable Bowel Syndrome

Many patients who complain of constipation have enhanced rectal sensitivity and anorectal reactivity that indicates an irritable rectum. A careful history reveals that although these patients complain of constipation, they often have a frequent desire to defecate, but are unable to expel the small pellets that they produce from the rectum. Studies from our laboratory have shown that as the size of a simulated spherical hard fecal pellet is reduced, higher pressures and more prolonged straining are required to expel it through the anus.[137] Presumably, patients with a hypersensitive rectum, unlike normal subjects, feel a desire to defecate when a small fecal pellet enters the rectum, but like normal subjects, have great difficulty trying to expel it.

Disturbances in Anorectal Function After Hysterectomy

From a gastroenterologist's viewpoint, disturbances in bowel function, particularly constipation and pain, appear to be common consequences of hysterectomy. It was therefore surprising to the authors to find in a recent survey that more women experienced improvement rather than exacerbation in abdominal symptoms after hysterectomy.[138] Nevertheless, women often date the onset of their bowel disturbances to previous hysterectomy. Studies on selected patients with severe posthysterectomy constipation[139] show a reduction in rectal sensation and sigmoid motor activity, suggesting damage to the autonomic nerves supplying the distal colon. In a recent prospective study of 26 women, however, the only significant finding after hysterectomy was an increase in rectal sensitivity.[138] These changes, however, were not necessarily related to the appearance of bowel symptoms.

Conclusions

Since constipation can be caused by a disturbance in colonic propulsion as well as by a disturbance of defecation, and the pathophysiologic mechanisms are poorly understood, anorectal function tests are arguably less useful than they are in incontinent patients. Their most important application is to distinguish between the causes of internal sphincter dysfunction, to identify those patients with evidence of Hirschsprung's disease and occult spinal lesions, and to distinguish between hemorrhoids and solitary rectal ulcer syndrome. Table 8B-2 lists the various clinical conditions which anorectal manometry may help to differentiate and the treatment for each condition.

The Use of Anorectal Function Tests in the Diagnosis of Severe Perianal Pain

These patients are a particularly troublesome group to manage. Anorectal manometry has a role in the differentiation of hemorrhoids from solitary rectal ulcer syndrome, a distinction which can cause much confusion clinically. It can identify those patients who have the hypersensitive and hyperreactive rectum of IBS. A few patients may experience pain as a result of hypertrophy of the IAS. This still leaves many patients without a diagnosis. *Proctalgia fugax* is a sudden severe pain in the anal area, lasting several seconds or minutes, then disappearing completely. It is assumed to be caused by spasm of the pelvic floor muscles, but there are no established manometric or electrophysiologic correlates.

Anorectal function tests therefore are not useful when evaluating perianal pain, but are very useful when evaluating obstructed defecation and fecal incontinence.

SUMMARY

Disorders of defecation and continence are common, and the mechanisms of defecation and continence each have several component parts. The combination of multiport manometry with electrophysiologic recordings and sensory testing can in theory identify different causes of incontinence or obstructed defecation and provide a useful guide to treatment. This combination of measurements allows a detailed assessment of different components of the continence mechanism under resting conditions and during provocative maneuvers that could lead to incontinence, such as rectal distention and increases in intraabdominal pressure. In constipated patients, these tests can differentiate between an occult spinal disorder, anismus, first degree hemorrhoids, solitary rectal ulcer syndrome, and adult short segment Hirschsprung's disease.

REFERENCES

1. Harris LD, Pope CE. The descending perineum syndrome. *The Practitioner.* 1964;203:612–619.
2. Harris LD, Winnans CS, Pope CE. Determination of yield pressures: a method for measuring anal sphincter competence. *Gastroenterology.* 1966;50:754–760.
3. Katz LA, Kaufman HJ, Spiro HM. Anal sphincter pressure characteristics. *Gastroenterology.* 1967;52:513–518.
4. Dent JA. A new technique for continuous sphincter pressure measurement. *Gastroenterology.* 1976;71:263–267.
5. Duthie HL, Watts JM. Contribution of the external anal sphincter to the pressure zone in the anal canal. *Gut.* 1965;6:64–68.
6. Varma JS, Smith AN. Anorectal profilometry with the microtransducer. *Br J Surg.* 1984;71:867–869.
7. Miller R, Bartolo DCC, James D, Mortensen NJMcC. Air-filled microballoon manometry for use in anorectal physiology. *Br J Surg.* 1989;76:72–75.
8. Schuster MM, Hookman P, Hendrix TR, Mendeloff AI. Simultaneous manometric recording of internal and external anal sphincter reflexes. *Bull. Johns Hopkins Hosp.* 1965;116:79–88.
9. Bubrick MP, Godec CJ, Cass AJ. Functional evaluation of the rectal ampulla with ampullometrogram. *J Royal Soc Med.* 1980;73:234–237.
10. Sun WM, Read NW, Prior A, Daly J, Cheah SK, Grundy D. The sensory and motor responses to rectal distention vary according to rate of balloon inflation. *Gastroenterology.* 1990;99:1008–1015.
11. Akervall S, Fasth S, Nordgren S, Oresland T, Hulten L. Manovolumetry—a new method for investigation of anorectal function. *Gut.* 1988;29:614–623.
12. Miller R, Bartolo DCC, Roe AM, Mortenson NJMcC. Assessment of microtransducers in anorectal manometry. *Br J Surg.* 1988;75:40–43.
13. Loening-Baucke V. Anorectal manometry: experience with strain gauge pressure transducers for the diagnosis of Hirschsprung's disease. *J Paediat Surg.* 1983;30:999–1006.
14. Rosenberg AJ, Vela AR. A new simplified technique for pediatric anorectal manometry. *Paediatrics.* 1983;71:240–245.
15. Kumar D, Williams NS, Waldron D, Wingate DL. Prolonged manometric recording of anorectal motor activity in ambulant human subjects: evidence of periodic activity. *Gut.* 1989;30:1007–1011.
16. Diamant NE, Harris LD. Comparison of objective measurement of anal sphincter strength with anal sphincter pressures and levator ani function. *Gastroenterology.* 1969;56:110–116.
17. Read NW, Harford WV, Schmulen AC, Read MG, Santa Ana C, Fordtran JS. A clinical study of patients with fecal incontinence and diarrhea. *Gastroenterology.* 1979;76:747–756.
18. Kerremans R. *Morphological and Physiological Aspects of Anal Continence and Defecation.* Brussels: Editors Arscia; 1969.
19. Gibbons CP, Bannister JJ, Trowbridge GA, Read NW. An analysis of anal sphincter pressure and anal compliance in normal subjects. *Int J Colorect Dis.* 1986;1:231–237.
20. Duthie HL, Kwong NK, Brown B. Adaptability of the anal canal to distention. *Br J Surg.* 1970;57:388.
21. Collins CD, Brown BH, Whittaker GE, Duthie HL. New method of measuring forces in the anal canal. *Gut.* 1969;10:160–163.
22. Taylor BM, Beart RW, Phillips SF. Longitudinal and radial variations of pressure in the human anal sphincter. *Gastroenterology.* 1984;86:693–697.
23. Shafik A. A new concept of the anatomy of the anal sphincter mechanism and the physiology of defecation. The external anal sphincter: a triple-loop system. *Invest Urol.* 1975;12:412–419.
24. Sun WM, Read NW. Reflex anal dilatation; the effects of parting the buttocks on anal function in normal subjects and patients with anorectal and spinal disease. *Gut.* 1990;32:670–673.

25. Sun WM, Read NW. Anorectal function in normal subjects: the effect of gender. *Int J Colorect Dis.* 1989;4:188–196.
26. Haynes WG, Read NW. Anorectal activity in man during rectal infusion of saline: a dynamic assessment of the anal continence mechanism. *J Physiol.* 1982;330:45–56.
27. Hancock BD, Smith K. The internal sphincter and Lord's procedure for hemorrhoids. *Br J Surg.* 1975;62:833–866.
28. Bouvier M, Gonella J. Nervous control of the internal anal sphincter of the cat. *J Physiol.* 1981;310:457–469.
29. Brindley GS. Neurobiology of incontinence. In: *Ciba Foundation Symposium 151.* Chichester: John Wiley and Sons; 1990:137.
30. Hancock BD. Measurement of anal pressure and motility. *Gut.* 1976;17:645–651.
31. Penninckx F, Kerremans R, Beckers J. Pharmacological characteristics of the nonstriated anorectal musculature in cats. *Gut.* 1973;14:393–398.
32. Hancock BD. Internal sphincter and the nature of hemorrhoids. *Gut.* 1977;18:651–656.
33. Sun WM, Read NW, Shorthouse AG. Hypertensive anal cushions as a cause of high anal pressure in patients with hemorrhoids. *Br J Surg.* 1990;77:458–462.
34. Hancock BD. The internal sphincter and anal fissure. *Br J Surg.* 1977;64:92–95.
35. Gibbons CP, Read NW. Anal hypertonia in fissures: cause or effect. *Br J Surg.* 1986;73:443–445.
36. Frenckner B, Von Euler C. Influence of pudendal block on the function of the anal sphincters. *Gut.* 1975;16:482–489.
37. Lestar B, Penninckx F, Kerremans R. The composition of anal basal pressure. An in vivo or in vitro study in man. *Int J Colorect Dis.* 1989;4:118–122.
38. Bannister JJ, Read NW, Donnelly C, Sun WM. External and internal anal sphincter responses to rectal distention in normal subjects and in patients with idiopathic fecal incontinence. *Br J Surg.* 1989;76:617–621.
39. Bennett RC, Duthie HL. The functional importance of the internal sphincter. *Br J Surg.* 1964;51:355–357.
40. Meunier P, Mollard P. Control of the internal anal sphincter (manometric study with human subjects). *Pflugers Arch.* 1977;370:233–239.
41. Frenckner B, Ihre T. Influence of autonomic nerves on the internal anal sphincter in man. *Gut.* 1976;17:306–312.
42. Gunterberg B, Kewenter J, Petersen I, Stener B. Anorectal function after major resection of the sacrum with bilateral or unilateral sacrifice of sacral nerves. *Br J Surg.* 1976;63:546–554.
43. Denny-Brown D, Robertson EG. An investigation of the nervous control of defecation. *Brain.* 1935;58:256–310.
44. Frenckner B. Function of the anal sphincters in spinal man. *Gut.* 1975;16:638–644.
45. MacDonagh R, Sun WM, Read NW. Anorectal function in patients with complete supraconal spinal cord lesions. Submitted for publication, 1991.
46. Langley JN, Anderson HK. On the innervation of the pelvic and adjoining viscera. Part I. The lower portion of the intestine. *J Physiol Lond.* 1895;18:67–105.
47. Rankin FW, Learmonth JS. Section of the sympathetic nerves of the distal part of the colon and rectum in the treatment of Hirschsprung's disease and certain types of constipation. *Ann Surg.* 1930;92:710–720.
48. Schuster MM. Motor activity of rectum and anal sphincter in continence and defecation. In: Code CF, ed. *Handbook of Physiology.* Washington, DC: American Physiological Society; 1968;4:2121–2139.
49. Garrett JR, Howard ER, Jones W. The internal anal sphincter in the cat: a study of nervous mechanisms affecting tone and reflex activity. *J Physiol Lond.* 1974;243:153–166.
50. Rayner W. Characteristics of the intestinal anal sphincter and the rectum of the velvet monkey. *J Physiol Lond.* 1979;286:383–399.
51. Burleigh DE, D'Mello A. Physiology and pharmacology of the

internal anal sphincter. In: Henry MM, Swash M, eds. *Colpo-proctology and the Pelvic Floor*. London: Butterworth's; 1985; 22–41.

52. Lubowski DZ, Nicholls RI, Swash M, Jordan MJ. Neural control of internal anal sphincter function. *Br J Surg.* 1987;74:668–670.

53. Carlstedt A, Nordgren S, Fasth S, Appelgren L, Hutten L. Sympathetic nervous influence on the internal anal sphincter and rectum in man. *Int J Colorect Dis.* 1988;3:90–95.

54. Shepherd JJ, Wright PG. The response of the internal anal sphincter in man to stimulation of the presacral nerve. *Am J Dig Dis.* 1968;13:421–427.

55. Floyd WF, Walls EW. Electromyography of the sphincter ani externum in man. *J Physiol.* 1953;122:599–609.

56. Parks AG, Porter NH, Melzak J. Experimental study of the reflex mechanism controlling the muscles of the pelvic floor. *Dis Colon Rec.* 1962;5:407–414.

57. Matheson DM, Keighley M. Manometric evaluation of rectal prolapse and fecal incontinence. *Gut.* 1981;22:126–129.

58. Read MG, Read NW. Role of anorectal sensation in preserving continence. *Gut.* 1982;23:345–347.

59. Nivatvongs S, Stern HS, Fryd DS. The length of the anal canal. *Dis Col Rect.* 1981;24:600–601.

60. Connell AM. The motility of the pelvic colon. *Gut.* 1961;2:175–186.

61. Scharli AF, Keisewetter WB. Defecation and continence: some new concepts. *Dis Col Rect.* 1970;13:81–107.

62. Whitehead WF, Engel BT, Schuster MM. Irritable bowel syndrome. *Dig Dis Sci.* 1980;25:404–413.

63. Orkin BA, Hanson RB, Kelly KA. The rectal motor complex. *J Gastroint Motil.* 1989;1:5–8.

64. Prior A, Read NW. Intermittent rectal motor activity: a rectal motor complex? *Gut.* 1991;32:1360–1363.

65. Hertz AF, Newton A. The normal movements of the colon in man. *J Physiol Lond.* 1913;47:57–65.

66. Connell AM, Avery-Jones F, Rowlands GN. The motility of the pelvic colon. IV-abdominal pain associated with colonic hypermotility after meal. *Gut.* 1965;6:105–112.

67. Duthie HL. Colonic response to eating. *Gastroenterology.* 1978; 75:527–529.

68. Sun EA, Snape WJ, Cohen S, Renny A. The role of opiate receptors and cholinergic neurons in the gastrocolonic response. *Gastroenterology.* 1982;82:689–693.

69. Soffer EE, Wingate DL. Colonic motility; a new technique for prolonged ambulatory recording. *Gastroenterology.* 1988; 94:A435.

70. Wright SH, Snape WJ, Battle W, Cohen S, London RL. Effect of dietary components on the gastrocolonic response. *Am J Physiol.* 1980;238:G228–232.

71. Brown S, Cann PA, Read NW. The effect of coffee on distal colonic function. *Gut.* 1990;31:450–453.

72. Ahran P, Faverdin C, Persoz B, et al. Relationship between viscoelastic properties of the rectum and anal pressure in man. *J Appl Physiol.* 1976;41:677–682.

73. Bannister JJ, Abouzekry LA, Read NW. Effect of aging on anorectal function. *Gut.* 1987;28:353–357.

74. Glick ME, Meshkinpour H, Haldeman S, Hoehler F, Downey N, Bradley WE. Colonic dysfunction in patients with thoracic spinal cord injury. *Gastroenterology.* 1984;86:287–294.

75. Sun WM, Read NW, Donnelly TC. Anorectal function in incontinent patients with spinal disease. *Gastroenterology.* 1990;99: 1372–1379.

76. White JC, Verlot MG, Ehrentheil O. Neurogenic disturbances of the colon and their investigation by the colonmetrogram. *Ann Surg.* 1940;112:1042–1057.

77. Ahran P, Faverdin C, Thouvenot J. Anorectal motility in sick children. *Scand J Gastroenterol.* 1972;7:309–314.

78. Garry RC. The responses to stimulation of the caudal end of the large bowel in the cat. *J Physiol.* 1933;78:208–224.

79. Horgan PG, O'Connell PR, Shinkwin CA, Kirwan WO. Effect of anterior resection on anal sphincter function. *Br J Surg.* 1989; 76:783–786.

80. Schuster MM, Hendrix TR, Mendeloff AI. The internal anal sphincter response: manometric studies on its normal physiology, neural pathways and alteration in bowel disorders. *J Clin Invest.* 1963;42:196–207.

81. Naudy B, Planche D, Monges B, Salducci J. Relaxations of the internal anal sphincter, elicited by rectal and extrarectal distentions in man. In: Roman C, ed. *Gastrointestinal Motility.* London: MTP Press; 1984:451–458.

82. Porter NH. Physiological study of the pelvic floor in rectal prolapse. *Ann Roy Coll Surg Engl.* 1962;31:379–404.

83. Ihre T. Studies on anal function in continent and incontinent patients. *Scand J Gastroenterol.* 1974;9(suppl):25.

84. Goligher J, Hughes F. Sensibility of the rectum and colon: its role in the mechanism of anal incontinence. *Lancet.* 1951;1:543–548.

85. Whitehead WE, Orr WC, Engel BT, Schuster MM. External anal sphincter response to rectal distention: learned response or reflex? *Psychophysiology.* 1982;19:57–72.

86. Sun WM, Read NW, Miner PB. The relationship between rectal sensation and anal function in normal subjects and patients with fecal incontinence. *Gut.* 1990;31:1056–1061.

87. Blunberg H, Haupt P, Janig W, Kohler W. Encoding of visceral noxious stimuli in the discharge patterns of visceral afferent fibers from the colon. *Pflugers Archiv.* 1983;398:33–40.

88. Morrison JFB. Splanchnic slowly-adapting mechanoreceptors with punctate receptive fields in the mesentery and gastrointestinal tract of the gut. *J Physiol.* 1973;233;349–361.

89. Read NW, Haynes WG, Bartolo DCC, et al. Use of anorectal manometry during rectal infusion of saline to investigate sphincter function in incontinent patients. *Gastroenterology.* 1983;85: 105–113.

90. Edwards CA, Brown S, Baxter AJ, Bannister JJ, Read NW. Effect of bile acid on anorectal function in man. *Gut.* 1989;30: 383–386.

91. Womack NK, Morrison JFB, Williams NS. Impaired recruitment of the pelvic floor musculature by intraabdominal pressure in fecal incontinence. *Gut.* 1985;26:26–31.

92. Melzack JO, Porter NH. Studies of the reflex activity of the external sphincter ani in man. *Paraplegia.* 1964;1:277–296.

93. Nivatvongs S, Stern HS, Fryd DS. The length of the anal canal. *Dis Colon Rectum.* 1981;24:600–601.

94. Gibbons CP, Bannister JJ, Trowbridge GA, Read NW. An analysis of anal sphincter pressure and anal compliance in normal subjects. *Int J Colorect Dis.* 1986;1:231–237.

95. Gibbons CP, Trowbridge GA, Bannister JJ, Read NW. The mechanisms of the anal sphincter complex. *J Biomechanics.* 1988;21:601–604.

96. Read MG, Read MW, Haynes WG, Donnelly TC, Johnson AG. A prospective study of the effect of hemorrhoids on sphincter function and fecal continence. *Br J Surg.* 1982;69:396–398.

97. Duthie HL, Bennett RC. The relations of sensation on the anal canal to the functional anal sphincter: a possible factor in anal continence. *Gut.* 1963;4:179–182.

98. Salducci J, Planche D, Nandz B. Physiological role of the internal anal sphincter and the external anal sphincter during micturition. In: Weinbeck M, ed. *Motility of the Digestive Tract.* New York: Raven Press; 1982;513–520.

99. Sun WM, Donnelly TC, Read NW. The utility of a combined test of anorectal manometry/electromyography and sensation in determining the mechanisms of idiopathic faecal incontinence. *Gut.* 1992. In press.

100. Neill ME, Swash M. Increased motor unit fiber density in the external anal sphincter muscle in anorectal incontinence; a single fiber EMG study. *J Neurol Neurosurg Psych.* 1980;43:343–347.

101. Kiff ES, Swash M. Slowed conduction in the pudendal nerves in idiopathic (neurogenic) fecal incontinence. *Br J Surg.* 1984;71: 614–616.

102. Snooks SH, Swash M. Electromyography and nerve latency stud-

ies. In: Gooszen HG, et al, eds. *Disordered Defecation: Current Opinion and Diagnosis and Treatment.* Lancaster, England: Martimus Nijhoff Publishers; 1987:17–30.

103. Sun WM, Donnelly TL, Read NW. Impaired internal anal sphincter in a subgroup of patients with idiopathic fecal incontinence. *Gastroenterology.* 1989;97:130–135.

104. Aaronson I, Nixon HH. A clinical evaluation of anorectal pressure studies in the diagnosis of Hirschsprung's disease. *Gut.* 1972;13:138–146.

105. Faverdin C, Dornic C, Ahran P. Quantitative analysis of anorectal pressures in Hirschsprung's disease. *Dis Colon Rec.* 1981;24: 422–427.

106. Meunier P, Marechal JM, Jaubert de Beaujeu M. Rectoanal pressures and rectal sensitivity in child constipation. *Gastroent.* 1979;77:330–336.

107. Baldi F, Ferrarini F, Corinaldesi R, et al. Function of the internal anal sphincter and rectal sensitivity in idiopathic constipation. *Digestion.* 1982;24:14–22.

108. Lennard-Jones JE. Constipation: pathophysiology, clinical features and treatment. In: Henry MM, Swash M, eds. *Coloproctology and the Pelvic Floor, Pathophysiology and Management.* London: Butterworth's; 1985;350–375.

109. Gonella J, Bouvier M, Blanquet F. The extrinsic innervation of motility of the small and large intestines and related sphincters. *Physiol Rev.* 1987;67:902–961.

110. Christensen J, Rich GA. The distribution of myelinated nerves in the ascending nerves and myenteric plexus of the cat colon. *Am J Anat.* 1987;178:250–258.

111. Sun WM, Read NW, Miner PB, Kerigan DD, Donnelly TC. The role of transient internal sphincter relaxation in fecal incontinence. *Int J Colorect Dis.* 1990;5:31–36.

112. Monges HO, Salducci J, Nandy B, Ranieri F, Gonella J, Bouvier M. The electrical activity of the internal anal sphincter: a comparative study in man and in cats. In: Christensen J, ed. *Gastrointestinal Motility.* New York: Raven Press; 1980;495–501.

113. Callaghan RP, Nixon NH. Megarectum physiology observation. *Arch Dis Child.* 1984;39:153–157.

114. Narducci F, Bassotti G, Gaburri M, Morelli A. Twenty-four hour manometric recording of colonic motor activity in healthy man. *Gut.* 1987;28:17–25.

115. Bassotti G, Gaburri M, Imbimb BP, et al. Colonic mass movements in idiopathic chronic constipation. *Gut.* 1988;29:1173–1179.

116. Wald A, Tunuguntla AK. Anorectal sensation dysfunction in fecal incontinence in diabetes mellitus. *N Eng J Med.* 1984;310: 1282–1287.

117. Read NW, Abouzekry L, Read MG, Ottewell PH, Donnelly TL. Anorectal function in elderly patients with fecal impaction. *Gastroenterology.* 1985;89:959–966.

118. Buser WD, Miner PB Jr. Delayed rectal sensation with fecal incontinence. Successful treatment using anorectal manometry. *Gastroenterology.* 1986;91:1186–1191.

119. Prior A, Sun WM, Read NW. Rectal sensitivity: a rational means of categorizing patients with the irritable bowel syndrome. Submitted for publication, 1991.

120. Sun WM, Read NW. Anorectal manometry and rectal sensation in patients with irritable bowel syndrome. *Gastroenterology.* 1988;94:A450.

121. Prior A, Maxton DG, Whorwell PJ. Anorectal manometry in irritable bowel syndrome: differences between diarrhea and constipation predominant patients. *Gut.* 1990;31:458–462.

122. Rao SSC, Holdsworth CO, Read NW. Anorectal sensitivity and reactivity in patients with ulcerative colitis. *Gastroenterology.* 1987;83:1270–1275.

123. Sun WM, Read NW, Donnelly TL, Bannister JJ, Shorthouse AJ. A common pathophysiology for full thickness rectal prolapse, anterior mucous prolapse and solitary ulcer. *Br J Surg.* 1989;76: 290–295.

124. Cann PA, Read NW, Holdsworth CD, Barends D. The role of loperamide and placebo in the management of the irritable bowel syndrome (IBS). *Dig Dis Sci.* 1984;29:239–247.

125. Brown DL, Lauder JC, Foon FW, Finley IG. Outlet obstructive constipation (obstructed defecation)—a failure of the posterior pelvic floor? *Gut.* 1988;29:A734.

126. Mahieu P, Pringot J, Bodart P. Defecography. I. Description of a new procedure and results in normal patients. *Gastroint. Radiol.* 1984;9:247–251.

127. MacDonagh R, Sun WM, Smallwood RH, Read NW. Sacral anterior root stimulation and defecation. *Br Med J.* 1990;330: 1494–1497.

128. Barnes PRH, Hawley PR, Preston DM, Lennard-Jones JE. Experience of posterior division of the puborectalis muscle in the management of chronic constipation. *Br J Surg.* 1985;72:475–477.

129. Preston DM, Lennard-Jones JE. Anismus in chronic constipation. *Dig Dis Sci.* 1985;30:413–418.

130. Bannister JJ, Lawrence W, Thomas DG, Smith ARB, Read NW. Urological abnormalities in patients with slow transit constipation. *Gut.* 1988;29:17–20.

131. Kamm MA, Hawley PR, Lennard-Jones JE. Lateral division of the puborectalis muscle in the management of severe constipation. *Br J Surg.* 1988;75:661–663.

132. Hallan RI, Williams NS, Melting J, Waldron DJ, Womack NR, Morrison JFB. Treatment of anismus in intractable constipation with Botulinum A-toxin. *Lancet.* 1988;ii:714–717.

133. Bleijenberg G, Kuijpers HC. Treatment of the spastic pelvic floor syndrome with biofeedback. *Dis Colon Rect.* 1987;30:108–111.

134. Devroede G. Idiopathic constipation and colonic dysfunction: relationship with personality and anxiety. *Dig Dis Sci.* 1989;34: 1428–1436.

135. Kamm MA, Law PJ, Hoyle C, et al. A newly identified condition; hereditary internal anal sphincter myopathy. *Gut.* 1989;30:A1466.

136. Read NW, Abouzekry L. Why do patients with fecal impaction have fecal incontinence? *Gut.* 1986;27:283–287.

137. Bannister JJ, Davison P, Timms JM, Gibbons CG, Read NW. Effect of the stool size and consistency on defecation. *Gut.* 1987; 28:1246–1250.

138. Prior A, Stanley K, Smith ARB, Read NW. The effect of simple hysterectomy on anorectal and urethrovesical symptoms. *Gut.* 1992; 33:264–267.

139. Varma JS, Smith AN. Abnormalities of colorectal function in intractable constipation following hysterectomy. *Gut.* 1985;26: 581–582.

Pelvic Floor Neuropathy

9A   Neurophysiology and Neuroanatomy

J. Thomas Benson

INTRODUCTION

Current concepts of intracellular and intercellular nerve conduction are discussed in this chapter, emphasizing the role of neurotransmitters. The guiding of the peripheral and the autonomic nervous systems by the central nervous system and their application to the urinary tract are discussed.

Neuroanatomy is described to gain a clearer comprehension of pathophysiology of pelvic floor neuropathy. New evidence of the significance of such neuropathy in pelvic floor dysfunction is presented.

RELATIONSHIP OF NEUROPATHY TO PELVIC FLOOR DISORDERS

The significant relationship of pelvic floor neuropathy with pelvic floor disorders, including urinary incontinence and fecal incontinence, was recently highlighted by combined efforts of colorectal specialists and neurologists at St. Mark's Hospital in London, England. In 1984, urinary incontinence in patients with coexisting fecal incontinence was shown to be related to a disturbance in the pudendal and/or pelvic nerves.[1] For the first time it was documented that stress urinary incontinence was caused by damage in the nerve supply of the urethral striated sphincter. The neuropathy in these patients was diagnosed by electrophysiologic studies principally involving "single fiber" density determinations and conduction studies. Histological and histochemical studies of muscle sections from patients with pelvic floor prolapse and with urinary stress incontinence confirmed the electrophysiologic studies demonstrating evidence of neuropathy.[2] Further electrodiagnostic studies were performed in Manchester, England in 1989,[3] supporting the previous findings. These studies concluded that women with pudendal nerve conduction time to the urethral sphincter of > 2.4 msec had a 97% chance of experiencing urinary incontinence with stress. This clearly establishes the link between pudendal nerve and pelvic plexus damage with women's pelvic floor disorders, including stress urinary incontinence.

How does such damage to the pudendal nerve happen? In a landmark 1986 article, Snooks and coworkers[4] reported a carefully controlled prospective study analyzing the risk factors in childbirth that cause damage to pelvic floor innervation. They found that multiparity, forceps delivery, increased duration of the second stage of labor, third degree perineal tears, and high birth weight are important factors leading to pudendal nerve damage. Of utmost importance is the fact that there was no pudendal nerve damage in patients who delivered by cesarean section, demonstrating that delivery and not pregnancy caused the pudendal nerve damage.

In patients with pudendal nerve damage who had not experienced delivery, it was suggested that stretch injuries to the pudendal nerve could occur with excessive Valsalva efforts at defecation, leading to perineal descent and stretch injuries of the pudendal nerve.

Pelvic nerve damage may be produced by surgery in the area of the pelvic plexus, or by excessive stretch with pronounced pelvic floor prolapse, or by the multitude of pathologic processes which may involve the cauda equina.

With these factors contributing to neuropathy in pelvic floor disorders, it is important to understand the anatomic and physiologic nerve supply to the pelvic floor to learn how neuropathy can be prevented.

NEUROPHYSIOLOGY

Current Concepts of Neurophysiology

To understand how electrodiagnosis is useful for determining neuropathy, some current concepts in nerve conduction will be considered. The nervous system must be appreciated as a dynamic entity. Apparently by genetic, predetermined signals, the cytoskeleton is constantly reorganizing so that with damage, coincident reorganization and reinnervation simultaneously occurs. The active system functions to transport electric signals, doing so first by intracellular conduction followed by intercellular conduction of the signal.

Intracellular Conduction

The nerve cell and its extensions are bounded by membranes consisting of lipoprotein bilayers, which are semipermeable and maintain an irregular distribution of ions on either side. The intracellular side has high concentrations of organic anions and inorganic cations, especially potassium, whereas the extracellular fluid has higher concentrations of sodium and chloride ions. Thus in the relatively quiescent state, there is a difference in the electrical potential across the membrane with the inside of the cell strongly negative compared to the outside. This difference in the electrical potential is referred to as the resting potential. The nerve cell can conduct changes in these potentials and thereby transmit impulses resulting from the changes along the course of its membrane. This transmitted impulse is referred to as the action potential (Fig. 9A-1) and its ionic current flow is recordable.

Myelin sheathing produces capacitance, which limits the flow of the ionic current. As the current flows across interruptions of the myelin sheath known as nodes of Ranvier (see Fig. 9A-1), concentrated voltage-dependent sodium channels augment the ongoing current

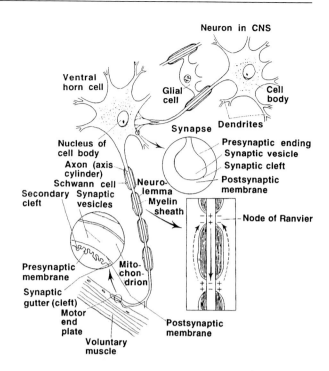

Fig. 9A-1 Neurons of central nervous system (CNS). Inset, **A**, e = Action potential (solid arrow), flow of action current (dashed arrows). (Reprinted from Manter JE. *Essentials of Clinical Neuroanatomy and Neurophysiology,* 7th ed, Philadelphia: FA Davis; 1987, with permission.)

flow, a process referred to as saltatory conduction. Nerves without myelin have no such arrangement and action potentials are propagated by a less efficient process of continuous conduction. Velocities of conduction then, are proportionate to the amount of myelinization and hence the size of the nerve. Conditions that disrupt myelin interfere with saltatory conduction and cause slowing of the conduction times, whereas axonal neuropathies affecting axonal loss and replacement have little effect on conduction velocity. Most pathologic processes cause both demyelinization and axonal degeneration.

Within the nerve cells, ionic conduction is modulated by calcium and intracellular messengers such as cyclic nucleotides, inositol phospholipid, and arachidonic acid. The study of these modulators is in its infancy.

Intercellular Conduction

Intercellular communication occurs at nerve synapses and neuroeffector junctions by electrical or chemical activity. Electrical communication is performed by low resistance connections between the membranes of two cells and is found extensively in invertebrates, but only at selected sites in mammals.

Chemical communications involve transmitting substances called *neurotransmitters,* which either excite (depolarize) or inhibit (hyperpolarize) the postsynaptic membrane. These responses are graded, not all or none as in intracellular communication.

Neurotransmitters

Acetylcholine and monoamines have long been recognized classes of neurotransmitters, to which large groups of neuropeptides and amino acids have been added. These chemical compounds are:

1. Synthesized in the presynaptic neuron.
2. Transported in the axon.
3. Stored and released at presynaptic endings.
4. Bound to specific receptor proteins, thereby opening a channel for passage of current flow.
5. Undergoing postsynaptic inactivation.

Acetylcholine and monoamine tend to act more efficiently in neurotransmission than do the neuronal peptides because presynaptic synthesis is more rapid, utilizing readily available substrates (acetyl CoA and choline) rather than requiring a de novo process in the cell body. Also, the release at the presynaptic endings in which synaptic vesicles fuse and release neurotransmitter into synaptic clefts requires shorter time for acetylcholine and the amines than for the neuropeptides.

Specific receptor proteins for each neurotransmitter exist in the presynaptic and postsynaptic membranes. The binding rate with the receptors is influenced by the cellular messengers, including those mentioned above as well as prostaglandin E. The number of receptors in certain locations is increased by estrogen. Various identified neurotransmitters and receptors are listed in Table 9A-1.

The pelvic floor and the inherent structures of the lower urinary tract, reproductive tract, and the colorectum are all under complex nervous system control. Local innervation is modulated by the central nervous system and consists of autonomic and somatic motor and sensory systems.

The Autonomic Neurophysiology

The autonomic system is a division of the peripheral nervous system which innervates cardiac muscle, smooth muscle, and glands. The autonomic nervous system consists of general visceral efferent and afferent fibers that ordinarily function at a subconscious level.

Table 9A-1

Electrodiagnosis in Pelvic Floor Disorders: Known Neurotransmitters and Receptors

	Neurotransmittors	Receptors
Ganglia	Acetylcholine Norepinephrine Neuropeptides, esp. enkephalin	Muscarinic and nicotinic alpha-adrenergic receptors, specific receptors
Detrusor	A noncholinergic, nonadrenergic transmitter	Nonmuscarinic (atropine resistant)
	Acetylcholine	Muscarinic-body
	Norepinephrine	Alpha receptors (more near base?) Beta receptors (more in body)
	Neuropeptide vasoactive intestinal polypeptide substance P Histamine and purine	Specific receptors (more in base)
Trigone	Norepinephrine	Alpha receptors (affected by higher dose) Beta receptors (affected by lower dose)
	Prostaglandin	Messenger for relaxation
Urethra	Acetylcholine Substance P Vasoactive intestinal polypeptide Histamine Norepinephrine	Rich in alpha-adrenergic receptors

Unlike the somatic motor system, the peripheral fibers reach the effector organ by a two neuron chain. The preganglionic neuron arises in the intermediolateral cell column of the brain stem, or spinal cord, and terminates at an outlying ganglion where the postganglionic neuron continues the impulse transmission to the end organ. Fibers arising from the intermediolateral gray column of the twelve thoracic and first two lumbar segments of the spinal cord constitute the sympathetic division of the autonomic system. The parasympathetic division consists of fibers arising from the second through fourth sacral segments as well as cranial outflows. The sympathetic versus parasympathetic systems are differentiated by their anatomic, physiologic, and pharmacologic properties.

Sympathetic nerves to the pelvic cavity originate in cord levels T5 to L2 and pass via white rami communicators to or through the sympathetic trunk (chain ganglia lateral to the vertebral column) to ganglia located at roots of arteries for which they are named. (For example, lumbar splanchnic nerves terminate in inferior mesenteric and hypogastric ganglia.) Postganglionic fibers from these ganglia follow the visceral arteries to the organs of the lower abdomen and pelvis.

Pelvic parasympathetic system preganglionic fibers originate in spinal segments S2 through S4, join the hypogastric plexus to form the pelvic plexus, and extend to ganglia located within or very near the organs they supply, thus having very short postganglionic fibers.

Ganglia

The parasympathetic ganglia are located within the wall of the bladder or colorectal system, a location quite vulnerable to end organ disease, such as overstretch or infection. Norepinephrine acts as a neurotransmitter conveyed principally by the sympathetic system to alpha adrenergic receptors at the parasympathetic ganglia. The action of this tends to stop transmission of parasympathetic activity by interfering with the nicotinic receptor of the presynaptic acetylcholine.

In the urinary tract, postganglionic parasympathetic detrusor nerve fibers diverge and store neurotransmitter agents in axonal varicosities termed synaptic vesicles. The agent is diffused to neuromuscular bundles of 12 to 15 muscle fibers enclosed in a collagen capsule acting similarly to the tendon insertion of a muscle. Stimulating electrical pulses produce two episodes of depolarization, suggesting the release of two neurotransmitters.

The trigone is a separate anatomic and embryologic region where muscle fibers have an almost exclusively adrenergic innervation.[5] Alpha adrenergic receptors in smooth muscle cause contraction whereas beta adrenergic receptors tend to cause relaxation. Alpha receptors tend to be located more at the bladder base whereas beta receptors are more prevalent in the bladder fundus.

The autonomic system, then, generally acts through the parasympathetic division to promote emptying of the viscera and through the sympathetic division to prevent such emptying. Illustrations of this are shown in Figs. 9A-2 and 9A-3, referring to the lower urinary tract. The colorectal system is somewhat more complex, somewhat less understood, and has an intrinsic neuronal mechanism going on as well. There is some spatial separation of neurons concerned with parasympathetic efferent bladder and colon control, neurons innervating the bladder being larger and situated more laterally. The autonomic effects are aided in the local innervation by somatic muscular effects.

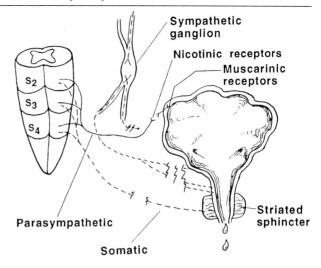

Fig. 9A-2 Parasympathetic system bladder emptying.

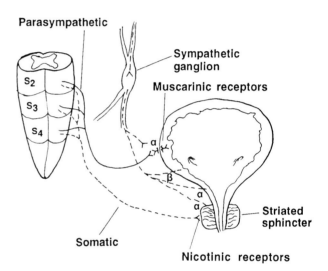

Fig. 9A-3 Sympathetic system bladder storage. α = alpha adrenergic receptors; β = beta adrenergic receptors.

Somatic Nerve Physiology

The somatic component, composed of the 12 paired cranial nerves and 31 spinal nerves, comprises the balance of the peripheral nervous system and functions to innervate skeletal muscle. This is done as a segmental skeletal reflex (Fig. 9A-4), with nerves that activate large extrafusal muscle fibers and others activating muscle spindles. Muscle spindles are muscle stretch receptor organs that can alter the sensitivity of the receptor to the muscle length.

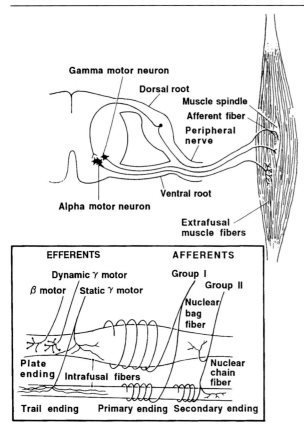

Fig. 9A-4 Cross section of spinal cord. Ia afferent fiber originates in muscle spindle, through peripheral nerve to dorsal root and synapses with alpha motor neuron that emerges through ventral root, through peripheral nerve to extrafusal muscle fibers. Inset shows enlarged view of the intrafusal fibers within the muscle spindle. (Reprinted from Manter JE, *Essentials of Clinical Neuroanatomy and Neurophysiology*, 7th ed, Philadelphia: FA Davis; 1987, with permission.)

Alpha motor neurons are the largest and their efferent axons go to the motor end plates near the center of the extrafusal muscle fiber. They are affected by afferent nerves from the muscle spindles which deliver stretch impulses without intermediate neurons. They are also affected by efferent fibers from Golgi (neurotendinous) organs connecting via intermediate neurons. Supraspinal afferent fibers similarly affect alpha motor neurons. Alpha motor neurons also innervate interneurons in the ventral horn (Renshaw cells), which act to inhibit other alpha motor neurons, a negative feedback response allowing more rapid firing.

The gamma motor neurons innervate the intrafusal fibers within the muscle spindles. They are strongly influenced by the reticular system, cerebellum, and basal ganglia.

Typically, motor neuron size correlates with muscle fiber types. Smaller motor neurons innervate smaller motor units to activate slower, less fatigable muscle fiber used for tonicity; larger ones activate the fast twitch response muscle fibers. The motor neurons in the sacral cord which innervate the urethral anal striated sphincter arise from Onuf's nucleus of anterior horn cells. There is a fundamental difference between Onuf's anterior horn cells and those innervating skeletal muscle because the former frequently remain unaffected in motor neuron disease.

In both urethral skeletal sphincter mechanisms, as well as anal sphincter mechanisms, there is double innervation. In the urethra the intramural component of the urethral striated muscle is probably innervated by somatic efferent branches of the pelvic nerves, a component of the pelvic plexus.[5] The periurethral skeletal muscle, however, is innervated by the pudendal nerve, as is the skeletal muscle of the external anal sphincter, perineal muscles, and urogenital diaphragm. (The pudendal nerve also has autonomic nerve components, as do the pelvic nerves.) A dual innervation frequently exists for the puborectalis, adding to speculation about its debated embryonic origin, that is, whether it is a part of the levator ani complex or the external anal sphincter. Embryologic speculation is that pelvic caudal muscles (tail-waggers) composing the levator group in humans are supplied from the pelvic plexus on the pelvic surface side, whereas the sphincter cloacal derivatives are supplied from the perineal aspect by the pudendal nerve.

In both the urethra and anal sphincters, the skeletal muscles are composed mostly of slow twitch fibers (type I) with an approximate concentration of 35% fast twitch (type II). Constant tonus, then, is effected with emergency reflex activity available.

The neurotransmitter at the periurethral and external anal sphincter neuromuscular junction is acetylcholine and receptors are primarily nicotinic type. There is an intimate adherence of the neuromuscular junction to the striated muscle fibers that convey a resistance to neuromuscular blocking agents.

Sensory Innervation

Proprioceptive endings in detrusor and, probably, colon exist as nerve endings in collagen bundles, being stimulated by stretch or contraction. These visceral afferents have cell bodies in the sensory ganglia of cerebrospinal nerves as do somatic sensory fibers, and do not constitute a morphologically independent system. The modalities of sensation are vague compared to somatic ones. It is well known that the ability to differentiate gas, liquid, and solid in the anal canal is mediated by nerve endings outside of the anal wall itself, and probably associated with levator ani musculature. Pain and temperature nerve endings in the urinary tract are free in the mucosa and submucosa. It is postulated[6] that there are two types of sensations in the bladder, the first sensor being the trigone, the second being stretch receptors in the bladder body. Loss of the first sensor may lead to urge incontinence as the bladder is ready to contract before sensation is noted.

Urethral and lower anal canal sensation is carried principally by the pudendal nerve, although the pelvic nerve also contributes sensation. The sensation is conveyed through both smooth and skeletal muscle components in both contralateral and ipsilateral nerve supply.

Central Nervous System Modulation

The central nervous system is involved in modulation of the autonomic and somatic regulation of colorectal, reproductive, and lower urinary tract activities. (The only exception to central nervous system involvement in autonomic regulation is the enteric plexus.) This leads to conscious control over largely autonomic functions. Postulations regarding central nervous system involvement in the urinary tract are extensive and will be discussed here.

The detrusor and the periurethral striated muscle mechanisms have separate cortical and other higher center regulation.[7,8] The detrusor is regulated by a micturition center in the brain stem, and the periurethral mechanisms are regulated by the sacral spinal cord.

Cortical-reticular axons, originating from pyramidal detrusor cells in the supramedial portion of the frontal lobes and the genu of the corpus callosum, traverse the basal ganglia and terminate in the pontomesencephalic reticular formation of the brain stem on detrusor motor nuclei in the nucleus lateralis dorsalis.[9] "Loop one" in Bradley's concept provides volitional control for the micturition reflex and is alterable by local brain disease that produces detrusor instability and small bladder capacity. Incontinence resulting from disease in this area is usually of a coordinated type; that is, the detrusor contraction is coordinated with urethral relaxation. The integrity of this circuit is demonstrated by the patient's volitional suppression of detrusor contractions. These brain-stem detrusor motor nuclei (the "micturition center") receive suppressive afferents from basal ganglia, coordinating afferents from the cerebellum and sensory cord afferents from tension receptors in the detrusor muscle, which synapse here to constitute the

so-called "long-routing" detrusor reflex. Fibers from the raphe nuclei of the reticular formation may function to moderate responsiveness to different phases of the sleep-wake cycle or emotional states.

Efferents of the brain stem detrusor motor nuclei go to detrusor motor neurons in the intermediolateral cell column from T10 to L1 and the S2 to S4 segments of the cord. Bradley postulates this as Loop 2 with efferents originating in the brain stem reticular formation and terminating in the sacral micturition area of detrusor motor neurons. The afferent arm of this loop originates in the detrusor sensory fibers, which form "long routes" to the brain stem. This long routing provides for temporal gain (increased duration) of the detrusor reflex. Partial interruption, such as occurs with cord disease, produces low threshold detrusor reflexes and more residual urine. These symptoms may mimic stress incontinence and may be produced as a response to a stimulation such as a cough. Complete interruption produces detrusor areflexia and urinary retention initially and, after chronic complete interruption, segmental reflex pathways lead to an "automatic" bladder, with spontaneous emptying with bladder filling. Local bladder disease and pelvic plexus disease may affect this pathway by acting on the sensory arm.

In the sacral cord, the pudendal motor nuclei act as a segmental skeletal muscle reflex to the periurethral striated muscle. Coordination of the detrusor motor neurons and the periurethral striated muscle innervation involves the rich interplay between the detrusor and the pudendal sacral nuclei for coordinating relaxation of the tonically contracted periurethral skeletal muscle with detrusor contraction. Such innervation involves the conus medullaris and connecting neurons. These areas comprise Bradley's Loop 3. Patients with abnormalities here may show detrusor sphincter dyssynergia or uninhibited sphincter relaxation. Central reflex connection loss can lead to atonic bladder, frequently associated with sensory deficit of corresponding dermatomes and flaccid motor loss in perineal and lower limb muscles.

Bradley's Loop 4 is the cerebral pyramidal sacral pathway, whereby upper neuron control of the lower pudendal motor axons lead to volitional control of the external striated sphincters. The clinical test of the pathway is the patient's ability to contract and relax the sphincter on command. Disruption may lead to loss of volitional sphincter control, associated with exaggerated reflexes and positive extensor plantar response. The pudendal cortical pathways involved in this affect periurethral striated muscle innervation by directly sending impulses originating in the central vertex of the pudendal cerebral cortical area and going to the puden-dal nuclei in the ventromedial portion of gray matter of the S2 to S4 cord segments. At this level the pudendal motor nuclei act as a segmental muscle reflex.

Ascending axons from the periurethral striated mus-cle go to the pudendal cortical area, possibly synapsing in the nucleus ventralis posterolateralis of the thalamus, the brain's chief relay station. Sensory afferents from both pudendal and detrusor pelvic nerves send input to the anterior vermis of the cerebellum, which then origi-nates an axon relay to the cortex and the dentate nu-cleus. Fibers for both detrusor and pudendal proprio-ception and exteroception (pain, temperature, and touch) ascend in the posterior column and spino-thalamic tracts, respectively.

Relationships of the central nervous system to the lower urinary tract are diagrammatically illustrated in Figure 9A-5.

Other Higher Centers

Basal ganglia clearly have an effect, which is probably suppressive, on detrusor reflex control. One million pa-tients suffer from Parkinson's disease with dopamine exhaustion and 45% to 75% of these patients have detrusor hyperreflexia. Temporal lobe limbic systems affect all autonomic function and are frequently in-volved in epileptiform activity. Such activity may lead to coordinated detrusor hyperreflexia. Disease in the area of the cerebellum produces spontaneous, high am-plitude bladder hyperreflexia. The brain stem's impor-tance in lower urinary tract function has been known since 1921, when Barrington[10] ablated this area in cats and caused permanent urinary retention.

NEUROANATOMY

Neuroanatomic considerations are vital in appreciat-ing how neuropathies leading to pelvic floor dysfunc-tion may occur. The following discussion will consider the neuroanatomy of the central nervous system, conus medullaris, cauda equina, pelvic plexus, and pudendal nerve.

Central Nervous System

The central nervous system includes the brain and spinal cord. Pathologic processes involving these areas are myriad and the effects of such processes are alluded to in neurophysiology.

A prime area of pelvic floor innervation is in the

terminal portion of the spinal cord, the conus medulla-ris. The adult conus medullaris is quite short and con-tains the entire S1 to S5 segment. Although the thoraco-lumbar functions are important in sympathetic autonomic influence on pelvic viscera, the conus medul-laris has greater significance because autonomic nuclei as well as somatic nuclei are housed in the intermedi-olateral and ventromedial anterior gray matter, respec-tively. The conus medullaris houses neurons involved in defecation, urination, and sexual function with relays for cortical separation of these visceral functions (ence-phalization) developing after birth. Through this highly compact area, then, many disease effects are produced. For example, multiple sclerosis affects the conus medul-laris as well as the exiting neurons, causing signs of both upper and lower motor neuron disorder as well as auto-nomic abnormality. So, a small amount of pathology can do a large amount of damage.

This area involves the interrelationship of many in-teractive reflexes. In the urinary tract urine storage and evacuation reflexes are classified by Mahoney and col-leagues[11] and are presented in Table 9A-2. These are conceptualized reflex pathways that have not been demonstrated in humans. In experimental animals three pathways were demonstrated. The first is the proximal urethra to the detrusor for facilitation of detrusor re-flex. This may be important when considering proximal urethral relationships to bladder instability. The second is periurethral striated muscle to the detrusor for detru-sor inhibition. This pathway is utilized in biofeedback therapy for unstable conditions. The third is sacral cord afferent fibers to lumbar cord efferent fibers for depres-sion of ganglion transmission.

The anal rectal reflex, with lowering of intra-anal pressure with rectal filling, is not dependent on the conus medullaris being an intrinsic gastrointestinal re-flex. The enteric plexus is the only portion of the vis-ceral system that seems to carry out reflex responses without involving the central nervous system.[12]

Cauda Equina

By adolescence, disparity in the growth of the spinal cord and the vertebral column leads to the cord's ter-minating around the first lumbar vertebrae. The cauda equina is thus formed by nerve roots leaving the spinal cord and exiting the vertebral column at their respective intervertebral foramina (Fig. 9A-6). It can be ap-preciated that the lowermost nerve roots, comprising those from the conus medullaris, occupy a central loca-tion in the cauda equina. That is, when pathologic

Table 9A-2
Proposed Reflexes

Reflexes	Actions
Bladder storage reflexes	
1. Sympathetic detrusor to detrusor	Inhibits detrusor in response to increased detrusor
2. Detrusor–urethral stimulating	Increased detrusor tension stimulates urethral smooth muscle
3. Perineal–detrusor inhibition	Inhibits detrusor in response to perineal sphincter muscles
4. Urethrosphincter guarding	Contracts external striated sphincter in response to trigone tension
Micturition initiation reflexes	
5. Perineodetrusor facilitative	Decreasing pelvic floor muscle tone; stimulates detrusor
6. Detrusor–detrusor facilitative	Increased detrusor tension; stimulates detrusor
Reflexes to maintain micturition	
7. Detrusor urethral inhibiting	Detrusor to segmental inhibition of urethral smooth muscle
8. Detrusor sphincter inhibiting	Detrusor to segmental inhibition of external striated sphincter
9. Urethrodetrusor facilitative	Proximal urethra segmental reflex to stimulate detrusor
10. Urethrobulbar detrusor facilitative	Proximal urethra reflex to stimulate detrusor via brain stem
11. Urethrosphincteric inhibiting	Urethra to external striated sphincter; segmental reflex
Micturition cessation reflex	Pelvic floor afferent fibers to brain stem to inhibit detrusor

processes occur in the vertebral column in the lumbosacral area, disruption of the centrally located fibers of the cauda equina can occur. Such lumbosacral disorders are extremely common in the erect human female and may give rise to neuropathy involving both the pelvic plexus and the pudendal nerve. Electrodiagnostic testing is helpful in evaluating a peripheral nerve disorder originating in this area.

Cauda equina lesions have features of lower motor neuron injury (that is, some degree of muscle paralysis and sensory loss in the myotomes and dermatomes in-

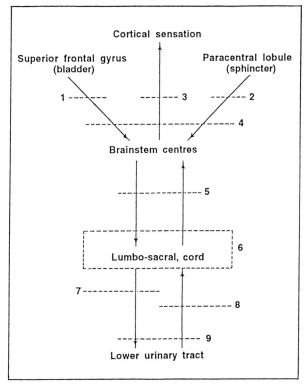

Fig. 9A-5 Simplified scheme of interaction of various levels of the nervous system in micturition. The locations of certain possible nervous lesions are denoted by numbers and explained as follows.

1. Lesions isolating the frontal gyrus prevent voluntary postponement of voiding. If sensation is intact this produces urge incontinence. If the lesion is larger there will be additional loss of social concern about incontinence.

2. Lesions isolating the paracentral lobule, sometimes associated with a hemiparesis, will cause spasticity of the urethral sphincter and retention. This will be painless if sensation is abolished. Minor degrees of this syndrome may cause difficulty in the initiation of micturition.

3. Pathways of sensation are not known accurately. In theory, an isolated lesion of sensation above the brain stem would lead to unconscious incontinence. Defective central conduction of sensory information would explain nocturnal enuresis.

4. Lesions above the brain stem centers lead to involuntary voiding that is coordinated with sphincter relaxation.

5. Lesions below brain stem centers but above the lumbosacral spinal cord lead, after a period of bladder paralysis associated with spinal shock, to involuntary reflex voiding that is not coordinated with sphincter relaxation (detrusor/sphincter dyssynergia).

6. Lesions destoying the lumbosacral cord or the complete nervous connections between the central and peripheral nervous system result in a paralyzed bladder which contracts only weakly in an autonomous fashion because of its remaining ganglionic innervation. However, if the lumber sympathetic outflow is preserved in the presence of conus and/or cauda equina destruction then there may be some residual sympathetic tone in the bladder neck and urethra which may be sufficient to be obstructive.

7. A lesion of the efferent fibers alone leads to a bladder of decreased capacity and decreased compliance associated experimentally with an increased number of adrenergic nerves.

8. A lesion confined to the afferent fibers produces a bladder which is areflexic with increased compliance and capacity.

9. As there are ganglion cells in the bladder wall it is technically impossible to decentralize the bladder completely, but congenital absence of bladder ganglia may exist producing megacystis.

(Reprinted from Torrens M, Morrison JFB. *The Physiology of the Lower Urinary Tract.* New York: Springer–Verlag; 1987:335, with permission.)

volved). Thus a herniated intervertebral disc may cause detrusor areflexia, saddle anesthesia, and reduced anal tone when severe. Mild effects may produce only a decreased detrusor contractility that may in turn cause decreased urine flow, which can contribute to recurrent cystitis. The effect on peristalsis in colonic activity is to decrease contractility in the colorectal tract.

Pelvic Plexus

As previously stated, the pelvic plexus is composed of both autonomic and somatic pathways. The autonomic portion consists of both sympathetic and parasympathetic divisions (Fig. 9A-7). Pelvic sympathetic neurons originate in cord levels from T5 to L2 and pass through

Fig. 9A-6 The cauda equina of the spinal cord showing the conus medullaris.

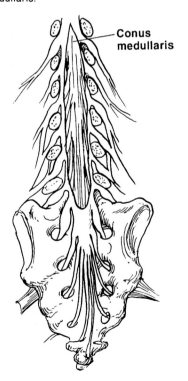

Conus medullaris

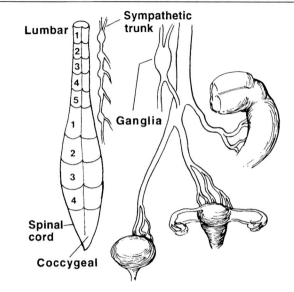

Fig. 9A-7 Autonomic nerve supply of pelvis.

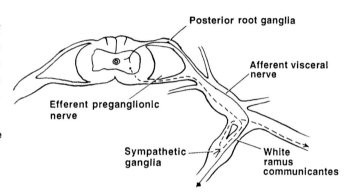

Fig. 9A-8 Spinal nerve conveying sympathetic nerve fibers.

the intervertebral foramen in the primary division of the spinal nerve. Soon after emerging, the fibers pass through the white ramus communicantes to the sympathetic chain and thus the roots of the sympathetic ganglia (Fig. 9A-8). Sympathetic ganglia supplying the pelvis are usually four in number and located between the vertebral body, psoas muscle and aorta (left), or vena cava (right) (Fig. 9A-9), extending from L2 to the aortic bifurcation (Fig. 9A-10). From the sympathetic ganglia, neurons travel through inferior mesenteric ganglia via the lumbar splanchnic nerves and continue through the hypogastric plexus to the presacral fascia, across the upper posterior lateral pelvic wall, 1 to 2 cm behind and below the ureter. After these neurons join the pelvic parasympathetic nerves, the pelvic plexus is formed running below and medial to the internal iliac vessels overlying the anterolateral lower rectum near the anal rectal junction. The plexus spreads in the lat-

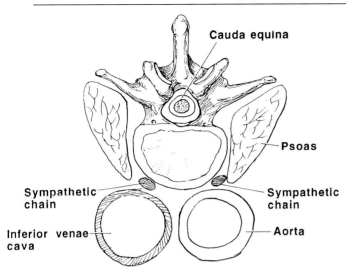

Fig. 9A-9 Diagramatic relationship of sympathetic chain.

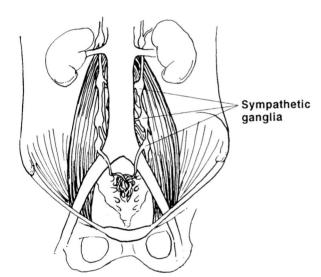

Fig. 9A-10 Outline of lumbar sympathetic ganglia.

eral wall of the upper one third of the vagina, beneath the uterine artery, medial to the ureter, and 2 cm inferolateral to the cervix. Within the vesico vaginal septum the plexus supplies the upper vagina, bladder, proximal urethra, and lower ureter components of the lower urinary tract. Smooth musculature and glands of the reproductive and colorectal systems are supplied similarly by visceral fibers generally following vessels.[13] Hence, pelvic plexus branches extend through hypogastric and inferior mesenteric plexuses to the descending and sigmoid colon and rectum, and uterovaginal plexuses send branches to the uterus and vagina.

Somatic peripheral innervation occurs by somatic efferent branches of the pelvic nerves, constituting a component of the pelvic plexus. The levator musculature is supplied from the pelvic plexus on the pelvic surface side, with supply to the puborectalis being somewhat variable. The intramural component of the urethral striated muscle is chiefly innervated by somatic efferent branches of the pelvic nerves.

The periurethral skeletal muscle as well as the skeletal muscle of the external anal sphincter, perineal muscles, and urogenital diaphragm are supplied by branches of the pudendal nerve. The pudendal nerve passes between the coccygeus and piriformis muscles, leaving the pelvis through the greater sciatic foramen, crossing the ischial spine and re-entering the pelvis through the lesser sciatic foramen. Here, the nerve accompanies the pudendal vessels along the lateral wall of the ischiorectal fossa in a tunnel formed by a splitting of the obturator fascia, Alcock's canal. At the urogenital diaphragm the nerve divides into the inferior rectal nerve, supplying the external anal sphincter and the perineal nerves, splitting into a superficial branch to the labia and a deep branch to the periurethral striated muscle. It is at the area of the Alcock's canal that the nerve is relatively trapped. Stretching of the nerve can then occur when there is a descent of the pelvic floor because of its trapped position in the canal.

The pudendal nerve can be damaged by excessive use of the Valsalva maneuver. Stretching of the nerve by as little as 12% of its length can cause nerve injury. With excessive straining at defecation or at second stage of labor, movement of the pelvic floor can cause stretching of up to 20% of the pudendal nerve length beyond its relative fixation in the canal. Such neuropathy was demonstrated to be an etiologic factor in urinary and anal incontinence.[1,14] The pelvic plexus nerves are particularly subject to damage with extensive dissection lateral to the cervix or anterior and lateral to the rectum. Dissection superior to Waldeyer's fascia may afford greater nerve protection than dissection inferiorly.

SUMMARY

Neuropathy is intimately related to pelvic floor disorders including prolapse, urinary incontinence, and fecal incontinence. Neuropathies may originate in the central nervous system or in the peripheral nervous system, including the autonomic and somatic areas through the pelvic plexus and the pudendal nerve.

Diagnosing these neuropathies is facilitated by understanding neurophysiology of intracellular and intercellular nerve conduction. The rapidly evolving information regarding neurotransmitters allows increased understanding and improved methodologies of treatment.

Understanding the physiology of the autonomic system, sensory innervation, central nervous system modulation, and peripheral nervous system as it relates to the pelvic floor is fundamental. The neuroanatomy of these areas helps us to understand the possible defects involved in pelvic surgery, obstetric delivery, and stretch injury to the peripheral nervous system in this area. Any patient presenting with pelvic floor dysfunction should be examined for possible neurologic disturbances.

REFERENCES

1. Snooks SH, Swash M. Abnormalities of the innervation of the urethral striated sphincter musculature in incontinence. *Br J Urol.* 1984;56:401–405.
2. Gilpin SA, Gosling JA, Smith ARB, Warrell DW. The pathogenesis of genitourinary prolapse and stress incontinence of urine. A histological and histochemical study. *Br J Obstet Gynaecol.* 1989;96:15–23.
3. Smith ARB, Hosker GL, Warrell DW. The role of pudendal nerve damage in the aetiology of genuine stress incontinence in women. *Br J Obstet Gynaecol.* 1989;96:29–32.
4. Snooks SJ, Swash M, Henry MM, Setchell M. Risk factors in childbirth causing damage to the pelvic floor innervation. *Int J Colorect Dis.* 1986;1:20–24.
5. Gosling JA, Dixon JS. The structure and innervation of smooth muscle in the wall or the bladder neck and proximal urethra. *Br J Urol.* 1975;47:549.
6. Klein LA. Urge incontinence can be a disease of bladder sensors. *J Urol.* 1988;139:1010.
7. Bradley WE, Timm GW, Scott FB. Innervation of the detrusor muscle and urethra. *Urol Clin North Am.* 1974;1:3.
8. Bradley WE, Timm GW, Scott FB. Cystometry. II. Central nervous system organization of detrusor reflex. *Urology.* 1975;5:578.
9. Bradley WE. Cerebrocortical innervation of the urinary bladder. *Tohoku J Exp Med.* 1980;131:7.
10. Barrington FJF. The relation of the hindbrain to micturition. *Brain.* 1921;44:23.
11. Mahoney DT, Laberte RO, Blais DJ. Integral storage and voiding reflexes: neurophysiologic concept of continence and micturition. *Urology.* 1977;10:95.
12. Kuntz A. *The Autonomic Nervous System.* 4th ed. Philadelphia: Lea & Febiger; 1953:605.
13. Gosling JA, Dixon JS. The structure and innervation of smooth muscle in the wall of the bladder neck and proximal urethra. *Br J Urol.* 1975;47:549.
14. Kiff E, Swash M. Slowed conduction in the pudendal nerves in idiopathic (neurogenic) fecal incontinence. *Br J Surg.* 1984;71:614–616.

Pelvic Floor Neuropathy

9B Partial Denervation in Pelvic Floor Prolapse

D. W. Warrell

INTRODUCTION

It is well recognized that childbirth is the leading cause of genital tract prolapse and urinary stress incontinence, for it is rare to find these conditions in nulliparous women. Until recently the mechanisms by which childbirth damaged the pelvic floor and genital tract supports was the subject of clinical rather than scientific study. This chapter outlines the historic concepts of the causes of genital tract prolapse and describes recent work suggesting that neuromuscular damage is an important cause of pelvic floor damage and urinary and fecal incontinence.

Role of Pelvic Floor Muscle and Fascia

Throughout this century there has been debate as to the respective roles of pelvic floor muscle and pelvic fascia in support of the genital tract and, consequently, the nature of the tissue damage leading to prolapse of the genital tract. Fothergill,[1] one of the pioneers of vaginal reconstructive surgery, writes that the muscles of the pelvic floor do not provide support for the pelvic viscera and are not useful in prolapse repair operations. He goes on to write "the cervix uteri does not rest on the pelvic diaphragm any more than the bottom of a hansom cab rests on the ground." Mengert,[2] in a classic cadaver dissection, demonstrated that the uterus would not descend until the fascial supports of the upper va-

gina and lower half of the uterus had been cut. Those who considered muscle damage to be important in the support of the genital tract have based their case on the failure to demonstrate fascial tissue on histologic examination. Though uterine supports such as the cardinal ligament are easily recognized clinically, when studied histologically they are found to consist of blood vessels, elastic tissue, collagen, and smooth muscle.[3] However, Malpas[4] stated that the differentiation between fascia and muscle was artificial when considering the etiology of prolapse, and stated that "the pelvic cellular tissue constitutes a fibrous framework of skeleton upon whose integrity the effective action of the muscle depends." He amplified this statement and suggested that in uterovaginal prolapse the distribution of damage involved fascia, as opposed to generalized prolapse in which pelvic floor muscle weakness was the dominant feature. This concept that pelvic fascia and the pelvic floor were complementary in function was supported by an important contribution on the functional anatomy of the pelvic floor by Berglas and Rubin.[5] They reported that in healthy nulliparous women in the erect position the vaginal axis is close to horizontal and the pelvic viscera are supported by the levator plate. In women with genital prolapse the levator plate sags, inclining the axis of the vagina toward vertical and widening the introitus. The mechanical effect of this change is to increase the strain on the so-called "fascial" supports of the pelvic viscera. This concept does not preclude fascial damage as a factor leading to prolapse but does explain how pelvic floor muscle damage may adversely affect the position of a pelvic organ immediately supported by smooth muscle, blood vessels, collagen, and elastic tissue.

The Pelvic Floor

The conventional textbook description of the pelvic floor is of two muscles.[6] These are the coccygeus, a triangular sheet of muscle and fibrous tissue that lies posteriorly and arises from the ischial spine and the sacrospinous ligament (which may be a degenerate part of it); and the levator ani, a broad muscle consisting of the iliococcygeus and the pubococcygeus (Fig. 9B-1). The latter arises in continuity across the obturator fascia and pubis to the ischial spine, forming the white line. Iliococcygeus arises from the posterior half of this insertion and crosses to insert in the side of the coccyx and anococcygeal raphe, which is formed by the interdigitation of muscle fibers from either side. The pubococcygeus is considered to be in two parts: the posterior flat portion inserted into the tip of the coccyx and the anococcygeal raphe and partially overlying ileococcygeus; and the thicker anterior part whose fibers, by swinging medially and joining those from the opposite side, form U-shaped slings around the midline effluents with the anal canal positioned at the apex and the vagina and urethra placed anteriorly. The part of the muscle passing around the anorectal junction is described as the puborectalis muscle, the posterior fibers of which are in communication with the fibers of the external anal sphincter. Similarly the medial fibers of pubococcygeus run alongside and are attached to the vagina. This interlacing of the pelvic floor with the effluent passages is important for the prevention of pro-

lapse and coordinated activity of adjacent structures. Thus, contraction of the pelvic floor muscle will lift the pelvic floor and perineum upwards, which is important for continence with maintenance of the angulation of the bladder with urethra and the rectum with the anal canal. Prolapse of the pelvic viscera may be accompanied by loss of these angles (anorectal urethrovesical, and uterovaginal) secondary to failure of the pelvic floor. Descent of the perineum is also seen in pelvic floor damage.[7] Parks[8] argues that despite the various labels given to different parts of the pelvic floor muscles they should be considered as an anatomic physiological unit. He likened the region to two tubes, one within the other. The inner visceral tube consists of mucosa, submucosa, circular, and longitudinal smooth muscle, and the outer funnel-shaped tube consists of striated muscle of the levator ani and external anal sphincter. To this description the striated muscle of the perineum and external urethral sphincter should be added. The pelvic floor muscle is a mixture of slow and fast twitch fibers enabling it to maintain tone for prolonged periods, with additional rapid increased muscle activity when needed.[9,10]

Nerve Supply of the Pelvic Floor, Anal Sphincter, and Urethral Sphincter

The pelvic floor is thought to derive its nerve supply from two sources: the pudendal nerve, and a direct branch from the S3 and S4 motor routes. The pudendal nerve arises from ventral divisions of S2, S3, and S4 in the sacral plexus. As the pudendal nerve passes with the pudendal vessel through the lesser sciatic foramen into the pudendal canal it gives off the inferior rectal nerve that supplies the external anal sphincter, the lining of the lower part of the anal canal, and the skin around the

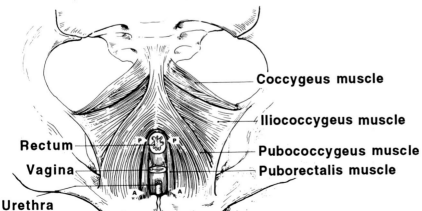

Coccygeus muscle

Iliococcygeus muscle

Rectum

Vagina

Pubococcygeus muscle

Puborectalis muscle

Urethra

Fig. 9B-1 The pelvic floor from above. (Reprinted from *Br J Obstet Gynaecol* 1989;96:16, with permission.)

anus, and then divides into the perineal nerve and the dorsal nerve of the clitoris. The perineal nerve supplies the sphincter urethrae and the anterior parts of the levator ani together with the superficial perineal muscles. Muscular branches from S4 supply the levator ani, coccygeus, and sphincter ani. Percy and coworkers[11] demonstrated by electrophysiologic techniques that the puborectalis is supplied by branches of the sacral nerves S3 and S4 above the pelvic floor rather than by the pudendal nerve. There is uncertainty on the innervation of the striated muscle of the urethral sphincter. Gosling,[12] using anatomical techniques, demonstrated that the striated muscle of the urethral sphincter is innervated by branches of the pelvic nerve rather than the pudendal nerve. However, Vodusek and Light,[13] using electrophysiologic techniques, demonstrated that the urethra is innervated by the pudendal nerve. It is possible that the striated urethral sphincter has a double innervation.

Neuromuscular Damage Leading to Urinary Incontinence, Fecal Incontinence, and Genital Tract Prolapse

Peterson and colleagues[14] investigated 24 women with normal urinary control. This group contained 13 parous women and 11 nulliparous women. They performed electromyography (EMG) of the urethral sphincter and in some cases the pubococcygeus muscle. In the urethral sphincter they found reduced electrical activity in the dorsal portion (5 to 7 o'clock) in multiparous women. The reduction in activity tended to vary directly with parity and was attributed to trauma during delivery. He found no fundamental electromyographic difference between the pubococcygeus and urethral sphincter muscle.

Anderson[15] studied patients with genuine stress incontinence and performed single fiber EMG on the anal sphincter of 35 women with stress incontinence and compared the results with those from 14 continent women. He found an increasing motor unit fiber density with advancing age in the continent women. There was increased fiber density in the incontinent group of women compared to the continent controls. This finding was consistent with damage to the motor nerve supply. Snooks and Swash[16] performed perineal nerve transcutaneous spinal cord stimulation and anal sphincter EMG on 17 patients with idiopathic anorectal fecal incontinence, of whom 12 suffered from urinary incontinence. Of these, 15 patients were parous and 9 gave a history of difficult labor. They found significant in-

creases in spinal, perineal, and pudendal nerve motor latencies in all patients, suggesting damage to the nerve supply of the intramural striated sphincter muscle and the perianal sphincter muscles.

Smith and coworkers[17] performed single fiber EMG on the pelvic floor (pubococcygeus muscle), histochemistry of pelvic floor muscle biopsy, and pudendal nerve terminal motor latency in women with stress incontinence of urine and/or genital tract prolapse. In agreement with Anderson, they found increasing motor unit fiber density with increasing age. The women with stress incontinence, prolapse, or both, have a higher motor unit fiber density than women with no prolapse and normal urinary control. Women with stress incontinence and/or prolapse had prolonged pudendal nerve conduction times to the pelvic floor and urethral sphincter. These results together with muscle histochemistry confirm the presence of partial denervation of the pelvic musculature in women with stress incontinence and/or genital tract prolapse. Parks[18] studied sphincter denervation in anorectal incontinence and rectal prolapse. This involved taking biopsies of the external anal sphincter, puborectalis, and levator ani muscles in 27 patients with anorectal incontinence. Idiopathic anorectal incontinence occurs mainly in women and their study included 24 women. The biopsy material showed histological evidence of denervation, most prominent in the external anal sphincter muscles.

Henry and Swash[19] studied the anal reflex in idiopathic fascial incontinence. The technique involved inserting a concentric needle electrode into the superficial portion of the external sphincter complex. This recorded the response when the perianal skin 1 to 2 cm from the anus was stimulated supramaximally with a bipolar surface stimulating electrode. They found an increased latency and a reduced amplitude of response in patients with idiopathic fecal incontinence. Snooks and coworkers[20] investigated women with idiopathic anorectal incontinence using nerve conduction studies. Of the 30 women studied, 25 were parous, 8 of whom reported difficult childbirth. The study involved the use of transcutaneous spinal stimulation at L1 and L4, pudendal nerve stimulation, and single fiber EMG. This combination of stimulation enabled direct assessment of the puborectalis muscle, which is thought to be innervated mainly by direct branches from S3 and S4 motor routes in the pelvic plexus. The external anal sphincter is thought to be innervated by the pudendal nerve. Their results suggested that the majority of patients with so-called idiopathic anal rectal incontinence had damage to the distal part of the innervation of the external anal sphincter and the puborectalis muscle.

The fact that genital tract prolapse and urinary and fecal incontinence occur mainly in parous women suggests that the (neuromuscular) damage observed in these conditions is initiated by childbirth. Allan and colleagues[21] report a neurophysiologic study of the effect of childbirth on the pelvic floor of 96 primiparous women. They report that changes indicating neuromuscular damage were found in 80% of women who delivered vaginally. Most did not have associated loss of urinary or bowel control. However, the six patients with the most severe degree of damage lost urinary control as a consequence of delivery. One may speculate that some of the women with lesser degrees of neuromuscular damage will deteriorate with age and repeated childbirth. However, this group needs to be studied for years before a causal relationship between neuromuscular damage sustained at childbirth and that found in women with genital tract prolapse and stress incontinence can be established.

The association between urinary and fecal incontinence and genital tract prolapse and neuromuscular damage is strong. However, this does not preclude the possibility that fascial damage may also be a factor leading to these conditions, because few studies have been conducted on the nature of endopelvic fascia in genital tract prolapse. However, there are hints of a fascial abnormality in both stress incontinence and genital tract prolapse, because hypermobility of joints was reported in genital prolapse[22] and Ulmsten and coworkers[23] report decreased collagen in the round ligaments and skin of women with stress incontinence. So it may well be that genital tract prolapse and stress incontinence are caused by combinations of muscle and fascial damage.

SUMMARY

There is clear neurophysiological evidence that the pelvic floor is partially denervated in women with urinary stress incontinence, genital tract prolapse, and anorectal incontinence. The gradual denervation of the striated muscle and pelvic floor with age in primiparous women is similar to that found in other striated muscles of the body. Childbearing in primiparous women commonly causes pelvic floor denervation but infrequently to the degree seen in women with urinary stress incontinence or genital tract prolapse. Partial denervation of the pelvic floor with subsequent reinnervation is a normal accompaniment of aging and is likely to be increased by repeated childbirth. Women with urinary stress incontinence, fecal incontinence, and/or genital

tract prolapse have a significant increase in denervation of the pelvic floor and the visceral sphincters compared with asymptomatic women.

REFERENCES

1. Fothergill WE. The supports of the pelvic viscera: a review of some recent contributions to pelvic anatomy with a clinical introduction. *J Obstet Gynec Brit Emp.* 1908;13:18–23.
2. Mengert WF. Mechanics of uterine support and positional factors influencing support: an experimental study. *Am J Obstet Gynec.* 1936;1:775.
3. Koster II. On the supports of the uterus. *Am J Obstet Gynec.* 1900;25:07.
4. Malpas P. *Genital Prolapse and Allied Conditions.* London: Pub Harvey & Blythe; 1955:45.
5. Berglas N, Rubin IC. Study of the supportive structures of the uterus by levator myography. *Surg Gynec Obstet.* 1955;97:677.
6. Warwick R, Williams PL, ed. *Gray's Anatomy.* 35th ed. London: Longman; 1973.
7. Henry MM, Parks AG, Swash M. The pelvic floor musculature in the descending perineal syndrome. *Br J Surg.* 1982; 69:470.
8. Parks AG. Anorectal incontinence. *Proc Royal Soc Med.* 1975; 68:681–690.
9. Parks AG, Swash M, Urich H. Sphincter denervation in anorectal incontinence and rectal prolapse. *Gut.* 1977;18:656.
10. Gosling JA, Dixon JS, Critchley HOD, Thompson A. Comparative study of the human external urethral sphincter muscle and periurethral levator ani muscles. *Br J Urol.* 1981;53:35.
11. Percy JP, Swash M, Neill ME, Parks AG. Electrophysiological study of the motor nerve supply of the pelvic floor. *Lancet.* 1981; 1:16.
12. Gosling J. Structure of the lower urinary tract and pelvic floor. In: Raz S, ed. *Clinics in Obstetrics and Gynaecology.* WB Saunders Co; 1985;285–294.
13. Vodusek DB, Light JK. The external urethral sphincter innervation: an electrophysiological study. *Proc Intern Cont Soc.* 1983; 108–110.
14. Peterson I, Franksson C, Danielson GO. Electromyography of the pelvic floor and urethra in normal females. *Acta Obstetrics Gynecol Scan.* 1955;34:273–285.
15. Anderson RS. A neurogenic element to genuine stress incontinence. *Br J Obstet Gynaecol.* 1984;91:41–45.
16. Snooks SJ, Swash M. Abnormalities of the urethral striated muscle sphincter in incontinence. *Br J Urol.* 1983;56:401–405.
17. Smith ARB, Hosker GL, Warrell DW. The role of partial denervation of the pelvic floor in the etiology of genitourinary prolapse and stress incontinence: a neurophysiological study. *Br J Obstet Gynaecol.* 1989;96:24–28.
18. Parks AD. Anorectal incontinence. *Proc R Soc Med.* 1975;8:81–90.
19. Henry MM, Swash HM. Assessment of pelvic floor disorders and incontinence by electrophysiological recording of the anal reflex. *Lancet.* 1978;1:1290–1291.
20. Snooks J, Swash M, Henry MM. Abnormalities in central and peripheral nerve conduction in patients with anorectal incontinence. *J Roy Soc Med.* 1985;78:294–300.
21. Allen RE, Hosker GL, Smith ARB, Warrell DW. Pelvic floor damage and childbirth: a neurophysiological study. *Br J Obstet Gynaecol.* 1990;97:770–779.
22. Norton P, Baker J, Sharpe H, Warrenski S. Genitourinary prolapse: relationship with joint mobility. *Neurol Urodyn.* 1990;9: 311–317.
23. Ulmsten U, Ekman G, Giertz G, Malmstrom A. Different biochemical composition of connector tissue in continent and stress incontinent women. *Acta Obstet Gynecol Scand.* 1987;66:455–457.

CHAPTER 9

Pelvic Floor Neuropathy

9C   Electrodiagnosis

J. Thomas Benson

INTRODUCTION

This chapter describes the methodology of electrodiagnosis in pelvic floor neuropathy with case discussions used to show clinical applications.

ELECTRODIAGNOSIS IN PELVIC FLOOR DISORDERS

Surface Electrodes

Surface electrodes measure gross electrical activity across relatively large areas and are widely used in urodynamic and defecation studies. They are helpful in gross diagnosis of particular syndromes and in biofeedback therapies. They are helpful in pelvic floor and sphincter studies not requiring needle precision and are available as anal plug electrodes, perineal skin surface electrodes, catheter mounted ring electrodes, and vaginal electrodes.

Needle Electromyography (EMG)

A single motor neuron and the muscle fibers innervated by its branches are termed a motor unit. The electrical activity of motor units in a muscle (motor unit action potentials, or MUAPs) is recordable by inserting a needle connected to amplifiers (Fig. 9C-1). Changes in established normal values for the amplitude, duration, and number of phases of MUAPs may suggest neuropathy or myopathy. Using concentric needles, the characteristic motor unit from the urethral sphincter and the anal sphincter has a duration of less than 6 msec, and amplitude of 0.10 to 0.5 mV. Unlike skeletal muscle that can be voluntarily relaxed to the point of complete electrical silence, the striated muscle of the urethral and anal sphincter show continuous motor unit activity.

With denervation there is increased muscle surface membrane sensitivity to neurotransmitters, leading to increased activity with needle insertion, recognized as

Fig. 9C-1 Schematic representation of motor unit action potential (MUAP).

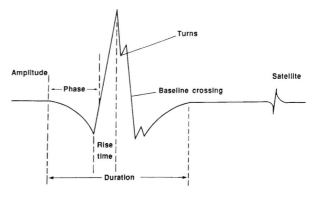

fibrillation potentials and positive waves. These occur 12 to 21 days after denervation and are short duration (0.5 to 2 msec), low amplitude (50 to 100 µV), diphasic or triphasic potentials that need complete electrical background silence to be detected; therefore, they are difficult to find in the tonically active anal and urethral sphincters. With denervation, concomitant reinnervation occurs with axonal sprouting from adjacent nerves causing bunching of fibers. The single-fiber EMG needle, having a very small pick-up diameter (300 micrometers) measures this bunching of fibers or fiber density. This single fiber electrode study is of particular interest in pelvic floor disorders as a relatively precise method of measuring sphincter denervation (Fig. 9C-2). An amplifier with 350 Hz low frequency filter setting and a trigger delay are required. Five fields of activity are observed for each of four needle insertions. The 20 fields' "fiber number" are averaged for a "fiber density." To be counted, the potential must have an amplitude of 100 mV and all observed potentials must be counted. In our laboratory, the normal value for external anal sphincter single fiber density is 1.6 ± .39. The density is known to slightly increase beyond age 60.

Recruitment is another needle EMG determination based on the principle that when a voluntary effort is increased, firing rates of acting motor units increase to a given level, at which level new motor units discharge. In neuropathies, a frequency greater than expected is obtained before enlisting new motor units. In myopathies, because of reduced force per motor unit, recruitment occurs when the acting motor units are discharging at lower frequencies than expected.

Nerve Conduction Studies

Stimulating a nerve depolarizes it and induces a propagated action potential, which may be recorded directly from the nerve or from the innervated muscle as a compound muscle action potential (CMAP). Neuropathies affecting the myelin (for example, diabetes, compression, stretch injury) affect the speed of conduction.

Sensory nerve conduction may be determined directly by measuring the propagation rate and dividing by the length of the nerve from stimulus to the recording area. Motor nerve studies recording the CMAP involve neuromuscular transmission in addition to the nerve conduction time, the sum being termed the motor terminal latency. Exemplifying the value of such studies is the increased awareness of pudendal nerve injury's significance in urinary incontinence. Kiff and Swask described a method wherein the stimulus is applied rectally over the pudendal nerve at each ischial spine and recorded at the anal sphincter using the St. Mark's pudendal electrode (Fig. 9C-3). The resulting right and left pudendal nerve motor terminal latency (Fig. 9C-4) has a normal value in our laboratory of 2.1 ± 0.2 msec. The recording may be done with a ring electrode about a Foley catheter, just below the inflated bulb, and on stimulation of the pudendal nerve at the ischial spine, a right and left perineal nerve motor terminal latency is obtained (Fig. 9C-5). The normal value for this in our laboratory is 2.29 ± .30. Technical factors, such as skin resistance and stimulation parameters, must be painstakingly monitored and standardized in conduction studies and evoked potentials.

Evoked Potentials

Evoked potentials are specific, time-locked electrical by-products of peripheral and central neuropathways occurring in response to an external stimulus. They are recorded by a computerized system that averages signals to reveal the evoked signal, which is otherwise hidden in the body's electrical activity. The presence and the timing of the evoked response are adjunctive evidence of the neuronal status.

Evoked response may be used to evaluate the entire

Fig. 9C-2 Single fiber needle EMG—areas of pick up (1,2,3) with recorded responses; 1 and 2 in normal muscle, 3 in muscle with reinnervation.

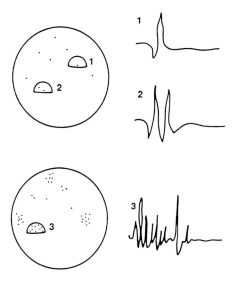

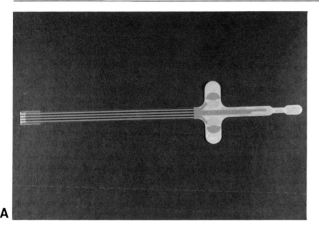

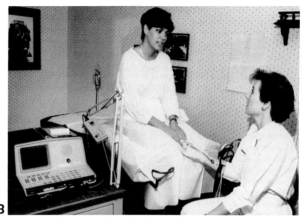

Fig. 9C-3   A, St. Mark's pudendal nerve conductor, a disposable conductor that is placed over examination glove. **B**, Stimulating electrodes (anode, cathode) at finger tip and receptor electrodes at base of finger.

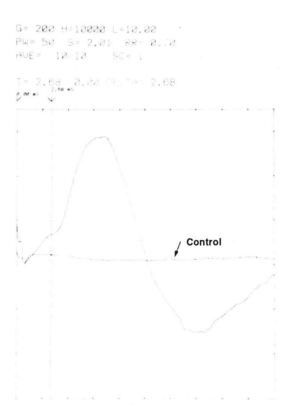

Control

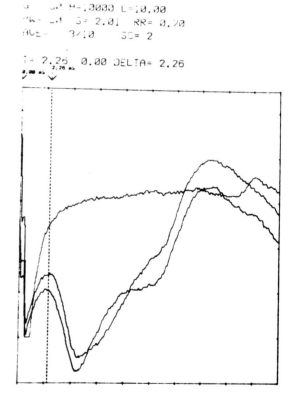

Fig. 9C-4   Right pudendal motor terminal latency. The normal mean and standard deviation is 2.1 ± 0.2 ms. G = gain = amplitude (V); H = high frequency filter setting (Hz); L = low frequency filter setting (Hz); PW = pulse width of stimulus (MS); S = sweep speed (MS); RR = repetition rate per second; SC = scale; AVE = number of averaged stimuli; T = time to receptor of L1, cortex; $DELTA$ = difference in the two times.

Fig. 9C-5   Right perineal motor terminal latency (Abbreviations as for Fig. 4.)

peripheral and central nervous system transmission as is done with posterior tibial somatosensory-evoked re-

sponse to the spine at L1 and to the cerebral cortex (Fig. 9C-6). Evoked responses to the spinal cord may also be obtained from the pudendal nerve with stimulation at the ischial spine as indirect evidence of disorder proximal to the ischial spine (Fig. 9C-7). Evoked pudendal responses over the spine and cortex are much more

G= ~5~   2 H= 500/ 500 L=10.00/10.00

PW=100 S=10.00 RR= 2.82
AVE= 200/200   SC= 1

T=22.24 39.52 DELTA=17.47

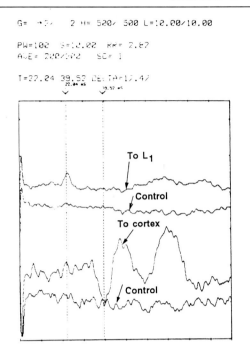

Fig. 9C-6 Posterior tibial somatosensory evoked response to spine at first lumbar vertebra (L1) and to cerebral cortex (cortex). The mean and standard deviation for our laboratory of L1 is 21.75 with an SD of 1.24 and the mean of cortex is 38.02 with an SD of 2.34. (Abbreviations as for Fig. 4.)

Fig. 9C-7 Evoked response over L1 vertebra with stimulation at pudendal nerve at ischial spine. Mean and standard deviation for our laboratory is 5.80 ± .99. (Abbreviations as for Fig. 4.)

G=   5 H= 500 L=10.00
PW= 50 S= 2.01 RR= 2.82
AVE= 18/200   SC= 1

T= 4.28 0.00 DELTA= 4.28

G= 200 H=10000 L=10.00
PW= 50 S= 5.00 RR= 0.70
AVE= 25/10   SC= 1

T=18.51   7.28 DELTA=11.23

Fig. 9C-8 F wave with pudendal nerve stimulation. (Abbreviations as for Fig. 4.)

easily obtained in women with stimulation of the pudendal nerve in the area of Alcock's canal compared to stimulation over the clitoris. Another method to attempt study of the pudendal nerve proximal to Alcock's canal is by "f wave" studies (Fig. 9C-8). This is a way to look at proximal segments of peripheral nerves. The f wave is produced by antidromic conduction in the stimulated motor fiber rebounding off the anterior horn cell and going back on itself orthodromically to produce another action potential. When obtainable, indirect estimation of conduction velocity can be performed. Indirect evidence of the status of the pelvic plexus can be obtained by the stimulation of the bladder base when picking up the response at L1 (Fig. 9C-9).

Finally, electromyelography may be utilized. As described by Bradley and colleagues[2] this evoked response is obtained at the anal sphincter with stimulation at the bladder base. Afferents at the bladder base through the pelvic plexus to the cord are transmitted to the pudendal nerve efferents to the external anal sphincter. The timing of this response, as well as the amplitude, may indicate disease processes involving the cauda equina

G=   5 H= 500 L=10.00
PW=150   S=20.00   RR= 2.80
AVE= 104/20   SC= 1

T=85.69   0.00 DELTA=85.69

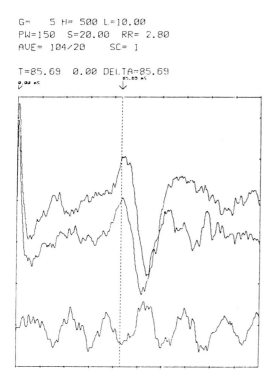

G=   20 H=10000 L=10.00
PW=150   S=20.00   RR= 2.80
AVE=   20/20   SC= 1

T=59.90   0.00 DELTA=59.90

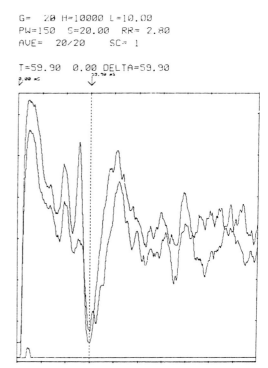

Fig. 9C-9 Evoked response over first lumbar vertebra with stimulation at bladder base. Mean and standard deviation for our laboratory is 20.24 ± 0.5. (Abbreviations as for Fig. 4.)

Fig. 9C-10 Electromyelography. Stimulation at bladder base and recording at anal sphincter. Mean and standard deviation of 44.56 ± 0.58 is for latency. Mean amplitude is 53.27 ± 15.25 microvolt. (Abbreviations as for Fig. 4.)

(Fig. 9C-10). Direct cauda equina stimulation with recording at sphincter areas would be a more precise means of assessing pelvic floor innervation than reflex latencies but awaits further development of the magnetic stimulator for painless spinal cord stimulation.

CLINICAL CONSIDERATIONS

Clinical Applications

The field of electrodiagnostic study of female pelvic floor neuropathy is still new. Possible clinical applications are not yet appreciated, although some clinically significant parameters are already evident. Diagnostic applications may be made in genuine stress urinary incontinence. Swash, Henry, and Snooks[3] state that urinary incontinence is not found when the fiber density is less than 1.9 and the pudendal nerve motor nerve terminal latency is less than 2.5, except in patients in whom

the denervation is situated in the cauda equina or pelvic nerves. Thus, a diagnosis of genuine stress urinary incontinence made in the patient who has normal physiologic studies is very likely in error. Cases of overlapping or confusing diagnoses may thus be assisted by this electrophysiologic parameter.

Localization of neurologic disturbance may be assisted with these methodologies, as illustrated in the following cases showing lesions progressing from cerebral cortex to the perineal branch of the pudendal nerve.

Case 1: M.B.; 42-year-old, white female with petit mal epilepsy (Fig. 9C-11). A fortuitous epileptiform attack occurred while undergoing cystourethrometric study showing episodic incontinence of coordinated nature, with urethral relaxation followed by detrusor contraction. Such coordinated detrusor hyperreflexia is typical of lesions above the brain stem micturition center.

Case 2: Patient with Brown-Séquard syndrome,

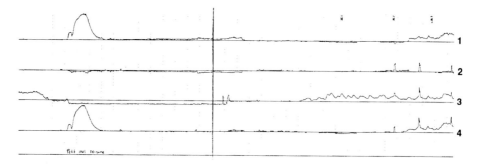

Fig. 9C-11 Cystourethrometric study when patient had a petit mal seizure. Lines: *1* = true detrusor pressure; *2* = intraabdominal pressure (through rectal lead); *3* = intraurethral pressure; *4* = intravesical pressure. Filling water, at a rate of 30 cc/minute, upright position, room temperature.

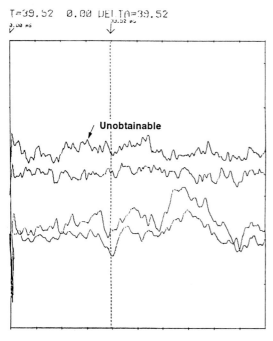

Fig. 9C-12 Posterior tibial somatosensory evoked response to cortex. Top line stimulation on right, bottom line stimulation on left. *T* = time to receptor of cortex, *Delta* = difference in the two times.

Fig. 9C-13 Evoked response at first lumbar vertebrae with stimulation over pudendal nerve at Alcock's canal on left and right sides. (Abbreviations as for Fig. 4.)

hemisection of the spinal cord at the C3 to C4 level resulting in ipsilateral spastic paralysis and contralateral loss of pain and thermal sense. There is absent posterior tibial evoked response to the head on the side of the defect (Fig. 9C-12). Cystometrics indicated hyperreflexia and the patient had increased residual urine.

Case 3: J.S.; 31-year-old, professional, former athlete. Patient developed inability to empty the bladder and on testing (Fig. 9C-13) was found to have a virtually absent response from the left pudendal nerve to L1. The patient's symptoms progressed until there developed left leg and thigh signs and at operation was found to have inoperable lipoma involving S2, S3, and S4 nerve roots on the left.

Case 4: J.U.; Nulliparous, 74-year-old, white female with complete inversion of the vagina. Because of this unusual condition in a nulliparous patient she was studied electrophysiologically and the evoked response from

```
G=   2 H= 500 L=10.00
PW= 50  S= 5.00  RR= 2.80
AVE=  56/500    SC= 1
```

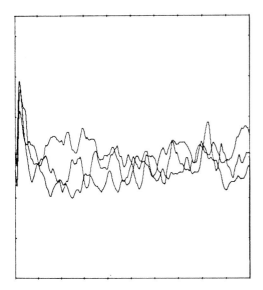

Fig. 9C-14 Unobtainable response over first lumbar vertebra with stimulation at bladder base. (Abbreviations as per Fig. 4.)

```
G=    5 H=1000 L=10.00
PW=200  S=10.00  RR= 2.80
AVE=  23/500    SC= 1
```

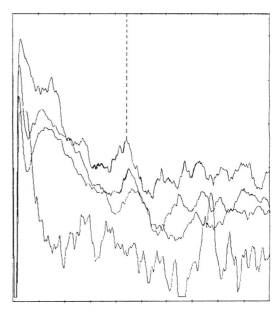

Fig. 9C-16 Electromyelography (stimulation at bladder base and recording at anal sphincter). Response is virtually absent. (Abbreviations as per Fig. 4.)

bladder base to L1 (Fig. 9C-14) was seen to be completely unobtainable. Magnetic resonance image (MRI) at lumbosacral spine shown in Fig. 9C-15*A* compared with a normal MRI (Fig. 9C-15*B*). This was caused by metastatic carcinoma and the patient's pelvic floor problem was not operated on, as treatment was directed toward the metastatic neoplasm.

Case 5: N.H.; 62-year-old, obese white female with advanced diabetes and pelvic floor prolapse. Bladder base to external anal sphincter electromyelography reflex was absent (Fig. 9C-16). Patient's uroflow shows

Fig. 9C-15 **A**, Lumbosacral magnetic resonance image in patient of Fig. 14. Note damaged spinal cord. **B**, Normal lumbosacral magnetic resonance image.

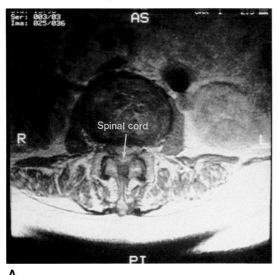

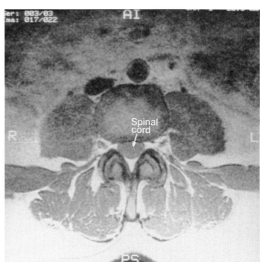

A   B

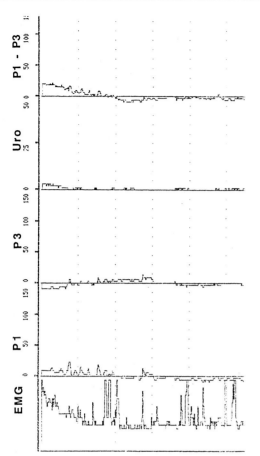

Fig. 9C-17 Instrumented uroflow: *P1 − P3* = true detrusor pressure; *Uro* = uroflow; *P3* = intraabdominal pressure; *P1* = intravesical pressure; *EMG* = perineal surface electrode EMG.

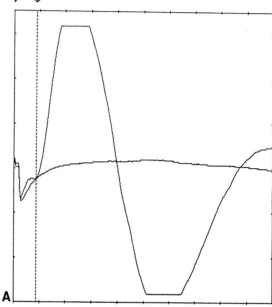

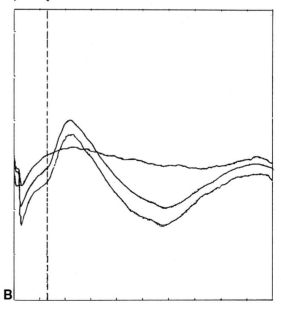

inadequate type of flow associated with poor detrusor function and poor synergy between detrusor and urethra (Fig. 9C-17). The patient had loss of sensation over S2 and S3 dermatomes and a low pressure urethra. The patient had surgery for the prolapse with prompt recurrence of a pulsion type cystocele.

Case 6: L.S.; 17-year-old female with her first pregnancy with pudendal nerve motor terminal latency studies before and after delivery (Fig. 9C-18 *A* and *B*). This patient developed stress urinary incontinence following this delivery.

Fig. 9C-18 **A,** Pudendal nerve motor terminal latency before and **B,** after delivery. (Abbreviations as per Fig. 4.)

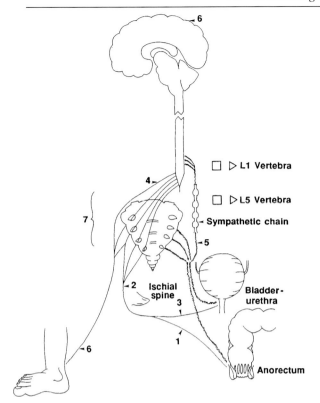

Fig. 9C-19   Schematic representation of pelvic floor electrodiagnosis: *1* pudendal nerve motor terminal latency; *2* pudendal nerve to L1 evoked response; *3* perineal nerve motor terminal latency; *4* posterior tibial evoked response to L1; *5* bladder base evoked response to L1; *6* posterior tibial evoked response to cortex; *7* electromyelography.

SUMMARY

Pelvic floor electrodiagnosis may help to anatomically locate lesions (Fig. 9C-19). Patients being operated on for anal incontinence with sphincter deficiencies may have electrodiagnostic studies. The amount of pudendal neuropathy may be appreciated and with needle studies the area of sphincter disruption can be ascertained. Intraoperative needle electromyography may be useful in pelvic floor surgery to help in the choice of vital musculature in various supportive operations.

Prognostic implications may be obtained with neurophysiologic studies. Finding severe denervation may indicate less likelihood of a surgical cure and may influence choice of therapy to provide medical management in lieu of surgery.

Preventive aspects may be important. Evidence of pudendal neuropathy after delivery of an infant and knowledge that such pudendal neuropathy may be accentuated by subsequent vaginal delivery may lead to cesarean delivery as a preventive measure.

The research parameters now open for consideration in electrophysiologic studies are virtually unlimited. Knowledge of obstetric events and their importance in pelvic floor neuropathy, better understanding of pelvic surgery effects on pelvic floor neuropathy, and studies on the effects of excessive straining with defecation are a few of the areas to be considered.

REFERENCES

1. Kiff ES, Swash M. Slowed conduction in the pudendal nerves in idiopathic (neurogenic) faecal incontinence. *Br J Surg.* 1984;71:614–616.
2. Bradley WE, Timm GW, Rockswold GL, Scott FB. Detrusor and urethral electromyelography. *J Urol.* 1975;114:69.
3. Swash M, Henry MM, Snooks SJ. Unifying concept of pelvic floor disorders and incontinence. *J R Soc Med.* 1985;78:906–911.

CHAPTER 10

Histological and Biochemical Studies

Peggy A. Norton

INTRODUCTION

Although some evidence exists that pelvic floor dysfunction is neurologic in origin, deficiencies in connective tissue and muscular components of the pelvic floor are equally suspect as the underlying cause. Connective tissue forms the cement of the body and allows stretching of tissue without loss of original form as well as remodeling in response to injury. Connective tissue has long been hypothesized as an important cause of genitourinary prolapse. Nichols and Randal[1] wrote:

> Of utmost importance is an appreciation of individual variation, particularly when recognized in terms of the relative strength of muscular and connective tissue components of the individual's pelvic supporting tissues.

To facilitate pregnancy and parturition, the connective tissue of the female reproductive tract undergoes profound changes unequaled anywhere else in the body. The amount of collagen in the uterus increases eight to tenfold to accommodate an expanding fetus and placenta, yet is rapidly resorbed postpartum.[2] Maintenance of pregnancy depends on cervical strength, largely due to collagen; however, the connective tissue of the cervix must soften and "ripen" to allow sufficient effacement and dilatation for parturition. These changes in collagen, elastin, and the other components of connective tissue are controlled by hormones and prostaglandins.

The ligaments and fascial planes of the pelvic floor are in close juxtaposition to the uterus and cervix. The conditions that cause softening and stretching of the cervical connective tissue to facilitate delivery may act on the connective tissue of the pelvic floor, making these ligaments and fascia prone to detrimental changes at the time of delivery.

Childbirth injuries and chronic straining with bowel movements may cause neurologic damage of the pelvic floor (see Chapter 9B), but may also stretch the connective tissue beyond recovery, tearing these fibers and causing scar formation. Errors in deposition of new connective tissue after such injuries or errors in the manufacture of any one element of connective tissue may greatly compromise the strength and resilience of ligaments and fascial planes of the pelvic floor.

Unfortunately, the histopathology of the pelvic floor has not been well studied except to describe the muscular fiber changes associated with neurologic dysfunction.[3] However, the role of connective tissue in disease was investigated in several other areas of medicine. In the study of parturition, researchers discovered that a relative deficiency of collagen may result in an incompetent cervix[4] and that prostaglandins initiate cervical ripening through the breakdown of collagen.[5] Research in the area of general surgery has identified abnormalities of collagen synthesis causing weak vascular walls, leading to abdominal aortic and cerebral aneurysms.[6]

Inexplicable differences between individuals in the

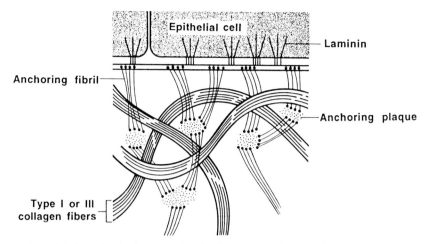

Fig. 10-1 A schematic drawing of the hypothesized extended anchoring network of fibrils. Collagen interacts with laminin and other connective tissue components to provide strength in the dermis. (From *Acta Obstet Gynecol Scand* 1989;148:13. Redrawn with permission.)

development of genitourinary prolapse (i.e., severe prolapse in a young nulliparous woman versus no prolapse or incontinence in a multiparous woman after many vaginal deliveries) continue to puzzle gynecologists. In the future, abnormalities in the synthesis and remodeling of connective tissue may explain these individual differences.

This chapter will review the pelvic floor from the histologic and biologic point of view: What holds these tissues together? How might abnormalities lead to clinical dysfunction? Where may the interested student of the pelvic floor begin to study connective tissue dysfunction?

COMPONENTS OF THE PELVIC FLOOR

The levator ani evolved from a "pelvic wall" with a primary function of tail-wagging, into the pelvic floor of bipeds with a primary function of maintaining continence despite gravity and intraabdominal pressure. Instead of undergoing hypertrophy, the muscles of the pelvic floor were converted to connective tissue.[7] Thus, a major component of the pelvic floor became ligamentous and fascial; the strength of this tissue is due to the various fibers that constitute the connective tissue.

Connective Tissue

Connective tissue is composed of three fibrous proteins (collagen, elastin, and reticulin), which provide the mechanical strength and ground substance that serves as the cement between these fibers. The three fibrous proteins are largely produced by fibroblasts and smooth muscle cells in all parts of the body. The term "extracellular matrix" refers to ground substance together with collagen, elastin, and reticulin.

Collagen

Collagen provides most of the mechanical strength of connective tissue (Fig. 10-1). As much as 25% of the body's protein is collagen, and in repair tissue collagen accounts for 50% of the total protein.[8] Although collagen was thought to be a single protein until 1968, we now recognize at least 12 different types of collagen—all with individual theoretical roles. The most important types of collagen in the pelvic floor are types I and III.

Type I collagen is ubiquitous, and large amounts are found in skin, tendon, cartilage, and ligaments. Composed of two alpha-1 (I) chains and one alpha-2 (I) chain, it is the form of collagen found in most mature structures (Fig. 10-2).

Type III collagen is formed from three alpha-1 (III) chains and is found in the aorta, lungs, skin, uterus, and ligaments. It is the major component in the skin at birth and is replaced by type I collagen with maturation.[9] In addition, type III collagen is the initial collagen laid down in wound healing and is usually then replaced over several months by type I collagen.[10] Type III collagen has disulfide cross-links in addition to hydrogen bonding, which facilitates differentiating the two in

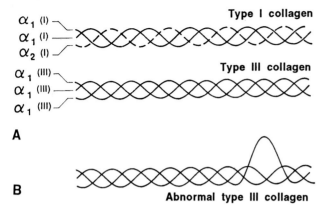

α_1 (I)
α_1 (I)
α_2 (I)

Type I collagen

α_1 (III)
α_1 (III)
α_1 (III)

Type III collagen

A

B

Abnormal type III collagen

Fig. 10-2 **A**, Type I collagen consists of two alpha 1 (I) chains and one alpha 2 (I) chain. Type III collagen is a trimer of alpha 1 (III) chains. **B**, An abnormal region in any one chain of the tropocollagen compromises the otherwise tight configuration, affecting strength or making the structure prone to enzymatic degradation.

vitro; type III requires reduction prior to denaturation in order to separate the three alpha-1 (III) chains. Although type III is generally found in lesser amounts than type I, it seems to be more important in the control of fibril formation.[11]

Collagen chains form a trimer in a right-handed helix known as tropocollagen. The tropocollagen molecules, which in vivo exist only momentarily, then aggregate to form long chains commonly referred to as collagen. Three right-handed chains are joined together to form a left-handed "superhelix" bonded by hydrogen bonds. Heat or mild urea break the weak hydrogen bonds and allow separation into individual, randomly coiled chains (as occurs when gelatin is formed). The mechanical strength is helped by the aggregation of tropocollagen and overlapping bundles. Most of the studies on the strength of collagen have been done with type I; very little is known about the formation of type III into large superhelices. Recently, the use of specific anticollagen probes has demonstrated that collagen helices can contain more than one collagen type.[12]

Why are there so many collagen types? Burgeson[12] believes that by varying the ratios of these collagen types, cells can control the parameters of fibril formations, such as rate of length extension versus diameter expansion, ultimate fibril diameter, and perhaps even fibril orientation.

Collagen is converted from a procollagen form. Since the precursor forms for collagen types I, II, and III are similar,[13] a large amount of collagen can be made quickly through conversion of the procollagen to collagen. Likewise, collagenase exists in a proform that facilitates the rapid breakdown of collagen for parturition.

Cross-linking of collagen occurs at different rates and may account for the variability of strength of newly synthesized tissues. Anything that disrupts the strength or number of cross-linkage will affect the integrity of tissue. This is illustrated by a condition called lathyrism caused by eating the seeds of the sweet pea, *Lathyrus odoratus*. Lathyrism results from the inhibition of the enzyme lysyl oxidase that interrupts cross-linking in the alpha chains and between molecules. With loss of cross-linking, the connective tissue of lathyritic animals loses its tensile strength, leading to skeletal deformation, aneurysms, and herniation.

Elastin

Elastin permits distention and allows tissue to stretch to a limited degree and to return to its original contour. When stretched, elastin fibers orient in the direction of the stretch. This restricts the amount of stretch in any one individual tissue. When released from the distentional forces, the fibers allow restoration of the original structure along the same orientation. Fibroblasts produce elastin at a relatively constant rate, so response to injury is not as profound as with collagen synthesis. With aging, elastin fibers undergo fragmentation, illustrated by the decreasing elasticity of the skin in the fifth and sixth decades.[14] Because scar tissue has very little elastin, the collagen fibers in wounds can only orientate along the lines of repair, resulting in very little stretch in scar tissue. This may have important implications for the injuries to ligaments and fascia during childbirth.

Elastin fibers contain the protein elastin in association with microfibrils, which interweave among collagen bundles. Elastin protein is synthesized from a soluble precursor, tropoelastin. During transcription, alternative splicing of gene copies of tropoelastin results in isoforms of the elastin fiber. The function of multiple isoforms of tropoelastin probably relates to a tissue-specific assembly of elastin.[15] Unfortunately, elastin is difficult to study because it is insoluble in ordinary solvents and is not susceptible to trypsin.

Reticulin

Reticulin forms a background matrix. Because reticulin is rather difficult to study, little is known about the abnormalities associated with this substance.

Ground Substance

Ground substance consists of the "filler or cement" between fibrous proteins. It consists largely of mucopolysaccharides in which 95% of the structure is polysaccharide, either *proteoglycans* (polysaccharides attached to protein in which 95% of the structure is polysaccharide) or *glycoproteins* (polysaccharides attached to protein in which the protein component predominates). Proteoglycans have special glycosaminoglycans (GAGs) which are negatively charged, repelling one another, causing the entire structure to become stiff and rigid (Fig. 10-3). Glycosaminoglycans are one class of mucopolysaccharides (the "muco" means that these molecules were first isolated from mucin, the slippery lubricating proteoglycan of mucus). The alteration in the kind and proportion of glycosaminoglycans in proteoglycans produces different properties. For example, chondroitin sulfate maintains a rigid structure and is found in cartilage, while hyaluronic acid is highly viscous and jellylike. Dermatan sulfate is a more flexible glycosaminoglycan found in skin proteoglycans, and keratan sulfate is found in cornea and fetal skeleton. *Fibronectin* is a high molecular weight glycoprotein that may be responsible for interactions between cells and other components of the extracellular matrix.[16] *Laminin* is an adhesive glycoprotein which may modulate smooth muscle growth.[17] Besides mucopolysaccharides and glycoproteins, ground substance contains many ions and a considerable amount of bound water, which further influences the strength of the tissue. Ground substance may be important in the stabilization of collagen fibrils through electrostatic bonding with a protein-polysaccharide.

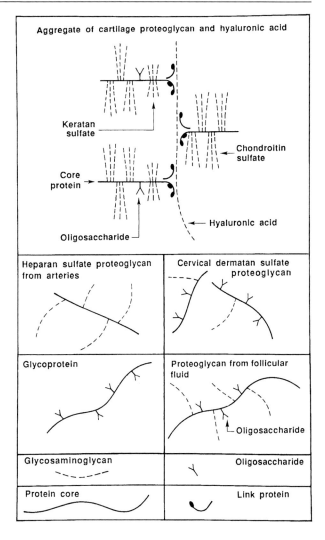

Fig. 10-3 A schematic diagram of different proteoglycans and a glycoprotein. (Reprinted from *Acta Obstet Gynecol Scand* 1989; 148:15 with permission.)

Muscle

In the pelvic floor, muscle is either smooth or striated. Loss of fast twitch muscle fibers with denervation has been described by Bierseck and coworkers.[18] The remaining cells hypertrophy to assume the role of fibers lost from denervation.

Voluntary muscle is important in studying the pelvic floor because maintenance of continence involves the ability to recruit additional motor units. The slow twitch muscles are responsible for the continuous pressure that the pelvic floor must exert against intraabdominal pressures, and against gravity. Slow twitch fibers are also called type I muscle fibers, and fast twitch are called type II fibers and are not to be confused with the types of collagen fibers. Unfortunately, little has been done in histological study of the effectiveness of pelvic floor exercise training.

Pelvic Tissue

Research to determine the ways in which connective tissue affects function of the pelvic floor is in progress. More is known about the uterus and cervix because of the extraordinary changes that occur in these organs with pregnancy. In the human uterus during pregnancy, the total amount of collagen increases eight to tenfold, while the total amount of elastin increases eightfold.[19] The loss of collagen in the postpartum mammalian uterus is the most rapid process of collagen removal known. Collagenase and elastase are produced in large amounts in a latent form and appear to be quickly activated in the postpartum uterus and cervix. In the involuting rat uterus, smooth muscle is the major cell type involved in the production of collagenase. If this is more than a local phenomenon, then the pelvic fascia and ligaments may undergo the same breakdown found in the nearby uterus and cervix.

The proportion of type I to type III collagen in the uterus is approximately 2:1. In abdominal aortic aneurysm, the vascular wall shows an increase in the proportion of type I collagen to type III. This may be due to a relative increase in type I or a decrease in type III. The proportion of type I to type III collagen and similar characteristics of the collagen itself may have equally important implications in the uterus, pelvic ligaments, and fascial structures.

Hormones have important effects on collagen and elastic. Stenback[21] demonstrated that in estrogen-deficient mucosa and in proliferative endometrium, collagen deposition is increased, with subsequent decreases of collagen in secretory endometrium. He also found that hyperplastic glands showed a dense deposition of collagen and that patients treated with medroxyprogesterone acetate had sparse amounts of type III collagen. On the other hand, Ryan and Woessner[22] demonstrated that estradiol inhibits collagen breakdown in the involuting rat uterus. It is possible that the wide fluctuations in hormone levels at the time of parturition and after the menopause may explain some of the changes that take place in women during these specific times of their lives. In a study by Brincat and colleagues,[23] skin collagen content and skin thickness were found to decrease proportionately with years after the menopause and to be reversed by estrogen replacement therapy (Fig. 10-4).

Aging seems to affect connective tissue in significant ways. In the skin, the proportion of collagen types is age-dependent.[24] Type III collagen represents between 10% and 50% of the collagen in the fetal dermis, depending on fetal age. In mature skin, about 85% of the collagen is type I.

The solubility of collagen in tissue gives us clues about the function of the connective tissue in a specific organ. In a human pregnancy at term, the solubility of collagen, particularly type I collagen, in the cervix is significantly increased.[25] Since other collagen in the pel-

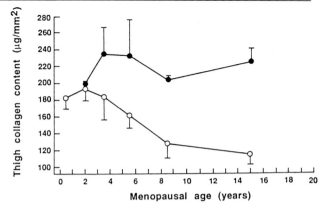

Fig. 10-4 The relationship between thigh skin collagen content and menopausal age in 52 patients treated with a sex hormone implant (●) and in 77 untreated patients (○). (Reprinted from Brincat[23] with permission.)

vis may be subject to the same hormonal changes, it is possible that collagen in the fascia and ligaments is also more soluble, and therefore subject to alteration.

Abnormalities in connective tissue may have profound effects on muscle function. Connective tissue interacts with muscle in many ways and is found between muscle fibers and cells in varying degrees. Moreover, muscles exert energy on a bony structure through ligaments, which are composed primarily of connective tissue.

CLINICAL CORRELATIONS

In gynecology and other specialties, deficiencies or abnormalities in connective tissue have been linked to clinical syndromes.

Connective Tissue Disorders

Ehlers-Danlos syndrome is a heterogeneous group of inherited connective tissue disorders characterized by joint hypermobility, easy bruisability, and cutaneous hyperextensibility.[26] There are now at least ten types identified that differ in the severity of organ involvement. Patients with Types II and III Ehlers-Danlos have subclinical disease with joint hypermobility, herniation of many fascial planes, and excessive skin elasticity. Patients with Type IV Ehlers-Danlos have severe deficiencies in vascular walls, joints, and lens; the high mortality is associated with aortic rupture. The abnormality is felt to be a deficiency of type III collagen.[27] Surprisingly, herniation of the pelvic floor is rarely mentioned in these patients; no evaluation seems to have been carried out. Although obstetric complications of patients with Ehlers-Danlos have been reviewed recently,[27] no evaluation for genitourinary prolapse was made.[28] Abnormal type I collagen seems to be the defect in osteogenesis imperfecta.[29] The specific connective tissue abnormality for the Marfan syndrome has not been identified but is suspected to be a defect in either collagen or elastin.[30]

Joint Hypermobility and Prolapse

Marshman and coworkers[31] reported that patients with rectal prolapse had excessively mobile ("double-jointed") joints compared with controls who did not have rectal prolapse. More recently, Norton and colleagues[32] reported that women with hypermobile joints had a significantly higher prevalence of pelvic relaxation compared to women with normal joints; this relationship was more significant with higher degrees of prolapse (Fig. 10-5). Newborns with congenital hip dislocations were found to have more type III collagen in their umbilical cords compared to normal newborns.[33] Because ligaments are composed largely of collagen and elastin, patients with hypermobile joints may have an abnormal composition of these connective tissues—that is, a different proportion of collagen types or elastin, abnormalities in structure, or alterations in the total amount of connective tissue. If alterations enable ligaments to stretch, allowing joint hypermobility, the same phenomenon may account for pelvic relaxation and rectal prolapse.

Fig. 10-5 Joint hypermobility and rectocele. In this population of middle-aged caucasion women attending a routine gynecologic clinic, patients with joint hypermobility had a higher prevalence of rectocele, especially the higher grade 2 (descent to the introitus) and grade 3 (descent beyond the introitus) compared to patients without joint hypermobility.

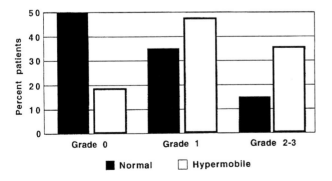

Stress Incontinence

Ulmsten and associates[34] biopsied the skin of women undergoing benign gynecologic surgical procedures and found a 40% decrease in the total collagen content in those subjects with stress incontinence compared to continent women. However, Landon and coworkers[35] were unable to demonstrate differences in the biomechanical properties of the fascia of women with stress incontinence. In Norton and coworkers'[32] study of women with joint hypermobility, no relationship was evident between joint hypermobility and stress urinary incontinence.

Pregnancy

Many groups have described a decreased collagen-to-smooth muscle ratio in the cervix of women with an incompetent cervix. This may be caused by decreased collagen or more probably decreased smooth muscle.

Cervical ripening seems to be an action of eicosanoids (prostaglandins) on the connective tissue of the cervix. Rechberger and colleagues[4] reported that collagen in the cervix undergoes changes detectable by biochemical studies; primiparas with higher levels of collagen and hyaluronic acid had long cervical dilatation times, suggesting a physiologic importance. Although softening and breakdown of connective tissue in the cervix and uterus is crucial to parturition, the same changes may be occurring in other pelvic tissue, that is, the pelvic ligaments and fascia, resulting in pelvic relaxation. Granstrom[5] demonstrated that women delivered by cesarean section due to protracted labor had a significantly higher concentration of collagen in the uterine isthmus and cervix compared to normal women, as well as a decrease in solubility of the collagen. Granstrom concluded that insufficient remodeling of uterine tissue during pregnancy may contribute to protracted labor, as did Uldbjerg (Fig. 10-6).

Aneurysm

Patients with cerebral aneurysm and abdominal aortic aneurysm reportedly have abnormally high ratios of type I collagen to type III collagen, producing weakness and subsequent aneurysm of the vascular wall.[20,36] This increased ratio could be due to: (1) increased type I and normal amounts of type III; (2) normal type I and decreased type III; or (3) abnormal collagen that is not recognized by biochemical methods, and therefore not totally measured. If abnormal in structure, this same

Prediction Interval (95%)

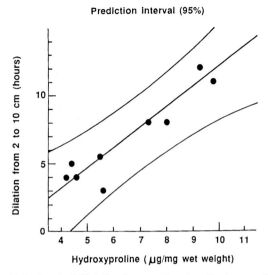

Fig. 10-6 Cervical dilatation time as a function of hydroxyproline concentration. Hydroxyproline is a rough quantitation of the total amount of collagen present, and time for cervical dilatation was directly related to the amount of collagen present in the cervix. (Reprinted from *Am J Obstet Gynecol* 1983;147:662 with permission.)

collagen may be equally abnormal in function. Recently, Deak and coworkers[37] found that the deficiency is actually abnormal type III collagen made in appropriate amounts but with an abnormal carboxyl end that affects function. This is due to a single-base deletion that causes a shift in the reading of the codon from that point to the end of the molecule.

Other Clinical Correlates

In both animal models and patients with benign prostatic hypertrophy, the urinary bladder responds to obstruction with moderate smooth muscle hypertrophy and excessive collagen deposition. The significance and function of these changes are not clearly understood. Reports of patients with mitral valve prolapse show a striking absence of type III collagen and normal amounts of type I in the valve.[38] Mitral valve prolapse is a common finding in patients with Ehlers-Danlos syndrome. Abnormalities in the ratio of synthesized type I to type III collagen from the cultured fibroblasts of woman with severe gential prolapse[39] and men with recurrent inguinal hernias[40] have also been reported.

SPECIFIC LINES OF INVESTIGATION

Abnormalities in the proportion of collagen types, nature of cross-linking, and proportion of collagen in the smooth muscles can cause abnormal tissue function in other organ systems. An examination of the investigative techniques used in these areas suggests possible applications to the study of the pelvic floor. Table 10-1 summarizes the individual techniques available.

Histopathology Methods

In 1949, Danforth[41] published his landmark paper on the connective tissue composition of the cervix and its relationship to the isthmic segment in gravid and nongravid uteri. He found that fibrous connective tissue (collagen) was the basic structural element of the cervix, and its smooth muscle accounted for very little of the total cervical tissue. Elastin also played only a minimal role in the cervix except between muscle fiber groups. Since then, Rechberger and coworkers[4] demonstrated an association between a decrease in the proportion of collagen to smooth muscle in the cervix and cervical incompetence.

Methods for evaluating the histopathology of the pelvic floor may include standard H and E stains, elastin, and collagen stains (Fig. 10-7), immunofluorescent studies, and ATPase studies.

Fig. 10-7 A biopsy of the levator ani. In color, Masson's trichrome and Verhoeff's stain would show the muscle as red and the collagen present between muscle fibers and fibrils as blue. The little elastin present here would stain black.

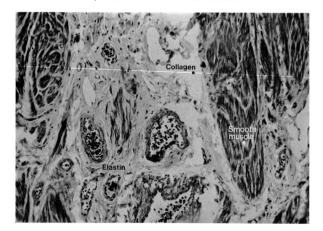

Biochemical Methods

Hydroxyproline is a unique bond between collagen fibers not found anywhere else in the body. The standard measurement of the total amount of collagen is performed by hydroxyproline assay.[43] Although more sophisticated techniques now exist that can differentiate type I and type III, the hydroxyproline content acts as an internal standard for quantitating collagen, since with many of these methods there is significant loss of collagen with progressive extraction. The other biochemical techniques are summarized in Table 10-1.

Other Lines of Investigation

Cell Culture

Fibroblasts and smooth muscle produce collagen, elastin, and ground substance. Although fibroblasts are easier to grow, smooth muscle cell lines can also be readily produced.[49] The two cell lines may appear somewhat similar under light microscopy but can be differentiated using actin stains. In tissue culture, such cell lines are useful to study the effects of hormones and other drugs on collagen production and to examine how cytokines, prostaglandins, and other intracellular

Table 10-1

Investigative Techniques Used to Determine Abnormal Tissue Structure and Function

Technique	Methodology	Advantages
Histologic		
Masson's trichrome and Verhoeff's stain[42]	Simultaneous staining of smooth muscle (red) collagen (blue-green) and elastin (black)	Can semiquantitate relative amounts of connective tissue with computer analysis
Immunohistochemical stain[18]	Antibodies to Type I and Type III collagen adhere to the collagen and can be visualized with fluorescein or other labels	Semiquantitation of amount of collagen types in tissue
ATPase stain[18]	Stains type I myofiber light brown type II myofiber dark brown	Quantitates the relative proportion of slow twitch to fast twitch fibers
Biochemical		
Hydroxyproline[23,43,44]	Protein unique to collagen which links fibers	Estimate total amount of collagen in tissue. Can also act as internal standard to estimate collagen lost during analysis
Extraction: pepsin or acetic acid[45] Polyacylamide gel electrophoresis[44] Cyanogen bromide High pressure liquid chromatography[47]	All take advantage of different physical properties of type I and type III in order to separate the two for quantitation	Quantitate type I vs type III
Immunoassay		
ELISA (enzyme-linked)[48]	Uses antibodies against type-specific collagen. A second antibody directed at the first can be measured with spectrophotometry	Indirectly measures type-specific collagen, even in very small amounts
Other		
Tissue culture (fibroblasts, smooth muscle)[49]	In vitro studies possible on the cell types that produce collagen	Study effects of hormones, cell damage, and drugs
Biomechanical[50,51]	Tensile strength of connective tissue, either by stretching or dilating (i.e., balloon in cervix)	Study the end result: strength and elasticity
Genetics (RFLP, DNA sequencing)[52,53]	Identify single base errors in genes for connective tissue	Study of major errors may lead to identification of common, more subtle errors

mediators affect the production of the different parts of the extracellular matrix.

Biomechanical Studies

Biomechanical studies can reveal differences in the tensile strength of different pelvic tissues. Oxlund[50] has analyzed many of the chemical properties of individual connective tissue components in smooth muscle, skin, muscle tendon, and aorta. Kiwi and colleagues[51] measured the elasticity of the uterine cervix using a 3 or 4 cm compliant balloon to determine the pressure-volume relationship while filling the balloon. Their findings showed a correlation between high elasticity and a diagnosis of incompetent cervix compared to normal controls.

Genetic Studies

Patients with homozygous genes for osteogenesis imperfecta have a known collagen abnormality which expresses itself in multiple connective tissue abnormalities. The abnormality defect is in collagen proportion, either excess type III collagen or lack of type I collagen. Parents of patients with osteogenesis imperfecta show a 50% production of the enzymes (not enough to produce clinical symptoms but to suggest a heterozygous gene).[52]

Type VII Ehlers-Danlos syndrome is characterized by extreme joint hypermobility associated with bilaterally dislocated hips at birth, but only minimal skin fragility. Type VII Ehlers-Danlos syndrome was found to have a splicing defect that causes abnormal type I collagen.[53] This was established by a DNA-cloning technique in which DNA grown from fibroblast cultures was amplified and the collagen and DNA separated by polyacrylamide gel electrophoresis (PAGE). The extra fraction of protein found in the electrophoresis was isolated and characterized by chromatography. In the case studied, 25% of the patient's type I collagen contained an abnormal chain, causing defective cross-linking; the responsible enzyme defect appeared to be temperature dependent. If a single base deletion can produce such alterations, many individuals in the population may carry genetic deficiencies in connective tissue genes that produce minor abnormalities in the strength and elasticity of their connective tissue.

SUMMARY

Because connective tissue and muscular fibers are responsible for the strength and integrity of the pelvic floor, they may be equally responsible for dysfunction of the pelvic floor. There are clinical syndromes in gynecology and other fields to support this hypothesis. Although most of the current research in connective tissue has focused on other organ systems, these same techniques may apply to the study of the pelvic floor.

REFERENCES

1. Nichols D, Randal C. *Vaginal Surgery*. Baltimore: Williams & Wilkins; 1976.
2. Woessner J, Brewer T. Formation and breakdown of collagen and elastin in the human uterus during pregnancy and postpartum involution. *Biochem J*. 1963;89:75–82.
3. Swash H. Histopathology of the pelvic floor muscles. In Henry M, Swash M, eds. *Coloproctology and the Pelvic Floor*. London: Butterworths; 1985;129–149.
4. Rechberger T, Uldbjerg N, Oxlund H. Connective tissue changes in the cervix during normal pregnancy and pregnancy complicated by cervical incompetence. *Obstet Gynecol*. 1988;7(4);563.
5. Granstrom L, Ehrman G, Ulmsted U, et al. Changes in the connective tissue of corpus and cervix uteri during ripening and labor in term pregnancy. *Br J Obstet Gynaecol*. 1989;96:1198–1202.
6. McCullough K, Balien C. Collagen characterization and cell transformation with human atherosclerosis. *Nature*. 1984;258:73.
7. Lansman H. The evolution of the pelvic floor. *South Carib J Obstet Gynecol*. 1988;5:9–18.
8. Prockop D, Kivirikko, K, Tuderman L, et al. The biosynthesis of collagen and its disorders. *N Eng J Med*. 1979;301(1):13–24.
9. Epstein E. Human skin collagen. *J Biol Chem*. 1974;249:3225–3231.
10. Bailey A, Bazin S, Selauney A. Change in the nature of the collagen during development and resorption of granulation tissue. *Biochem Biophys Res Commun*. 1973;66:1160–1169.
11. Keene D, Sakai L, Bachinger H, et al. Type III collagen can be present on banded collagen fibrils regardless of fibril diameter. *J Cell Biol*. 1987;105:2393–2402.
12. Burgeson R. New collagens, new concepts. *Ann Rev Cell Biol*. 1987;4:551–577.
13. Kuhn K. The classical collagens: types I, II, and III. In: Mayne R, Burgeson R, eds. *Structure and Function of Collagen Types*. New York: Academic; 1987;1–42.
14. Braverman I, Fonfuko E. Studies in cutaneous aging. I. The elastic fiber network. *J Invest Dermatol*. 1972;58:347–361.
15. Parks W, Deak S. Tropoelastin heterogeneity: implications for protein function and disease. *Am J Respir Cell Mol Biol*. 1990;2:399–406.
16. Isomura M, Sato N, Yamguchi Y, et al. Isolation and characterization of fibronectin-binding proteoglycan carrying both heparin sulfate and dermatan sulfate chains from human placenta. *J Biol Chem*. 1987;262(18):8926–8933.
17. Hedin U, Bottger B, Forsberg E, et al. Diverse effects of fibronectin and laminin on phenotypic properties of cultured arterial smooth muscle cells. *J Cell Biol*. 1988;107(1):307–319.
18. Bierseck F, Parks A, Swash M. Pathogenesis of anorectal incontinence: a histometric study of the anal sphincter musculature. *J Neuro Sci*. 1979;42:111–127.
19. Blair H, Teitelbaum S, Ehlilch L, et al. Collagenase production by smooth muscle: correlation of immunotractive with functional enzyme in the myometrium. *J Cell Physiol*. 1986;129:111–123.
20. Neil-Dwyer G, Bartlett J, Nichols A, et al. Collagen deficiency in ruptured cerebral aneurysms. *J Neurosurg*. 1983;59:16.
21. Stenback F. Collagen type III formation and distribution in the uterus: effects of hormones and neoplasm development. *Oncology*. 1989;46:326–334.

22. Ryan J, Woessner J. Oestradiol inhibits collagen breakdown in the involuting rat uterus. *Biochem J.* 1972;127:705–715.

23. Brincat M, Moniz C, Studd J, et al. The long-term effects of the menopause and of administration of sex hormones on skin collagen and skin thickness. *Br J Obstet Gynaecol.* 1985;92:256–259.

24. Woessner J. Age-related changes in the human uterus and its connective tissue framework. *J Gerontol.* 1963;18:220–225.

25. Ito A, Kitamura K, Mori Y, et al. The change in the solubility of type I collagen in human uterine cervix in pregnancy at term. *Biochem Med.* 1979;21:262–265.

26. McKusick V. *Heritable Disorders of Connective Tissue.* 4th ed. St. Louis: CV Mosby; 1972;61–223.

27. Pope F, Martin G, Lichtenstein J, et al. Patients with Ehlers-Danlos syndrome type IV lack type III collagen. *Proc Nat Acad Sci.* 1987;72(4):1314–1316.

28. Johnson M, Sorokin Y, Rogowski N, et al. Obstetric and gynecologic dysfunction in the Ehlers-Danlos syndrome. *Proceedings of the Society for Gynecologic Investigation.* 1990;72.

29. Byers P, Cohn D, Starman B, et al. Nature and location of mutations in the collagen alpha 1(I) and alpha 2(I) gene products predicts clinical phenotype in osteogenesis imperfecta. In: Prockop D, ed. *Proceedings of the Second International Conference on Molecular Biology and Pathology of Matrix.* Univ Penn; 1988.

30. Hollister D, Godfrey M, Sakai L, et al. Immunohistologic abnormalities of the microfibrillar-fiber system in the Marfan syndrome. *N Eng J Med.* 1990;323(3):152–157.

31. Marshman D, Pereyra J, Fielding F, et al. Rectal prolapse and joint laxity. *Aust NZ J Surg.* 1987;57:827–829.

32. Norton P, Baker J, Sharp H, Warenski H. Genitourinary prolapse: relationship with joint mobility. *Neuro Urodyn.* 1990;9(4):321–322.

33. Jensen B, Reimann I, Fredensborg N. Collagen type III predominance in newborns with congenital dislocation of the hip. *Acta Orthop Scand.* 1986;57:362–365.

34. Ulmsten U, Ekman G, Giertz G, Malstrom A. Different biochemical composition of connective tissue in continent and stress incontinent women. *Acta Obstet Gynecol Scand.* 1987;66:455–457.

35. Landon C, Smith A. Crofts C, et al. Biomechanical properties of connective tissue in women with stress incontinence of urine. *Neuro Urodyn.* 1989;8(4):369–370.

36. Hanson A, Bentley J: Quantitation of type I to type III collagen ratios in samples of human tendon, blood vessels, and atherosclerotic plague. *Analyt Biochem.* 1983;130:32–40.

37. Deak S, Ricotta J, Mariani T, et al. Abnormalities in the biosynthesis of type III procollagen in patients with multiple aneurysms. *Matrix.* In press.

38. Hammer D, Leier C, Baba N, et al. Altered collagen composition in a prolapsing mitral valve with ruptured chordae tendinae. *Am J Med.* 1979;67:863–868.

39. Norton PA, Friedman D, Boyd C, Deak S. Reduced type I and type II collagen ratio in women with genital prolapse. *Proceedings of the Society for Gynecologic Investigation.* March 20–23, 1991: 192–193.

40. Friedman D, Norton PA, Boyd C, MacKenzie J, Deak S. Abnormal collagen synthesis associated with recurrent inguinal hernia. *Ann Surg.* In press.

41. Danforth D. The fibrous nature of the human cervix and its relation to the isthmic segment in gravid and nongravid uteri. *Obstet Gynecol.* 1949;4:541–547.

42. Goodfellow B, Mikat E. A stain for the simultaneous demonstration of collagen, muscles, and elastin elements in mammalian tissue. *Lab Med.* 1988;219(4):243–244.

43. Stegeman H, Stalder K. Determination of hydroxyproline. *Clinica Chemica Acta.* 1969;18:267–273.

44. Buckley A, Hill K, Davidson J. Collagen metabolism. *Meth. Enzymol.* 1988;163:674–693.

45. ChandaRajan J. Separation of type III collagen from type I collagen and pepsin by differential denaturation and renaturation. *Biochem Biophys Res Common.* 1978;8(1):180–186.

46. Sykes B, Tuddle B, Francis M, et al. The estimation of the two collagens from human dermis by interrupted gel electrophoresis. *Biochem Biophys Res Common.* 1976;72:1472–1480.

47. Macek K, Deyl Z, Conpek J, et al. Separation of collagen types I and III by high-performance column liquid chromatography. *J Chromatog.* 1981;222:284–290.

48. Rennard S, Berg R, Martin G, et al. Enzyme-linked immunoassay (ELISA) for connective tissue components. *Analyt Biochem.* 1980;104:205–214.

49. Casey L, MacDonald P, Mitchell M, et al. Maintenance and characterization of human myometrial smooth muscle cells in monolayer culture. *In Vitro.* 1984;20(5):396–403.

50. Oxlund H. Relationship between the biomechanical properties, composition, and molecular structure of connective tissues. *Connect Tiss Res.* 1986;15:65–72.

51. Kiwi R, Neuman M, Merkatz I, et al. Determination of the elastic properties of the cervix. *Obstet Gynecol.* 1971;71(4):568–574.

52. Francis M, Smith R, MacMillan D: Polymeric collagen of skin in normal subjects and in patients with inherited connective tissue disorders. *Clin Sci.* 1973;44:429–438.

53. Weil D, D'Alessio M, Ramirez F, et al. Temperature-dependent expression of a collagen splicing defect in the fibroblasts of a patient with Ehlers-Danlos syndrome type VII. *J Biol Chem.* 1989;264(28):16804–16809.

CHAPTER 11

Urinary Incontinence

11A   Psychosocial Factors

Henry A. Thiede

INTRODUCTION

To appreciate the magnitude of the problem of urinary incontinence, one must understand its prevalence. Urinary incontinence is most prevalent in institutionalized, elderly women and, among community-dwellers, is more common in women than in men.[1,2] Table 11A-1 depicts some contemporary studies of the incidence of this disorder in various countries.[1,3–8] Discrepancies in the rates result from varying definitions of "significant incontinence" and ages of the population studied; the use of subjective versus objective evidence of incontinence; retrospective versus prospective data sources; and from the use of different instruments. Other factors affecting study results are cultural differences in the willingness to discuss the subject openly, and increased awareness of the problem among health professionals and clients in the more recent studies.

These variables notwithstanding, it is safe to conclude that urinary incontinence is a common problem, especially in women, and is usually aggravated by vigorous physical activity. Fecal incontinence often coexists, especially in the elderly. Loss of bladder and/or rectal control to any significant degree has a devastating impact on wellness and the quality of life.

ECONOMIC IMPACT

Incontinence is costly for the individual affected as well as society as a whole. It is estimated that at least 10 million adult Americans suffer from incontinence at an estimated annual cost of $10.3 billion.[9] Incontinent, community-living women spend a great deal to replace ruined clothes and to purchase protection products. Brink and colleagues,[10] in their evaluation of 200 community-living women, found that 62% wore protection, usually menstrual pads. Among the incontinent women seen in our urodynamic laboratory, more than 80% wore protection of some kind at least occasionally. The approximate cost of a single menstrual pad is $.13. If it is changed just twice a day the annual cost to a woman

Table 11A-1
Prevalence of Urinary Incontinence
in Women

Country	Age Group	Residence	% Incontinent
Sweden	75–79	Institution	33
New Zealand	75+	Community	30
Wales	75+	Community	59
Canada	85+	Home care	25
USA	85+	Nursing home	55
Japan	80+	Community	31
USA	60+	Community	38

is close to $100. The unit cost of special products developed for the incontinent woman differs some, but using an average unit cost of $.50 and two changes a day, roughly $365 per year is needed for protection.

Government studies[11] indicate there are now 3 million persons age 85 or older and that in another decade the number could nearly double. A very substantial number of these people will need daily assistance with basic functions such as eating, bathing, dressing, transferring, and toileting. Along with immobility, dementia, depression, and physical frailty, incontinence is a leading reason for admission to some type of long-term health facility.[12] Of current nursing home patients, 30% to 60% are incontinent.[7,13,14] The Surgeon General's office once estimated the cost of diapering incontinent women in institutions to be $8 billion.[15] Consider, also, the nursing time and medications used in treating skin breakdown and urinary infections as well as the materials and personnel time consumed in changing bed linens. The projected dramatic increase in the aged population, compounded by anticipated inflation, will have a profound impact on this already astronomic cost.

A recently published stratified random sampling of nursing homes in Maryland revealed that 9% of the women sampled had catheters, and that 83% of all catheter users were women.[16] The authors calculated from this that nearly 100,000 residents of nursing homes nationwide were using chronic urethral catheterization to manage urinary problems. Complications such as stones, cystitis, pyelonephritis, bacteremia, and death are associated with long-term catheter use. The cost of treating these complications is not known, but is surely substantial.

A brochure from Blue Cross/Blue Shield in 1989 indicated that at some point in their lifetime, one out of two Americans will need long-term care of some kind and that the average length of stay in a nursing home is 2½ years, with expenses averaging more than $35,000 per year in New York. Much of this cost burden is borne by the patients' families, as most nursing home residents spend virtually all their savings in less than a year.

Medicare has strict medical requirements that exclude many occupants of even skilled nursing facilities from coverage. The charges in such institutions are $100 per day or more, and most third-party payors don't provide adequate coverage for domiciliary care in spite of the extremely high premiums charged.

Though it varies from state to state, the limited availability of nursing home beds and inadequate reimbursement rates exclude a large number of people needing extended-care admission. Many languish 6 months or more in acute-care hospital beds awaiting placement in nursing homes. Moreover, the financial restrictions for Medicaid eligibility often result in a spend-down of nearly all the family's resources before coverage is available.

Since incontinence is a major reason for institutionalization and is a significant cost factor for people in care facilities, finding the means for prevention and better management of urinary incontinence is a high national priority, especially for those interested in geriatric problems.

PSYCHOLOGICAL IMPACT

While many different causes for urinary incontinence have been identified, the underlying pathophysiology for most is often poorly or, at best, incompletely understood. Nearly half of patients with detrusor instability are still labeled as idiopathic for lack of comprehending the cause. Children with severe developmental anomalies or mental retardation and individuals of any age or gender with damage to the central or peripheral nervous system or urogenital pathology are susceptible to urinary incontinence. The primary pathology carries a significant emotional burden of its own; the added problem of coping with urinary and/or fecal incontinence can sometimes be overwhelming.

Control of bowel and bladder function is an emotionally charged issue which begins in infancy. Toilet training is an early objective for most parents of newborns. Changing diapers is unpleasant and tiresome, to say nothing about the associated expense. The behavioral modification involved leaves an indelible mark on the infant's psyche. Usually this is unrecognized, although a spectrum of voiding problems might be attributed to toilet training, ranging from inability or difficulty with voiding in public restrooms to detrusor-sphincter dyssynergia of an obscure nature. The stage is therefore set in early life for an emotional backlash to loss of control of bodily functions in later years.

Since toilet training is a learned behavior as a conditioned reflex, emotional or psychologic turmoil which inhibits this reflex may play a role in the development of incontinence. Part of the examination of any patient with incontinence is to determine mental impairment or emotional disturbance. Dementia is a major cause of chronic, progressive loss of intellectual function in the elderly, and such cognitive loss is often associated with urinary incontinence. Additionally, Sutherland[17] found rebellion, attention-seeking, dependency and insecurity, as well as sensory deprivation to be associated with urinary incontinence. Like the reproductive tract in women, the bladder also seems to be the focus of psychosomatic disturbances. Frewen[18,19] has written extensively about his observations on the effect of life's stresses on bladder function, especially with respect to complaints of urgency/frequency and urge incontinence. Severe situational problems, chronic depression, and hysterical personality traits were common psychogenic factors found by Stone and Judd[20] in a series of patients with urge incontinence.

While it is easy to ascribe many urinary symptoms to disturbed affective and cognitive states, there are many confounding variables involved which preclude an unqualified acceptance of these concepts as either cause or effect until further, more definitive studies are completed. That aside, there are many psychologic problems associated in some fashion with urinary incontinence involving not only the patient, but family, friends, and care providers. Box 11A-1 lists several psychologic responses of the incontinent patient that were culled from literature on the subject.[21–24] One or more of the items in this list are likely to be encountered daily in any busy urodynamic laboratory.

Some of these psychologic manifestations are in response to the organic disease process causing the incontinence. Even in the absence of other associated disease states, however, urinary incontinence itself is associated with many problems. Vulvar irritation, sleep deprivation, recurrent urinary infection with its accompanying symptoms and risk of sepsis and death, decubitus ulcers in those who are bedridden, fluid and dietary restrictions, and side effects from drugs prescribed for treatment of the incontinence all have an impact on the patient's mental health.

Box 11A-1
Psychological Responses to Incontinence

Shame
Depression
Withdrawal
Guilt
Denial
Regression
Anxiety
Indignation
Secretiveness
Fear
Preoccupation

Management of the patient's incontinence should include early identification and intervention of emotional problems. When the incontinence is part of another disease process, counseling becomes even more vital. Giving the patient time and encouragement to ask questions and discuss her complaints and concerns can be therapeutic; too often there is no one with whom she is comfortable in sharing this emotionally charged information. Reassurance and encouragement from an informed professional can be immensely supportive. Insight as to the underlying problem, when it is known, can help the patient cope. Open and thorough presentation of alternative approaches to managing the problem, including realistic expectations of short-term and long-term outcome, and explanation of potential side effects, of course, are basic. Repeated office visits and reinforcement are often required. On occasion, use of antidepressants is indicated.

Emotional stress is placed on the family when they are responsible for care of an incontinent member of the household. The potential for conflict is enormous and the dynamics are often complex and intense. The household members may perceive the patient as less appealing, demanding, attention seeking, unappreciative of their sacrifices made on her behalf, and as an extreme financial burden. Unless the patient has significant cognitive impairment, she will detect these attitudes and the stage will be set for dissension and hardship for all. The patient may feel guilty for being a burden; she may react to any perceived indifference or hostility from the family with anger, withdrawal, self-pity, or fear of being rejected or abandoned by the family and placed in an institution. This scenario is being played out more often as the bed shortage and cost of long-term facilities increase in response to our aging population.

There is clearly a psychologic impact on health care workers as well. The hospitalized or institutionalized incontinent patient, who frequently is incontinent of both urine and feces, requires more nursing time, is aesthetically unpleasant, and is more likely to spread certain pathogens. This creates ambivalence: caregivers may experience negative reactions to the patient followed by guilt feelings, depression, or frustration as a result. Some may overcompensate for their guilt by being excessively attentive. Erosion of staff morale, excessive fatigue, and deterioration of care on the unit can result. Since the nursing shortage continues to be a significant problem in most parts of the United States, awareness of these issues is an important first step to finding appropriate solutions.

If one accepts that control of urinary continence has significant psychological overtones, then it is logical to consider using behavioral therapy in the management of some cases. Biofeedback, prompted voiding, bladder drill, peri-vaginal muscle exercises, psychotherapy, and hypnosis fall into this broad category and are discussed in more detail elsewhere in this volume. Suffice it to say that some of these techniques have been studied in some depth and show considerable promise for at least short-term improvement, and, with periodic reinforcement, possibly long-term improvement as well.

SOCIAL IMPACT

Urinary incontinence of any significant degree can have a major influence on a woman's life. The complaints are many and varied and seldom trivial. Some of those more commonly offered are listed in Box 11A-2. The largest group of patients is age 65 or older; this generation often finds it difficult to discuss such personal and private matters as sex and loss of control of body waste with anyone, including their husbands and children. This contributes to the sense of isolation many patients often feel. Change is slowly occurring thanks to the help of the lay press, professional media, and various support groups; people are now becoming more comfortable, open, and assertive in discussing the problem. Also, physicians and nurses are addressing their patients more proactively by including direct questioning about incontinence in their interviews and by being more attentive to patients who mention incontinence.

Box 11A-2
Common Complaints from Women with Urinary Incontinence

I can't go on trips with my family.
I'm afraid I will smell of urine.
I have to plan ahead so I can be near a bathroom.
I don't go anywhere anymore.
I'm always in the bathroom.
We don't have sex anymore.
I have to wear clothes I can get off in a hurry.
I can't do aerobics or any sports or even dance.
I have to be careful of what I wear in case it shows.
I'd like to be able to walk without a pad.
I leave puddles on the floor and wet the chairs.
My boss wonders why I'm in the toilet all the time.
I always feel dirty.

Consider the plight of a young, attractive dental hygienist who had urge incontinence. Before she left for the shopping mall she emptied her bladder, and on arriving she sought out the restrooms and emptied again. If, despite these precautions, she had an urge to void again while shopping, she learned that by squatting on her heel pretending to tie her shoelace she could suppress the detrusor contraction and avoid a major accident. One can't do that often without raising suspicion among one's friends that something is amiss. As a result, our hygienist made few friends. Only her mother knew of her problem and that was partly because there were also some episodes of nocturnal enuresis. Her dentist employer found it annoying that she made so many trips to the toilet every day. She met a young man with whom she became emotionally involved; he invited her to spend the night with him. She stayed awake all night after their lovemaking, while he slept peacefully, because she was afraid she might have an accident and wet the bed. After several weekends like that, she finally sought medical help.

Interestingly, the young woman in our story did not have incontinence with sexual intercourse. However, this is certainly an underreported and little recognized problem for many women. Patients seldom volunteer this information, but, when asked directly, most are quick to admit this is an embarrassing problem and a source of difficulty in their sexual relationship. For some of the women seen in our urodynamic laboratory this was the reason they finally sought medical advice, although they did not present it as their major complaint. The incidence of incontinence associated with coitus in 235 patients we queried was 27%. This is similar to Hilton's[25] findings of 24% loss with sexual activity among 324 women. Within our group of patients losing urine during or after intercourse, 57% had genuine stress incontinence; 14% had detrusor instability; 29% had both. This distribution is not significantly different from the type of incontinence in all 358 patients seen during that same period. Moreover, among those with genuine stress incontinence, there was no significant difference between those losing and those not losing urine with coitus, in the degree of pelvic relaxation, parity, age, residual urine, maximum bladder capacity, and functional area of the urethral pressure profile. Hilton's findings were similar except for a smaller cystometric capacity in his index cases as compared with his control group.

One senior citizen widow was an active bowler and regional pinochle champion. She enjoyed a beer or two and the companionship of her card partners and bowling team. One morning she slipped on the ice in her employer's parking lot. Although she was bruised and sore after the fall, x-ray films revealed no evidence of any fractures. Within several weeks she began having urgency, frequency, and then urge incontinence. She had never had any significant incontinence before. Her local medical doctor's work-up showed nothing abnormal in the genitourinary tract, but her symptoms persisted. Lifting at work precipitated incontinence, bowling was out of the question, and a single beer aggravated her symptoms. One evening while at a friend's house playing cards she had a coughing spell and left a large wet spot on her friend's upholstered chair. She was mortified. She became reclusive and depressed.

The two preceding, true vignettes are illustrative of the way in which urinary incontinence can affect the lives of otherwise healthy community-living people. While all medical histories are not this dramatic, the impact on the happiness and well-being of many men and women is often just as considerable. Among those employed, it tends to be a bigger problem because they cannot always manipulate conditions to suit their needs. The teacher can't leave the classroom; the lawyer can't leave the courtroom; assembly workers can't leave the line to empty their bladders frequently enough to prevent urge incontinence. Those whose work involves physical activity soon learn that frequent emptying doesn't prevent them from leaking. Their problem then becomes getting free to change protection often enough to avoid odor and discomfort.

The odor of urine is pervasive and offensive. It implies uncleanliness. For the patient, it promotes paranoia, isolation, and withdrawal. Women who enjoy travel, participate in sports, or go camping, to name just a few examples, find particular difficulty staying dry and have the added problem of unavailable facilities for changing their protection and washing in order to minimize the risk of odor. Most patients who are not demented are very aware and sensitive to the risk of smelling of urine; some wash themselves raw to avoid offending others.

For those close to the patient, the unpleasant odor promotes only superficial contact, disengagement and, often, ultimate rejection from friends, family, and even health care providers. And for the patient with other medical problems, especially the bedridden, such isolation can compromise health and recovery.

Incontinence, therefore, can be a major preoccupation adversely affecting all aspects of public and personal life for the patient and everyone with whom she interacts. For all concerned, the ultimate happiness is dryness.

SUMMARY

There is much we don't know about the prevention, causes, and the effects of urinary incontinence. It is apparent, however, that the incidence of incontinence increases universally with age. Given the rapidly enlarging population of elderly men and women, and a prevalence of incontinence that approaches 50% in the aged, the social implications and the economic impact of the problem attains considerable importance.

Data in hand suggest that the related direct and indirect health care costs are already significant and may become staggering. The social issues surrounding incontinence are just beginning to unfold, but it is already clear that they are enormously complex and have a major impact on the well-being of the unfortunate patients, their loved ones, and their caregivers.

REFERENCES

1. Diokno AC, Wells TJ, Brink CA. Urinary incontinence in elderly women: urodynamic evaluation. *J Am Geriatr Soc.* 1987;35:940.
2. Palmer MH. Incontinence: the magnitude of the problem. *Nurs Clin N Am.* 1988;1:139.
3. Ekelund P, Rundgren A. Urinary incontinence in the elderly with implications for hospital care consumption and social disability. *Arch Gerontol Geriatr.* 1987;6:11.
4. Holst K, Wilson PD. The prevalence of urinary incontinence and reasons for not seeking treatment. *NZ Med J.* 1988;101:756.
5. Yarnell JWG, Voyle GJ, Richards CJ, Stephenson TP. The prevalence and severity of urinary incontinence in women. *J Epidemiol Community Health.* 1981;35:71.
6. Mohide AE, Pringle DM, Robertson D, Chambers LW. Prevalence of urinary incontinence in patients receiving home care services. *Can Med Assoc J.* 1988;139:953.
7. Ouslander JG, Kane RL, Abrass IB. Urinary incontinence in elderly nursing home patients. *J Am Med Assoc.* 1982;248:1194.
8. Koyano W, Shibata H, Haga H, Suyama Y. Prevalence and outcome of low ADL and incontinence among the elderly: five year follow-up in a Japanese urban community. *Arch Gerontol Geriatr.* 1986;5:197.
9. NIH Consensus Conference. Urinary incontinence in adults. *J Am Med Assoc.* 1989;261:2685.
10. Brink CA, Wells TJ, Diokno AC. Urinary Incontinence in Women. *Pub Health Nurs.* 1987;4:114.
11. Special Committee on Aging, United States Senate. *Aging America: Trends and Projections.* US Government Printing Office. Publication 1986-498-116-814/42395.
12. Solomon DH, Judd HL, Sier HC, Rubenstein LZ, Morley JE. New issues in geriatric care. *Ann Intern Med.* 1988;108:718.
13. Tobin GW, Brocklehurst JC. The management of urinary incontinence in local authority residential homes for the elderly. *Age Aging.* 1986;15:292.
14. Starer P, Libow LS. Obscuring urinary incontinence. *J Am Geriatr Soc.* 1985;33:842.
15. Brazda JF. In Washington Report. *Nation's Health.* 1983;13:3.
16. Warren JW, Steinberg L, Hebel RJ, Tenney JH. The prevalence of urethral catheterization in Maryland nursing homes. *Arch Intern Med.* 1989;149:1535.

17. Sutherland SS. The psychology of incontinence. In: Willington FL, ed. *Incontinence in the Elderly*. New York: Academic Press; 1976.
18. Frewen WK. Urgency incontinence. *J Obstet Gynaecol Brit Commonw*. 1972;79:77.
19. Frewen WK. An objective assessment of the unstable bladder of psychosomatic origin. *Brit J Urol*. 1978;50:246.
20. Stone CB, Judd GE. Psychogenic Aspects of Urinary Incontinence in Women. *Clin Obstet Gynec*. 1978;21:807.
21. Newman JL. Old folk in wet beds. *Brit Med J*. 1962;1:1824.
22. Willington FL. Incontinence: psychologic and psychogenic aspects. *Nurs Times*. March 13, 1975.
23. Blaivas JG, Raz S, Resnick NM, Whelan J. When the problem is incontinence. *Patient Care*. January 15, 1988:1.
24. Ory MG, Wyman JF, Yu L. Psychosocial factors in urinary incontinence. *Geriatr Med*. 1986;2:657.
25. Hilton P. Urinary incontinence during sexual intercourse: a common but rarely volunteered symptom. *Brit J Obstet Gynaecol*. 1988;95:377.

CHAPTER 11

Urinary Incontinence

11B Pathophysiology

Jay B. Hollander   Ananias C. Diokno

INTRODUCTION

This chapter will discuss the pathogenesis of various types of incontinence in women. It is estimated that at least 8.5% of females suffer from some form of urinary incontinence.[1] The prevalence of incontinence may be as high as 37% in elderly females.[2] There are many different ways that incontinence can develop. As such, the type of incontinence and its cause may vary from one woman to another. In some instances abnormalities of the female pelvic floor may be responsible for incontinence. In others, the pelvic floor may be entirely normal and intact yet incontinence occurs. In order to approach the pathophysiology of urinary incontinence in an organized fashion, we first discuss normal bladder and urethral function. We then incorporate urodynamic findings which are essential for normal continent storage and voiding of urine. The chapter will then go on to describe causes for incontinence using, when appropriate, urodynamic models to illustrate specific conditions in which incontinence occurs. It will become clear that in many instances the cause for incontinence may be multifactorial. The diagnosis and treatment, however, should be simplified by knowing the wide spectrum of causes for incontinence in the female.

NORMAL ANATOMY AND FUNCTION OF BLADDER AND URETHRA

Gross Anatomy and Function

The female bladder and urethra function only to provide for continent storage and controlled release of urine. Though the neurophysiology is complex, the urodynamic findings during normal function are quite easy to understand.

Urine is delivered to the bladder via the ureters on a continuous basis with the volume delivered dependent primarily on the state of hydration. Once in the bladder, the urine loses its contact with the upper urinary tract because of the nonrefluxing nature of the ureteral orifices in the normal bladder. Urine is stored until it is expelled with voiding. Storage of urine in the bladder is done under low pressures. The bladder wall muscle is referred to as the detrusor and has elastic properties, allowing it to expand during filling without increasing the pressure within its lumen up to a certain capacity, at which time the pressure increases as filling continues because the bladder wall is stretched to its limit. This ability to enlarge as the bladder fills without increasing the pressure within is referred to as accommodation. As the bladder accommodates its volume of urine, the outlet spout, the urethra, remains closed. The unique bladder mucosa (transitional epithelium) and the elastic nature of the smooth muscle wall allow for low pressure storage and bladder accommodation. Abnormalities in the bladder wall can alter the bladder's ability to accommodate urine and change the pressures inside the bladder as urine is stored. Should the pressure within the bladder lumen exceed the pressure within the urethral lumen, urine will leak out the spout. Normally, the urethra opens in coordination with contraction of the bladder when voiding occurs. If the void can be controlled to occur only when desired, a person is continent.

The female urethra is a conduit with sphincteric properties to provide for closure, facilitating urinary continence. The sphincter is composed of an internal smooth muscle component which is continuous with the bladder at the vesicourethral junction and extends throughout the proximal two thirds of the female urethra. At the mid urethra, skeletal muscle surrounds the internal smooth muscle and is referred to as the external striated portion of the urethral sphincter or simply "external sphincter." The female urethra is divided into a proximal and distal portion. The external sphincter and the portion of internal smooth muscle adjacent represents the distal portion of the urethral sphincter. The smooth muscle surrounding the urethra at the vesicourethral junction or "bladder neck" and proximal one third of the urethra is referred to as the proximal sphincter (Fig. 11B-1). If a cystoscope is passed under direct vision via the external urethral meatus with water flowing, the very distal urethra appears patent. Destruction of this area, as occurs with resection of urethral prolapse, will not alter continence. As the scope is passed proximally, the mid urethra appears closed with longitudinal mucosal folds coapting against each other, separating from the force of the advancing scope sheath rather than from the irrigant via the scope. This is the region of the distal urethral sphincteric mechanism. It is heavily influenced by the external sphincter. The striated muscle of the external urethral sphincter is under voluntary control. If the patient is asked to squeeze the urethra, this region can be seen to tighten endoscopically. Destruction of this area can occur with radical vulvectomy and can result in some degree of incontinence.[3] As the scope is passed further, the proximal urethral sphincter is seen and represents the region of the proximal one third of urethra and the vesicourethral junction. This area appears as a sphincter attempting to close against the force of the advancing scope.

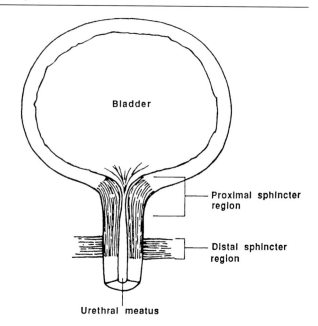

Fig. 11B-1 Schematic illustration of sphincteric regions of the female urethra.

The proximal sphincter itself is under indirect voluntary control. If the patient is asked to "squeeze to hold your urine," the area will elevate from tightening of the pelvic floor musculature to which it is connected via supporting fascial attachments. The sphincter itself which is continuous with the bladder neck musculature is composed of smooth involuntary muscle and does not itself contract voluntarily, as occurs with the striated portion of the distal sphincteric mechanism. On the other hand, if the patient is asked to void, the sphincter opens in coordination with the voiding contraction, thus the proximal sphincter is closed without any voluntary input necessary while the bladder is filling and storing urine. During a bladder contraction it opens in coordination with the contraction, appearing as funneling of the vesical neck and proximal urethra if viewed fluoroscopically (Fig. 11B-2). The status of the distal urethral mechanism at this time determines whether continence or voiding occurs. If the distal sphincter relaxes, voiding ensues. If the sphincter tightens during a bladder contraction, continence is determined by which pressures are greater, intraurethral or intravesical.

Neural Anatomy and Function

The precise mapping of neuropathways involved in bladder and urethral function are not yet completely

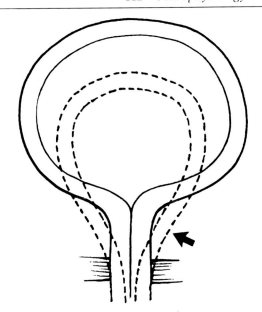

Fig. 11B-2 During bladder filling the bladder neck and proximal urethra are closed. With bladder contraction the region appears to funnel *(arrow).*

bladder neck or urethral sphincter may not relax or open properly in conjunction with the bladder contraction. This may result in high pressures in the bladder during voiding, intermittent stream, and poor bladder emptying. This is termed detrusor sphincter dyssynergia or voiding with an uncoordinated sphincter. The sacral area S2 to S4 serves as a reflex center resulting in spontaneous bladder contractions which can be reflexly stimulated by afferent proprioceptive or sensoreceptive nervous input from the bladder such as stretching with filling or irritation with infection. If the sacral reflex center is destroyed, then no messages may be transmitted to or received from the bladder and urinary retention can result. Likewise, peripheral nerves subserving the bladder and urethra must be intact for central neurologic control to be effective.

Though the peripheral innervation of the bladder and urethra is still being studied, generalizations can be made which are clinically useful. Sacral parasympathetics originating in S2 to S4 and running in the pelvic nervous plexus are thought to be responsible for bladder contractions via cholinergic neurotransmitters to the bladder smooth muscle. Lumbar sympathetics traveling in the presacral nervous plexus are thought to be

defined. A full discussion is beyond the scope of this chapter. Nevertheless, clinical findings in neurologically injured or diseased individuals allow us to make useful conclusions regarding neuroanatomy relative to normal bladder and urethral function.[4] A simplified clinically useful representation of pertinent neuroanatomy is represented in Fig. 11B-3. The intact cerebrum is necessary for all voluntary actions regarding bladder and urethral function. Perceiving a full bladder, holding one's urine, and initiating voiding at the appropriate time are all voluntary activities requiring cerebral function. Without the cerebral control, voiding may occur but there is no voluntary control. This is what occurs in infants. The brain stem has a voiding center likely located in the pons that is responsible for allowing voiding to occur in a coordinated fashion, such that the bladder outlet and urethral resistance is reduced while bladder contractions are stimulated.[5]

In experimental models on decerebrate animals, urodynamically normal voiding occurs. If a complete central neurologic lesion occurs below this pontine micturition center, bladder contractions still occur as long as the sacral micturition center, located in the spinal segments S2 to S4, is intact along with the peripheral nerves to the bladder and urethra. Voiding, however, may not be normal because the pontine micturition center can no longer coordinate it. That is to say the

Fig. 11B-3 Neuroanatomy involved in normal bladder and urethral function.

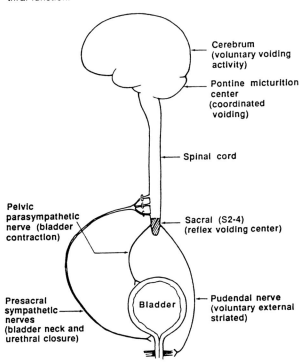

responsible for vesical neck and proximal urethral smooth muscle contraction via alpha-adrenergic neurotransmitters. The bladder outlet is thus closed when the bladder is storing urine and inhibition of this alpha-adrenergic influence is important in voiding in a coordinated fashion. Perhaps as important in coordinated voiding is the pudendal nerve somatic input to the skeletal muscle of the pelvic floor and the striated component of the distal urethral sphincter. This is the voluntary sphincter used to interrupt or cut off the urinary stream. This must relax for voiding to occur and is normally under voluntary control.

Normal bladder storage and emptying thus requires the sophisticated coordination of multiple neurostimuli and inhibitors. In addition, normal bladder and urethral anatomy and anatomic relationships are also necessary.

TYPES OF URINARY INCONTINENCE

Urge Urinary Incontinence

If a voiding contraction occurs despite the person's desire not to void, incontinence occurs if the urinary sphincter cannot tighten enough to stop the flow of urine. The patient may feel the sense of urgency at this time and this type of incontinence is referred to as *urge urinary incontinence*. When the patient cannot sense the urgency (as in spinal cord injury), the incontinence resulting from the involuntary detrusor contraction is termed *reflex urinary incontinence*.

Stress Urinary Incontinence

If the bladder storing urine normally under low pressures is subjected to external pressures such as occurs with a cough or a sneeze, incontinence occurs if the bladder pressure exceeds urethral pressure. When this occurs it is referred to as *stress urinary incontinence*. The bladder is at rest storing urine without contracting during stress urinary incontinence. Conditions which reduce the urethra's ability to remain closed predisposes to stress urinary incontinence.

Overflow Incontinence

If the bladder fills to capacity, the pressure within the bladder will rise as the bladder continues to fill as previously discussed. The pressure can rise to greater than resting urethral pressure. When this occurs, urine will leak from the urethra and is referred to as *overflow incontinence*.

Total Urinary Incontinence

If the resting urethral pressure is so low that it provides no resistance for passage of urine, the bladder is not able to store urine, and incontinence is continuous. This is referred to as *total urinary incontinence*.

Functional Incontinence

Incontinence can occur despite normal bladder and urethral function in every other respect. Such would be the case in patients who void in inappropriate circumstances due to disorientation or dementia. Psychologic problems and medication side effects can also manifest themselves with symptoms of incontinence. The diagnosis is one of exclusion.

Miscellaneous

Leakage of urine from acquired conditions such as vesicovaginal fistula or congenital conditions such as ectopic ureter is difficult to categorize but must always be considered in the differential diagnosis of urinary incontinence, as will be discussed.

The types of incontinence refer to general divisions based on physical mechanisms of incontinence. Combinations of the different types are a common clinical reality. The pathophysiology of each type can vary and involve dysfunction of bladder, urethra, or both. For simplicity the following discussion is divided initially into detrusor dysfunction and urethral dysfunction.

URINARY INCONTINENCE SECONDARY TO DETRUSOR FACTORS WITH INTACT URETHRAL SPHINCTER MECHANISM

Detrusor Instability

When a child is born, incontinence is expected. The bladder fills until a voiding contraction occurs and urination results. If viewed fluoroscopically, the voiding mechanism appears identical to normal adult voiding with opening of the vesical neck and proximal urethra as the bladder contracts. The difference is that the infant is unaware of the voiding and unable to inhibit the voiding contraction. Among continent females the urge

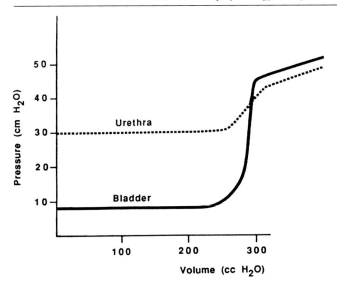

Fig. 11B-4 Cystometrogram with simultaneous urethral pressure monitoring showing detrusor instability. Patient has bladder contraction despite trying not to void. Incontinence occurs when bladder pressure exceeds urethral pressure *(arrow)*.

to void or the sensation of bladder fullness is perceived and cerebral perception results in inhibitory messages that are transmitted to the brain stem micturition center and sacral reflex voiding center to inhibit efferent stimulation of nerves that would otherwise result in voiding. If the female is unable to inhibit these impulses that stimulate a voiding contraction, urination occurs unless she is able to squeeze her urethra closed with pressure greater than that within the bladder. This is precisely what occurs with urinary urgency and urge urinary incontinence. If there is a neurologic lesion that is responsible for the inability to inhibit a bladder contraction (such as stroke), the condition is referred to as an uninhibited neurogenic bladder or detrusor hyperreflexia. More commonly, however, urge incontinence can occur without any defined neurologic lesion identified. This is referred to as detrusor instability and can be idiopathic or result from a number of irritative bladder conditions. Detrusor hyperreflexia and instability are basically the same entity when studied urodynamically and can result in incontinence (Fig. 11B-4).

Idiopathic detrusor instability is a diagnosis of exclusion, after proving uninhibited bladder contractions are occurring and identifying no specific source. It occurs at any age and is a common cause of incontinence in the elderly.[6] Many times, however, a source for detrusor instability is found. Irritative sources for urinary urgency and urge urinary incontinence include urinary tract infections and noninfectious conditions of the bladder wall, such as interstitial cystitis, carcinoma in situ of the bladder, and radiation cystitis. Conditions distorting or displacing the bladder can also irritate the

bladder and result in urinary incontinence. These conditions include pelvic tumors or inflammatory processes, distal ureteral stones, and pregnancy. Detrusor instability can even be caused by procedures to correct vaginal prolapse or stress urinary incontinence.[7]

Low Bladder Compliance

The normal bladder has the ability to accommodate urine in such a way as to store urine at low pressures. If the bladder wall is damaged, its ability to accommodate urine can be diminished, resulting in low bladder compliance. When bladder compliance is lowered, urine is stored with higher pressures at a lower volume. There can be discomfort with low volume of urine in the bladder. Incontinence results if urine is stored at pressures greater than the urethral sphincters can maintain (Fig. 11B-5). Incontinence can be of any type: stress, urge, overflow, or a combination. Many of the conditions which cause detrusor instability can also lead to low bladder compliance.

MISCELLANEOUS CONDITIONS WHICH CAN CAUSE DETRUSOR INSTABILITY OR LOW BLADDER COMPLIANCE

Urinary Tract Infection

The classic triad of urinary frequency, urgency, and dysuria describes the symptoms of simple urinary tract infection. Not infrequently, infection can be present in

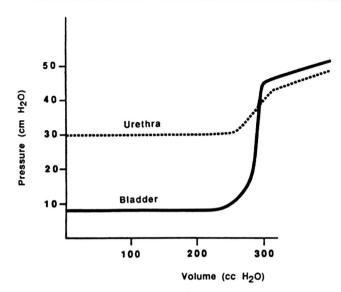

Fig. 11B-5 Cystometrogram with simultaneous urethral pressure monitoring showing low bladder compliance. Bladder stores urine under high pressures and at low volumes. Bladder pressure can exceed resting urethral pressure *(arrow)* where incontinence will occur.

the absence of frequency and dysuria. Treatment of the infection can resolve the urinary urgency and urge urinary incontinence it may have caused. It is, therefore, important that infection be ruled out or treated in all cases of incontinence. Severe bacterial or fungal cystitis can involve the entire bladder wall and occasionally result in scarring with loss of bladder compliance. In addition to increasing the risk for incontinence, such bladders are prone to recurrent urinary tract infection.

Interstitial Cystitis

Interstitial cystitis is a condition much more common than is clinically apparent. It presents with symptoms including irritative voiding symptoms such as urinary frequency and urgency along with suprapubic discomfort. Dysuria and dyspareunia are not infrequent symptoms. Symptoms can wax and wane over years. The urinalysis is normal and urine cultures are negative. The diagnosis is made by clinical history and cystoscopy usually under anesthesia. The bladder is often small and noncompliant. On distention under anesthesia fine punctate submucosal hemorrhages can be seen.[8] Pathologic features are nonspecific.[9] Stress urinary incontinence and urge urinary incontinence can be associated symptoms along with the much more common presenting feature of frequency and discomfort.[10] There is no

known etiology for interstitial cystitis. The clinical course is highly variable. Treatment is directed at relieving symptoms and includes oral medications, intravesical installations, and bladder distention.[11]

Carcinoma in Situ

Carcinoma in situ is a nonpapillary malignant change of the urothelium. It can present with irritative voiding symptoms and in some cases incontinence. Although microhematuria is not uncommon, urine analysis may not show any abnormalities. Cystoscopy may be unremarkable.[12] The diagnosis is made by urine cytology and bladder biopsy. If severe, bladder compliance can be reduced.

Radiation and Chemical Cystitis

Radiation cystitis should be familiar to all physicians dealing with pelvic malignancies. The condition results from radiation changes to the bladder that result in reduced vascularity and damage to bladder tissues. Radiation cystitis can reduce the bladder capacity, diminishing the bladder's ability to accommodate urine. It can cause irritative voiding symptoms including frequency, urgency, and incontinence. The diagnosis is made by history and cystoscopy with biopsy. The urethra may also be affected, contributing to incontinence, but isolated radiation cystitis alone can result in incontinence.

Chemical cystitis can occur after medical treatment with drugs that can be toxic to the bladder. Cytoxan is one such medication that can cause cystitis to the point of severe hematuria. The bladder wall can lose its compliance and ability to store urine at low pressures.

Radical Pelvic Surgery

Radical procedures such as anteroposterior (A-P) resection for rectal cancer or radical hysterectomy can occasionally denervate the bladder. This can result in a neurogenic bladder that is unable to contract and may eventually become very small and noncompliant. Incontinence is often the result.

NEUROGENIC INCONTINENCE

Disruption of neuropathways can result in incontinence. The bladder suffering from such disrupted neuropathways is referred to as a *neurogenic bladder*. Many neurogenic bladder patients suffer from incontinence, although the mechanisms may differ. Lapides[13] developed a classification of neurogenic bladder that is still in use today and useful in understanding different types of neurogenic incontinence.

Any lesions involving the cerebrum which could prevent inhibition of bladder contractions can result in incontinence. This type of neurogenic bladder is referred to as an *uninhibited neurogenic bladder*. If the patient is alert, she gives a history similar to a patient with detrusor instability. Because the inability to inhibit a bladder contraction is from a defined cerebral lesion such as a stroke or tumor, the condition is referred to as detrusor hyperreflexia denoting a neurogenic source.

The mechanism of incontinence in spinal cord injured paraplegics or quadriplegics (whose lesion is above the sacral reflex center) would be from reflex neurogenic contractions. In this case, the patient can neither perceive nor inhibit the bladder contraction and incontinence is the norm. This type of bladder is referred to as a *reflex neurogenic bladder*. If a person is neurologically injured in the sacral cord, the reflex micturition center can be destroyed. Messages to contract the bladder cannot be transmitted. The bladder stores urine until the pressure within the bladder overrides the urethral closure pressure and incontinence ensues. This bladder is autonomous of efferent and afferent input. It cannot contract without neurostimulation and is referred to as an *autonomous neurogenic bladder*. This lesion is common in myelodysplastics and in lower cord trauma patients. If peripheral motor fibers to the bladder are injured, as can happen in radical pelvic surgery, urinary retention occurs. Incontinence could result if the bladder is allowed to fill and overflow. Bladder discomfort occurs before that point, however, if sensory nerves are intact. This type of neurogenic bladder is referred to as a *motor paralytic bladder*. If, on the other hand, sensory nerves serving the bladder are damaged, as can occur in diabetes, and more rarely syphilis, the bladder fills without sensation of fullness. Overflow incontinence can result. The bladder muscle can eventually stretch to the degree of decompensation and overflow incontinence occurs. This is referred to as a *sensory paralytic bladder*. Although the neurogenic bladder can be a source for incontinence, many times the lesion can also affect the urethra, thus contributing to the problem. This is discussed later.

DECOMPENSATED BLADDER

The bladder can decompensate from chronic infrequent voiding and gradual stretching of the bladder to accommodate volumes much greater than it was meant to hold. At first, the bladder capacity enlarges. Next, the bladder does not completely empty with each void. Postvoid residuals are high and eventually the detrusor musculature loses its ability to effectively contract. Patients void by straining and carry high postvoid residuals. If the volume within the bladder is such that pressures can override the urethral sphincter mechanism, overflow incontinence results (Fig. 11B-6). In this case, the bladder muscle itself has lost its ability to effectively contract in response to neurostimuli.

DETRUSOR HYPERREFLEXIA WITH INCOMPLETE CONTRACTILITY

Combinations of the above conditions can occur resulting in incontinence. Such is the case of the recently

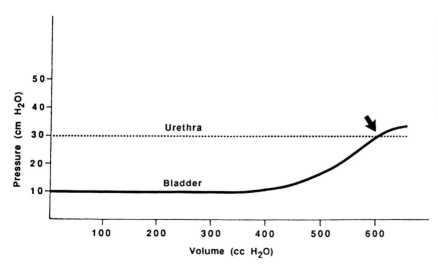

Fig. 11B-6 Cystometrogram with simultaneous urethral pressure monitoring showing overflow incontinence. Bladder is full to capacity and never completely empties. At maximum capacity pressures within the bladder may exceed that of resting urethral pressure *(arrow)* and incontinence will occur.

described entity of detrusor hyperreflexia with impaired contractility (DHIC).[14] In this case, bladder contractions cannot be inhibited but when they occur the bladder muscle itself may be partially decompensated, thus unable to completely empty the bladder. Patients have high residual urine, resulting in more frequent urinary urgency and incontinence. The condition is common in the elderly.[15]

In all of the above examples, the urethra and supporting structures can be entirely normal. The female pelvic floor in a person with urge urinary incontinence may therefore be identical to the normal continent female. Any effort to improve incontinence by altering or "restoring pelvic floor anatomy" will be futile and not in the best interest of the patient.

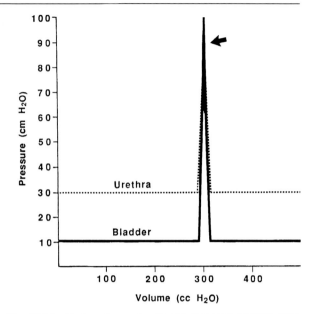

Fig. 11B-7 Cystometrogram with simultaneous urethral pressure monitoring showing stress incontinence. Sudden intraabdominal pressure increases, as in coughing or sneezing, can increase bladder pressure above that of resting urethral pressure *(arrow)* and incontinence will occur.

URINARY INCONTINENCE SECONDARY TO URETHRAL SPHINCTER FACTORS WITH NORMAL DETRUSOR MECHANISM

The previous section discussed the mechanisms of incontinence in which the urethra itself was not the primary factor in the pathogenesis of the abnormal urinary leakage. A woman with urge urinary incontinence secondary to an acute urinary tract infection has an entirely normal female pelvic floor and urethra grossly and histologically. In contrast, this section deals with disorders of the female pelvic floor and urethra which can result in incontinence despite otherwise normal bladder storage and emptying mechanisms.

PRIMARY (GENUINE) STRESS URINARY INCONTINENCE

The human female is an upright being, consequently the pelvic structures spend most of their time sitting on the pelvic floor. With age and childbearing, the pelvic floor can weaken, resulting in common physical findings such as cystocele, rectocele, vaginal, and uterine prolapse.[16] Similar weaknesses in urethral supporting structures can occur altering urethral closure mechanisms such that storage of urine may be faulty in certain circumstances resulting in incontinence. Such is the case in genuine stress urinary incontinence (SUI). In SUI the bladder fills and stores urine normally. When the bladder is subjected to sudden pressure increases as

occurs with coughing or straining, the urethra is unable to maintain a closed seal against the pressure within the bladder, and urine leaks. The pressure within the bladder lumen is temporarily greater than that of the urethral lumen and incontinence is demonstrable (Fig. 11B-7). The pathophysiology of such occurrence can be multifactorial and has been debated and discussed for decades, with our understanding still not complete. This section discusses the current thinking on the pathophysiology of stress urinary incontinence so as to be useful and logical to the clinician in treating this condition.

Poor Urethral Support

The importance of urethral support with regards to stress urinary incontinence was demonstrated decades ago with the advent of the chain or lateral cystogram. Findings before and after urethral suspension procedures gave visual proof "that urethral support was lacking during stress urinary incontinence" and that restoration of support could cure this.[17] Chapters were written on lateral straining cystograms and how proper interpretation could predict which suspension procedures would be advised depending on the degree of changes seen.[18] It is now commonly accepted that if intrinsic urethral closure mechanisms are intact (i.e., the proximal and distal sphincters are normal), then resting urinary continence is maintained. If, however, this otherwise normal urethra were to lose its urethral suspension (i.e., its attachments to pelvic floor and pubis which maintain it in a normal retropubic position), stress urinary incontinence results despite otherwise normal intrinsic urethral anatomy.

The most common explanation for why loss of urethral suspension results in stress urinary incontinence despite an otherwise normal urethra is as follows: normally the bladder neck and proximal female urethra lie above the female pelvic floor, well suspended behind the pubis. So positioned, the proximal urethra lies in an intraabdominal position. Activities and actions resulting in sudden increases in intraabdominal pressures result in both bladder and proximal urethra increasing their intraluminal pressures equally. If the urethral pressure is greater than the bladder pressure at rest, it remains so during stress activities and no incontinence occurs. With relaxation of the female pelvic floor the urethra can fall, such that its axis rotates posteriorly away from the pubis and its position migrates caudally with the weak pelvic floor. The portions of the urethra that were intraabdominal are moved. With stress activities the bladder increases its pressure as before but the urethra is no longer subjected to these increased pressures from the outside. Its resistance is not increased by these external pressures as before and its intrinsic resting pressure is not enough to provide for continence (Fig. 11B-8).

There have been numerous studies to support this theory. The concept was first supported with the research of Einhorning.[19] Multiple studies in humans before and after continence surgery with urethral pressure profilometry show that suspension procedures allow for transmission of intraabdominal pressure increases to the proximal urethra after surgery where such transmission was not possible prior to surgery.[20–23] Dogs studied under anesthesia with the urethral sphincter paralyzed were found to have passive increases in urethral pressure coinciding with similar increases in intraabdominal pressure.[24] McGuire and Herlihy[25] performed a similar study in cats under anesthesia with the same findings; however, when they opened the abdomen and placed pressure directly on the bladder, no such similar increases in intraurethral pressure occurred and urinary leakage occurred at much lower pressures than would be expected with the abdomen closed. Clinical studies show that any procedure which suspends

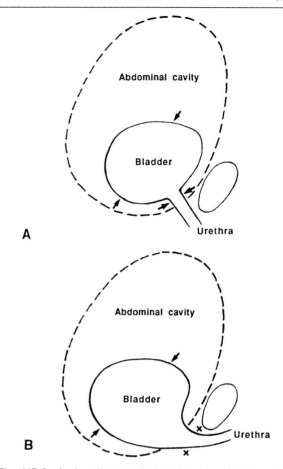

Fig. 11B-8 A, A well-suspended urethra is subjected to the same extrinsic intraabdominal pressures *(arrows)* as the bladder during coughing or sneezing. **B,** With poor support the urethra may no longer be subjected to the intraabdominal pressures experiencd by the bladder and stress incontinence can result.

the bladder neck to subject its proximal portion to intraabdominal pressure results in a high rate of success.[26–29]

As plausible as such a theory is for the mechanism of stress urinary incontinence with relaxation of the female pelvic floor and periurethral supporting structures, questions still exist. Loss of periurethral support and suspension measured by urethral axis on lateral cystography cannot predict incontinence.[30] There are many women whose proximal urethra is below the urogenital diaphragm and yet are totally continent. When a continent woman is in the process of voiding, the Valsalva maneuver can increase flow. If this increased pressure is transmitted to the proximal urethra one might think the flow would decrease or at least not change. An explanation would be that the vesical neck and proximal urethra is actively opened during the process of voiding and therefore its intraluminal pressure would not be equally affected by increases in intraabdominal pressure as in its passive closed state. Delancey[31] suggests that rather than intraabdominal positioning, it is the mechanical closure of the urethra by virtue of strong ligamentous connection to the pubis and toned pelvic floor (of which the levator ani is the major component) which provides for closure during stress activities. During voiding the pelvic floor relaxes and assists with urethral opening rather than compression, thus urine flow may increase with the Valsalva maneuver. This theory would best explain why pelvic floor exercise as first suggested by Kegel and modified by others can improve SUI.[32,33] Both theories are consistent with the clinical finding that procedures which restore the urethra and vesical neck to the position elevated and fixed behind the pubis are successful in treatment of classic stress urinary incontinence if pelvic floor relaxation is the etiology for the incontinence.

The question arises as to what is the pathophysiology of pelvic relaxation itself. We have already mentioned that aging can result in weakening of all muscular and fascial structures and that dependency of pelvic organs in the upright female may contribute to this weakening. Obesity can subject the female pelvic floor to increased weakening. Stress incontinence is more common in heavy women.[34] Pregnancy and vaginal delivery may also contribute. There is data to support peripheral nerve injury to the pelvic floor in patients with prolapsed pelvic structures and genuine SUI.[35–39] Some suggest that pregnancy is the source of this denervation.[38,40] Whether the pelvic floor has lost its strength through atrophy, stretching, or denervation, the urethra being intimately involved with the muscles of the pelvic floor and vagina can lose its ability to withstand increased bladder pressures and maintain its watertight seal. Furthermore, the weak or denervated skeletal muscle of the pelvic floor is intimately involved with the external sphincter, which may lose its ability to reflexly tighten at the instant of coughing. Magnetic resonance cross-sectional urethral imaging has further substantiated the importance of urethra relations to the pubis and levator sling via urethropelvic ligaments in maintaining a position advantageous for continence.[41]

Urethral Neuromuscular Deficiency

Stress incontinence also can occur when the bladder is normal and urethral position and support is normal. As discussed earlier, the urethra has proximal and distal sphincteric regions. Damage to both of these regions could result in total urinary incontinence, where urine leakage is continuous and urine is never stored in the bladder. Lesser degrees of damage could result in continence at rest but not during stress activity.

Neurologic Deficiency

The internal sphincter can be compromised from denervation during radical hysterectomy or pelvic exenteration. The presacral nerve which carries sympathetic input to the vesical neck can be disturbed during such surgery, resulting in lost alpha-adrenergic tone to the vesical neck at rest. In such a case, the vesical neck and proximal urethra is opened at rest, weakening the overall urethral resistance and increasing the risk of incontinence. In reality, events which injure the presacral nerve usually compromise the pelvic nervous plexus that carries parasympathetics to the bladder, therefore, concomitant bladder emptying problems can occur. The resulting injury may appear as overflow incontinence. Patients with myelodysplasia involving the lower cord can present similarly with an open bladder neck and neurogenic bladder emptying difficulties with overflow incontinence.

Injuries to the sacral cord alone, as discussed earlier, can result in an autonomous neurogenic bladder that is unable to empty. At the same time the pudendal nerve that originates in the sacral cord may be affected, resulting in paralysis of the external striated sphincter, which can diminish the maximal urethral pressure the patient is able to generate and, therefore, contribute to urinary incontinence.

Urethral instability is a urodynamic finding which may be related to stress and/or urge incontinence.[42] It is described by urethral pressure variations which may allow for urine to enter the urethra or precipitate urinary urgency and thus predispose to incontinence. It is thought to be caused by a nervous factor. Its actual role in urinary incontinence is still unknown.

Muscular Deficiency

Repeated urethral or bladder suspension procedures can result in poor intrinsic urethral sphincter function from scarring of the muscle itself in a fixed or open position.[43,44] Such a urethra might appear as an open pipe on cystoscopy and would not be improved by standard suspension procedures. The urethra in this case, ironically, is often well suspended but in an open position. Procedures to squeeze the urethra closed such as the artificial urinary sphincter or sling procedure are required.[45,46] Surgical procedures involving the urethra obviously risk damage to the sphincteric mechanisms if the procedure involves the proximal two thirds of urethra. Chronic urethral inflammatory conditions can lead to scarring and risk to the intrinsic continence mechanism. Infected urethral diverticula and radiation urethritis can predispose to this entity.

Deficient Mucosal Seal

We have discussed the significance of proper urethral positioning and normal urethral neuromuscular status of the sphincters as important in preventing incontinence. A final intrinsic factor necessary for maintenance of continence is the urethral mucosal seal. The female urethral mucosa is richly vascular and appears pliable with redundant longitudinal folds on urethroscopy. The mucosal folds coapt forming a watertight mucosal seal in the normal female. Conditions which can jeopardize this mucosal seal can lead to incontinence despite normal urethral positioning and neuromuscular sphincteric properties. The importance of this mucosal seal was emphasized by Zinner and coworkers.[47] Placing a grooved probe in the urethra he was able to show that normal females were able to maintain continence despite the groove in the probe.[48] In normal females the urethral mucosa was able to fold into the groove and seal it, preventing incontinence. He was able to show a correlation between age and the ability of the urethral mucosa to fold into the groove. Postmenopausal women were less able to seal the urethra closed than younger ones. The female urethral mucosa and its richly vascular submucosa were shown to have a high concentration of estrogen receptors.[49] Postmenopausal women lack circulating estrogen and their urethra mucosa may develop deficiencies in its vascularity or its pliability. This may contribute to incontinence in elderly females. Replacement of estrogen may improve mucosa thickness and pliability and improve incontinence in certain women.[50] An analogy can be drawn to the response of atrophic vaginitis to estrogens in postmenopausal women. The contribution of the urethral mucosal seal to female urinary continence can be significant. Raz and colleagues[51] suggested that the female urethral mucosa is responsible for up to one third of resting urethral closure pressure, but their data was based on animal studies. Recent work, however, has challenged the ability of estrogen replacement to improve postmenopausal women with SUI.[50] Perhaps more important than the role of estrogens in increasing urethral closure pressures is the finding that estrogens may play a role in relieving irritative voiding symptoms

in postmenopausal females, including urge urinary incontinence.[52] The role of estrogens (or lack of estrogens) in female urinary incontinence is still unclear, but the role of the urethral mucosal seal is widely accepted.

Radiation changes to the urethra can cause deficiencies in the urethral mucosal seal resulting in incontinence. The mechanism again may be diminished submucosal vascularity and mucosal pliability. This type of mucosal deficiency does not respond to estrogen therapy.

MISCELLANEOUS CAUSES OF FEMALE URINARY INCONTINENCE

Epispadias

Congenital failure of the urethra to be closed on the dorsal aspect is referred to as epispadias. The anomaly is most commonly associated with exstrophy of the bladder, in which case the bladder abnormality is clearly of primary significance. Rarely, however, epispadias occurs in absence of exstrophy. The incidence in females is 1 in 481,000 according to Dees.[53] Incontinence is obviously secondary to deficiency in the urethral sphincter and the urethral wall itself. Surgical correction is required and even after surgical correction, stress urinary incontinence is sometimes a persistent problem.[54]

Urethral Diverticula

Diverticula of the female urethra presents with dribbling incontinence. During voiding the diverticulum fills with urine. After voiding the diverticulum can empty, depending on patient position and pressures placed on the diverticulum. This results in intermittent dribbling incontinence. Associated symptoms may include urethral discharge, dysuria, and dyspareunia. The diagnosis can be made by palpation of the urethra during physical examination and at the time of urethroscopy, where at times contents of the diverticulum empty into the urethral lumen. Voiding cystourethrogram and retrograde urethrography may image the diverticulum. The treatment is surgical.

Urinary Fistulae

Fistulae between the female urinary system and genitalia are not uncommon and can be postsurgical or caused from disease including tumor, inflammation, and irradiation. Fistulae can occur between the ureter, bladder, or urethra and vagina. Vesicouterine fistulae can also occur and result in incontinence. In the case of fistulae to the vagina the incontinence is usually continuous. Rare vesicouterine fistulae may result in intermittent incontinence, the source of which may be difficult to diagnose unless it is included in the differential diagnosis and looked for. A more thorough discussion is presented elsewhere in this text. The possibility of fistulae must always be considered during the workup of urinary incontinence in the female or it can be easily missed.

Ectopic Ureter

When the ureter opens into the vesical neck, urethra, or structures other than the bladder it is referred to as ectopic. The incidence of ectopic ureter is 1 in 1,900.[55] The upper pole ureter of a complete ureteral duplication is the source of the ectopic orifice 80% of the time. The ureteral ectopy is from a single ureter and collecting system 20% of the time. The ectopic ureter can cause female incontinence if it empties distal to continent sphincteric mechanisms in the urethra. Ectopic ureters can also empty into the cervix or the vagina, resulting in incontinence. One third of ectopic ureters in the female empty at the level of the vesical neck. These women are usually continent, but can suffer from other urologic problems including ureteral obstruction, reflux, and infection. Another one third of ectopic ureters open into the mid and distal urethra and incontinence occurs. Another 25% empty into the vagina and 5% into the cervix or the uterus.[56] Incontinence can be continuous or infrequent, depending on the location of the ureteral orifice relative to the proximal urethral sphincter. The diagnosis requires careful urologic work-up. Many times the ectopic ureter serves a poorly functioning kidney or renal segment. In this case, excretory urography may not be diagnostic. Cystourethroscopy, vaginoscopy, retrograde ureterography, and voiding cystourethroscopy may be required to make the diagnosis. Intravenously administered dye such as indigo carmine can also be useful to color the urine during the examination, assisting in locating the orifice. The treatment is surgical.

Functional Incontinence

Patients who are incontinent of urine despite entirely normal urodynamic, anatomic, and neurologic vesicourethral status are considered functionally incontinent.

Patients with confused mental status or psychiatric disease are incontinent because of a lack of awareness that incontinence is undesirable or inappropriate. The elderly are prone to this especially when medicated. Such medications include antidepressants, antipsychotics, sedative hypnotics, and narcotic analgesics. Removal of medications and improvement of mental status can cure the problem.[15,57]

Many patients have complaints of incontinence associated with urinary urgency and frequency yet no incontinence is documented and no abnormality is found after complete urologic evaluation. Psychologic counseling can help.[58, 60]

Diuretics can cause increased urine formation and predispose to detrusor instability or bladder distention and SUI. Fecal impaction can interfere with bladder emptying and result in overflow incontinence. In most of these cases the patient is predisposed to incontinence, but incontinence is improved or cured by removing the precipitating factor. Functional incontinence is often reversible and therefore termed *transient incontinence*. When precipitating factors are identified, incontinence improves.

Patients confined to bed who are unable to ambulate may void in bed if there is no one to assist them with a bed pan or urinal. Likewise, patients hospitalized after operations may not be able to ambulate without assistance and incontinence occurs. This is especially common in restrained patients. It is a temporary situation that puts the patient at risk for incontinence, and the term *situational incontinence* is used. Bedside commode, nursing assistance, and other measures improve incontinence. The mnemonic DIAPPERS has been suggested to remember causes of transient or situational incontinence[15]:

D — Delirium/confusion state
I — Infection
A — Atrophic urethritis/vaginitis
P — Pharmaceuticals
P — Psychological
E — Endocrine (i.e., diabetes with polyuria)
R — Restricted mobility
S — Stool impaction

SUMMARY

It should be clear from this chapter that there are multiple conditions that are responsible for urinary incontinence. These conditions may be unrelated and be specific sources for incontinence, or they can coexist, such that the pathophysiology of incontinence is multifactorial. Abnormal bladder and/or urethral function can occur, resulting in incontinence despite an otherwise entirely normal female pelvic floor. On the other hand, weakness of the female pelvic floor can result in incontinence despite otherwise normal bladder and urethral function. Congenital anomalies and acquired fistulae can also result in incontinence. A specific diagnosis is required in order to determine appropriate treatment. A careful history and physical examination is required in order to tailor the diagnostic work-up such that the source for incontinence is diagnosed and properly managed.

REFERENCES

1. Thomas TN, Plymat KR, Blannin J, Meade TW. Prevalence of urinary incontinence. *Br Med J.* 1980;281:1243.
2. Diokno AC, Brock BM, Brown MB, Herzog AR. Prevalence of urinary incontinence and other urologic symptoms in the noninstitutionalized elderly. *J Urol.* 1986;136:1022.
3. Reid GC, DeLancey JL, Hopkins MP, Roberts JA, Morley GW. Urinary incontinence following radical vulvectomy. *Obstet Gynecol.* 1990;75:852.
4. Blaivas JG. The neurophysiology of micturition: a clinical study of 550 patients. *J Urol.* 1982;127:958.
5. Carlsson CA. The supraspinal control of the urinary bladder. *Acta Pharmacol Toxicol.* 1978;43:8.
6. Diokno AC, Brown MB, Brock BM, Herzog AR, Normolle DP. Clinical and cystometric characteristics of continent and incontinent noninstitutionalized elderly. *J Urol.* 1988;140:567.
7. Langer R, Ron-El R, Newman M, Herman A, Caspi E. Detrusor instability following colposuspension for urinary stress incontinence. *Br J Obstet Gynaecol.* 1988;95:607.
8. Hanno P, Levin RM, Monson FC, et al. Diagnosis of interstitial cystitis. *J Urol.* 1990;143:278.
9. Holm-Bentzen M, Lose G. Pathology and pathogenesis of interstitial cystitis. *Urology.* 1987;29:8.
10. Jenson H, Nielsen K, Frimodt-Moller C. Interstitial cystitis: review of the literature. *Urol Int.* 1989;44:189.
11. Parivar F, Bradbrook RA. Interstitial cystitis. *Br J Urol.* 1986;58:239.
12. Althausen AF, Prout GR, Daly JJ. Noninvasive papillary carcinoma of the bladder associated with carcinoma in situ. *J Urol.* 1976;116:575.
13. Lapides J. The Lapides classification. In Gillenwater JY, Grayhack JT, Howards SS, Duckett JW, eds. *Adult and Pediatric Urology.* Chicago: Year Book Medical Publishers, Inc; 1987;882–883.
14. Resnick NM, Yalla SV. Detrusor hyperactivity with impaired contractility. *JAMA.* 1987;257:3076.
15. Resnick N. Diagnosis and treatment of incontinence in the institutionalized elderly. *Sem Urol.* 1989;7:117.
16. Staskin DR. Age-related physiologic and pathologic changes affecting the lower urinary tract. *Geriat Clin North Am.* 1986;2:701–710.
17. Jeffcoate T, Roberts H. Observations on stress incontinence of urine. *Am J Obstet Gynecol.* 1952;64:721.
18. Green TH. Urinary stress incontinence: pathophysiology, diagnosis, and classification. In: Buchsbaum HJ, Schmidt J, eds. *Gynecologic and Obstetric Urology,* 2nd ed. Philadelphia: WB Saunders Co; 1982;199–224.
19. Einhorning G. Simultaneous recording of the intravesical and intraurethral pressures. *Acta Chir Scand.* 1961;276:1.
20. Bump R, Fantl A, Hurt G. Dynamic urethral profilometry pressure transmission ratio determinations after continence surgery: understanding the mechanism of success, failure, and complications. *Obstet Gynecol.* 1988;72:870.
21. Bump R, Copeland W, Hurt W, Fantl J. Dynamic urethral pressure/profilometry pressure transmission ratio determinations in stress-incontinent and stress-continent subjects. *Am J Obstet Gynecol.* 1988;159:749.
22. Constantinou C, Govan DE. Contribution and timing of transmitted and generated pressure components in the female urethra. In: Zinner NR, Sterling M, eds, *Female Incontinence.* New York: Alan R. Liss; 1980:113–120.
23. Constantinou, CA. Impact of bladder neck suspension on mode of distribution of abdominal pressure on urethra. *Prog Clin Biol Res.* 1981;78:121–132.
24. Graber P, Laurent G, Tanagho E. Effect of abdominal pressure rise on the urethral profile: an experimental study on dogs. *Invest Urol.* 1974;12:57.
25. McGuire E, Herlihy E. The influence of urethral position on urinary continence. *Invest Urol.* 1977;15:205.
26. Bergman A, Ballard C, Koonings P. Comparison of three different surgical procedures for genuine stress incontinence: prospective randomized study. *Am J Obstet Gynecol.* 1990;160:1102–1106.
27. Bergman A, Koonings P, Ballard C. Primary stress urinary incontinence and pelvic relaxation: prospective randomized comparison of three different operations. *Am J Obstet Gynecol.* 1989;161:97.
28. Geelen J, Theeuwes A, Eskes T, Martin C. The clinical and urodynamic effects of anterior vaginal repair and Burch colposuspension. *Am J Obstet Gynecol.* 1988;159:137.
29. Karram M, Bhatia N. Transvaginal needle bladder neck suspension procedures for stress urinary incontinence: a comprehensive review. *Obstet Gynecol.* 1989;73:906.
30. Fantl J, Hurt W, Bump R, Dunn L, Choi S. Urethral axis and sphincteric function. *Am J Obstet Gynecol.* 1986;155:554.
31. DeLancey JO. Anatomy and physiology of urinary continence. *Clin Obstet Gynecol.* 1990;33:298.
32. Kegel A. Physiologic therapy for urinary stress incontinence. *JAMA.* 1952;10:915.
33. Olah K, Bridges N, Denning J, Farrar D. The conservative management of patients with symptoms of stress incontinence: a randomized, prospective study comparing weighted vaginal cones and interferential therapy. *Am J Obstet Gynecol.* 1990;162:87.
34. Dwyer P, Lee E, Hay D. Obesity and urinary incontinence in women. *Br J Obstet Gynaecol.* 1988;95:91.
35. Varma J, Fidas A, McInnes A, Smith A, Chisholm G. Neurophysiological abnormalities in genuine female stress urinary incontinence. *Br J Obstet Gynaecol.* 1988;95:705.
36. Smith A, Hosker G, Warrell D. The role of pudendal nerve damage in the etiology of genuine stress incontinence in women. *Br J Obstet Gynaecol.* 1989;96:29.
37. Gilpin S, Gosling J, Smith A, Warrell D. The pathogenesis of genitourinary prolapse and stress incontinence of urine. A histological and histochemical study. *Br J Obstet Gynaecol.* 1989;96:15.
38. Smith A, Hosker G, Warrell D. The role of partial denervation of the pelvic floor in the etiology of genitourinary prolapse and stress incontinence of urine. A neurophysiological study. *Br J Obstet Gynaecol.* 1989;96:24.
39. Snooks S, Badenoch D, Tiptaft R, Swash M. Perineal nerve damage in genuine stress urinary incontinence. *Brit J Urol.* 1985;57:422.
40. Tapp A, Cardozo L, Versi E, Montogomery J, Studd J. The effect of vaginal delivery on the urethral sphincter. *Br J Obstet Gynaecol.* 1988;95:142.

41. Klutke C, Golomb J, Barbaric Z, Raz S. The anatomy of stress incontinence: magnetic resonance imaging of the female bladder neck and urethra. *J Urol*. 1990;143:563.

42. Vereecken RL, Das J. Urethral instability: related to stress and/or urge incontinence?. *J Urol*. 1985;134:698.

43. McGuire E. Urodynamic findings in patients after failure of stress incontinence operations. *Prog Clin Biol Res*. 1981;78:351.

44. Blaivas J, Salinas J. Type III stress urinary incontinence: importance of proper diagnosis and treatment. *Surg Forum*. 1984;35: 473.

45. Appell RA. Techniques and results in the implantation of the artificial urinary sphincter in women with type III stress urinary incontinence by a vaginal approach. *Neuro Urodyn*. 1988;7: 613.

46. McGuire E, Lytton B. Pubovaginal sling procedure for stress incontinence. *J Urol*. 1978;119:82.

47. Zinner N, Sterling A, Ritter R. Role of inner urethral softness in urinary continence. *Urology*. 1980;16:115.

48. Zinner N, Sterling A, Ritter R. Evaluation of inner urethral softness: part II clinical study using new grooved probe device. *Urology*. 1983;22:446.

49. Iosif C, Batra S, Ek A, Astedt B. Estrogen receptors in the human female lower urinary tract. *Am J Obstet Gynecol*. 1981;141:817.

50. Cardozo L. Role of estrogens in the treatment of female urinary incontinence. *J Am Geriatr Soc*. 1990;38:326.

51. Raz S, Caine M, Zeigler M. The vascular component in the production of intraurethral pressure. *J Urol*. 1972;108:93.

52. Walter S, Wolf H, Barlebo H, Jensen H. Urinary continence in postmenopausal women treated with estrogens: a double-blind clinical trial. *Urol Int*. 1978;33:135.

53. Dees JE. Congenital epispadias with incontinence. *J Urol*. 1949; 62:513.

54. Jordan G, Gilbert D. Operative procedures of epispadias and exstrophy of the bladder. *Sem Urol*. 1987;5:243.

55. Campbell MF. Anomalies of the ureter. In: Campbell MF, Harrison JH, eds. *Campbell's*, 3rd ed. Philadelphia: W. B. Saunders Co.; 1970;1487–1670.

56. Snyder HM. Anomalies of the Ureter. In: Gillenwater JY, Grayhack JT, Howards SS, Duckett JW, eds. *Adult and Pediatric Urology*, Chicago: Yearbook Medical Publishers, Inc; 1987;1642–1646.

57. Psychosocial factors in urinary incontinence. *Geriat Clin North Am* 1986;659.

58. Macaulay A, Stern R, Holmes D, Stanton S. Micturition and the mind: psychological factors in the etiology and treatment of urinary symptoms in women. *Brit Med J*. 1987;294:540.

59. Rees D, Farhoumand N. Psychiatric aspects of recurrent cystitis in women. *Brit J Urol*. 1977;49:651.

60. Stone C, Judd G. Psychogenic aspects of urinary incontinence in women. *Clin Obstet Gynecol*. 1978;21:807.

CHAPTER 11

Urinary Incontinence

11C Nonsurgical Therapies

11C1 Pharmacologic Therapy

Hilary J. Cholhan   Alfred E. Bent

INTRODUCTION

An epidemiologic survey by Diokno and colleagues[1] estimated that the prevalence of urinary incontinence in noninstitutionalized women was 38%. Although this figure may be inflated due to the liberal inclusion of all patients with any degree of involuntary loss of urine within the previous twelve months, nonetheless, this study corroborates the findings of others[2] that urinary incontinence is a problem confronting a substantial portion of the female population.

The prevalence of female urinary incontinence potentially will mushroom in the near future because of the prolongation of the life span in our society, principally as a result of modern medicine. Since the incidence of female urinary incontinence increases with age,[3] the cost to society of managing urinary incontinence parallels the prolonged life expectancy and has been estimated to approximate $10 billion yearly, according to the National Institutes of Health-sponsored Consensus Development Conference of 1988.

For many patients with urinary incontinence surgical intervention may not represent the optimal approach for management of their incontinence. Just as other medical disorders are controlled pharmacologically, so too many causes of urinary incontinence respond positively to medical intervention. However, in some instances drug therapy may be overly risky to the patient or ineffectual for the diagnosed condition, and thus would not be appropriate.

Many members of the geriatric population use multiple medications to control an assortment of acute and chronic conditions. Adding pharmacologic agents to the patient's existing regimen may increase the risk of drug interactions and compound the inconvenience of taking numerous drugs. Thus, the overall effect of pharmacotherapy directed toward urinary incontinence may be diminished by a lack of compliance, or by being physiologically compromising.

The intent of this chapter is to familiarize the clinician with possible indications and contraindications for the pharmacologic management of female urinary incontinence and to review the various medications currently in usage or under investigation.

Prior to examining the particular pharmacologic agents and their applications, the etiology of female urinary incontinence is reviewed, since it is of utmost importance to understand the cause of the incontinence before pharmacotherapy can be useful. All terminology utilized in this chapter is in agreement with the definitions proposed by the International Continence Society,[4] unless specified otherwise.

NEUROPHYSIOLOGY OF LOWER URINARY TRACT

Since the bladder and urethra are related anatomically and functionally, it would be inappropriate to isolate one structure from the other in a discussion of urinary incontinence. Controversy still exists regarding the intricacies of lower urinary tract neurophysiology, neuropharmacology, and neuroanatomy. However, authorities agree universally that accommodation permits the bladder to function as a reservoir during the filling/storage phase, and when appropriate, the bladder empties its urinary contents. The urethral sphincteric mechanism complements the bladder's functions by maintaining increased pressure (positive urethral closure pressure) during the storage phase, and permits micturition by a drop in closure pressure during the emptying phase. Effecting these precise complementary actions of the bladder and urethra are the synergistic functions of the parasympathetic/sympathetic components of the peripheral nervous system.[5] Modulation of this local innervation is achieved by the central nervous system.

By way of the pelvic nerve, which provides the principal motor supply to the detrusor muscle, the parasympathetic nervous system (PNS) causes evacuation of urine from the bladder. Fibers of the pelvic nerve originate in the spinal cord roots S_2 to S_4. These preganglionic fibers coalesce to form the pelvic nerve, which synapses in the ganglia of the autonomic pelvic and bladder wall plexuses. The detrusor muscle responds to this direct PNS stimulation by contracting. Effecting the transmission of stimulatory information from the preganglionic to the postganglionic sides is the neurotransmitter acetylcholine, which traverses the synapse and triggers the acetylcholine-specific receptors on the postganglionic side. The smooth muscle component of the bladder neck and urethra, however, does not respond to this parasympathetic stimulation to any significant degree, and thus remains relaxed as the bladder contracts during normal voluntary micturition.

The principal role of the sympathetic nervous system (SNS) is maintenance of continence by effecting the dual action of relaxation of the bladder and contraction of the smooth muscle component of the urethral sphincter. The fibers of the SNS stem from spinal nerve roots T_{10} to L_2. These preganglionic fibers pass through the splanchnic nerves, and most synapse at the superior hypogastric plexus. Postganglionic fibers continue their course to 'the bladder where they terminate in the smooth muscle cells and blood vessels of the bladder. A small fraction of these postganglionic fibers cross over and terminate on the ganglionic cells of the PNS in the immediate vicinity of the bladder wall. This crossing over is testimony to the synergistic relationship of the PNS and SNS in the control of bladder-urethral functions.

Alpha- and beta-adrenergic receptors have been identified in the lower urinary tract.[6] Beta receptors are distributed predominantly in the body and fundus of the bladder, whereas the alpha receptors are clustered in the bladder base and urethra. Beta stimulation causes relaxation of the bladder, thus promoting storage of urine. Alpha activation results in contraction of the internal urethral smooth muscle and aids in maintenance of continence.

DETRUSOR INSTABILITY

Vesical instability involves uncontrolled bladder activity as demonstrated objectively by cystometry. The bladder may contract with provocation (e.g., coughing, heel bouncing, Valsalva maneuver) or without provocation during the filling phase, while the patient is trying to inhibit micturition. Traditionally, a bladder contraction is required to generate a rise in intravesical pressure of at least 15 cm/H_2O; however, more recently subthreshold instability has been recognized as clinically relevant in symptomatic patients.[7] It is important to realize that not all patients with detrusor instability (DI) experience urinary incontinence. In fact, the small percentage of those with DI who are not incontinent may suffer from other symptoms which may be exceedingly uncomfortable. These symptoms include sensory urgency, frequency, suprapubic pressure, pelvic pain, and others.

Before considering phamacotherapy for the control of bladder instability, it is imperative for the clinician to eliminate the less common causes of this disorder. Neurologic and locally irritative conditions, including cystitis/urethritis, urolithiasis, and intravesical lesions (polyps, malignancies) must be ruled out. Although most of these conditions would respond somewhat to drugs commonly used for DI, the primary cause ought to be addressed with properly selected antibiotics, surgical or nonsurgical stone elimination, or lesion extirpation, respectively.

Once the presence of DI has been established unequivocally via cystometry and an attempt has been made to pinpoint the underlying cause, the clinician has a relatively substantial menu of options for the management of this condition (Box 11C1-1). Among the more commonly employed and successful therapeutic strategies are bladder retraining drills with or without the addition of pharmacologic agents. Fantl and associates[8] demonstrated that statistically there was no difference

---

Box 11C1-1
Alternative Modes of Therapy for Detrusor Instability

Acupuncture
Biofeedback
Bladder retraining drills
Functional electrical stimulation
Pharmacotherapy
Surgical denervation
Transvesical phenol instillation

Box 11C1-2
Pharmacologic Agents for Management of Detrusor Instability

Anticholinergics
Musculotropic relaxants
Calcium-antagonists
Tricyclic antidepressants
Prostaglandin synthetase antagonists
Beta-adrenergic agonists
Other

---

in results for groups practicing bladder drills alone or adding a drug.

In patients who are recalcitrant to more conservative forms of therapy, use of medications that can help achieve bladder quiescence is appropriate. Innumerable pharmacologic agents have been evaluated and/or applied in the management of DI; nevertheless, the efficacy of most has been less than stellar. In addition, many patients find the side effects of these agents to be quite problematic. Often this results in poor patient compliance or cessation of drug therapy altogether.

The vast array of drugs utilized for detrusor muscle relaxation alter bladder overactivity by affecting the synthesis, storage, release, and transportation of the neurotransmitters of the PNS/SNS or their inactivation, reuptake, and degeneration. In addition, other drugs exert direct influence on the smooth muscle cells (musculotropic) or inhibit transmembrane transport of extracellular calcium ions, which are necessary for the contractility of those smooth muscle cells.

Because their mechanisms of action are multiple and frequently overlap, medications to control the unstable bladder cannot be packaged neatly in discrete categories. However, for the sake of simplicity we have grouped the more commonly used drugs in categories based on their predominant activity (Box 11C1-2).

ANTICHOLINERGIC AGENTS

Anticholinergic medications target receptors specific for the postganglionic neurotransmitter of the PNS, acetylcholine. As such, these drugs are sometimes known as antimuscarinic agents. They exert influence by competitively blocking the acetylcholine receptors, thereby not permitting the neurotransmitter to stimulate the receptors, thus they effect bladder quiescence.

Since most anticholinergic agents are nonspecific, they have influence on most of the body's acetylcholine receptors. Because of this lack of specificity it is not surprising that most of these pharmacologic agents are fraught with numerous side effects, many of which patients find difficult to tolerate. Often this intolerance results in cessation of drug usage.

Propantheline

Propantheline bromide affects the PNS by directly interfering with the synaptic transmission of the neurotransmitter acetylcholine. This interference prevents contraction of the detrusor muscle. It has been shown that administration of this medication decreases the frequency and amplitude of bladder contractions or eliminates them altogether without significantly increasing the residual volume.[9] In the United States propantheline (Pro-Banthine) is available for oral administration only and is usually prescribed in doses of 15 mg to 30 mg two to four times a day. It is suggested that the tablets be ingested approximately one-half hour before meals. The onset of action occurs at 30 minutes and the duration of action is about 4 hours.[10]

We recommend starting at a dosage of 15 mg twice daily and titrating upward as necessary until the desired effect is achieved. Most patients cannot tolerate regimens in excess of 30 mg four times a day. Anticholinergic side effects, the most prominent of which are dryness of the mouth, blurred vision, mydriasis, drowsiness, constipation, and tachycardia, mitigate against higher dosage. Due to the anticholinergic action, propantheline should be used with great caution in patients with a cardiac condition, and must be avoided altogether in patients with narrow-angle glaucoma, my-asthenia gravis, and in conditions which include compromised gastrointestinal motility and urinary obstruction. Propantheline may interfere with bladder emptying to the point of complete urinary retention.[11]

Emepronium

Emepronium bromide (Cetiprin) is another agent with predominantly anticholinergic and antinicotinic (ganglion-blocking) properties. Usual dosages are 100 mg to 200 mg three or four times daily. However, poor gastrointestinal absorption of the oral form has cast doubts on its efficacy as an agent for DI.[12] Favorable reports included an increase in bladder capacity, decreasing intravesical pressure, and suppression of uncontrolled bladder contractions.[13]

Adverse side effects include all of those mentioned for propantheline, predominantly antimuscarinic effects. Moreover, mucosal alterations have been reported,[12] at times resulting in oral ulcers and/or esophagitis. At present this agent is not available in the United States.

MUSCULOTROPIC AGENTS

By a nonspecific and not yet fully understood mechanism,[14] musculotropic drugs act directly on the smooth muscle cells and cause deactivation and relaxation of these muscle cells. Since most of the agents in this category exhibit antimuscarinic cross-reactivity to variable degrees, they often precipitate anticholinergic side effects.

Oxybutynin

Oxybutynin chloride (Ditropan®) exerts action primarily directly against smooth muscle cells. In addition, it provides moderate anticholinergic as well as anesthetic activity. Besides its well-documented effect on idiopathic bladder instability, oxybutynin is useful in the management of DI which develops after incontinence surgery, or DI associated with lower urinary tract infection or irradiation to the pelvic region or after removal of an intravesical catheter.

Cystometric studies[15,16,17,18] demonstrated that oxybutynin effects a decrease in the amplitude and frequency or complete obliteration of uncontrolled bladder contractions. Oxybutynin is available as a scored 5 mg tablet. Usual dosages that produce desired clinical results range from 5 mg two to four times a day.

Although, in theory, oxybutynin's anticholinergic ef-

fect is less profound than that of propantheline, at times the side effects are so severe they lead to discontinuation of this drug even though the patient's DI may have improved as a result of its usage. Cardozo and associates[17] reported recently that 8 of the 20 patients who were included in their study ceased using oxybutynin because of intolerable side effects. Thus, for patients who develop bothersome side effects, the clinician should attempt to titrate the dosage downward in an effort to achieve a balance between mitigated, yet tolerable, side effects and the desired clinical effect.

Contraindications to the usage of oxybutynin include glaucoma, myasthenia gravis, gastrointestinal hypomotility conditions, and outflow obstruction of the urinary tract. In patients with suspected or known cardiac conditions, oxybutynin should be used only with great caution.

Dicyclomine

Dicyclomine hydrochloride (Bentyl) is a musculotropic/antimuscarinic agent that has been used more commonly for the management of functional bowel/irritable bowel syndrome. However, this agent has proved its usefulness in the treatment of vesical instability. The response rate is reportedly similar to that of oxybutynin.[19] Besides improvement in involuntary bladder contractions, dicyclomine has caused increases in bladder capacity.[20]

Dicyclomine is available in 10 mg capsules or 20 mg tablets. Gastrointestinal absorption is rapid and complete. Plasma half-life is short (less than 2 hours), requiring more frequent administration. The recommended regimen for adults is 10 to 20 mg four times daily.

Since dicyclomine is a less potent anticholinergic than oxybutynin, adverse side effects are less prominent. Thus, this medication deserves consideration in instances where oxybutynin is determined to be intolerable, despite tries at downward titration. Furthermore, as with other agents for bladder instability, dicyclomine may be used in conjunction with another agent to achieve the desired effect. Contraindications, absolute and relative, are similar to those for any medication with anticholinergic action (Box 11C1-3)

Flavoxate

Flavoxate hydrochloride (Urispas) is a synthetic agent with a direct relaxant effect on the smooth muscle cells of the bladder and urethra and has mild anesthetic

Box 11C1-3
Contraindications to Usage of Agents with Anticholinergic Properties

Obstructive uropathy
Gastrointestinal disorders
obstructive/hypomotility
reflux esophagitis
ulcerative colitis
Glaucoma
Myasthenia gravis
Cardiovascular disease
unstable
Hypersensitivity

properties. It is primarily intended to mitigate irritative symptoms (e.g., dysuria, urgency, frequency, suprapubic pressure, nocturia, etc.) associated with the inflammatory/infectious conditions of the lower urinary tract. However, it might be considered for use in patients for whom side effects, the anticholinergic ones in particular, are overly bothersome.[21] The recommended dosage is 100 mg to 200 mg orally three to four times daily.

As mentioned, the side effects are relatively mild; they include visual disturbances, drowsiness, and dry mouth.[22] Despite mild side effects, flavoxate has not yielded the same positive clinical results as have other agents,[23] and thus has not achieved a prominent position in the management of DI.

TRICYCLIC ANTIDEPRESSANTS

Since 1968 antidepressants have been studied and found to be effective in managing bladder instability.[24] Tricyclic antidepressants (TCA) exert their action by one or a combination of three modes[25]: (1) anticholinergic actions, both central and peripheral; (2) direct interference with the presynaptic reuptake mechanism for the neurotransmitters serotonin and norepinephrine; and (3) central sedative effect.

Imipramine

Imipramine hydrochloride (Tofranil) is the pharmacologic agent in the TCA category that has demonstrated the greatest applicability in patients with DI.

Imipramine is a dibenzazepine compound which has been used for childhood enuresis.

In spite of its relatively weak antimuscarinic effect on the bladder, imipramine's primary mode of action is a direct musculotropic relaxant effect,[26] which is neither anticholinergic nor adrenergic. It does, however, stimulate alpha- and beta-adrenergic receptors indirectly. Sustained use of this agent can increase intraurethral pressure and decrease detrusor tone.

Recommended starting dosage is 25 mg two to three times daily and can be given as a single dose at bedtime. Maximum dose is 150 mg/day, but this is seldom used.[27] Caution must be exercised when prescribing this medication to older patients and patients with a history of cardiovascular disease, because orthostatic hypotension, hypertension, or ventricular dysrhythmias may ensue. Also, imipramine is contraindicated in patients using a monoamine oxidase inhibitor, since these agents combined can cause a hypertensive crisis.

PROSTAGLANDIN SYNTHETASE INHIBITORS

When initially studied several types of pharmacologic agents showed promise in the management of DI. These agents included the prostaglandin antagonists (PGA), bromocriptine, and pure beta-adrenergic agents.

Several investigators[28,29] demonstrated that prostaglandins can induce contractions of the human detrusor muscle. But to what degree do prostaglandins contribute to the development of involuntary bladder contractions in DI? Prostaglandins may sensitize (i.e., lower the threshold) the afferent component so that the involuntary contractions occur at smaller bladder volumes. Thus, a role for PGA might be envisaged, at least theoretically, in the management of DI. However, clinical studies have not borne out this role for PGAs.

Indomethacin (Indocin) and flurbiprofen (Ansaid) are the two PGAs which were hoped to mitigate or abolish involuntary bladder contractions. Cardozo and coworkers[30] conducted a double-blind, controlled study on 30 patients using flurbiprofen, currently approved in the United States as an antiarthritis medication, in dosages of 50 mg three times a day. Although this agent was shown to afford significant symptomatic relief (i.e., decreased urgency, diurnal/nocturnal frequency, and urge incontinence), it did not abolish abnormal bladder activity. Since 43% of the participants showed an assortment of side effects, predominantly gastrointestinal, the authors concluded that increasing the dosage in the hope of eliminating bladder activity would not be feasible.

Cardozo and Stanton[31] also evaluated indomethacin, another PGA, in oral doses of 50 to 200 mg daily. It would be difficult to draw objective conclusions from the results of this study because the sample size was small (32 completed the study) and urodynamic assessments were not conducted. Nonetheless, indomethacin did afford subjective improvement in diurnal/nocturnal frequency. No improvements were noted in urgency or urge-related incontinence. These observations, in conjunction with the high incidence of side effects, have not helped to popularize indomethacin in the treatment of the unstable bladder.

CALCIUM ANTAGONISTS

In order to initiate and sustain contractile activity, smooth muscle cells require an influx of calcium ions from the extracellular environment and/or release of these ions from intracellular depots. If direct interference can be established to inhibit calcium ion influx, passive relaxation of the smooth muscle occurs.

The calcium antagonists (CA), which are commonly used in North America, are geared principally toward the management of cardiovascular disease. For instance, nifedipine (Procardia) is used widely for angina because it produces dilatation of the coronary as well as systemic arteries, thereby improving coronary blood flow and decreasing cardiac afterload, respectively. Diltiazem (Cardizem) has similar mechanisms of action and is applied in much the same way as nifedipine, while verapamil is more useful in the control of paroxysmal supraventricular tachycardias.

Although calcium-channel blockers tend to be nonspecific with regard to site of action (i.e., organ), particular CAs exhibit greater affinity for, and affect the function of, certain structures. Nifedipine, as an example, has demonstrated a relatively high affinity for the smooth muscle of the bladder and thus has promise in the management of bladder overactivity.[32]

Urodynamically, nifedipine is shown to effect a decrease in the amplitude and frequency of involuntary bladder contractions, as well as improving the patient's bladder capacity.[32] Dosage is 10 mg twice daily to a maximum of 120 mg/day to obtain therapeutic efficacy.

Nifedipine's major drawback is its predominant selectivity for the cardiovascular system. Thus, while it has shown positive effects on the bladder, unwanted and potentially dangerous cardiovascular reactions should be anticipated. These include transient facial flushing, hypotension, tachycardia, cardiac palpitations, dysrhythmias, and/or heart block. Of less concern are side effects such as headache, dizziness, abdominal discomfort, and weakness.

Since the early 1980s increasing interest has been focused on another CA. Terodiline (Micturin) has been studied extensively and approved for usage in Europe, the Middle East, and Far East for almost a decade.[33,34,35] More recently very positive results were reported by Tapp and colleagues[36] in a prospective, double-blind, multicenter, placebo-controlled study. Of the patients who received terodiline, 62% reported subjective improvement in terms of decreased total diurnal frequency and number of incontinent episodes. Furthermore, bladder capacity and bladder volume at first urge were increased. Interestingly, 42% of the placebo controls reported significant improvement as well. Terodiline is a secondary amine that has dual mechanisms of action. The calcium-blocking and anticholinergic properties function synergistically, with the former predominating. In addition, a mild anesthetic effect is present.[37] A relatively long plasma half-life of approximately 60 hours permits a less frequent dosing schedule, which translates into greater convenience for the patient and thus enhances compliance. Usual doses are 25 mg twice daily; however, 12.5 mg is recommended for debilitated, elderly (over age 75) and very young (less than age 16) patients.

Side effects are mostly anticholinergic with dry mouth, tremor, blurred vision, and tachycardia reported most frequently. Only 6.5% of the patients enrolled in the study found it necessary to discontinue terodiline because of side effects.

Terodiline is absorbed rapidly and completely in the intestine due to its lipophilic nature. As opposed to oxybutynin and propantheline, bioavailability is exceptionally high (90%).[38] This agent is metabolized in the liver and excreted by the kidneys.

Major contraindications include those for anticholinergic medications (Box 11C1-3), especially glaucoma and a host of gastrointestinal conditions with decreased motility, since terodiline may exacerbate the motility problem. In areas where elevated ambient temperatures are commonplace, terodiline ought to be administered cautiously, since this agent suppresses sweating. This may cause fever or heat prostration.

Currently terodiline is undergoing a multicenter, prospective, double-blind, placebo-controlled study in North America. It is hoped that this agent will attain Federal Drug Administration approval in the near future, because it offers an attractive alternative in the

Table 11C1-1
Pharmacologic Agents for Detrusor Instability

Class	Agent	MOA	Dosage/Frequency	Side Effects
Anticholinergic	Propantheline	Competitive inhibition of acetylcholine	15–60 mg BID-TID	Anticholinergic: ++ blurred vision dry mouth mydriasis tachycardia constipation
Musculotropic	Oxybutynin Dicyclomine Flavoxate	Direct relaxation of bladder smooth muscle cells	2.5–5 mg BID-QID 10–40 mg BID-QID 100–200 mg BID-QID	Anticholinergic +++ Anticholinergic ++ Anticholinergic +
Tricyclic depressants	Imipramine	Beta-adrenergic stimulation	25–75 mg BID	Anticholinergic +
Calcium antagonists	Nifedipine	Competitive inhibition of Ca^{+2} ion influx	10–120 mg BID	Facial flushing, headache, dizziness, hypotension, tachycardia, palpitations, dysrhythmias, heart block
	Terodiline		12.5–25 mg BID	Anticholinergic +

MOA = principal mechanism of action; BID = twice daily; TID = three times daily; QID = four times daily; + = relative severity.

pharmacologic management of DI. It offers excellent absorption and bioavailability, relatively fewer side effects and, above all, high selectivity for the detrusor muscle and resultant good therapeutic efficacy. Table 11C1-1 summarizes the pharmacologic agents used in the management of detrusor instability.

ADRENERGIC STIMULANTS

Adrenergic agonists can provide improvement in patients with incontinence associated with bladder instability by stimulating the beta receptors in the bladder and/or the alpha receptors found in the smooth muscle component of the urethra. As mentioned previously, beta stimulation results in bladder quiescence whereas alpha stimulation can bring about an increase in intraurethral pressure.

Ephedrine

Ephedrine sulfate directly stimulates alpha and beta receptors and causes a peripheral release of endogenous adrenergic substances.[39] Usual adult dosages are 25 to 50 mg four times daily. Side effects include anxiety, nervousness, tachycardia, palpitations, dry mouth, constipation, and increase in intraocular pressure and psychologic dependence.[40]

The plethora of drugs currently utilized and, even more, once-studied, underscores the lack of a universally efficacious agent that can render the bladder quiescent during the filling phase and be relatively free of untoward side effects, allowing for patient acceptance. The search continues for just such an agent.

GENUINE STRESS INCONTINENCE

The most prevalent form of urinary incontinence in the female patient is genuine stress incontinence (GSI). This condition is characterized by a demonstrable loss of urine concurrent with an abrupt rise in intraabdominal pressure as might be precipitated by coughing, sneezing, lifting, straining, or stooping. During such activities the urethral sphincteric mechanism cannot resist the sudden rise in intravesical pressure, which is caused by transvesical transmission of the increased intraabdominal pressure. In such instances the intraurethral pressure is exceeded by the intravesical pressure, thereby creating a urethral closure pressure of zero or less, which results in loss of urine. It is important to recognize that there is no detrusor contraction present when pressure equalization and urine loss occur.

Several factors contribute to the maintenance of a positive urethral closure pressure and urinary continence. Within the urethra three major contributors, of approximately equal significance, are: (1) the sealing capacity of the urethral mucosa, (2) the extensive vascular plexus of the urethral wall, and (3) the muscular component of the urethral sphincteric mechanism. This muscular component is divided into an internal smooth muscle complex and an external striated sphincter network. With the exception of the external periurethral sphincter, all of the aforementioned components are estrogen dependent. A number of investigative teams demonstrated the presence of high-affinity estrogen receptors primarily within the urethra, and in the bladder base to a lesser degree. Batra, Iosif, and their co-workers[41,42] were able to corroborate what many clinicians had observed previously: the status (i.e., the degree of suppleness or atrophy) of the urethral lining parallels that of the vaginal mucosa.

The development of GSI can be attributed to three main factors: (1) derangement of pelvic floor anatomy, (2) peripheral neuropathy, and (3) alterations of the urethra associated with the aging process.

Despite the contribution of these three causative factors, surgery continues to be the most widely accepted and used approach to the management of GSI. The primary objective of surgery is to reestablish the pelvic anatomy in order to enhance transmission of increases in intraabdominal pressure to the proximal urethra and bladder base.[43]

In a select subset of patients in whom anti-incontinence surgery is inadvisable, not feasible, or unacceptable, nonsurgical measures can be employed. Box

---

Box 11C1-4
Nonsurgical Approaches to Management
of GSI

Pelvic floor exercises (Kegel)
Biofeedback
Functional electrical stimulation
Pharmacotherapy

11C1-4 contains a list of possible alternatives, including pharmacotherapy.

Pharmacologic intervention for GSI is directed toward the poorly functioning urethra. To bolster the steadily sagging intraurethral pressures seen in aging postmenopausal female patients,[44] improvement is necessary in the integrity of the urethral mucosa, submucosal vascular plexus, as well as stimulation of the urethral smooth muscle component. Theoretically, such improvements should be attainable with the administration of estrogen and/or an alpha-adrenergic stimulant (Table 11C1-2).

Estrogen Therapy

Teleologically the vagina and urethra share a common source—the urogenital sinus. Thus, it should come as no surprise that, as mentioned above, the state of the vaginal and urethral mucosa mirror each other. It was

---

Table 11C1-2
Pharmacologic Agents for Stress Incontinence

Class	Agent	MOA	Dosage/Frequency	Side Effects
Alpha-adrenergic agonists	Pseudoephedrine Ephedrine Phenylpropanolamine Ornade Entex-LA Imipramine	Urethral smooth muscle stimulation	15–30 mg TID 25–50 mg TID-QID 75 mg BID One capsule BID One tablet BID 25–50 mg TID	Headache Tachycardia Hypertension Palpitation Dry mouth Change mentation Cardiac conduction disturbances*
Transvaginal estrogen cream	Premarin Estrace Dienestrol Ogen	↑ Urethral mucosa ↑ Submucosal vasculature ↑ Urethral blood flow ↑ Connective tissue bulk ?↑ Number/sensitivity of alpha-receptors	*Initial:* ⅓–½ appl. 3 × /wk *Maintenance:* ⅓–½ appl. 1–2 × /wk	Breast tenderness Weight gain Hypertension Cholelithiasis Endometrial cancer

*Imipramine only; MOA = mechanism of action; BID = twice daily; TID = three times daily; QID = four times daily; ↑ = improvement/increased.

not until the late seventies that Bayard and coworkers[45] identified estrogen receptors in the female genital tract. Thereafter, a number of investigators discovered the presence of estrogen receptors in the lower urinary tract, as mentioned above.

Atrophy of the mucosa of the vagina and urethra are commonly seen, to varying degrees, in postmenopausal women,[46] especially in the absence of estrogen replacement. In spite of the generally accepted beneficial effects of systemic estrogen replacement with regard to minimizing the risks of cardiovascular disease and retardation of the osteoporotic process, it is our experience that oral estrogen replacement therapy (ERT) alone or in combination with a progestin (hormone replacement therapy, or HRT) is most often inadequate in achieving the localized vaginal/urethral tissue levels of estrogen necessary to exert an anabolic effect on the mucosa and submucosal components of these two structures. A host of investigators[47–49] found that exogenous ERT/HRT results in improvement of chronic irritative lower urinary tract symptoms; however, no studies[50,51] demonstrated consistent improvements in objective urodynamic parameters (i.e., urethral closure pressures, at rest or during stress).

Nonetheless, ERT may be of benefit to the patient with GSI. We prefer to use vaginal application of estrogen for the reasons outlined above. Dienestrol vaginal cream 0.01%, 1/3 to 1/2 applicator, is administered transvaginally. Initial management consists of 2 to 3 applications weekly. As the atrophic vaginal (and urethral) mucosa improves, the dosing frequency is changed to maintenance dosage once or twice weekly. In some postmenopausal patients, mild GSI may be completely cured in this manner. However, GSI of moderate severity or worse is less frequently responsive to ERT. Other transvaginal creams are available for patients who may prefer one product over another. These include Premarin vaginal cream (conjugated estrogen 0.625 mg/g), Ogen (estropipate 1.5 mg/g) or Estrace (estradiol 0.01%).

It must be remembered that estrogens delivered transvaginally are absorbed systemically. Although it is generally agreed that systemic delivery of estrogen, in oral, parenteral, or transcutaneous form, achieves predictable serum levels, transvaginal delivery affords less predictable levels.[52] Thus, the transvaginal route ought to be reserved solely for localized effect (vaginal/urethral) and should not be intended to substitute for the other forms of ERT. Furthermore, estrogen delivered transvaginally in a patient already on systemic ERT may precipitate excessively high serum levels with attendant side effects (Table 11C1-2).

Alpha-Adrenergic Agonists

As mentioned previously, alpha-adrenergic receptors are concentrated in the bladder base and urethra. Stimulation of these receptors by sympathomimetic agents results in increased tone of the urethral sphincteric mechanism.[40]

Phenylpropanolamine

Phenylpropanolamine hydrochloride (PPA) is a direct stimulant of alpha receptors, thus effecting contraction of the internal urethral sphincter.[53] This drug is available in oral form only and is contained in Ornade and Entex-LA (Table 11C1-2). Ornade spansules permit twice daily dosing and contain 75 mg of PPA combined with the antihistaminic chlorpheniramine. Contraindications to its usage include severe hypertension, coronary artery disease, GI, or urinary tract obstruction and concurrent use with a monoamine oxidase inhibitor. Entex-LA also contains 75 mg of PPA in conjunction with guaifenesin (400 mg). This agent is intended for upper or lower respiratory tract inflammation and congestion. The contraindications to use of Entex-LA are similar to those of Ornade.

It was reported that a regimen of a PPA-containing agent coupled with estrogen yields better results[54,55] than the use of either agent alone. Kinn and Lindskogg[54] found estrogen to increase the number of alpha adrenoreceptors two- to threefold, and this finding may substantiate the increased efficacy of combined PPA/ERT.

Imipramine

Imipramine-hydrochloride (Tofranil) has been mentioned before in the management of DI. Besides its beta-receptor stimulation, imipramine is an alpha-adrenergic agonist as well. Prolonged use of this agent may help patients with GSI by increasing intraurethral pressures.[53]

MIXED INCONTINENCE

Approximately 15% to 20% of patients with involuntary urinary loss have mixed incontinence (MI). This condition by definition contains components of both GSI and DI. The degree to which each component contributes to the patient's urinary incontinence varies. Nonetheless, in most instances, one factor predominates. After the clinical and urodynamic identification of the overriding component, it is this component that must be addressed initially. Karram and Bhatia[56] concluded that for patients with MI, where bladder instability is the more significant contributor, the unstable bladder should be controlled, in most cases medically, before embarking on surgical correction of the GSI. For instance, imipramine may be used alone for MI, or in combination with other medications. Evaluation is vital in these cases in order to have exact diagnoses and specific indications for drug therapy.

SUMMARY

As the longevity of the female population continues to increase, so too will the prevalence of urinary incontinence. Pharmacotherapy for vesical instability will continue to play a leading role in the management of this condition and, in all probability, newer agents will be accompanied by increasingly fewer side effects, making medical treatment more acceptable to the patient with bladder instability. The role of pharmacotherapy for GSI may be expanded as well, as a result of several factors: increased selectivity and efficacy of new agents, overwhelming patient numbers requiring prioritization of candidates for surgery, and reluctance of medical insurance companies to provide reimbursement for anti-incontinence surgery as first-line treatment for GSI.

REFERENCES

1. Diokno AC, Brock BM, Brown MB, Herzog AR. Prevalence of urinary incontinence and other urologic symptoms in the noninstitutionalized elderly. *J Urol.* 1986;136:1022.
2. Yarnell JWG, Voyle GJ, Richards CJ, Stephenson TP. The prevalence and severity of urinary incontinence in women. *J Epidemiol Comm Health.* 1981;35:71.
3. Thiede, HA. The prevalence of urogynecologic disorders. *Obstet Gynecol Clin North Am.* 1989;16:709.
4. Abrams P, Blaivas JG, Stanton SL, et al. The standardization of terminology of lower urinary tract function. *Scand J Urol Nephrol.* 1988;114(suppl):5.
5. Benson JT. Neurophysiologic control of lower urinary tract. *Obstet Gynecol Clin North Am.* 1989;16:853.
6. Awad SA, Bryniak S, Downie JW, Bruce A. The treatment of the uninhibited bladder with dicyclomine. *J Urol.* 1977;117:161.
7. Bent AE. Etiology and management of detrusor instability and mixed incontinence. *Obstet Gynecol Clin North Am.* 1989;16:853.
8. Fantl JA, Hurt WG, Dunn LJ. Detrusor instability syndrome: the use of bladder retraining drills with and without anticholinergics. *Am J Obstet Gynecol.* 1981;140:885.
9. Finkbeiner AE, Bissada NK. Drug therapy for lower urinary tract dysfunction. *Urol Clin North Am.* 1980;7:3.
10. Thompson IM, Lavretz R. Oxybutynin in bladder spasm, neurogenic bladder, and enuresis. *Urology.* 1976;8:452.
11. Wein AJ. Pharmacology of the bladder and urethra. In: Stanton SL, Tanagho EA, eds. *Surgery of Female Incontinence.* New York: Springer; 1980:185.
12. Ritch AES, George CF, Castleden CM, Hall MRP. A second look

13. Wein, AJ. Pharmacologic treatment of lower urinary tract dysfunction in the female patient. *Urol Clin North Am.* 1985;12:259.
14. Finkbeiner A, Welch L, Bissada N. Uropharmacology: IX. Direct-acting smooth muscle stimulants and depressants. *Urology.* 1978; 12:231.
15. Diokno AC, Lapides J. Oxybutynin: a new drug with analgesic and anticholinergic properties. *J Urol.* 1972;108:307.
16. Moisey C, Stephenson T, Brendler C. The urodynamic and subjective results of treatment of detrusor instability with oxybutynin chloride. *Br J Urol.* 1980;52:472.
17. Cardozo LD, Cooper D, Versi E. Oxybutynin chloride in the management of idiopathic detrusor instability. *Neurourol and Urodyn.* 1987;6:256.
18. Bradley D, Cazort R. Relief of bladder spasm by flavoxate: a comparative study. *J Clin Pharmacol.* 1970;10:65.
19. Mundy AR. The unstable bladder. *Urol Clin North Am.* 1985;12: 317.
20. Fischer C, Diokno A, Lapides J. The anticholinergic effects of dicyclomine hydrochloride in uninhibited neurogenic bladder dysfunction. *J Urol.* 1978;120:328.
21. Gilman AG, Goodman LS, Rall TW, et al. *The Pharmacologic Basis of Therapeutics.* 7th ed. New York: MacMillan Publishing Co; 1985.
22. Stanton SL. A comparison of emepronium bromine and flavoxate hydrochloride in the treatment of urinary incontinence. *Urology.* 1973;110:529.
23. Scalambrino S, Milani R, Maggioni A, et al. High dose flavoxate versus oxybutynin in the treatment of urge syndrome. *Urogynecol J.* 1988;1:36.
24. Milner G, Hills N. A double-blind assessment of antidepressants in the treatment of 212 enuretic patients. *Med J Aust.* 1978;1:943.
25. Wein AJ. Drug therapy for detrusor hyperactivity; where are we? *Neurourol and Urodyn.* 1985;4:337.
26. Benson G, Sarshik S, Raezer D, Wein A. Comparative effects and mechanisms of action of atropine, propantheline, flavoxate, and imipramine on bladder muscle contractility. *Urol.* 1977;9:31.
27. Castleden CM, George CF, Renwick AG, Asher MJ. Imipramine—a possible alternative to current therapy for urinary incontinence in the elderly. *J Urol.* 1981;125:318.
28. Andersson KE, Forman A. Effects of prostaglandins on the smooth muscle of the urinary tract. *Acta Pharmacol Toxicol.* 1978;43(suppl II):90.
29. Abrams PH, Fenely RCL. The action of prostaglandins on the smooth muscle of the human urinary tract, in vitro. *Br J Urol.* 1976;48:631.
30. Cardozo L, Stanton S, Robinson H, Hole D. Evaluation of flurbiprofen in detrusor instability. *Br Med J.* 1980;280:281.
31. Cardozo L, Stanton S. A comparison between bromocriptine and indomethacin in the treatment of detrusor instability. *J Urol.* 1979;123:399.
32. Rud T, Andersson KE, Ulmsten U. Effects of nifedipine in women with unstable bladders. *Urol Int.* 1979;34:421.
33. Rasmussen WF. Evaluation of long-term safety and clinical benefit of terodiline in women with urgency/urge incontinence. A multicenter study. *Scand J Urol Nephrol.* 1989;87(suppl):35.
34. Rud T, Andersson K, Boye N, Ulmsten U. Terodiline inhibition of human bladder contractions: effects in vitro and in women with unstable bladder. *Acta Pharmacol Toxicol.* 1980;46:39.
35. Ulmsten U, Ekman G, Andersson KE. The effect of terodiline treatment in women with motor urge incontinence: results from a double-blind study and long-term treatment. *Am J Obstet Gynecol.* 1985;153:619.
36. Tapp A, Fall M, Norgaard J, et al. A dose-titrated, multicenter study of terodiline in the treatment of detrusor instability. *Neurourol and Urodyn.* 1987;6:254.
37. Gahlin K, Strindlund U. Local anesthetic action of terodiline in conscious guinea pigs. 1982; Technical Report No. 8298110.

38. Andersson KE. Clinical pharmacology of terodiline. *Scand J Urol Nephrol*. 1984;87(suppl);13.

39. Weiner N. Norepinephrine, epinephrine and the sympathomimetic amines. In: Gilman AG, Goodman LS, Gilman A, eds. *The Pharmacological Basis of Therapeutics*. 6th ed. New York: MacMillan Publishing Co; 1980.

40. Beck RP. Neuropharmacology of the lower urinary tract in women. *Obstet Gynecol Clin North Am*. 1989;16:4.

41. Iosif CS, Batra S, Ek A, Astedt B. Estrogen receptors in the human female lower urinary tract. *Am J Obstet Gynecol*. 1981;141:817.

42. Batra SC, Iosif CS. Female urethra: a target for estrogen action. *J Urol*. 1983;129:418.

43. Cholhan HJ, Ostergard DR. Vaginal vs abdominal surgery for genuine stress incontinence. *Obstet/Gynecol Report*. 1990;2:323.

44. Asmussen M. Static and dynamic pressures of the lower urinary tract as measured by simultaneous urethral cystometry. In: Ostergard DR, ed. *Gynecologic Urology and Urodynamics*. 2nd ed. Baltimore: Williams & Wilkins; 1985:133.

45. Bayard F, Damilano S, Robel P, Baulieu EE. Cytoplasmic and nuclear estradiol and progesterone receptors in human endometrium. *J Clin Endocrinol Metab*. 1978;46:635.

46. Smith P. Age changes in the female urethra. *Br J Urol*. 1972;44:667.

47. Salmon UJ, Walter RI, Geist SH. The use of estrogens in the treatment of dysuria and incontinence in postmenopausal women. *Am J Obstet Gynecol*. 1941;42:845.

48. Furuhjelm M, Karlgren E, Carstrom K. Intravaginal administration of conjugated estrogens in premenopausal and postmenopausal women. *Int J Gynecol Obstet*. 1980;17:335.

49. Hilton P, Stanton S. The use of intravaginal estrogen cream in genuine stress incontinence. *Br J Obstet Gynaecol*. 1983;90:940.

50. Rud T. The effects of estrogens and gestagens on the urethral pressure profile in urinary continent and stress incontinent women. *Acta Obstet Gynecol Scand*. 1980;59:265.

51. Fantl JA, Wyman JF, Anderson RL, et al. Postmenopausal urinary incontinence: comparison between nonestrogen-supplemented and estrogen-supplemented women. *Obstet Gynecol*. 1988;71:823.

52. Rigg LA, Hermann H, Yen SSC. Absorption of estrogens from vaginal creams. *N Eng J Med*. 1978;298:195.

53. Ostergard DR. Effects of drugs on lower urinary tract. In: Ostergard DR, ed. *Gynecologic Urology and Urodynamics*. 2nd ed. Baltimore: Williams & Wilkins, 1985:347.

54. Kinn AC, Lindskaag M. Estrogens and phenylpropanolamine in combination for stress urinary incontinence in postmenopausal women. *Urology*. 1988;23:273.

55. Beisland HO, Fossberg E, Moer A, Sander S. Urethral sphincteric insufficiency in postmenopausal females: treatment with phenylpropanolamine and estriol separately and in combination. *Urol Int*. 1984;39:211.

56. Karram MM, Bhatia N. Management of coexistent stress and urge urinary incontinence. *Obstet Gynecol*. 1989;73:4.

CHAPTER 11

Urinary Incontinence

11C Nonsurgical Therapies

11C2 Biofeedback Therapy

Kathryn L. Burgio

INTRODUCTION

Biofeedback is a training technique soundly based on the principles of human behavior and learning and supported by considerable evidence derived from years of experimental investigation. The technique aims to reverse urinary incontinence by teaching patients to alter physiologic responses of the detrusor and pelvic floor muscles that mediate urine loss. Using biofeedback, patients can learn new skills for maintaining continence or relearn previous control of urination.

In 1988 the National Institutes of Health held a Consensus Conference on Urinary Incontinence in Adults. Regarding the staging of treatment, the consensus panel concluded that: "As a general rule, the least invasive or dangerous procedure should be tried first," and that "for many forms of incontinence, behavioral techniques meet this criterion." Biofeedback is not a treatment in itself. It is a training technique that, appropriately used, is one component in a behavioral training program. It facilitates acquisition of desired responses, such as pelvic floor muscle contraction and other continence skills. Biofeedback is one among many behavioral techniques that have been shown to be effective, practical, efficient, and acceptable to patients.

The purpose of this chapter is to familiarize the reader with various methods of biofeedback training and their practical implementation in office practice. Techniques of bladder biofeedback, pelvic floor muscle biofeedback, and combined bladder-sphincter biofeed-back are reviewed as well as procedures to help patients practice their skills at home.

THE PROCESS OF BIOFEEDBACK

Using biofeedback, physiologic change is possible by means of operant conditioning in which learning occurs as a result of feedback or the knowledge of the consequences of one's behavior. For example, speech is acquired by hearing the sounds that are uttered. Learning to write is made possible by visualizing one's attempts to form letters. In biofeedback a physiologic response is identified and measured. The measured response is amplified, processed, and immediately a form of the response is fed back to the subject by means of visual display, auditory signal, or other sensory modality. In this way biofeedback makes it possible to control responses of which, ordinarily, we may have little or no knowledge or awareness, and consequently little ability to control. It can be used to modify responses that usually are easily regulated, but for which control has been lost,[1] as well as responses that were once thought to be involuntary, such as heart rate or blood pressure. It is not necessary to make a major distinction between voluntary and involuntary responses.

For biofeedback to be useful, four conditions must be met. First, there must be a readily detectable and measurable response, such as bladder pressure or pelvic floor muscle activity. Second, there must be variability in that response, a detectable change as opposed to total paralysis. Third, there must be a perceptible cue such as the sensation of urgency that indicates to the patient when control should be performed. Fourth, because biofeedback is based on learning, it requires the active involvement of a motivated patient.

Central to understanding biofeedback is the acceptance of physiologic responses as behavior. When a behavioral analysis is made of bladder and sphincter physiology, incontinence can be characterized as a behavioral deficit. Incontinence occurs when an individual (1) fails to inhibit reflex bladder contractions voluntarily, or (2) fails to adequately contract the striated muscles of the pelvic floor, which obstruct bladder emptying. Both bladder inhibition and sphincter contraction are acquired physiologic responses that preserve continence.

The goals of the training are different depending on whether the patient has stress incontinence or urge incontinence. For stress incontinence, the primary goal of training is to enable the patient to contract the periurethral muscles selectively while inhibiting contraction of abdominal muscles. For urge incontinence, the goals are to train the patients to inhibit detrusor contraction voluntarily and to contract periurethral muscles selectively in order to prevent urine loss until detrusor inhibition can be achieved.

Patients acquire these self-control skills in outpatient training sessions. Through repeated practice and implementation of skills, they improve muscle strength and control over responses that affect continence.

Bladder Biofeedback

The earliest reported use of a biofeedback procedure for urge incontinence was described in 1948 by Wilson.[2] He reported that 10 of 23 elderly patients with precipitancy or incontinence were improved or completely continent following a diagnostic cystometrogram. During cystometrograms, bladder pressure readings were available to his patients and may have provided a mechanism for feedback that allowed them to acquire better control. Wilson referred to his method as inhibitory re-educative training, but he clearly described a form of intervention that would now be termed biofeedback.

Willington[3] has also described a method of biofeedback in which a patient's catheter is attached to a vertical tube and the fluid level is visible to the patient. The fluid level remains low as long as the bladder remains relaxed, but rises noticeably when bladder contractions occur.

Cardozo and colleagues[4,5] reported on a bladder

pressure biofeedback procedure for treating urge incontinence associated with detrusor instability. This method provides both auditory and visual feedback of bladder pressure during repeated bladder filling. Auditory feedback was a tone emitted through a loudspeaker that increased in pitch as bladder pressure rose, and decreased in pitch as bladder pressure fell. Visual feedback was provided by means of a mirror that reflected movement of the pens recording bladder pressure. Using the feedback, patients were asked to control bladder pressure by whatever means was helpful during bladder filling. Twenty-seven women ages 18 to 64 with bladder instability were treated in 4 to 8 1-hour sessions at weekly intervals. Of those, 81% were subjectively improved, including 41% who were judged to be cured. Five-year follow-up conducted with eleven subjects indicated that four (36%) had maintained subjective improvement.

Burgio and colleagues[6] used biofeedback in a behavioral training program for older men and women with urge incontinence. During training sessions, patients observed bladder pressure during retrograde filling and practiced keeping bladder pressure low. One patient's progress across three trials of bladder inhibition is depicted in Fig. 11C2-1. Note that on trial 1, infusion of 30 ml sterile water was followed immediately by detrusor contraction and bladder emptying. On trial 2, this

Fig. 11C2-1 Learned inhibition of detrusor contraction. Arrows show artifacts produced by infusion of sterile water.

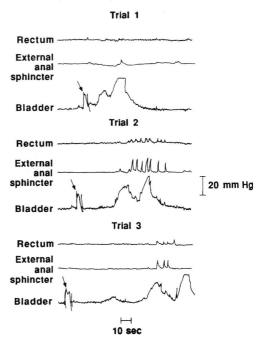

patient was able to inhibit for approximately 30 seconds before she experienced detrusor contraction, and on trial 3, a small rise in detrusor pressure was suppressed and she was able to postpone detrusor contraction for 60 seconds.

Pelvic Floor Muscle Biofeedback

Several approaches have been taken to measure pelvic floor muscle activity to provide biofeedback.

Vaginal Manometry

As early as the 1940s, Arnold H. Kegel, a gynecologist, asserted that stress incontinence in women was a result of a lack of awareness of function and coordination of pelvic floor muscles.[7] He developed and used the perineometer, an instrument now regarded as a biofeedback device. It consisted of an intravaginal balloon attached to an external pressure gauge which registered the pressure exerted on the balloon by circumvaginal muscles, specifically the pubococcygeal, or PC muscle. The gauge could be held by the patient, providing visual feedback of the strength of pelvic floor muscle contractions during daily exercises. In an early report of biofeedback for stress incontinence, Kegel reported a 90% improvement rate among 455 women who were trained with this method.[8]

Vaginal Electromyography

Following vaginal manometry, another methodology emerged in which vaginal electromyography (EMG) is recorded instead of pressure. Surface electrodes may be placed inside the vaginal introitus, but it has become more popular to use a vaginal probe with electrodes embedded. Feedback is provided by means of an auditory signal or visual display such as lights or any number of computerized graphic displays.

The vaginal probe has the advantage that it is easy to insert and remove, it is comfortable, and most patients are able to place it themselves. Thus, portable models or "home trainers" offer the possibility of guided daily practice at home. A disadvantage of the home trainer method is that patients who are dependent on the biofeedback to be assured of correct practice may lose interest in the instrument as the novelty wears off and before they have gained the ability to exercise independently. Nevertheless, there are anecdoctal reports that the instrument enhances the effectiveness of training.

The usefulness of vaginal EMG biofeedback was tested as an integral part of behavioral training programs for urinary incontinence. Henderson and Taylor[9] conducted a small study of pelvic floor muscle strengthening using vaginal EMG biofeedback in nine women ages 55 years or older and five women under the age of 55 who were experiencing simple stress incontinence. All participants were self-selected, noninstitutionalized, ambulatory, and without neurogenic bladder problems. Subjects were trained using biofeedback in eight weekly clinic visits and instructed in a detailed program of daily pelvic muscle exercise. All women reported improvement in the frequency or amount of incontinence on a self-assessment of continence questionnaire. Eighty percent of the younger group and 67% of the older group reported no incontinence in the final week of the program.

Baigis-Smith and colleagues[10] studied a larger series of 54 subjects (45 women and 9 men) ages 60 to 86 years (mean = 70 years). All were cognitively intact volunteers with stress, urge, or mixed urinary incontinence. An EMG perineometer was used to provide both visual and auditory biofeedback of pelvic floor muscle activity (vaginal or anal). Biofeedback was conducted at 2-week intervals. Between training sessions, subjects were instructed in a daily exercise program including 50 pelvic floor muscle exercises, relaxation techniques, and habit training. As a group, patients reduced the frequency of incontinence significantly from a mean 17.4 accidents per week to 4.2 at the end of treatment, and 3.3 at 1-month follow-up. The mean reduction was 78%; 50% of subjects were at least 90% improved.

Burns and colleagues[11] conducted a randomized clinical trial of vaginal EMG biofeedback in treatment of urinary incontinence. As part of this trial 40 elderly women (ages 55 or over) with stress or mixed urinary incontinence were assigned to eight weeks of biofeedback assisted pelvic floor muscle training. A no treatment control group was comprised of 38 subjects. Biofeedback combined with daily practice resulted in a mean 61% reduction in frequency of urine losses, significantly better than the mean 9% increase in incontinence demonstrated by the control group.

A drawback of vaginal manometry or electromyography is the distinct tendency among most incontinent women to contract incorrect or dyssynergistic muscles simultaneously with vaginal muscles. It is most common to observe tensing of the thighs, buttocks, or rectus abdominis muscles during pelvic floor muscle training. In particular, involvement of abdominal muscles appears to accompany most attempts at maximal pelvic floor muscle contraction. Tensing of abdominal muscles is counterproductive during attempts to prevent incontinence because it increases bladder pressure and consequently contributes to the forces that push urine out of the bladder.

In order to minimize inappropriate tensing it is helpful to train patients to keep these muscles relaxed when trying to prevent urine loss. Some patients can accomplish this by means of simple instruction, deep breathing and relaxation, or by feedback from placing a hand on the abdomen. However, others need some form of abdominal muscle biofeedback in order to acquire the appropriate selective contraction. Users of the vaginal probe have in some cases used a rectal balloon (measuring intraabdominal pressure) or surface electrodes on the abdomen (measuring rectus abdominis EMG) for this purpose.

Anal Sphincter Biofeedback

The external anal sphincter and the external urinary sphincter have similar innervation via branches of the pudendal nerve.[12,13] The activity of the anal sphincter is measured easily and provides a good index of urethral sphincter activity. Although there are conflicts in the literature about the issue of correspondence between the anal and urinary sphincters, several studies indicate that the sphincters act in concert,[14–18] and data indicate that training and controlling the anal sphincter results in urinary sphincter activity that corresponds in magnitude.[19]

Anal sphincter activity can be measured by means of surface electrodes placed in the perianal area or embedded in a rectal probe. Investigators at the National Institute on Aging have used the instrument illustrated in Fig. 11C2-2, developed originally by a gastroenterologist for manometric assessment of anorectal re-

sponses and used subsequently to provide biofeedback in the treatment of fecal incontinence.[20,21]

The anorectal assembly consists of a rectal tube with three small balloons attached which, once inserted, are inflated with air. One balloon positioned inside the rectum measures intraabdominal pressure. Measurement of intraabdominal pressure is included because of the counterproductive tendency displayed by many patients to tense abdominal muscles together with the sphincter. Another balloon positioned at the anal opening measures activity of the external anal sphincter, and a third balloon positioned at the internal anal sphincter stabilizes the recording apparatus, but provides no data when used for treatment of urinary incontinence.

Combined Bladder-Sphincter Biofeedback

Another approach to biofeedback for urinary incontinence combines bladder pressure and pelvic floor muscle biofeedback in a procedure that provides simultaneous visual feedback of bladder, external anal sphincter, and intraabdominal pressures[6] (Fig. 11C2-2). Using three-channel biofeedback, patients are taught to contract and relax pelvic floor muscles selectively without increasing bladder pressure or intraabdominal pressure.

The value of combined biofeedback can be seen in Fig. 11C2-3. Fig. 11C2-3A illustrates the response of a typical patient to instructions to contract pelvic floor muscles as if to hold back urine. Noteworthy is the small increase in sphincter pressure accompanied by maladaptive increases in intraabdominal pressure, which is transmitted to the bladder and reflected in increased bladder pressures. Patients can learn abdomi-

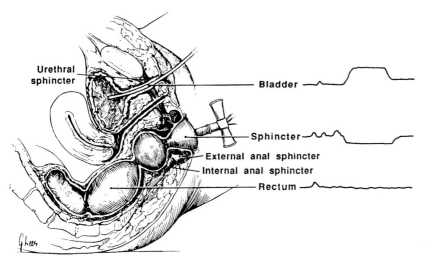

Fig. 11C2-2 Diagram of female pelvic anatomy showing anorectal assembly and catheter used for combined bladder-sphincter biofeedback.

Urethral sphincter

Bladder

Sphincter

External anal sphincter
Internal anal sphincter
Rectum

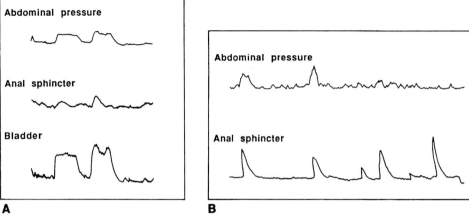

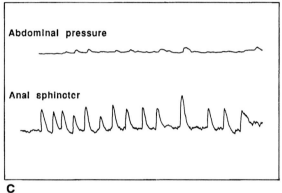

Fig. 11C2-3   A, Incorrect contraction of abdominal muscles during attempts at pelvic floor muscle contraction. **B,** Training selective contraction of pelvic floor muscles. **C,** Correct contraction of external anal sphincter coupled with abdominal relaxation.

nal relaxation by viewing either bladder pressure or intraabdominal pressure during attempts to contract the pelvic floor muscles selectively. Fig. 11C2-3*B* shows the continued process of training in which early attempts are accompanied by increased intraabdominal pressure, and in later attempts this pressure is eliminated. Eventually, with repeated practice most patients learn to minimize abdominal pressure, as depicted in Fig. 11C2-3C.

Once selective contraction is acquired, patients can learn techniques for sustaining pelvic floor muscle contraction. It is also useful to have them practice using their muscles to prevent urine loss under circumstances that are known to be associated with incontinence. For example, patients with stress incontinence induced by coughing may practice using active pelvic floor muscle contractions during voluntary coughing in the biofeedback session. They can observe the sharp increase in abdominal or bladder pressure that results from coughing and are often impressed with such a demonstration

that helps them understand the mechanism of their incontinence. To counteract these sudden increases in pressure, they can learn to contract their muscles just prior to and during increased abdominal pressure.

These procedures combined with a program of daily home practice were tested in a clinical series of 19 elderly patients with stress incontinence who were nondemented, ambulatory, and living independently in the community. An average of 3.3 training sessions resulted in a mean 82% reduction in the frequency of stress incontinence, with a 55% improvement being the poorest response and 7 patients achieving greater than 90% improvement.[6]

Combined biofeedback is also valuable in treatment of urge incontinence. In addition to learning voluntary inhibition of detrusor contraction by feedback of bladder pressure, patients can learn active, maximal contraction of pelvic floor muscles. This has two results: it can help inhibit detrusor contraction or it can occlude the urethra, preventing urine loss during uninhibited detrusor contraction.

As demonstrated in Fig. 11C2-4, detrusor contraction is usually accompanied by a reflex relaxation of pelvic floor muscles, allowing the urethra to open and urine to flow out. Observing a decline in sphincter pressure and a rise in bladder pressure, patients can be trained to respond with a strong sphincter contraction. This can help to inhibit detrusor contraction and maintain higher sphincter pressure, as depicted in Fig. 11C2-5.

Patients can also be taught to emit this contraction in response to perceived urgency even before the observation of increased bladder pressure. Bladder catheterization and filling is an important component in training because it allows teaching of the appropriate response under the circumstances that a patient will encounter after leaving the office. Practice in the clinic under simulated conditions should increase the patient's ability to

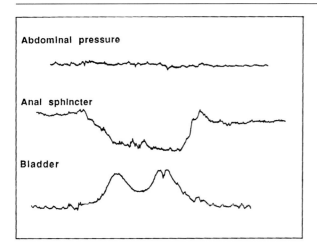

Fig. 11C2-4   Detrusor contraction accompanied by reflex sphincter relaxation.

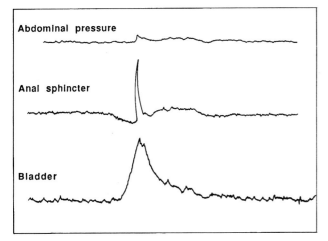

Fig. 11C2-5   Sphincter contraction accompanied by detrusor inhibition.

implement her newly acquired skills the next time she senses urgency.

These methods, combined with a program of home practice (described below) were tested in a group of 18 nondemented elderly outpatients with urge incontinence. Patients with detrusor instability reduced incontinence 39% to 100% with a mean 85% reduction in the frequency of accidents following an average of four training sessions. Those with symptoms of urge incontinence in the absence of documented detrusor instability ($n = 8$) achieved 84% to 100% improvement with a mean of 94%.[6]

The skills described here are acquired by some patients in a single session, whereas others require several treatments. Some women are able to identify pelvic floor muscles immediately, but many have had little awareness of these muscles or believe that they are not under voluntary control. For these reasons it is important to individualize treatment according to each woman's demonstrated abilities and progress.

Once the skills are demonstrated reliably, the issue of weaning from biofeedback can be addressed. The patient's ability to function without biofeedback can be assessed easily by recording one or more responses with eyes closed or feedback otherwise eliminated. Those whose performance is inadequate without biofeedback can be helped by alternating trials with and without feedback. During feedback trials patients are encouraged to pay attention to proprioceptive signals, and on trials without feedback to reproduce those sensations. This often brings the nonfeedback performance into greater correspondence to that with biofeedback assistance. Fig. 11C2-6 is an example of consecutive trials with and without biofeedback (eyes open and eyes closed). Note the diminished ability to sustain the sphincter contraction accompanied by small, but noticeable increases in intraabdominal and bladder pressure without biofeedback.

HOME PRACTICE

Once the ability to contract pelvic floor muscles selectively is established, it is crucial that patients are provided with a program of daily muscle exercise and active use of the muscles to prevent urine loss. Biofeedback assists in the acquisition of continence skills. For these skills to be mastered they must be practiced, and for them to be effective in preventing urine loss, they

Fig. 11C2-6   External anal sphincter contraction with and without visual biofeedback.

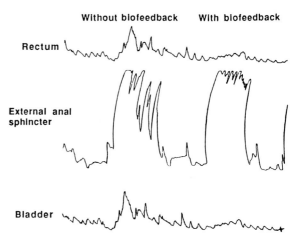

must be implemented at critical times. Between training sessions with repeated exercise and practice, patients aim to improve not only the strength of pelvic floor muscles, but voluntary control over responses that determine continence.

Although the optimal number of exercises has not been determined or agreed on, 45 to 50 exercises per day has yielded success in several studies. The exercises are usually divided among two or more sessions per day, for example 10 exercises at a time, 5 times per day, or 15 at a time, 3 times per day. Distribution of the exercises across the day helps to avoid problems with muscle fatigue and facilitates the frequent awareness and use of these muscles. It is important, in order to build muscle strength, that pelvic floor muscle contractions are sustained for up to 10 seconds with equal intervals of rest between contractions. Many patients are incapable at first of such a long duration of contraction, in which case it is possible to begin with the level of ability demonstrated by the patient (e.g., 3 seconds or 5 seconds) and increase duration gradually.

Patients may be taught to monitor abdominal tension by resting a hand on the abdomen. Interruption of the urinary stream can be recommended as a method to assist in identifying and improving control over other pelvic floor muscles at home.

In addition to strengthening pelvic floor muscles, patients with stress incontinence can be trained to contract the muscles voluntarily to prevent loss of urine during coughing, lifting, or whatever physical activities are known to produce incontinence. Although muscle exercise may increase resting tone, the goal of biofeedback and active contraction of pelvic floor muscles is to produce a transient rise in intraurethral pressure that is adequate to prevent urine loss with transient increases in intraabdominal pressures.

Patients with urge incontinence are also instructed to perform muscle strengthening exercises and to use their muscles actively to prevent urine loss during urgency or uninhibited detrusor contraction. Further, they are taught alternative strategies for managing urgency. Most patients with urge incontinence rush to the toilet in response to urgency, producing increased intraabdominal pressure, perhaps increasing the sensation of fullness, and potentially interfering with the ability to suppress detrusor contraction. Also, proximity to the toilet can function as a cue to urinate, triggering detrusor instability and making incontinence more likely the closer she gets to the toilet. Patients are instructed instead to stay away from the toilet and remain still and relaxed. They contract pelvic floor muscles several times to prevent urine loss and possibly inhibit bladder

contraction and practice suppressing the urgency. They wait until the urgency subsides before walking calmly to the bathroom.

These procedures for home practice are described in greater detail elsewhere in a step-by-step format appropriate for use by patients.[22]

THE ROLE OF BIOFEEDBACK

Over the years since Kegel introduced his perineometer and reported his results with stress incontinent women, pelvic floor muscle exercises have continued to be prescribed, but typically without the use of the perineometer. Instead, the patient is instructed to squeeze her vaginal muscles around the examiner's finger to learn the correct technique or simply given a pamphlet describing the exercises. Under these circumstances the exercises are seemingly less effective and their use, as well as enthusiasm with their benefits, have waned.

It is possible and, given our observations, quite likely that this has occurred because many women never locate the correct muscle group or they use wrong muscles together with pelvic floor muscles. Biofeedback assures that the exercises are being performed properly. Another possible explanation is that patients give up too soon without ongoing encouragement and feedback of their progress. Behavioral training usually results in gradual change and requires persistence and a long-term perspective on the part of both patient and therapist.

Certainly, many women have benefitted significantly from pelvic floor muscle exercises learned without biofeedback. What then is the role of biofeedback? Is it an essential component of behavioral training? Three studies have examined this issue in the treatment of stress incontinence.

Shepherd and coworkers[23] taught voluntary contraction of pelvic floor muscles to 22 stress incontinent women ages 23 to 67 years. One group of patients was trained using a vaginal perineometer similar to Kegel's; the control group was trained without the perineometer. Ninety-one percent of biofeedback patients, but only 55% of control patients were cured or improved. It should be noted, however, that the biofeedback group received a greater number of weekly treatments (mean = 5.7) than did the control group (mean = 3.5).

Burgio et al[24] treated 24 stress incontinent women ages 29 to 64 years for six weeks. One group received simultaneous bladder, sphincter, and abdominal pressure feedback using the methods described above; the control group received verbal feedback based on vaginal palpation. All patients in both groups received comprehensive training in 100 trials across four training sessions. Treatment sessions were separated by 2-week intervals during which patients practiced identically described programs of daily pelvic muscle exercises. Results were similar to those of Shepherd et al.[23] Ninety-two percent of the biofeedback patients and 55% of the control patients were cured or improved (at least 50% reduction of incontinence). The biofeedback group averaged 75.9% reduction in the frequency of incontinence, significantly greater than the mean 51% reduction shown by the verbal feedback group. The biofeedback group improved the strength and selective control of pelvic floor muscles; the control group did not. Together, these two studies indicate that although many patients can succeed without biofeedback, it improves the patient's ability to learn appropriate pelvic floor muscle contractions and increases the likelihood of successful outcome.

However, a larger randomized clinical trial conducted by investigators at the University of Buffalo reports a different conclusion.[11] This study compared the effects of pelvic floor muscle exercises with and without biofeedback to a no treatment control group. Subjects included 135 mentally competent, nondepressed women (55 years or older) who had documented stress (n = 123) or mixed (n = 12) urinary incontinence. Subjects in the two experimental groups were seen in eight weekly visits for evaluation and pelvic floor muscle training. The biofeedback group (n = 40) improved the strength of circumvaginal muscles significantly more than did the group trained without biofeedback (n = 43), as well as the control group (n = 38), and the latter two groups did not differ from each other. However, the subjects who underwent biofeedback did not differ significantly from those trained without biofeedback on the measure of urine loss reduction. The biofeedback group showed a mean 61% reduction in frequency of incontinence, similar to the 54% reduction demonstrated by the group trained without biofeedback. Both were significantly different from the control group (n = 38) which had a mean 9% increase in incontinence.

Because these studies yield contradicting results, this issue remains unresolved. Further investigation is needed to determine whether simply telling patients to exercise or teaching them to contract around the examiner's fingers will yield the greatest reductions in stress incontinence.

The role of biofeedback in treatment of urge incontinence is less clear. One small randomized study explored this issue in 20 elderly, nondemented subjects with well-established urge incontinence.[25] Eleven subjects trained without biofeedback responded as well to treatment as 9 subjects who were trained with bladder-sphincter biofeedback to contract pelvic floor muscles and inhibit detrusor contraction.

The number of subjects was small, however, and the groups were significantly different in severity of incontinence (i.e., frequency of accidents) at the beginning of the study. A larger study is needed to determine, with adequate power, whether biofeedback improves the response to behavioral training. Because the treatments for stress and urge incontinence focus on the training of different skills, it is possible that biofeedback is essential for one and not for the other.

PRACTICALITY OF BIOFEEDBACK

A salient concern about biofeedback-assisted behavioral training is its practicality for application by clinicians in office practice. Clinical experience indicates that such behavioral treatment can be administered with success by registered nurses, nurse practitioners, physical therapists, occupational therapists, psychologists, and social workers, indicating that there are many settings in which these treatments can be offered.

In a study initiated by investigators at the Johns Hopkins University School of Medicine, the bladder-sphincter biofeedback procedure was implemented by a nurse practitioner working with a geriatrician in an outpatient geriatric practice.[25] With approximately 72 hours of training, the nurse practitioner treated 27 elderly, nondemented ambulatory patients with well-established stress, urge, or mixed urinary incontinence. Every patient demonstrated improvement in continence status as measured by a bladder diary. After up to 6 training sessions, the group demonstrated an average 80% reduction in frequency of accidents.

Other methods of biofeedback, such as the perineometers, are no more difficult to implement and in many cases are easier. This approach has been used more widely and it is clear that it can be used effectively by nurses in office practice.

ADVANTAGES AND DISADVANTAGES

Biofeedback-assisted training, like other treatments for urinary incontinence, has distinct advantages and disadvantages. The data show clearly that training with biofeedback is an effective and practical method of reducing incontinence in most noninstitutionalized persons who comply with the procedures. Among its advantages are very low risk and absence of documented side effects. Whether or not patients are candidates for surgery or certain medications, behavioral treatment offers a safe alternative. This makes behavioral training particularly relevant to the elderly population.

One limitation of the approach may be the necessity of repeated instrumentation in many patients. It is our experience that most patients tolerate 3 or 4 treatment sessions without difficulty. In some patients, however, this repetition of training procedures may make the intervention unacceptable.

Another limitation is that training relies on the attention and active participation of a cooperative patient. Patients who are motivated and prefer to engage actively in their own health care are the most desirable candidates. Because the treatment is based on acquisition of new responses (i.e., learning) it requires a patient capable and ready to learn. This will limit its application in patients with cognitive impairment.

As a treatment based on a learning process through which new continence skills are acquired, change is not immediate. Reduction of incontinence is a gradual process that becomes evident as muscle control and other continence skills are practiced and applied. In selecting candidates for biofeedback, patients should be educated regarding these facts so that the nature of the intervention is understood. Those who can accept the intervention will have appropriate expectations about rate of improvement and will be prepared for active self-administration of the treatment procedures in daily home practice.

SUMMARY

In line with the recommendations of the 1988 Consensus Conference, biofeedback-assisted behavioral training is a rational and conservative treatment method appropriate for most motivated patients with stress or urge incontinence. Biofeedback facilitates skill acquisition and there is evidence that it improves the outcome of behavioral treatment for incontinence. The procedures described in this chapter are supported by research. They are practical and can be implemented with success by physicians or nurses in office practice.

REFERENCES

1. Blanchard EB, Epstein LH. *A Biofeedback Primer.* Reading, Mass: Addison-Wesley; 1978.
2. Wilson TS. Incontinence of urine in the aged. *Lancet.* 1948;ii:374–377.
3. Willington FL. Urinary incontinence: A practical approach. *Geriatrics.* 1980;35:41–48.
4. Cardozo LD, Abrams PD, Stanton SL, et al. Idiopathic bladder instability treated by biofeedback. *Br J Urol.* 1978;50:27–30.
5. Cardozo LD, Stanton SL, Hafner J, et al. Biofeedback in the treatment of detrusor instability. *Br J Urol.* 1978;50:250–254.
6. Burgio KL, Whitehead WE, Engel BT. Urinary incontinence in the elderly: bladder/sphincter biofeedback and toileting skills training. *Ann Intern Med.* 1985;103:507–515.
7. Kegel AH. Progressive resistance exercise in the functional restoration of the perineal muscles. *Am J Obstet Gynecol.* 1948;56:238–248.
8. Kegel AH. Stress incontinence of urine in women: physiologic treatment. *J Int Coll Surg.* 1956;25:487–499.
9. Henderson JS, Taylor KH. Age as a variable in an exercise program for the treatment of simple urinary stress incontinence. *JOGNN.* 1987;July/August:266–272.
10. Baigis-Smith J, Smith DAJ, Rose M, Newman DK. Managing urinary incontinence in community-residing elderly persons. *Gerontol.* 1989;29:229–233.
11. Burns PA, Pranikoff K, Nochajski T, Desotelle P, Harwood MK. Treatment of stress incontinence with pelvic floor exercises and biofeedback. *JAGS.* 1990;38:341–344.
12. Bradley WE, Timm GW, Scott FB. Innervation of the detrusor muscle and urethra. In: Lapides J, ed. *Symposium on Neurogenic Bladder.* Philadelphia: WB Saunders Co; 1974:3–27.
13. Schuster MM. Motor action of rectum and anal sphincters in continence and defecation. In: Code CF, ed. *Handbook of Physiology.* Washington, DC: American Physiological Society; 1968;IV:2121–2146.
14. Sundin T, Peterson I. Cystometry and simultaneous electromyography from the striated urethral and anal sphincters and from levator ani. *Investigative Urol.* 1975;13:40–46.
15. Rodriguez AA, Awad E. Detrusor muscle and sphincteric response to anorectal stimulation in spinal cord injury. *Arch Phys Med Rehabil.* 1979;60:269–272.
16. Scott FB, Quesada EM, Cardus D. Studies on dynamics of micturition: observations on healthy men. *J Urol.* 1964;92:455–463.
17. Lose G, Tanko A, Colstrup H, Andersen JT. Urethral sphincter electromyography with vaginal surface electrodes: a comparison with sphincter electromyography recorded via periurethral coaxial, anal sphincter needle, and perianal surface electrodes. *J Urol.* 1985;133:815–818.
18. Vereecken, RL, Verduyn H. The electrical activity of the paraurethral and perineal muscles in normal and pathological conditions. *Br J Urol.* 1970;42:457.
19. Burgio KL, Engel BT, Quilter RE, Arena VC. The relationship between external anal and external urethral sphincter activity in continent women. *Neurol Urodyn.* 1991;10:555–562.
20. Engel BT. The treatment of fecal incontinence by operant conditioning. *Automedica.* 1978;2:101–108.
21. Engel BT, Nikoomanesh P, Schuster MM. Operant conditioning of rectosphincteric responses in the treatment of fecal incontinence. *N Engl J Med.* 1974;290:646–649.
22. Burgio KL, Pearce KL, Lucco AJ. *Staying Dry: A Practical Guide to Bladder Control.* Baltimore: The Johns Hopkins University Press; 1989.
23. Shepherd AM, Montgomery E, Anderson RS. Treatment of genuine stress incontinence with a new perineometer. *Physiother.* 1983;69:113.
24. Burgio KL, Robinson JC, Engel BT. The role of biofeedback in Kegel exercise training for stress urinary incontinence. *Am J Obstet Gynecol.* 1986;154:58–64.
25. Burton JR, Pearce KL, Burgio KL, et al. Behavioral training for urinary incontinence in elderly ambulatory patients. *J Am Geriatr Soc.* 1988;36:693–698.

CHAPTER 11

Urinary Incontinence

11C   Nonsurgical Therapies

11C3   Electrical Stimulation

Bjarne Chr. Eriksen

INTRODUCTION

Encouraging experimental and clinical results have been achieved during the last two decades with functional electrical stimulation of the pelvic floor for various types of urinary incontinence.[1–6] The principle of electrostimulation is based on the restoration of normal physiological reflex mechanisms in abnormal nerves and muscles. It is potentially curative and has few side effects.

Functional neuromuscular electrostimulation has been used in medical practice since ancient times. The first bioelectric phenomenon that humans became aware of was the electric discharge of certain types of fish. Greek fishermen could feel the electric field surrounding their nets when a black torpedo fish was caught. Alive, this fish could produce electric energy up to 200 V.

One of the first Roman physicians, and the first known electrotherapist, Scribonius Largus, introduced the electrical power of the fish into clinical medicine in the year 46 AD. Thirty years later the Greek physician Pedanius Dioscorides recommended its use for hemorrhoids and prolapsus ani, which may have been the first intentional stimulation of muscles by artificial means. The torpedo fish was used for medical purposes until the 16th century. Studies of the fish in modern times have shown that electric discharge from the fish is analogous to the electric potentials arising in nerves and muscles during physical activity.[7]

The influence of electrostimulation on the pelvic floor was first described by Bors in 1952,[8] who presented the effect of pudendal nerve stimulation on the vesical neck. Caldwell et al.[9] was the first to show that anal and urinary incontinence could be controlled by implantable electrical stimulators. However, these systems were never widely used because of a high technical failure rate.

Alexander and Rowan[10] constructed the first nonimplantable stimulator using electrodes on a vaginal pessary in patients with urinary stress incontinence, and Suhel[11] presented the first integrated, automatic vaginal stimulator for female urinary incontinence.

GENERAL ASPECTS OF NEUROMUSCULAR ELECTRICAL STIMULATION

Excitation of nerve and muscle cells is produced by transport of ions across the cell membrane under the influence of an electrical field.[12] The excitation is generated in the peripheral nerve, rather than through the muscle directly. Using short pulses, the nerve has much lower threshold and therefore little direct activation of the muscle takes place. To cause an effective depolarization and elicit an action potential, the stimulus must be given rapidly and be of adequate intensity and duration. In addition, the membrane should be depolarized without introducing deleterious effects to the tissue or electrodes. A number of factors are critical in determining whether or not a stimulating current delivered through cutaneous electrodes is sufficient for neural excitation. These include the impedance, or sum of the resistive, capacitive and inductive components of tissue which resist current flow; the size and orientation of the electrodes that influence the current density; and electrical parameters.[13]

In biphasic stimulation, the ordering of the positive and negative pulse, the duration of each phase, and the timing between the application of each phase can either raise or lower the required stimulus for threshold excitation.[14] Threshold excitation is a function of nerve fiber diameter because the node spacing on an axon is related to the fiber diameter, and it depends on pulse duration and waveform.[15]

Impedance

Current flows more easily through tissue of low impedance than tissue of high impedance. High tissue impedance requires a high voltage to pass an equivalent amount of current.

Electrodes and Types of Stimulus

During stimulation, electron migration occurs in the electrode medium as well as in the tissue. At the electrode/tissue interface, oxidation and reduction processes occur to support the conversion of the charge carrier. These processes produce a change in the chemical composition of the tissue in the immediate vicinity of the stimulating electrode and may directly or indirectly damage the electrically activated cells. The choice of electrodes and type of stimulus is important to reduce these oxidation-reduction processes.[16] Small electrodes and high charge densities are desirable to avoid cell damage near the electrode, as well as corrosion of the electrode itself.[15] Monophasic negative pulses alone result in a local increase in pH near the electrode and may induce tissue damage. At very high levels of cathodic charge it is possible to exceed the local saturation limits for dissolved hydrogen, in which case gas bubbles will be generated and mechanically damage the cells. The hydrogen may also dissolve into the electrode and cause embrittlement, which can degrade the fatigue resistance of the electrode material. Dissolution processes result in oxidation, corrosion, and eventually electrode failure.

Biphasic pulses minimize these chemical changes. Ideally, in the positive pulse, the products of the ca-

thodic processes, primarily hydroxyl ions, are consumed by anodic reactions before they can diffuse away from the electrode. Hydrogen oxidation and oxide formation produce hydrogen ions or consume hydroxyl ions, and thus counteract the pH changes induced in the negative pulse. A ratio of anodic charge to cathodic charge less than one tends to increase the amount of cathodic products lost by diffusion away from the electrode.[15] By use of capacitor electrodes which charge and discharge the membrane without a net current flow, these reactions may be elicited.[16]

The degree of corrosion depends on the type of electrode material.[15] Certain good electrical conductors (copper, silver, etc.) can form products toxic to human tissue when they are involved in the ionization processes occurring at the electrodes. Thus, the electrode material must elicit minimal biologic reaction; it must be strong, fatigue and corrosion resistant, and have low impedance.

Stimulation Parameters

Current Amplitude

The amplitude (intensity) of the current pulse and its duration (pulse width), must be adequate to create membrane depolarization of the stimulated tissue. The nerve fibers closest to the electrode are excited first; among them, fibers of large diameter are excited before small fibers. Increasing the current amplitude results in the excitation of additional fibers.[13]

Pulse Width

The population of fibers excited can be controlled by maintaining a constant current amplitude and adjusting the pulse width. The amount of charge required to excite a nerve membrane decreases as the pulse width decreases.[13]

Pulse Rise Time

The rate of the rise of the current pulse is also important in causing depolarization. Due to membrane changes which are not well understood, a nerve or muscle fiber is capable of "accommodation," which implies a gradual elevation of the threshold of excitation in the presence of a slowly increasing stimulus. Accommodation effects are avoided when short pulse rise times are used.[13]

Pulse Repetition Rate (Frequency)

The fire rate of the nerve fibers depends on the pulse repetition frequency. The quality of the electrically evoked motor response is metabolically more expensive and fatiguing than normal physiologic activity.[13] Rapid neuromuscular fatigue, attributed to decreased transmitter release and failure of the synaptic junction, was shown to occur during stimulation at frequencies greater than 30 to 40 Hz.[17]

"On-Off" Duty Cycle

The duty cycle is the ratio between the time the stimulator is on and off. During the "on" time the stimulator delivers a train of individual pulses of prescribed amplitude, duration, and frequency. Each pulse in the train determines whether a motor response will be evoked, and the length of the pulse train determines how long the response will be maintained. The length of the "off" cycle defines the recuperative period for the stimulated tissue. A "soft-start" stimulator allows the stimulus intensity to be gradually increased during the initial part of the "on" cycle.

Type of Waveform

A wide range of stimulation waveforms has been used through the years to cause neural excitation (Fig. 11C3-1). The rectangular pulse current rises abruptly to a finite amplitude, is held constant for a determined period of time, and then falls abruptly. When the pulse starts at zero value and never crosses below this level it is called monophasic (Fig. 11C3-1B and C).

Asymmetric, balanced, biphasic pulses reduce this unidirectional ion transfer and allow the active electrode pulse to be greater in one direction than the other. The total current flow is the same in both directions, and thus the average flow is zero. This reduces the possibility of skin irritation, but some chemical reactions may still occur. These can be further reduced by using symmetric biphasic pulses with an equal current flow in both directions (Fig. 11C3-1A and D).[13]

Short square wave pulses are most efficient for nerve stimulation,[18] but any pulse configuration would be adequate provided that the stimulation equipment can deliver pulses of sufficient amplitude.[19] Very short pulse duration require very large amplitudes. A practical compromise may be 0.2 to 0.5 msec pulses.[18,20]

Regulated Current and Voltage

Electrical stimulators may provide constant voltage, constant current, or a combination of both. Constant voltage stimulators produce the same wave shape and pulse amplitude regardless of changes in tissue/electrode impedance. An increased impedance will thus reduce the current flow proportionally. A constant cur-

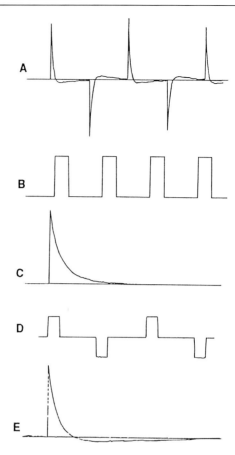

Fig. 11C3-1   Different types of electrical waveforms. **A**, Biphasic, capacitively coupled pulses. **B**, Monophasic square pulses. **C**, Monophasic spike pulses. **D**, Biphasic square pulses. **E**, Monophasic capacitively coupled spike pulses.

rent generator maintains the same current waveform regardless of changes in impedance or electrode contact. Consequently the clinical response is more consistent and easier to predict. However, a safety feature of voltage limitation must be present to avoid possible burns caused by increased current density when electrode contact with the tissue is not maintained.

Muscle Fatigue

Skeletal muscle is a heterogeneous tissue that is composed of both aerobic slow contracting motor units and anaerobic fast contracting units. The resistance to fatigue is inversely correlated to the aerobic oxidative capacity.

Muscle fatigue during electrically induced contractions is related primarily to the composition of the muscle fibers and the rate of stimulation. At high frequencies, the muscle fatigues rapidly due to impaired neuromuscular transmission and/or sarcolemmal excitation; at lower frequencies there is less fatigue due to impaired excitation-contraction coupling.[16,21] For fatigue resistant activity, the primary composition of the muscle should be slow twitch fibers.

Most striated muscles of the body are composed of three motor unit types, one with slowly contracting muscle fibers and two with fast.[22] The intramural urethral sphincter is composed exclusively of small, slow muscle fibers, whereas the paraurethral pelvic floor muscles contain all three types. The three motor unit types differ with respect to their maximal force development, fusion frequency, such as the activation frequency for a smooth sustained contraction, and resistance to fatigue.[19] The slow units develop little force, have fused contractions at about 10 Hz of activation, and can sustain the contraction for a long time. The fastest units produce 10 to 20 times more contraction force, have a fusion frequency of about 50 Hz or more, and fatigue rapidly. The intermediate fast units are somewhat weaker and considerably more fatigue resistant.[19] The intramural striated urethral sphincter may generate a well-sustained but rather limited increase in urethral pressure. This muscle is a main part of the passive continence mechanism. In provocative situations, it must be the fast motor units of the paraurethral pelvic floor muscles that provide most of the closing force on the urethra. During increase of the intraabdominal pressure, a central reflex mechanism induces muscle contraction in advance of the pressure rise, thus counteracting the latter. In normal situations, contraction of the pelvic floor muscles may create urethral pressures well above the maximal detrusor or intraabdominal pressure, and thus provide an adequate urethral closure during stress.[19] The pubourethral and pubovesical ligaments are connected to the pelvic floor muscle complex,[23,24] and one of the effects of pelvic floor contraction seems to be a reduction of urethral mobility.

Motor activity seems to be a basic regulator in the plasticity of metabolic and functional properties of muscle.[25] Following denervation, the various types of muscle fibers gradually lose their enzymatic differences. Immobilization induces atrophy of both types of muscle fibers,[26] the contraction times of slow muscles increase, and the muscles become faster.[27] In muscles atrophied by disuse, the muscle response is weak, and fatiguing is rapid.

Transformation of Skeletal Muscle by Chronic Electrical Nerve Stimulation

Electrically induced "exercise" has been employed to modify the physiologic and metabolic characteristics of normal muscle and muscle atrophied by disuse. The chronically stimulated muscles assume properties similar to those of the slow motor unit, with a marked increase in resistance to fatigue; they become slow contracting and slow relaxing and have approximately the same cross-sectional area as their unstimulated slow counterparts.[28,29]

Long-term electrical stimulation induces an almost complete transformation of fast to slow myosin subunits.[28,30,31] A fast muscle with an anaerobic metabolism is thus turned into a slow muscle with a high capacity for energy supply by aerobic oxidative processes which provide more efficient energy utilization in situations of prolonged activity.[32] The muscular transformation is manifest in alterations in sarcoplasmic reticulum, glycolytic and oxidation enzymes, parvalbumins, myosin light chains, and in twitch and fatigue characteristics.[33] The increase in tissue oxidative capacity is reflected by an increase in myoglobin and mitochondrial content,[34] a pronounced increase in volume density of mitochondria,[35] and an increase in capillary density which is attributed to capillary growth resulting from increased capillary flow.[36]

The progressive striated muscle transformation affects equally the three main functional systems of the muscle fiber: energy metabolism for ATP supply, the Ca^{2+}-releasing and sequestering membranes of the sarcoplasmic reticulum,[37] and the proteins of the contractile apparatus.[34] The transformation of the sarcoplasmic reticulum is evident from the marked decrease in Ca^{2+} uptake capacity.[29] Stimulation induces a rapid decrease in parvalbumin which is no longer detectable in the chronically stimulated fast twitch muscle after 28 days.[37]

The transformation of the sarcoplasmic reticulum is completed after 30 days of stimulation.[33] The enzyme pattern of the energy metabolism is complete before major changes are detectable in the myofibrillar proteins, indicating that the conversion of the muscle results from a transformation of the preexisting fibers.[34] However, some fibers degenerate and are replaced by newly formed fibers from satellite cell proliferation.[33] The basic mechanism seems to be a switch in gene expression due to profound changes in RNA transcriptional activity.[38]

The transformation of fast into slow twitch fibers is

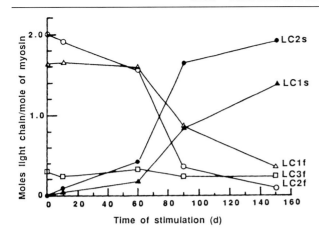

Fig. 11C3-2 Time dependent changes in the stoichiometry of fast and slow type of myosin light chains during chronic stimulation (10 Hz, 24 h/day) of rabbit tibialis anterior muscle. (Reprinted from Seedorf[39] with permission.)

progressive with the duration of the stimulation, and affects various functional systems of the muscle fiber in an orderly sequence.[33] The most extensive changes occur between 60 and 90 days (Fig. 11C3-2).[39] The total number of fibers remains constant during the transformation process.[40] Intermittent phasic, high frequency stimulation (40 to 60 Hz) induces fast to slow transition similar to the findings after low-frequency stimulation (10 Hz), suggesting that the transformation process is elicited by an increase in the total amount of contractile activity.[32] The reverse process may be brought about by inactivity, such as chronic immobilization.[41]

GENERAL PRINCIPLES OF PELVIC FLOOR STIMULATION

Electrical stimulation of the pelvic floor muscles induces a reflex contraction of the striated para- and periurethral muscles accompanied by a simultaneous reflex inhibition of the detrusor muscle.[42] This reciprocal response depends on a preserved reflex arc through the sacral micturition reflex center.[5] In order to obtain a therapeutic effect of pelvic floor stimulation in patients with urinary incontinence, a total or partial peripheral innervation of the pelvic floor muscles must be present.[5,43] No effect can be expected in patients with complete lower motor neuron lesions. Vaginal and clitoral stimulation elicits inhibitory bladder reflexes which are normally active during intercourse, while anal stimulation activates reflexes normally utilized during defecation.[19]

Neuronal Pathways

Urethral Closure

The urethral closure mechanism involved during pelvic floor stimulation is mainly due to a direct stimulation of efferent pudendal nerves, but activation of efferent hypogastric fibers with the contraction of smooth periurethral muscles may also contribute.[44] Efferent stimulation of the pelvic nerves seems to increase the intraluminal urethral pressure and increase the length of urethra. Stimulation of hypogastric nerves seems to give the same changes in the proximal part of the urethra.[45]

Some patients do not tolerate stimulation intensities high enough to induce motor nerve activation. Yet the stimulation may have a positive effect on stress incontinence.[19] This observation may be due to activation of pelvic floor afferents with reflex connections to the muscles. This reflex may be activated through afferent fibers from muscles and mucosa in the anogenital region.[19]

Bladder Inhibition

The bladder is equipped with a self-sustaining positive feedback system that ensures complete bladder emptying during the micturition contraction. Detrusor instability may be caused by ineffective inhibition of this feedback system. Intravaginal or pudendal nerve stimulation of sufficient intensity may cause a complete bladder relaxation. Electrical stimulation of clitoris or anal branches of the pudendal nerve also results in a profound detrusor inhibition, which is not the case when branches to the pelvic floor itself are stimulated.[19] The higher the intensity, the more efficient the bladder inhibition, which is caused by two spinal reflex mechanisms which have their afferent limb in the pudendal nerves and may operate without supraspinal control.[46]

The neurophysiologic basis of detrusor relaxation in response to pelvic floor stimulation is due to a long-lasting reflex discharge in the hypogastric nerves, which also provides a powerful central inhibition of the efferent activity in the pelvic nerves.[47] The hypogastric system alone may cause profound inhibition of the actively contracting bladder by directly inhibiting the detrusor muscle and the transmission of pelvic excitatory outflow through the vesical parasympathetic ganglia.

The hypogastric system is extremely sensitive to the frequency of stimulation. Both the central and peripheral parts of the system function optimally at about 5 Hz, which also has a pronounced effect on pelvic efferent activity.[47] In practice, alternating pulses of 10 Hz are recommended.

The threshold for reflex activation is close to the perception threshold in man. Maximal bladder inhibition is obtained at stimulation intensities two to three times the threshold intensity, which is painful in unanesthetized subjects.[19] Usually, the maximal tolerance level in humans is about 1.5 to 2 times the perception threshold,[48] which means that all clinical applications of electrical stimulation today utilize suboptimal intensities.[19] The optimal stimulation intensity differs considerably among individuals.

Relaxation of the detrusor muscle is accompanied by tightening of the detrusor sling fibers around the bladder neck that are important for passive continence. These fibers are lacking in women with stress incontinence.[49]

Pelvic floor stimulation probably reorganizes the system controlling detrusor activity either centrally or peripherally.[47] The effect of maximal stimulation in detrusor instability may be due to reinforcement of the intrinsic inhibitory mechanism within the detrusor by normalizing the disturbed balance between cholinergic and beta-adrenergic neurotransmission. Isolated strips of urinary bladder from rabbits were analyzed after maximal electrical stimulation. They showed a higher level of beta-adrenergic activity in the detrusor muscle, whereas the activity for cholinergic receptors was decreased. This may explain the persisting bladder inhibition observed after electrical stimulation.[50] However, it was impossible to draw a conclusion about the nature of these changes, whether an increased number of receptors or altered affinity to the receptors.

The possible role of central endorphin production, and peripheral vasoactive intestinal polypeptide (VIP) production and distribution within the detrusor after maximal stimulation is presently unknown. Injections of enkephalins into the sacral subarachnoid space inhibit bladder reflexes.[51] The parasympathetic reflex pathway to the bladder is probably subject to tonic enkephalinergic control.[52] It is reasonable to believe that the endogenous opiate system may be involved in the neuromuscular response observed after electrostimulation of the pelvic floor by the same mechanisms observed after transcutaneous electrostimulation for pain relief.[53]

Muscular Response

Single fiber electromyography has identified the following types of responses in the pelvic floor muscles during electrostimulation: a direct response due to stimulation of the motor axons; oligosynaptic reflex responses; polysynaptic reflex responses conducted through different numbers of interneurons; and recurrent responses of antidromically activated motorneurons.[54] Polysynaptic reflex responses comprise the largest proportion of the obtained motor effect. An increase in stimulation rate from 1 to 10 Hz frequently results in recruitment of additional motor units.

The advantages of reflex stimulation compared to direct motor nerve stimulation are obvious. The responses retain the physiological plasticity which is lost with direct stimulation, and the spinal reflex center can coordinate the contractions of the individual muscles; direct stimulation tends to activate a limited number of motor units, whereas a number of muscles can be activated from a single stimulation site; the position of the electrodes is less critical and, finally, the physiological protective mechanisms such as fatigue are not bypassed as is the case with direct stimulation.[54]

CLINICAL APPLICATION

Incontinence caused by detrusor instability and/or pelvic floor weakness may be corrected by long-term electrical stimulation of the pelvic floor.[4,5,55-58] Detrusor instability may also be relieved by acute maximal stimulation of the pelvic floor.[20,59,60]

Long-Term Stimulation (Chronic)

Electric long-term stimulation of the anal and urethral sphincters is based on daily application of relatively weak electrical impulses for a period of 3 to 12 months. The applied stimulation is so weak that it does not reach sensory threshhold in all the patients. The disadvantage is long, daily preoccupation with the treatment.

With this mode of stimulation, fast motor units are recruited first, as they have the largest axons with the lowest threshold for electrical stimulation. This effect is desirable because of the role these units play in the maintenance of continence in stressful situations.[19]

The changes in muscle fiber morphology, enzyme activity, and metabolism observed in striated skeletal muscles after experimental long-term electrical stimulation,[28,32] should theoretically be similar in human striated pelvic floor muscles. It was suggested that chronic pelvic floor stimulation increases the frequency of slow twitch fibers in the paraurethral region.[61] Slow and intermediate motor units are recruited first during reflex activation by electrical stimulation. The reinnervation of partly denervated pelvic floor muscles may be improved by accelerated sprouting of surviving motor axons.[19] Activation may promote the development of large motor units with many muscle fibers.[62] Repeated pelvic floor contraction may also strengthen the supportive ligaments. However, more studies are required to determine why pelvic floor stimulation has a positive effect on stress incontinence.[19] So far, it seems advisable to use high-frequency stimulation (25 to 50 Hz) in stress incontinence.

Transrectal stimulation produces the highest pressure rise in the urethra at low current intensity (12 to 24 mA) in experimental studies in dogs, and is claimed to be the optimal method of stimulation in the treatment of urethral sphincter weakness.[63]

Muscle fiber atrophy in the pelvic floor will cause a reduced muscular resting tone, reduced fatigue resistance to stress provocation, and reduced active contractile force. These processes may be reversed during long-term stimulation in animal models.[28,30,34] The recovered muscle is able to produce slower, less powerful, but more sustained contractions with less fatigue during stress. It is reasonable to believe that the same mechanism is involved in long-term electrical endurance training of the pelvic floor muscles of women with stress incontinence.

Re-education of the pelvic floor, implying a persistent remission of symptoms for several years after long-term stimulation (carry-over effect), was observed in stress, urge, and mixed urinary incontinence.[4] Until now, it was not possible to explain this phenomenon neurophysiologically.

Long-term pelvic floor stimulation also causes a reflex inhibition of detrusor activity, and may restore normal function in an overactive detrusor muscle.[3,42,64] Pelvic floor stimulation is therefore recommended in combined stress and motor urge incontinence.[3,4,64,65] If the urge component is effectively treated, the stress incontinence may be treatable with surgical repair.[4]

Technical Demands of a Long-Term Stimulation Device

The neuromuscular response of long-term stimulation is reflexogenic, and the stimulation may therefore be applied by implantable intramuscular electrodes,[1] by needle electrodes in the pudendal nerves,[66,67] or by plug and pessary devices located anally or vaginally.[4,11,57,64,68] The external methods have few complications and are equally effective as electrode implantation due to the principle of reflex stimulation.

An electrical device for anal and vaginal application must have a smooth surface, should be easy to clean, and should not become discolored or cause chemical or allergic tissue reactions. Because of the acid environment, the plastic material must be resistant to a low pH,

fragmentation must be avoided, expansion during temperature variation should be tolerated, and the material in the housing and the metal electrodes must match each other with regard to coefficient of thermal expansion. Polyphenyloxide (PPO) has satisfactory physical, chemical, and mechanical properties.[69] When symmetric electrical pulses are applied, acid resistant steel electrodes are used long-term without any problems.[69] Technical failure due to humidity and electrolysis must be avoided and penetration of fluid into the interior of the device should not occur, as it may destroy the electrical components.

Some long-term nonimplantable stimulators consist of a battery-operated external pulse generator that is connected to a vaginal or anal electrode by wire. The pulse generator has a knob to adjust current intensity. Other devices are fully integrated with battery and electronic circuit located within a plug device (Fig. 11C3-3). The stimulation parameters of the latter are fixed, but different models of the device are produced with "high" or "low" stimulation intensity, to be chosen individually for anal or vaginal application (Fig. 11C3-4). They start automatically after insertion, triggered by the humid mucosa.

Fig. 11C3-3 A fully integrated anal stimulator for long-term pelvic floor stimulation.

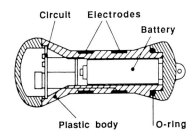

Fig. 11C3-4 Personal long-term pelvic floor stimulator for anal or vaginal application (PSA/PSV, Medicon, Trondheim, Norway).

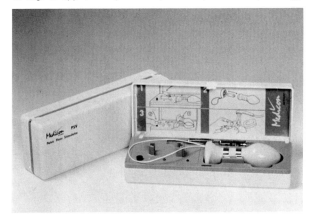

Selection of Electrical Parameters

When electrical stimulation is applied, the patient usually adapts to the current intensity within a few minutes. To allow for adaptation, the stimulation device may be constructed to increase current intensity gradually from zero to maximum within a few minutes. A pulse length of 0.5 to 1.0 msec is nearly optimal with regard to efficiency of muscle contraction.[11,70] To achieve optimal contraction of the anal sphincter, the pulse voltage has to exceed 3.75 V.[11]

The type of electric pulses is important in order to avoid tissue reactions and muscle fatigue.[13,71] It was stated that biphasic pulses (Fig. 11C3-1A and D) give 30% to 40% better therapeutic response than monophasic pulses.[11] In addition, capacitively coupled pulses (Fig. 11C3-1A and E) further prohibit tissue reactions at the tissue/electrode interface.[16]

The pulse repetition frequency in the pulse train may be of particular importance for the therapeutic response in pelvic floor stimulation. Different frequencies are claimed to give different effects on urethral closure and bladder relaxation.[43] In experiments on cats, maximum urethral closure was obtained using alternating pulses of 50 Hz.[44] Frequencies down to 20 Hz may be used without an increase in pulse power dissipation.[18] This may be clinically important in patients with combined bladder and urethral disturbances. Rottembourg and colleagues[70] found no difference in urethral closure within the range of 10 to 50 Hz in dogs. Maximum detrusor inhibition was obtained with a frequency of 5 Hz.[47] In clinical experiments, good therapeutic effect was observed both in stress and motor urge incontinence with a fixed frequency of 25 Hz.[64,65] Thus, the frequency is probably unimportant within the range of 5 to 50 Hz in human beings.

Intermittent stimulation appears to be superior to continuous stimulation,[70,72] and may be mandatory to avoid muscle fatigue during long-term stimulation. Less total electrical energy is then delivered to the muscle. The ratio of length of pulse train/rest period is also important for optimal stimulation. According to Racovec[73] the anal sphincter reaches maximum contraction in 0.5 sec during continuous stimulation. The most effective rest period is thought to be three times longer than the active one.

Clinical Results

URINARY INCONTINENCE

Successful pelvic floor stimulation was reported in 50% to 92% of women with various types of urinary incontinence.* Patient selection, application time of the device, and variation in the electrical parameters may explain this wide variation in therapeutic effect.

The best results were obtained in patients without previous incontinence surgery.[64] This could be expected because of formation of nonelastic scar tissue around the bladder neck and urethra after surgery. No increase in residual urine volume was observed, nor important changes in flow parameters or urethral resistance index.[65] A normal urethral closure mechanism may thus be restored without creating urethral obstruction.

In patients with genuine stress incontinence, no changes were observed in the cystometrograms. However, a significant increase was noted in the functional urethral length after long-term stimulation therapy.[64] This must be caused by elevation of the levator ani muscle as it strengthens during therapy.

A change in urethral closure pressure from negative to positive during stress provocation was reported in 94% of patients reporting cure of stress incontinence after long-term stimulation.[68] The changes in these urethral measurements, which are well correlated to clinical cure or improvement, may be explained by reduced muscle fatigue during stress, increased contractile force, improvement of resting tone, and restoration of normal reflex activity in the striated urethral and pelvic floor muscles after stimulation.

Patients with stress incontinence due to muscular sphincter weakness, which presents positive pressure transmission to the proximal urethra during stress provocation, respond excellently to long-term stimulation.[68] The primary etiologic factor in this group is probably a delayed reflex response in the pelvic floor after sudden increase of intraabdominal pressure, and a weak, easy-fatiguing urethral sphincter mechanism.

The same mechanisms are probably involved in genuine stress incontinence with insufficient pressure transmission to the urethra. Electrostimulation may also restore a normal urethral closure mechanism in this group, but some of these patients obviously need surgical correction to reposition the bladder neck and proximal urethra and its supportive tissue into the intraabdominal pressure zone. This may be due to severely damaged pubourethral ligaments that are less likely to be restored by muscular training.

FECAL INCONTINENCE

Few studies have been published on the subject of electrical stimulation of the pelvic floor in anal sphincter dysfunction. Collins and coworkers[74] applied long-

*References 4–6, 11, 57, 58, 64, 65, 68.

term stimulation on 12 patients with fecal incontinence. Poor subjective and objective results were obtained. They found the anal sphincter response to continuous stimulation to be the same whether the stimulus was bipolar, unipolar, with long or short pulse width, or of high or low frequency.

Larpent and colleagues[75] studied 13 patients with fecal incontinence, of whom 8 responded positively from electrical stimulation of the pelvic floor. The stimulation was applied 30 minutes per day for 10 days.

Electrostimulation is at present an interesting method for the treatment of fecal incontinence. A few encouraging results have been presented, but further, more extended studies are required for an adequate evaluation of the effect of pelvic floor stimulation in patients with anal sphincter dysfunction.

Clinical Strategy for Long-Term Stimulation

Before therapy is started, a detailed presentation of a long-term stimulator should be given by health personnel familiar with the principle of long-term stimulation. Thereafter the device should be tested by the patient under careful supervision in order to obtain maximum understanding and acceptance of the method. Trained, specialized nurses or continence advisors with patience, knowledge, and interest will probably fill this job best.

The device should be used daily for at least 6 to 8 hours, either anally or vaginally, depending on individual preference. Patients should be advised to contact the therapist immediately in case of technical problems, and should be informed that a treatment period of 3 to 6 months could be necessary to obtain a successful result. A follow-up visit should be arranged 1 to 2 weeks after the start of therapy to solve minor problems, and later every third month. It is important to encourage the patient to do Kegel exercises regularly when the stimulation is discontinued, in order to keep the pelvic floor muscles in optimal condition and thus prohibit disuse atrophy and reduce the recurrence rate to a minimum.

In women after menopause, vaginal application of a long-term device may cause mechanical irritation of the atrophic mucosa. Treatment combined with estrogen (estriol) therapy is therefore recommended to prohibit vaginal discharge and bleeding.

Short-Term Maximal Stimulation (Acute)

Various types of dysfunction of the lower urinary tract may be treated successfully by maximal stimulation of the pelvic floor.[59,60,72,76-79] The therapeutic effect in urinary stress incontinence has been debated,[59,76,80,81]

and successful results seem to depend on a significant number of repetitive stimulation sessions.[82] For the electrical stimulation to be successful, an at least partially intact reflex arc must be present.[59]

Maximal stimulation makes it possible to regain normal motor function in an overactive detrusor muscle.[59,60] Due to its inhibitory effect, maximal stimulation represents a therapeutic alternative in patients with detrusor instability and motor urge incontinence.[6,60,83,84] A current frequency of 5 to 10 Hz seems to give optimal inhibitory effect.[18,46]

Maximal stimulation is applied repetitively using needle electrodes, vaginal or anal plug electrodes.[20,59,60] The current intensity is adjusted individually on each electrode from a high-intensity stimulation device capable of producing currents up to 100 mA on each electrode. The current intensity is successively increased just below the pain level of the patient. The duration of each acute maximal application has been 15 to 25 minutes, and four to ten repetitions with two to three days between each application has been recommended.[59,60] The stimulation is repeated until a satisfactory effect is obtained.

In-clinic Treatment

An in-clinic stationary device for acute maximal pelvic floor stimulation is shown in Fig. 11C3-5 (Medicon MS-210). For maximum safety for the patient, a rechargeable 12V nickel-cadmium accumulator is chosen as power source for the stimulator with a capacity of at least ten treatments in sessions of 20 minutes before recharging is necessary. Two different output canals are built into the device. An anal and a vaginal plug could thus be operated separately and applied simultaneously in order to obtain a summation effect of the afferent

Fig. 11C3-5 In-clinic stationary device for maximal pelvic floor stimulation (MS-210, Medicon, Trondheim, Norway).

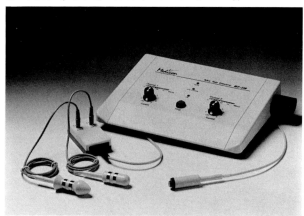

electrical input into the patient. The strength of stimulation was individually determined by the patient's level of pain tolerance.

The current intensity may be adjusted on each canal individually within the range of 0 to 100 mA, and after 20 minutes it was switched off automatically. For patient security, an emergency remote control unit enables the patient to interrupt the current at any time during the treatment.

Three different stimulation modes may be selected: continuous, monophasic square pulses with a frequency of 10 Hz for detrusor instability; intermittent, 25 Hz, biphasic pulses for stress incontinence; and continuous, 25 Hz, monophasic pulses for intravesical stimulation in patients suffering from hypotonic detrusor. After use, new disposable plug electrodes are connected.

The maximal stimulation device is easy to operate, safe for the patient, and technically reliable. The entire therapy may be performed by specialized nurses. It is at present the most inexpensive and purposeful method of regaining normal bladder function without side effects in female motor urge incontinence. Treatment in the outpatient clinic facilitates optimal patient compliance and continuous control of current intensity input during therapy.

In refractory cases, perineally inserted electrodes may be justified to stimulate the pudendal nerves directly.[85]

Home Treatment

Maximal stimulators for home treatment were recently developed and tested in clinical practice.[20] A one-channel maximal stimulator for home treatment emitting continuous, biphasic square pulses with a frequency of 10 Hz (Medicon MS-105), is shown in Fig. 11C3-6. Either disposable, permanent, and vaginal or anal electrodes are available.

Clinical Results

Successful maximal stimulation of the pelvic floor in female motor urge incontinence was reported in 52% to 92% of patients.[20,79,83,84,86,87] Phasic detrusor instability is most responsive to electrical stimulation.[19] The uninhibited overactive bladder is more refractory to treatment. Maximal stimulation, however, seems to be the therapy of choice in this group of patients.[85]

The effect of maximal stimulation cannot be predicted from the degree of detrusor instability before treatment. Nor can the effect of therapy be predicted by the urodynamic type of response of the bladder and urethra to initial stimulation.[60,88]

Some recurrences occur after treatment, necessitating

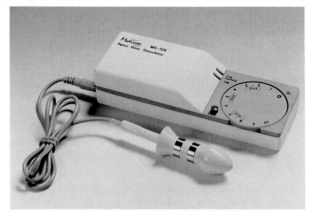

Fig. 11C3-6 Home-treatment device for maximal pelvic floor stimulation (MS-105, Medicon, Trondheim, Norway).

periods of repetitive stimulation to keep some patients continent. According to Kralj and Lukanovic,[84] a recurrence rate of about 25% may be expected after successful maximal stimulation in motor urge incontinence. Eriksen and coworkers[79] found a recurrence rate of 15% within 1 year after therapy in idiopathic detrusor instability. Kralj and colleagues[87] obtained therapeutic success in 75% of patients with recurrent urge incontinence. Repeat stimulation should be offered when recurrence occurs, before pharmacotherapy is started.

Acute maximal pelvic floor stimulation is recommended as primary therapy in cases of idiopathic detrusor instability[79] and in uninhibited overactive bladders.[19] In mixed stress and motor urge incontinence, a period of maximal stimulation may eliminate urge incontinence before long-term electrostimulation is started. Women suffering from motor urge incontinence during intercourse or postoperative urgency and urge incontinence after repair for stress incontinence may also profit from maximal pelvic floor stimulation (Eriksen, unpublished data).

Further studies are necessary to evaluate the potential therapeutic effect of maximal stimulation in diurnal and nocturnal enuresis, urge incontinence at intercourse, postoperative bladder disturbances, sensory dysfunction of the urinary bladder (pain conditions), nonulcerous interstitial cystitis, anal sphincter dysfunction, and in selected patients with neurogenic bladder and detrusor hyporeflexia.

CONTRAINDICATIONS TO PELVIC FLOOR STIMULATION

Electrical pelvic floor stimulation should not be used in patients with on-demand heart pacemakers, because

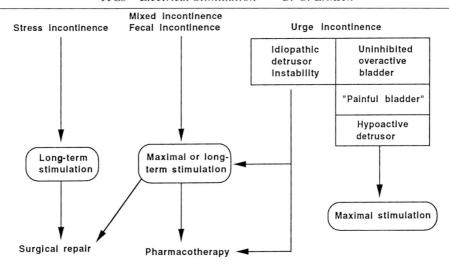

Fig. 11C3-7   Recommendations for the selection of the type of pelvic floor stimulation for disorders of the lower urinary tract and the pelvic floor.

disturbances in the heart rhythm may be provoked. At present, stimulation during pregnancy should also be avoided, as potential side effects have not yet been ruled out. Patients with extraurethral incontinence and "overflow" incontinence due to urethral obstruction require other therapy. In patients with complete peripheral denervation of the pelvic floor, no therapeutic effect of pelvic floor stimulation may be expected. Urinary infection must be excluded before therapy is started. Prolapse of uterus or vagina may prohibit vaginal application. However, improved muscular strength by anal stimulation may improve the prolapse. The patient must be able to cooperate and understand the instruction for use, as patient compliance depends on the understanding of practical use and mechanisms of action.

SUMMARY

Modern stimulators for long-term and acute maximal electrical stimulation of the pelvic floor have given us new and improved techniques for incontinence therapy in women. The method has great potential for the treatment of lower urinary tract disorders. They may be applied in the outpatient clinic at a low cost. They are nondestructive, have few side effects, and have a potential curative effect. Due to the simplicity of this therapy, information about both types of pelvic floor stimulation should be offered personnel in primary health care services. Doctors, nurses, physiotherapists, and midwives may easily learn the technique. Recommendations for selection of type of pelvic floor stimulation are shown in Fig. 11C3–7.

REFERENCES

1. Caldwell KPS, Cook PJ, Flack FC. Stress incontinence in females: report on 31 cases treated by electrical implant. *J Obstet Gynaec Br Commonw.* 1968;75:777.
2. Edwards L, Malvern J. Electronic control of incontinence. A critical review of the present situation. *Br J Urol.* 1972;44:467.
3. Fall M, Erlandson B-E, Nilson AE, Sundin S. Long-term intravaginal electrical stimulation in urge and stress incontinence. *Scand J Urol Nephrol.* 1977;44(suppl):55.
4. Fall M. Does electrostimulation cure urinary incontinence? *J Urol.* 1984;131:664.
5. Godec C, Cass AS, Ayala GF. Electrical stimulation for incontinence. Technique, selection and results. *Urology.* 1976;7:388.
6. Kralj B, Suhel P. The results of treatment of female urinary incontinence by functional electrical stimulation. *Proc First Vienna Intern Workshop Func Electrostim.* Vienna: Robidruck; 1983: 10.4.
7. Kellaway P. The part played by electric fish in the early history of bioelectricity and electrotherapy. *Bull Hist Med.* 1947;20:112.
8. Bors E. Effect of electric stimulation of the pudendal nerves on the vesical neck: its significance for the function of cord bladders: a preliminary report. *J Urol.* 1952;67:925.
9. Caldwell KPS, Flack FC, Broad AF. Urinary incontinence following spinal injury treated by electronic implants. *Lancet.* 1965;1: 846.
10. Alexander S, Rowan D. Electrical control of urinary incontinence by radio-implants. *Br J Surg.* 1968;55:358.
11. Suhel P. Adjustable nonimplantable electrical stimulators for correction of urinary incontinence. *Urol Int.* 1976;31:115.
12. Hodgkin AL, Huxley AF. Currents carried by sodium and potassium ions through the membrane of the giant axon of loligo. *J Physiol.* 1952;116:449.
13. Benton LA, Baker LL, Bowman BR, Waters RL. *Functional Electrical Stimulation—a Practical Clinical Guide.* Downey, California: Rancho Los Amigos Rehab Engineer Cntr; 1980:1–133.
14. Van den Honert C, Mortimer JT. The response of the myelinated nerve fiber to short duration biphasic stimulating currents. *Ann Biomed Engineer.* 1979;7:117.
15. Mortimer JT, Daroux ML. Electrode and nerve membrane processes during stimulation. *Proc Second Vienna Intern Workshop Func Electrostim.* Vienna: Robidruck; 1986;13.

16. Peckham PH. Functional neuromuscular stimulation. *Phys Technol.* 1981;12:114.
17. Brown GL, Burns BD. Fatigue and neuromuscular block in mammalian skeletal muscle. *Proc R Soc Lond (Biol).* 1949;136:182.
18. Ohlsson B, Lindström S, Erlandson B-E, Fall M. Effects of some different pulse parameters on bladder inhibition and urethral closure during intravaginal electrical stimulation: an experimental study in the cat. *Med Biol Eng Comput.* 1986;24:27.
19. Fall M, Lindström S. Electrical stimulation. A physiologic approach to the treatment of urinary incontinence. *Urol Clin North Am.* 1991;18:1.
20. Plevnik S, Janez J, Vrtacnik P, Trsinar B, Vodusek DB. Short-term electrical stimulation: home treatment for urinary incontinence. *World J Urol.* 1986;4:24.
21. Stokes, M, Edwards, RHT. Strategies for overcoming muscle fatigue caused by functional electrical stimulation. *Proc Second Vienna Intern Workshop Func Electrostim.* Vienna: Robidruck; 1986:87.
22. Burke RE, Levine DN, Tsairis P, et al. Physiological types and histochemical profiles in motor units of the cat gastrocnemius. *J Physiol.* 1973;234:723.
23. Zacharin R. The suspensory mechanism of the female urethra. *J Anat.* 1963;97:423.
24. DeLancey JOL. Pubovesical ligament: a separate structure from the urethral supports (pubourethral ligaments). *Neurourol Urodynam.* 1989;8:53.
25. Buchegger A, Nemeth PM, Pette D, Reichmann H. Effects of chronic stimulation on the metabolic heterogeneity of the fiber population in rabbit tibialis anterior muscle. *J Physiol.* 1984;350:109.
26. Karpati G, Engle WK. Correlative histochemical study of skeletal muscle after suprasegmental denervation, peripheral nerve section, and skeletal fixation. *Neurology.* 1968;18:681.
27. Vrbova G. The effect of motoneuron activity on the speed of contraction of striated muscle. *J Physiol.* 1963;169:513.
28. Peckham PH. *Electrical Excitation of Skeletal Muscle: Alterations in Force, Fatigue, and Metabolic Properties.* Cleveland, Ohio: Case Western Reserve University; 1972: Report EDC 4-72-32, ref. 73-6330.
29. Salmons S, Sreter FA. Significance of impulse activity in the transformation of skeletal muscle type. *Nature.* 1976;263:30.
30. Salmons S, Vrbova G. The influence of activity on some contractile characteristics of mammalian fast and slow muscles. *J Physiol.* 1969;201:535.
31. Carraro, U, Catani, C. Myosin heavy chain analyses as a tool for the study of electrostimulated muscle. *Proc Second Vienna Intern Workshop Func Electrostim.* Vienna: Robidruck; 1986;51.
32. Pette D. Activity-induced fast to slow transitions in mammalian muscle. *Med Sci Sports Exerc.* 1984;16:517.
33. Pette D, Vrbova G. Invited review: neural control of phenotypic expression in mammalian muscle fibers. *Muscle Nerve.* 1985;8:676.
34. Pette D. Transformation of skeletal muscle by chronic nerve stimulation. *Proc First Vienna Intern Workshop Func Electrostim.* Vienna: Robidruck; 1983:III.
35. Reichmann H, Hoppeler H, Mathieu-Costello O, von Bergen F, Pette D. Biochemical and ultrastructural changes of skeletal muscle mitochondria after chronic electrical stimulation in rabbits. *Pflügers Arch.* 1985;404:1.
36. Hudlicka O, Dodd L, Renkin EM, Gray SD. Early changes in fiber profile and capillary density in long-term stimulated muscles. *Am J Physiol.* 1982;243:H528.
37. Klug G, Wiehrer W, Reichmann H, Leberer E, Pette D. Relationships between early alterations in parvalbumins, sarcoplasmic reticulum, and metabolic enzymes in chronically stimulated fast twitch muscle. *Pflügers Arch.* 1983;399:280.
38. Heilig A, Pette D. Changes in transcriptional activity of chronically stimulated fast twitch muscle. *FEBS Lett.* 1983;151:211.
39. Seedorf K, Seedorf U, Pette D. Coordinate expression of alkali

40. and DTNB myosin light chains during transformation of rabbit fast muscle by chronic stimulation. *FEBS Lett.* 1983;158:321.
40. Pette D, Müller W, Leisner E, Vrbova G. Time dependent effects on contractile properties, fiber population, myosin light chains, and enzymes of energy metabolism in intermittently and continuously stimulated fast twitch muscles of the rabbit. *Pflüger Arch.* 1976;364:103.
41. Sreter FA, Pinter K, Jolesz F, Mabuchi K. Fast to slow transformation of fast muscles in response to long-term phasic stimulation. *Exper Neurol.* 1982;75:95.
42. Godec C, Cass AS, Ayala GF. Bladder inhibition with functional electrical stimulation. *Urology.* 1975;6:663.
43. Erlandson B-E, Fall M, Sundin T. Intravaginal electrical stimulation. Clinical experiments on urethral closure. *Scand J Urol Nephrol.* 1977;44(suppl):31.
44. Fall M, Erlandson B-E, Carlsson CA, Lindström S. The effect of intravaginal electrical stimulation of the feline urethra and urinary bladder. Neuronal mechanisms. *Scand J Urol Nephrol.* 1977;44(suppl):19.
45. Koinuma N, Tsuchida S, Nishizawa O, Moriya I, Wada I, Ebina K. Urethral responses to nerve stimulation measured by strain-gauge force transducer. *Proc Internat Cont Soc.* Lund, Sweden: Skogs Trelleburg; 1981:51.
46. Fall M, Erlandson B-E, Sundin T, Waagstein F. Intravaginal electrical stimulation. Clinical experiments on bladder inhibition. *Scand J Urol Nephrol.* 1977;44(suppl):41.
47. Lindström S, Fall M, Carlsson CA, Erlandson B-E. The neurophysiologic basis of bladder inhibition in response to intravaginal electrical stimulation. *J Urol.* 1983;129:405.
48. Ohlsson BL. Effects of some different pulse parameters on the perception of intravaginal and intra-anal electrical stimulation. *Med Biol Eng Comput.* 1988;26:503.
49. Tanagho EA, Smith DR. Mechanism of urinary continence. I. Embryologic, anatomic, and pathologic considerations. *J Urol.* 1968;100:640.
50. Janez J, Plevnik S, Korosec L, Stanovik L, Vrtacnik P. Changes in detrusor receptor activity after electric pelvic floor stimulation. *Proc Intern Cont Soc.* Lund, Sweden: Skogs Trelleborg; 1981;22.
51. Hisamitsu T, Roques BP, de Groat WC. The role of enkephalins in the sacral parasympathetic reflex pathways to the urinary bladder of the cat. *Soc Neurosci Abstr.* 1982;8:60.18.
52. Roppolo JR, Booth AM, de Groat WC. The effects of naloxone on the neural control of the urinary bladder of the cat. *Brain Res.* 1983;264:355.
53. Clement-Jones V, McLoughlin L, Tomlin S, Besser GM, Rees LH, Wen HL. Increased β-endorphin but not met-enkephalin levels in human cerebrospinal fluid after acupuncture for recurrent pain. *Lancet.* 1980;ii:946.
54. Trontelj JV, Janko M, Godec C, Rakovec S, Trontelj M. Electrical stimulation for urinary incontinence: a neurophysiologic study. *Urol Int.* 1974;29:213.
55. Doyle PT, Edwards LE, Harrison NW, Malvern J, Stanton SL. Treatment of urinary incontinence by external stimulating devices. *Urol Int.* 1974;29:450.
56. Glen ES. Effective and safe control of incontinence by the intra-anal plug electrode. *Br J Surg.* 1971;58:249.
57. Sotiropoulos A, Yeaw S, Lattimer JK. Management of urinary incontinence with electronic stimulation: observations and results. *J Urol.* 1976;116:747.
58. Suhel P, Kralj B, Plevnik S. Advances in nonimplantable electrical stimulators for correction of urinary incontinence. *TIT J Life Sci.* 1978;8:11.
59. Godec C, Cass A. Acute electrical stimulation for urinary incontinence. *Urology.* 1978;12:340.
60. Plevnik S, Janez J. Maximal electrical stimulation for urinary incontinence. *Urology.* 1979;14:638.
61. Bazeed MA, Thüroff JW, Schmidt RA. Effect of chronic electrostimulation of the sacral roots on the striated urethral sphincter. *J Urol.* 1982;128:1357.

62. Ridge RMAP, Betz WJ. The effect of selective, chronic stimulation on motor unit size in developing rat muscle. *J Neurosci.* 1984;4:2614.

63. Kiesswetter H. Wirkung von niederfrequenten strømen auf die beckenbodenmuskulatur. Urologie. *Fortschritte der Medizin.* 1985;103:63.

64. Eriksen BC, Bergmann S, Mjølnerød OK. Effect of anal electrostimulation with the "Incontan" device in women with urinary incontinence. *Br J Obst Gyn.* 1987;94:147.

65. Eriksen BC, Mjølnerød OK. Changes in urodynamic measurements after successful anal electrostimulation in female urinary incontinence. *Br J Urol.* 1987;59:45.

66. Janez J, Plevnik S, Vrtacnik P. Perineal percutaneous needle pudendal nerve stimulation for urinary incontinence. *Proc Intern Cont Soc: Aachen, Germany.* 1983:127.

67. Vodusek DB, Plevnik S, Janez J, Vrtacnik P. Detrusor inhibition on selective pudendal nerve stimulation in the perineum. *Proc Intern Cont Soc: Boston.* 1986:612.

68. Eriksen BC, Eik-Nes SH. Long-term electrostimulation of the pelvic floor. Primary therapy in female stress incontinence? *Urol Int.* 1989;44:90.

69. Bergmann S, Eriksen BC. Anal electrostimulation in urinary incontinence. Technical description of a new device. *Urol Int.* 1986; 41:411.

70. Rottembourg JL, Ghoneim MA, Fretin J, Susset JG. Study on the efficiency of electrical stimulation of the pelvic floor. *Invest Urol.* 1976;13:354.

71. Mortimer JT, Kaufman D. Intramuscular electrical stimulation: tissue damage. *Ann Biomed Engineer.* 1980;8:235.

72. Collins CD. Intermittent electrical stimulation. *Urol Int.* 1974;19: 221.

73. Racovec S. Reflex electrical stimulation for urinary incontinence. *Eur Urol.* 1975;1:24.

74. Collins CD, Brown BH, Duthie HL. An assessment of intraluminal electrical stimulation for anal incontinence. *Br J Surg.* 1969; 56:542.

75. Larpent JL, Cuer JC, Da Poigny M. Clinical and manometric results of electrical stimulation in patients with anal incontinence. *Colo-proctology.* 1987;9:183.

76. Moore T, Schofield PF. Treatment of stress incontinence by maximum perineal electrical stimulation. *Br Med J.* 1967;3:150.

77. Trsinar B, Plevnik S, Vrtacnik P, Drobnic J. Maximal electrical stimulation for enuresis. *Proc Intern Cont Soc.* Innsbruck, Austria: Buch Offsetdruck Plattner KG; 1984:495.

78. Eriksen BC. Painful bladder disease in women—effect of maximal electric pelvic floor stimulation. *Neurourol Urodynam.* 1989;8: 362.

79. Eriksen BC, Bergmann S, Eik-Nes SH. Maximal electrostimulation of the pelvic floor in female idiopathic detrusor instability and urge incontinence. *Neurourol Urodynam.* 1989;8:219.

80. Glen ES, Samuels BM, MacKenzie IM, Rowan D. Maximum perineal stimulation for urinary incontinence. *Urol Int.* 1976;31: 134.

81. Turner AG. An appraisal of maximal faradic stimulation of pelvic muscles in the management of female urinary incontinence. *Ann R Coll Surg Eng.* 1979;61:441.

82. Huffman JW, Osborne SL, Sokol JK. Electrical stimulation in the treatment of intractable stress incontinence. *Arch Phys Med.* 1952;33:674.

83. Kaneko S, Park YC, Yachiku S, Kurita T. Electrical control of urgency and urge incontinence. *Proc Intern Cont Soc: Aachen, Germany.* 1983:125.

84. Kralj B, Lukanovic A. Treatment of detrusor dysfunction with functional electrical stimulation (FES). *Proc Second Vienna Intern Workshop Func Electrost.* Vienna:1986:223.

85. Ohlsson BL, Fall M, Frankenberg-Sommar S. Effects of external and direct pudendal nerve maximal electrical stimulation in the treatment of the uninhibited overactive bladder. *Br J Urol.* 1989; 64:374.

86. Kralj B, Plevnik S, Janko M, Vrtacnik P. Urge incontinence and maximal electrical stimulation. *Proc Intern Cont Soc.* Portoroz, Yugoslavia: 1977;16.

87. Kralj B, Suhel P, Roskar E. The treatment of detrusor-hyperreflexia by Vagicon-AMFES. *Proc Third Medit Conf Med Biol Engineer.* Portoroz, Yugoslavia: 1983;10:4.

88. Nakamura M, Sakurai T, Sugao H, Sonoda T. Maximum electrical stimulation for urge incontinence. *Urol Int.* 1987;42:285.

Urinary Incontinence

11D   Surgical Therapies

11D1   Choice of Surgical Procedure for Stress Incontinence

Scott A. Farrell   Donald R. Ostergard

INTRODUCTION

Stress incontinence is a widespread problem among white North American women. Small degrees of stress incontinence should be considered normal because the incidence among both nulliparous and parous women is quite high.[1] Numerous studies have demonstrated an increased incidence of stress incontinence in association with increasing parity (vaginal births), advancing age, and postmenopausal status.[2] Current studies suggest that the anatomic defect that contributes to stress incontinence is a loss of the critical musculofascial attachments to both the pelvic sidewall and to the pubic symphysis.[3,4] The loss of these structural supports permits prolapse of the urethrovesical junction out of the abdominal cavity, with a resultant loss of pressure transmission to the proximal urethra. In addition, reflex tension on these support structures via levator muscle contraction may contribute to the urethral closure pressure at the time of stress. Neurophysiologic studies clearly demonstrate that in addition to the anatomic defects previously described, pelvic nerve damage as a consequence of vaginal birth results in denervation and prolonged nerve conduction times.[5,6] These neurologic abnormalities could result in a much less efficient external urethral striated sphincter mechanism, both at rest and with reflex contractions during stress.

The standard surgical approach to the correction of stress incontinence, regardless of the procedure chosen, strives to elevate and support the urethrovesical junction. The net result, then, is to correct the anatomic defect. Surgery cannot correct the neurologic problem and may actually exacerbate it as a consequence of dissection and further scarring.

Although the medical literature contains descriptions of more than 100 procedures to surgically correct stress incontinence,[2] a limited number of procedures are widely employed by urogynecologists in North America. The purpose of this chapter is to discuss the essential aspects of the preoperative urologic evaluation of patients with genuine stress incontinence (GSI), which leads to selection of an appropriate surgical procedure for correction.

PREOPERATIVE EVALUATION

The preoperative evaluation of a patient with stress incontinence should be designed to confirm the diagnosis of GSI while ruling out other causes of incontinence. Some of the more important causes of incontinence that must be ruled out include detrusor instability, overflow incontinence, vesicovaginal fistula, urinary tract infection, and the functionless drainpipe urethra. A systematic approach to patient evaluation is necessary.[7] Our approach includes the following basic steps:

1. Urine culture and sensitivity test to rule out urinary tract infection

2. Neurologic evaluation of the sacral segments
3. Pelvic examination
4. Demonstration of a correctable anatomic defect—the Q-Tip test
5. Residual urine test to exclude overflow incontinence
6. Cystometrogram to exclude detrusor instability
7. Cystourethroscopy to exclude drainpipe urethra
8. Urodynamic testing to determine urethral closure pressure

Neurologic evaluation permits any gross neurologic deficits to be discovered and confirms that the necessary nerve roots (S2, S3, S4,) required for the anocutaneous and bulbocavernosus reflexes are intact. This gives reassurance that the sacral reflex pathways are intact. Pelvic examination is an essential part of the evaluation to identify pelvic hernial defects such as cystocele, rectocele, enterocele, uterine prolapse, and vaginal vault prolapse. These structural alterations in pelvic support may impinge on the urethra, altering the continence mechanism and sometimes even enhancing continence. Knowledge of the presence of a cystocele or prolapse prompts careful urodynamic evaluation using a Sims' speculum to reduce the prolapse, looking for potential incontinence. Urethral diverticula or fistula as well as vesicovaginal fistula and pelvic masses of sufficient size to impinge on the bladder may be detected.

Once the diagnosis of genuine stress incontinence is made, the proper choice of a surgical procedure involves three basic criteria, including the presence or absence of (1) urethral hypermobility, (2) a urethral drainpipe, and (3) low urethral closure pressure.

Urethral Hypermobility

The Q-Tip test, when carefully performed, can provide essential reproducible evidence of an anatomic defect (Fig. 11D1-1). A straining angle of greater than 30° from the horizontal confirms a prolapsed urethrovesical junction which, if not scarred into a fixed location, can be surgically corrected. If there is no anatomic defect, standard surgical approaches to the correction of GSI will be ineffective and other alternatives must be considered.

Urethral Drainpipe

Dynamic cystourethroscopy permits visual assessment of the urethrovesical junction's mobility and function and permits the diagnosis of a functionless drainpipe urethra (Fig. 11D1-2). It also allows the exclusion

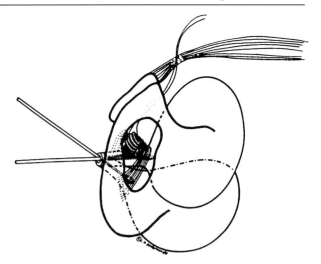

Fig. 11D1-1   The Q-Tip test. The end of the Q-Tip is placed at the urethrovesical junction. At rest it is horizontal. With straining, the urethrovesical junction descends and since the urethral meatus is fixed in location, the end of the Q-Tip ascribes an upward arc. (Reprinted from Ostergard DR, ed, *Gynecologic Urology and Urodynamics: Theory and Practice,* 2nd ed, Baltimore: Williams & Wilkins; 1985:535, with permission.)

of irritative factors such as cystitis, stones, urethritis, and diverticula.

Urethral Closure Pressure

Urodynamics is essential for most patients being evaluated for incontinence. Urodynamics serves two pur-

Fig. 11D1-2   The functionless drainpipe urethra. With the urethroscope at the external urethral meatus, the urethrovesical junction is seen. (Courtesy of JR Robertson, Las Vegas, Nevada.)

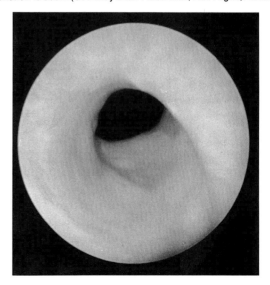

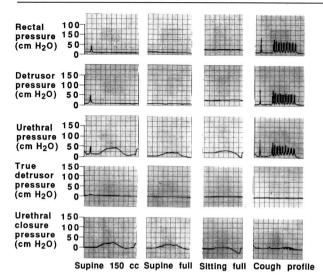

Rectal pressure (cm H₂O)
Detrusor pressure (cm H₂O)
Urethral pressure (cm H₂O)
True detrusor pressure (cm H₂O)
Urethral closure pressure (cm H₂O)

Supine 150 cc   Supine full   Sitting full   Cough profile

Fig. 11D1-3 Urethral pressure profiles. Urethral closure pressure is determined under three different conditions. When the bladder is full in the sitting position, the pressure is about 5 cm H₂O. The cough profile confirms pressure equalization with each cough. (Reprinted from Ostergard DR, ed, *Gynecologic Urology and Urodynamics. Theory and Practice*, 3rd ed, Baltimore: Williams & Wilkins; 1991:398, with permission.)

poses. The first is to exclude confounding causes of incontinence such as detrusor instability, urethral instability, and uninhibited urethral relaxation. The second is to allow the measurement of urethral closure pressures, an assessment of the functional integrity of the urethral sphincteric mechanism (Fig. 11D1-3).

With the data available from the above evaluations, the following questions can be answered:

1. Does this patient have a surgically correctable incontinence problem?
2. Is there hypermobility of the bladder base and urethrovesical junction?
3. Is the intrinsic urethral sphincteric mechanism intact?
4. What closure pressures are being generated by the urethral sphincteric mechanism?
5. Does the patient have a urethral drainpipe?

The standard surgical procedures used to correct anatomic stress incontinence have a single purpose: to elevate the bladder base and proximal urethra to their original intraabdominal location and to provide the necessary support to maintain them in that position permanently. For patients with a functionally intact sphincteric unit and hypermobility of the urethrovesical junction, three surgical options are available:

1. A needle suspension procedure[8]
2. Retropubic urethropexy[9]
3. Suburethral sling[10]

Each of these surgical procedures has within it a number of variations. Each variation has its advocates with data to support the claim that it gives the best results. Anterior vaginal repairs are no longer advocated for the surgical treatment of stress incontinence. Table 11D1-1 shows the algorithm which, applied to the clinical data concerning a patient, permits the selection of the most appropriate surgical procedure. After the clinical and urodynamic evaluation is complete and the diagnosis of GSI is made, the most important factor in determining specific recommendations for surgery is the condition of the urethra. A urethra with a fixed, nonmobile, urethrovesical junction is often scarred from previous surgery. This scarification often results in a rigid, "drainpipe urethra," which no longer can function as a sphincter to maintain continence. The only surgical options available to such a patient are to occlude the urethra by sling or by periurethral collagen injections, or with an artificial sphincter.[11]

The finding most commonly associated with GSI is just the opposite of that described above, a functionally intact sphincteric unit which is "hypermobile." These patients have an anatomic defect that can be corrected surgically by means of a needle suspension procedure, retropubic urethropexy, or a suburethral sling. Recent evidence suggests that long-term results with a needle suspension procedure are not as good as with a retropubic urethropexy[12,13] and are similar to results obtained with anterior vaginal repairs. The needle suspension procedure should be reserved for patients who undergo pelvic prolapse surgery and who have urodynamically proven potential incontinence. The diagnosis of potential incontinence is made when pressure equalization and/or urine loss is demonstrated during a dynamic urethral pressure profile with a Sims' speculum in the vagina to reduce the prolapse. The patient with potential incontinence does not experience urine loss under other circumstances.

When the diagnosis of genuine stress incontinence is made, the urethral closure pressure determines whether a retropubic urethropexy or a suburethral sling is recommended. McGuire[14] first noted an increased incidence of unsuccessful incontinence surgery among patients with a urethral closure pressure of <20 cm/H₂O. He classified these patients as having type III stress incontinence and noted that many did not have urethral hypermobility. In a retrospective review of failed ret-

Table 11D1-1
Selection of Appropriate Surgical Procedure

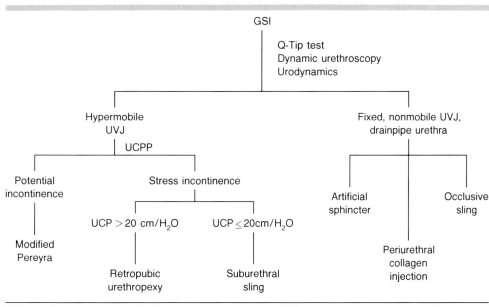

UVJ = urethrovesical junction; UCP = urethral closure pressure; UCPP = urethral closure pressure profile.

ropubic urethropexies, Sand and colleagues[15] found a threefold increased incidence of objective surgical failure in patients with urethral closure pressure of ≤20 cm/H_2O. Bowen and coworkers[16] conducted a retrospective, case-controlled study of the Burch retropubic urethropexy. Looking at the preoperative urethral closure pressure, he found that only 5 of 21 patients, 24%, who failed the Burch retropubic urethropexy had urethral closure pressure >20 cm/H_2O. In the group who experienced successful surgery, the incidence of closure pressure >20 cm/H_2O was 81%. A further study by Horbach and colleagues[17] compared the Burch retropubic urethropexy with the suburethral sling procedure in a case-controlled fashion in patients with low urethral closure pressure. The Burch procedure was successful only 35% of the time, whereas the sling produced a cure rate of 80%. Given these factors, if the maximum urethral closure pressure in the sitting position with a subjectively full bladder is greater than 20 cm/H_2O, a retropubic urethropexy, usually Tanagho's modification of the Burch procedure, is the procedure of choice.[9] If, on the other hand, the maximum urethral closure pressure is ≤ 20 cm/H_2O, a suburethral sling procedure is recommended. All other risk factors being equal, if excess risk for failure is present and the patient has chronic obstructive airway disease, is a chronic cougher or is a smoker with other pulmonary disease, a sling is recommended. Extreme obesity or an occupation that

demands heavy lifting may also necessitate the use of a suburethral sling.

In undertaking a surgical procedure to correct stress incontinence, regardless of the type of procedure being done, the surgeon should follow certain basic principles.

Principle I

There must be some means of determining that an appropriate amount of anatomic correction is achieved to ensure continence but avoid overcorrection and potential obstruction.

The authors have found that intraoperative urethroscopy permits a visual assessment of bladder neck closure. For a Pereyra or sling procedure, just prior to completing fixation of the urethrovesical junction in an elevated position, urethroscopy is undertaken. With the water running, the bladder neck should be 90% closed, and with the water off, it should be completely closed. Once the appropriate elevation is visually determined by urethroscopy, a Q-Tip can be placed at the urethrovesical junction and the angle noted. The Q-Tip then provides an objective means for the surgeon to adjust the urethrovesical junction elevation and complete the procedure. As a general rule, a Q-Tip angle of approximately + 5° with the patient anesthetized gives good results.

Principle II

There must be assurance that no damage occurs to either the bladder or the ureters.

Intraoperative cystoscopy performed after all the sutures are placed but before the final fixation occurs, allows the surgeon to verify that the bladder is intact. Indigo carmine dye injected intravenously is extruded via the kidneys in approximately 5 to 7 minutes, and is seen ejecting from the orifices of normally functioning ureters.

Principle III

There should be a systematic approach to the postoperative care of the patient. Postoperative instructions to the patient for activity limitations should be clear and a systematic means of ensuring normal voiding should be established.

Patients should limit their activities for at least three months following their surgery to allow enough time for collagen remodeling to form strong scars. Good scar tissue ensures a long-term result from the procedure. No heavy lifting, bending, stooping, or pushing should be undertaken during this time. The patient should be encouraged to walk for exercise but to avoid activities that require contraction of the abdominal muscles. Intercourse is forbidden during this interval.

A protocol to evaluate bladder function postoperatively is essential. Studies demonstrate that there is no advantage to the use of either "bladder training" or urecholine in the postoperative period.[18,19]

A suprapubic catheter permits evaluation of postvoid residuals. Residuals should be consistently 50 ml or less for 24 to 48 hours before the catheter is removed.

SUMMARY

As with most aspects of modern medicine, the various procedures outlined above are not perfect and clinical judgment must be used. This schema is derived from the available information in the medical literature and demonstrates the method of patient evaluation and selection of surgical procedure for genuine stress incontinence that seems most appropriate for an individual patient. This approach offers the patient the best chance of a long-term satisfactory result. Recent research efforts have made significant progress toward better understanding of the physical structures that contribute to continence mechanisms.[3] Approaches to urodynamic evaluation may change in the future[4] and nerve conduction studies may be added to our routine preoperative evaluation.[6] A thorough evaluation of the patient allows the urogynecologist to be as precise as possible in his surgical treatment of stress incontinence.

REFERENCES

1. Nemir A, Middleton RP. Stress incontinence in young nulliparous women. *Am J Obstet Gynecol.* 1964;68:1166.
2. Stanton SL. Stress incontinence: why and how operations work. *Urol Clin NA.* 1985;12(2):279–284.
3. DeLancey JOL. Structural aspects of urethrovesical function in the female. *Neurourol Urodyn.* 1988;7:509–519.
4. Constantinou CE. Urethrometry: considerations of static, dynamic, and stability characteristics of the female urethra. *Neurourol Urodyn.* 1988;7:521–539.
5. Smith ARB, Hosker GL, Warrell DW. The role of partial denervation of the pelvic floor in the etiology of genitourinary prolapse and stress incontinence of urine: a neurophysiologic study. *Brit J Obstet Gynecol.* 1989;96:24–28.
6. Snooks SJ, Badenoch DF, Tiptaft RC, Swash M. Perineal nerve damage in genuine stress urinary incontinence: an electrophysiological study. *Brit J Urol.* 1985;57:422–426.
7. Ostergard DR, Hodgkinson CP. Preoperative evaluation of patients for incontinence surgery. In:Ostergard DR, ed. *Gynecologic Urology and Urodynamics: Theory and Practice,* 2nd ed. Baltimore: Williams & Wilkins; 1985:187–198.
8. Pereyra AJ, Lebherz TB, Growdon WA, Powers JA. Pubourethral supports in perspective: modified Pereyra procedure for urinary incontinence. *Obstet Gynecol.* 1982;59:643–648.
9. Tanagho EA. Retropubic procedures: a physiologic approach to repair of genuine stress incontinence. In: Ostergard DR, ed. *Gynecologic Urology and Urodynamics: Theory and Practice.* Baltimore: Williams & Wilkins; 1985:503–510.
10. Horbach NS, Blanco JS, Ostergard DR, Bent AE, Cornella JL. A suburethral sling procedure with polytetrafluoroethylene for the treatment of stress incontinence in patients with low urethral closure pressure. *Obstet Gynecol.* 1988;71:648–652.
11. Scott FB, Bradley WE, Timm GW. Treatment of urinary incontinence by an implantable prosthetic urinary sphincter. *Urol.* 1974;112:75–80.
12. Karram MM, Bhatia NN. Transvaginal needle bladder neck suspension procedures for stress urinary incontinence: a comprehensive review. *Obstet Gynecol.* 1989;73:906–914.
13. Bergman A, Ballard CA, Koonings PP. Comparison of three different surgical procedures for genuine stress incontinence: prospective randomized study. *Obstet Gynecol.* 1989;160:1102–1106.
14. McGuire EJ. Urodynamic findings in patients after failure of stress incontinence operations. *Prog Clin Biol Res.* 1981;78:351–360.
15. Sand PK, Bowen LW, Panganiban R, Ostergard DR. The low pressure urethra as a factor in failed retropubic urethropexy. *Obstet Gynecol.* 1987;69:399–402.
16. Bowen LW, Sand PK, Ostergard DR, Franti CE. Unsuccessful Burch retropubic urethropexy: a case-controlled urodynamic study. *Am J Obstet Gynecol.* 1989;160:452–458.
17. Horback NS, Bent AE, Ostergard DR, Cornella JL. A comparison of retropubic urethropexy and suburethral sling procedure for the treatment of stress incontinence and the low pressure urethra. *Obstet Gynecol.* (Submitted for publication).
18. Bergman A, Matthews L, Ballard CA. Bladder training after surgery for stress incontinence: is it necessary? *Obstet Gynecol.* 1987;70:909–912.
19. Farrell SA, Webster RD, Higgins LM, Steaves RA. Duration of postoperative catheterization: a randomized, double-blind trial comparing two catheter management protocols and the effect of bethanechol chloride. *Internat Urogynecol J.* 1990;1:132–135.

Urinary Incontinence

11D   Surgical Therapies

11D2   Surgery for Stress Incontinence

J. Thomas Benson

INTRODUCTION

In the normal healthy female, the pelvic floor is a dynamic entity aiding physiologic control over urinary storage and elimination, reproductive and sexual function, and rectal accommodation and elimination. When a disturbance occurs in this dynamic entity allowing urinary incontinence, fecal incontinence, or vaginal dysfunction to become a problem severe enough to require surgery, the defect in the pelvic floor is usually not limited to just the obvious component. Therefore, surgeries for urinary incontinence must not be thought of as isolated procedures. Restorative surgery to structures to promote urinary continence, for example, will change directions of force vectors to the remaining pelvic floor so that a slight deficiency in another compartment existing at the time of the urinary incontinence surgery may well become a marked deficiency postoperatively, necessitating further surgery. More than 15% of patients having anterior urethropexy develop posterior compartment deficiency, and subsequently present with enterocele, rectocele, and vaginal vault prolapses.[1] Fig. 11D2-1 depicts the area of the cul-de-sac as seen with defecography and simultaneous vaginal opacification before (A), and after (B) anterior urethropexy. The area of the cul-de-sac is markedly increased in this patient, with clinically normal pelvic findings. In patients with defects already present posteriorly, the resultant defect is even more pronounced.

The entire pelvic floor function must be thoroughly investigated before a choice of surgical procedure for incontinence is made. Such investigation and application of the necessary surgical procedures to correct the patient's particular constellation of defects can reduce the number of subsequent surgeries the patient requires. To help identify the various pelvic floor defects, a system of defect recognition such as Baden and Walker's[2] may be used. The pelvic surgeon must be able to perform various types of urinary incontinence surgical procedures and to recognize the most appropriate surgeries for each particular set of pelvic floor problems. This chapter, after outlining an historical review of surgery for female urinary incontinence, defines modern anatomical considerations, mechanisms of successful surgery, and causes of surgical failure. Descriptions of abdominal retropubic cystourethropexies, transvaginal cystourethropexies, and urethral vesical sling procedures will follow.

HISTORICAL OVERVIEW OF SURGERY FOR FEMALE URINARY INCONTINENCE

J. Marion Sims must be mentioned as the "father" of surgery for urinary incontinence. In the middle 1800s, incontinence from obstetrically induced vesicovaginal fistula was considered surgically incurable. Dr. Sims

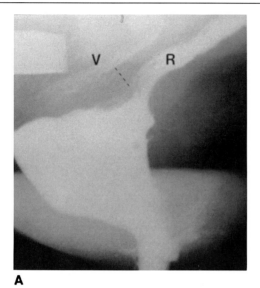 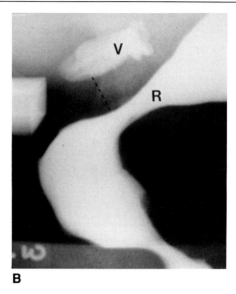

A   B

Fig. 11D2-1   **A**, Defecography with vaginal opacification before, and **B**, after anterior urethropexy. The increased distance of cul-de-sac between the vagina and rectum (*dashed lines*) signals an increased potential for enterocele development. *V* = vagina; *R* = rectum.

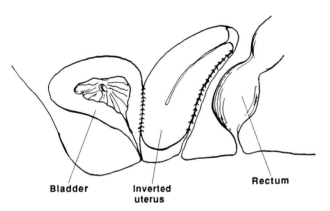

Bladder   Inverted   Rectum
                    uterus

Fig. 11D2-2   Watkins interposition operation. The bladder is elevated by the interposed uterus. Note the inverted uterus is stitched to the bladder and posterior vaginal wall.

incontinence began appearing in the late 1800s. Watkins[4] described his interposition operation before the Chicago Gynecological Society in September 1899. In this operation the bladder is supported by and rested upon the posterior wall of the uterus (Fig. 11D2-2). Donald[5] described the "Manchester Procedure" in the early 1900s, in which the bladder neck is elevated with an anterior colporrhaphy and the cardinal ligaments are attached to the anterior surface of the partially amputated cervix (Fig. 11D2-3). Near this same time,

Fig. 11D2-3   Manchester procedure. The cervical isthmus is preserved for augmented upper vaginal support. The cervix is amputated and the cardinal ligaments are brought to an anterior location.

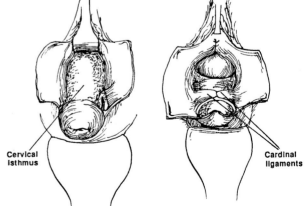

Cervical   **Cardinal**
Isthmus   **ligaments**

accidently realized how the fistulae could be approached from viewing the patient in the knee-chest, or "Sims" position, using a posterior retractor, the "Sims' speculum." His excitement in this approach was reflected in his writing as follows:

I thought only of relieving the loveliest of all God's creation of one of the most loathsome maladies that can possibly befall poor human nature . . . full of sympathy and enthusiasm, thus all at once I found myself running headlong after the very class of sufferers that I had all of my professional life most studiously avoided.[3]

Effective surgical correction for nonfistulous urinary

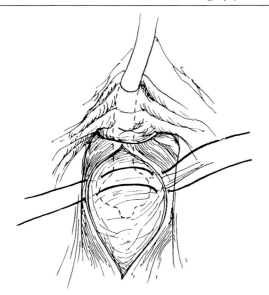

Fig. 11D2-4   The classic Kelly plication stitch.

Goebell[6] performed the earliest successful urethrovesical sling operation using the pyramidalis muscle, first in a child with myelomeningocele and hypospadias, and later in an adult.

In 1913, Howard Kelly[7] published a paper describing the Kelly plication in association with anterior colporrhaphy (Fig. 11D2-4) and this was subsequently modified by Kennedy. Shortly thereafter, sling operations became common. Stoeckel[8] reported the use of the pyramidalis muscle and sphincter plication in 1917. The use of fascia lata for this procedure was originally suggested by Price in 1933.[9] In 1942 Aldridge[10] combined some of the points of his various predecessors and developed strips of aponeurosis from the rectus sheath, which pass through the rectus muscle retropubically to encircle the urethra.

Throughout the remaining first half of this century, the Kelly-Kennedy plication became a standard therapy for the woman with stress urinary incontinence. There were many surgical failures which were then treated by one of the sling operations, until a new era was born following the efforts of Dr. Victor Marshall.

In 1946, Marshall corrected incontinence in a man who developed the symptom following transurethral prostatectomy after abdominal perineal resection of the rectum for carcinoma. Continence was restored with a retropubic urethrovesicopexy by attaching the bladder neck high on the back of the symphysis pubis. Marshall collaborated with Drs. Marchetti and Krantz to develop a remarkably effective similar procedure for treatment

of women with urinary incontinence.[11] The standard anti-incontinence surgery through the 1950s was one of operating vaginally first with anterior colporrhaphy and Kelly-Kennedy plication and, if that procedure failed, subjecting the patient to an abdominal repair using the Marshall-Marchetti-Krantz procedure.

In the 1960s, attempts were made to select patients who could more properly be treated with the abdominal procedure first. Prevalent at that time was the concept that constricting the urethra by making a more acute posterior urethrovesical angle was the mechanism by which continence was restored. Hodgkinson[12] and Green[13] developed preoperative criteria based on the posterior urethrovesical angle and the axis of inclination of the urethra to differentiate patients into "Type 1" and "Type 2" urinary incontinence. The suggestion was made by Green that Type 1 patients should be operated vaginally and Type 2 patients operated abdominally (Fig. 11D2-5).

Various modifications of the Marshall-Marchetti-Krantz procedure were developed because of the occasional complication of osteitis pubis resulting from placing sutures into the pubic bone. One widely used modification devised by Burch[14] suspended the periurethral tissue and bladder neck to Cooper's ligament. In the 1970s Tanagho[15] modified the Burch procedure by advocating no dissection within two centimeters of the urethra or vesical neck and removing the fatty tissue lateral to this area to stimulate fibrosis. He also carefully avoided unnecessary tension on the sutures to Cooper's ligament. The Tanagho modification of the Burch colposuspension is widely used today.

The physiologic principle that elevation of the urethrovesical junction allows transference of abdominal pressure to the urethra was established in 1961 by En-

Fig. 11D2-5   Classification of patients with stress urinary incontinence. Type 1 patients show a vertical axis of urethral inclination; Type 2 patients show a more horizontal axis of urethral inclination.

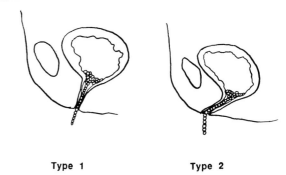

Type 1   Type 2

horning.[16] For the first time it was recognized that urinary loss associated with a sudden rise of intraabdominal pressure was due partly to lack of transmission of that increased force to the urethra. Operations were then designed more to elevate the urethrovesical junction to a level allowing transmission of abdominal forces to the urethra rather than concentrating on urethrovesical angles, opening the way for development of needle procedures.

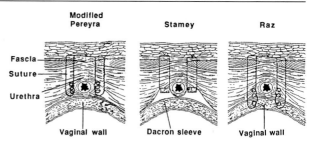

Fig. 11D2-6 Schematic representation of the mechanics of the modified Pereyra, Stamey, and Raz needle urethropexies.

NEEDLE PROCEDURES

Having observed that retropubic elevation of the urethrovesical junction was an effective means of treating urinary incontinence, a vaginal approach to the problem was developed by Pereyra in 1959.[17] In Pereyra's original description, wire sutures elevated the paraurethral tissue on each side of the bladder neck to the anterior rectus fascia. A specially devised needle was advanced through the abdominal fascia of the rectus muscle into the retropubic space, keeping the needle in contact with the posterior aspect of the pubic bone. An inner cannula and trocar were components of the needle so that when each was advanced, a paraurethral loop of wire would be placed in the vagina. These two wires were then tied together above the rectus fascia.

Pereyra and Lebherz's[18] first modification of the procedure consisted of combining bladder neck plication with the vaginal urethropexy and was prompted by failures occurring when the wire loop eventually cut through the anterior vaginal wall. A second modification[19] resulted in exposing the space of Retzius completely transvaginally so that each step of the operation could be performed under direct vision or palpation. Thus, the first description of entering the retropubic space through the vagina was made by Pereyra. His last revision[20] consisted of passing helical sutures through the paraurethral tissues before suspending the sutures abdominally.

Stamey[21] modified Pereyra's procedure by utilizing the cystoscope while placing heavy monofilament sutures on each side of the vesical neck. He used two separate one-inch transverse incisions on each side of the midline abdominally and a T-shaped vaginal incision beneath the urethra and trigone, passing the needle twice on each side. The vaginal end of the suture is threaded through a broad band of tissue along the vesical neck, and if the tissue quality is poor, the nylon suture is passed through a one centimeter length of a netted dacron arterial graft used to buttress the vaginal loop.

In 1981, Raz[22] modified the procedure by using an inverted U-incision in the vagina to allow the vaginal dissection to be lateral to the urethra and bladder neck. The suspension sutures were anchored laterally in whatever tissue was available. Although called the endopelvic fascia, the tissue is comprised of musculature and fascial vaginal attachment tissue or portions of the musculature components of the compressor urethrae and urethrovaginal sphincter (urogenital diaphragm) in conjunction with the fibromuscular layer of the vaginal wall.[23] Again, the use of cystourethroscopy is mandatory because permanent sutures are placed with this procedure. (Fig. 11D2-6)

In 1987, Gittes[24] modified Pereyra's procedure using no suprapubic incision other than two stab wounds and no vaginal incision. Thus, his procedure is similar to the original Pereyra procedure, the choice of suture material being the main difference. This procedure is now being used as an adjunct to other pelvic floor surgery.[25]

In 1987, Karram and Bhatia[26] described a needle vaginal approach for placing a patch of fascia lata to support the bladder base and urethra. In a similar procedure described by Raz, a portion of the vaginal wall itself is used as a patch which is suspended by four permanent monofilament sutures to the anterior abdominal wall.

Paravaginal repairs are being widely advocated today as therapy for stress incontinence. These procedures are more anatomically reconstructive, and although old, they are recently becoming popular again (see Chapter 12).

ANATOMIC CONSIDERATIONS

To the surgeon beginning to perform these procedures, understanding of the pelvic floor anatomy is complicated by different descriptions of the urethral supporting mechanisms.

A significant step forward in clarifying the anatomy of this area was made by Krantz[27] in his prize thesis at the American Association of Obstetricians and Gynecologists and Abdominal Surgeons Meeting in 1950. In his thesis Krantz defined the bladder and urethra as a functioning unit which is likened to a lever system of the first class—the bladder at one end and the external urethral meatus at the other—while the pubo-prostatic ligament acts as the fulcrum. Krantz also further developed concepts of paraurethral anatomy by describing the distal urethra as having muscle groups surrounding both the urethra and the vagina, and in fact he found the urethra to be inseparable from the vagina in this distal location.

Milley and Nichols[28] extended the description of the pubo-prostatic ligaments suggesting they be called pubourethral ligaments. They proposed that the anterior and posterior ligaments were formed by reflections of the inferior and superior fascial layers of the urogenital diaphragm.

Terms such as pubourethral ligament, pubourethroprostatic ligament, endopelvic fascia, urogenital diaphragm, deep transverse perineal muscle, cervical-vaginal fascia, and others were used by surgeons to describe this area in confusing and conflicting ways. The work of DeLancey[29,30] has since helped clarify the pelvic floor anatomy for the surgeon (see Chapter 2). In the distal components of the urethra as shown in Fig. 11D2-7, there is, as Krantz indicated, muscle tissue which surrounds both the urethra and the vagina and is properly called the urethrovaginal sphincter. This inserts into the perineal body and, in conjunction with the compressor urethrae, exerts a somewhat posterior force in this portion of the vagina. This musculature, previously referred to as the deep transverse perineal muscle, comprises a significant portion of the area referred to as the urogenital diaphragm. Combined with the striated muscle surrounding most of the urethra in the same region, it is found to be the area of greatest transference of pressure from the abdomen to the urethra. The urethra is relatively fixed here, forming a urethral "knee" above which there is more mobility to the urethra which can be voluntarily elevated to a more anterior position. There is more muscular tissue located anterior to the urethra than posterior, opposite to the concept underlying vaginal sphincter plication surgery.

The more superior attachments illustrated in Fig. 11D2-8 are based on studies above the vesical neck. The urethra is supported by vaginal wall attachments of both fascial and muscular nature. The fascial attachments extend to the arcus tendineus fasciae pelvis and the muscular attachments extend to the superior fascia

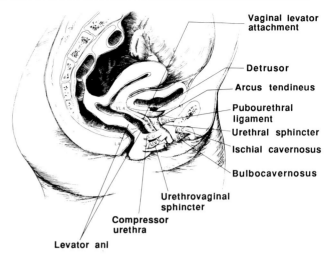

Fig. 11D2-7 Urethral supports. Reprinted with permission from The American College of Obstetricians and Gynecologists (*Obstet Gynecol* 1988; 72:296).

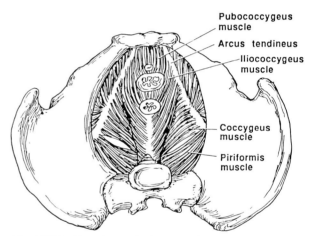

Fig. 11D2-8 Superior urethral structural supports.

of the pelvic diaphragm. The attachment to the fascia of the pelvic diaphragm is actually near the origin of the iliococcygeus muscle from the obturator internus fascia, the so-called arcus tendineus levator ani.

Urethral support can be thought of diagrammatically as having a spatial distribution of paraurethral structures (Fig. 11D2-9). The structures in the most superior portion of the urethra act voluntarily to elevate this area toward the symphysis. Muscles at the urogenital diaphragm represent the highest concentration of fast twitch muscle fibers to augment pressure transmission here. This is also the area where voluntary squeeze has the most effect on stopping urinary flow in the urethra.

In surgery for urinary incontinence, the area immediately lateral to the urethra, just inferior to the bladder, represents an angle where safe penetration can be made

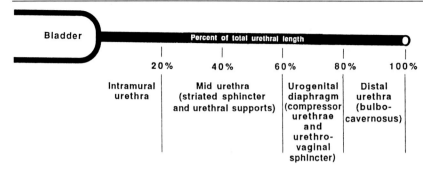

Fig. 11D2-9 DeLancey's concept of the spatial distribution of urethral support. Reprinted with permission from The American College of Obstetricians and Gynecologists (*Obstet Gynecol* 1988;72:-296).

to the space of Retzius. When vaginal tissue is incised here and the urethra and bladder reflected from the vaginal tissues, the remaining substance is principally the muscular wall of the vagina. Overlying endopelvic fascia is tissue of an areolar nature described by the anatomist and not useful in surgical support. Therefore, the fascia used by surgeons is more properly termed the "muscularis" of the vagina or the "fibromuscular" layer of the vagina. The strength of this tissue is quite variable, with many females having portions of the compressor urethrae and urethral-vaginal sphincter (urogenital diaphragm area) more developed. Sharp dissection is occasionally required to enter the space of Retzius from this area, although in many women, blunt dissection achieves penetration easily. Whether operating from above with an abdominal retropubic urethropexy or from below with a vaginal retropubic urethropexy, the same structures are encountered.

Understanding the paraurethral supports to the levator ani musculature (pelvic diaphragm) enables one to appreciate the dynamic effects of urethral closure. The levator ani dynamics are effected by both posterior and anterior groups of muscles. The posterior groups arise primarily from obturator fascia (the arcus tendineus of the levator ani group) and perform a diaphragmatic role. The anterior group arises from the symphysis pubis and is termed the pubovisceral muscles. The group of muscles act to dynamically support the viscera, and by active contraction draw the viscera upward and forward. These pubovisceral muscles are divided into pubourethralis, pubovaginalis, and puborectalis, which function to draw the urethra, vagina, and upper anal canal forward. By the attachment of their sling fibers through the levator plate and the perineal body, they help close the urethra, vagina, and anal canal.

The levator ani contains mostly type I (slow twitch) fibers acting in a tonic fashion, but type II (fast twitch) fibers are also present. Type II fibers act reflexly with sudden increases in muscle contraction and are more prevalent in the anterior (pubovisceral) levator, and

more in the perianal region than in the periurethral region.

Nerve supply to this region is important for the pelvic surgeon to understand. As depicted by Ingleman-Sundberg,[31] the infravesical nerves (inferior hypogastric plexus) are located in the coronal planes between the bladder floor and the levator ani (Figs. 11D2-10 and 11D2-11). Operations in this area should avoid the abundant nerve supply as much as possible so as not to alter bladder function secondary to nerve disruption. This consideration is not only important in urethropexy procedures but may also impact hysterectomy. Intrafascial and extrafascial hysterectomies may result in different nerve disruption (Fig. 11D2-12). Nerve fibers were demonstrated in regions lateral to the cervix and in the vesical vaginal septum where bundles of nerves occupy a mid-position between the vaginal and bladder mucosa. The neuroanatomy of this region is important not only in surgery, but as indicated in Chapter 9, also in the etiology of urinary incontinence.

MECHANISMS OF SUCCESSFUL SURGERY

The predominant pathophysiology of genuine stress urinary incontinence is sphincteric insufficiency. Evidence of a neurogenic origin as outlined in Chapter 9 is quite impressive. The classic urodynamic finding is that in association with a rise in intraabdominal pressure, pressure within the bladder exceeds the maximum within the urethra in the absence of detrusor contractions. The sphincteric insufficiency is, for the most part, secondary to abnormal urethral-trigonal anatomy characterized by increased mobility of the urethra as measured by a cotton tip, x-ray, or ultrasound. In fact, the patient most likely to be cured by urethropexy is one in whom the bladder neck distance from the pubic symphysis is horizontally greater at rest and moves toward the symphysis with straining. The best chance of surgi-

Fig. 11D2-10 Left hemipelvis revealing the inferior hypogastric nerve plexus.

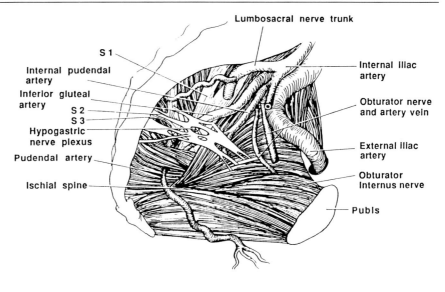

Fig. 11D2-11 Vaginal approach relationship to the inferior hypogastric nerve plexus.

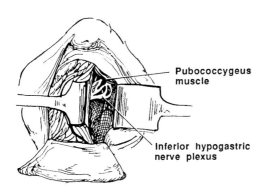

Fig. 11D2-12 Differing planes in intrafascial and extrafascial hysterectomies.

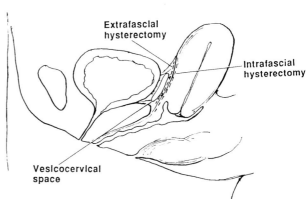

cal cure is with the first operation and surgical success is highly correlated with a postoperative decrease in bladder neck mobility, especially in the horizontal plane excursion.

Closure pressure is another factor in female incontinence. This pressure is created by a combination of the "sponge" effect of the submucosa vascular plexus (markedly affected by estrogen) and by pressures generated by smooth and skeletal musculature. This measurable parameter is, to a large degree, not affected by urethropexy. The sling procedures, on the other hand, do increase the closure pressure.

Urethral length is important in continence from both an anatomic and functional standpoint. While urethropexy may correct some funneling ("vesicalization" of the proximal urethra) and thereby indirectly increase urethral length, its general effect on urethral length is negligible.

The anatomic position of the urethrovesical junction is of extreme importance. When located retropubically, sudden changes in intraabdominal pressure are better transmitted to the intraabdominally located proximal urethra. Where a reflex component is significant the reflexes may thus be improved. The bladder to urethral pressure transmission ratio is markedly affected by urethropexy. Transmission ratios approaching 100% are ideal, as are present in normal continent females. Ratios significantly lower than 100% result in failed procedures, whereas ratios significantly higher may result in a degree of obstruction with a consequent increase in bladder instability. Abdominal urethropexies tend to show stabilization of the bladder neck in patients who are cured by the procedure. This finding is not reflected in vaginal urethropexy patients. More than half of the patients who are objectively and subjectively cured with vaginal urethropexy still have increased mobility as measured by the Q-Tip test.[32] The mechanism for continence with the vaginal procedure may then be other than stabilization of the bladder neck during stress. Beck and coworkers[33] suggested a urethral "kinking" effect with increasing resting intraurethral pressure, which may be a significant mechanism in both vaginal colporrhaphy and vaginal urethropexy procedures.

The bladder's most dependent portion should also be considered preoperatively. When the most dependent portion of the bladder is the bladder neck, all intraabdominal pressure forces are transmitted there directly. Proper surgical correction elevates the bladder neck so that the most dependent portion of the bladder becomes posterior to the urethrovesical junction, enabling forces to act posterior to, rather than on, the urethrovesical junction. This function may be measured by cystogram, videocystourethrography, or ultrasound.

Urethropexy is recognized as having an effect on bladder instability. It is postulated that creating an element of obstruction may increase a predisposition toward abnormal detrusor contractions. When the pressure transmission ratio is increased considerably over 100%, preexisting bladder instability may be increased in amount, or bladder instability not recognized preoperatively may appear subsequent to the surgery (de novo instability).[34] Conversely, bladder instability may be improved by urethropexy. McGuire and coworkers[35] suggested that the ability to surgically improve detrusor instability varies inversely with the degree of anatomic defect present. Bergman and colleagues[36] found that when doing preoperative cystourethrometrics, the group of patients whose detrusor instability was preceded by urethral relaxation was improved by medical or surgical management which stabilized the urethra. In patients with both genuine stress urinary incontinence and detrusor instability, preoperative cystourethrometrics may help forecast the surgical impact on detrusor instability.

CAUSES OF SURGICAL FAILURE

A prospective randomized study comparing surgical procedures for genuine stress incontinence has long been needed. Bergman and others[32] presented such a study using the same group of operators, suture types, and objective follow-up of the patients. In a comparison of 107 patients randomly operated with anterior colporrhaphy, revised Pereyra procedure, or Burch retropubic urethropexy, the three-month cure rates were 82%, 84%, and 92%, respectively, and the differences were statistically insignificant. However, at one year the

cure rates were 65%, 72%, and 91%. Failures in all three groups occurred mainly in patients with preoperative low urethral pressure (resting maximal urethral closing pressure of less than 20 cm/H_2O on urethral pressure profile performed in the supine position and at maximal cystometric capacity), a finding repeatedly documented by many investigators.[37–39]

Patient selection is an important element of cure. Diagnosis of surgically correctable conditions prior to operating is necessary. Patients with bladder instability should be treated medically first, as the need for surgery may be diminished when medical management, bladder training, and biofeedback are utilized (see Chapter 11C). When the patient is cured of the symptom of stress incontinence, but urgency and urge incontinence replace it, the patient is not pleased and the surgery is a failure. Hence, "de novo" detrusor instability may occur. It is particularly likely to occur with retropubic urethropexy wherein the bladder neck is lifted to higher levels than normal. Iatrogenic bladder instability also may be related to anterior colporrhaphy and hysterectomy and, at present, we are performing prospective studies to more carefully evaluate this.

The improper selection of surgical procedure is a cause of failure. The concept still exists that only when a standard urethropexy fails should a sling procedure be performed. It is becoming evident, however, that in patients with low urethral pressures, the sling procedure may properly be chosen as the primary procedure. Patients with both decreased bladder neck mobility and low urethral pressure may need another modality of therapy (see Chapter 11D1).

Another cause for surgical failure is improper location of the sutures. If the sutures are located above the urethrovesical junction, then suspension of the anterior portion of the bladder to the symphysis may occur without proper suspension of the urethra, and symptoms may actually increase. With sutures placed too far distally, obstructive phenomena may occur. Sutures placed too close to the urethra and involving the adventitia may produce paraurethral scarring, prohibiting elevation of the bladder neck.

Sutures placed into the muscularis of the urethra may later migrate through the urethral epithelium or bladder epithelium. Thus, any tenting effect of permanently placed sutures must be checked by cystourethroscopy at the time of the procedure. Should a movable tenting effect be observed, the sutures should be removed.

Transient urine retention lasting days to weeks is common with these procedures. If retention is prolonged, when does it become necessary to revise a procedure? For the most part, time is an ally and treatment with self-catheterization should be employed for at least 4 to 6 months. If symptoms still persist, an instrumented voiding study may be utilized to determine maximum detrusor pressure in centimeters of water and maximum urinary flow. The study should be repeated at least twice on separate occasions for consistency. Following a formula for urethral obstruction,[4] if the detrusor pressure divided by the flow rate squared is equal to or less than 0.25, there is probably not a significant obstructive element. Should this ratio be higher, obstruction should be considered and carefully selected patients may require "take down" procedures and replacement of the sutures. A vaginal approach under careful endoscopic control with complete lysis of adhesions and replacement by modified Pereyra procedure sutures is the preferred surgery.

Surgical Procedures

Anti-incontinence operations fall into three broad groups: abdominal retropubic cystourethropexies, transvaginal cystourethropexies, and urethrovesical sling procedures.

The paravaginal repair, either abdominal (Chapter 12A) or vaginal (Chapter 12B), has the advantage over other anti-incontinence surgeries of restoring normal anatomy, whereas the urethropexy procedures and slings overcorrect the defects. Because of this, postoperative voiding difficulties are more common with urethropexy than with paravaginal repairs. If long-term objective clinical cure of incontinence could be accomplished as well by restoring normal anatomy (paravaginal repair) as by obstructing (urethropexy), then this would be the preferred procedure. At this time, prospective randomized studies with long-term, objective follow-up are not available to answer this question.

The theoretical answer to this question depends on the etiology of the incontinence. If the incontinence is caused by a structural defect alone, such as a tear in the urethral support, then restoring normal musculofascial anatomy (paravaginal repair) would restore normal function (placing normal urethra in normal location). However, if there is a significant neuropathy present, restoring normal musculofascial anatomy may not be effective over long periods of time, because the defective urethral musculature does not have normal function (placing abnormal urethra in normal location). Therefore, overcorrection (e.g., urethropexy, sling, etc.) may be necessary to cure the incontinence, although necessitating the attendant voiding dysfunction. We are currently studying procedure selection based on the extent of preexisting neuropathy.

Abdominal Retropubic Cystourethropexy

The following description is the surgical procedure of choice for patients with genuine stress urinary incontinence, deficient pressure transmission ratios, increased bladder neck mobility (especially in the horizontal axis), normal urethral closing pressure, and the urethral egress at the bladder's most dependent portion. Other candidates may include those with a mixed pattern of unstable bladder and genuine stress urinary incontinence when medical management has not produced a satisfactory response, and especially when cystourethrometric studies show urethral pressure changes preceding bladder contractions.

The patient is placed in universal stirrups or in a frog-leg position and a Foley catheter is inserted to aid in identification of the vesical neck during surgery. The knees must be carefully supported in the frog position to prevent damage to the peroneal nerve. It is important that assistants not put pressure on the patient's legs in this position. The preferred incision is a Pfannenstiel type of transverse incision. A midline incision may be made in patients who have had them previously.

The space of Retzius is identified next (Fig. 11D2-13). A Balfour retractor is placed with the anterior blade directed posteriorly. Special landmarks of the space of Retzius which must be avoided are the obturator canal, obturator nerve, and obturator vessels. No dissection occurs near the urethra, and in fact, the complete avoidance of the area between the symphysis and the urethra with hand or instrument should be practiced. Going beyond 2 cm lateral to each side, fatty tissue is removed from the retropubic area. With the surgeon's nondominant hand in the vagina, the bladder is retracted medially until the white tissue of the muscularis of the vagina is identified. Lateral parts of the retropubic area are mobilized down to the muscularis of the vagina, again avoiding the area within 2 cm of the midline (Fig. 11D2-14).

Three sutures are placed with the preferred 0 polypropylene material. The first suture is at the ure-

Fig. 11D2-13 Space of Retzius.

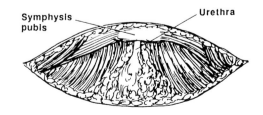

Symphysis pubis   Urethra

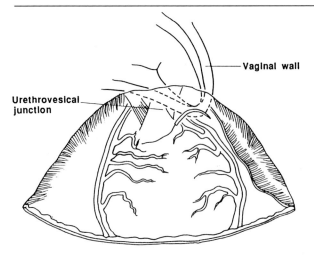

Fig. 11D2-14 Space of Retzius. The surgeon's finger, placed vaginally, is uplifting the vaginal wall lateral to the urethrovesical junction.

throvesical junction 2 cm from the midline with the vaginal finger placed in the lateral vaginal fornix. A mattress suture is placed through the vaginal wall's full thickness except the epithelium. The suture is then brought up to Cooper's ligament. A second suture is placed lateral to the first, and the third suture placed immediately inferior to the two preceding sutures. If there is a cystocele with lateral defects, further supporting sutures to the arcus tendineus are placed (see Chapter 12A). Then with the vaginal hand supporting the urethra and the table placed horizontally (as measured by a level), a cotton-tip applicator placed in the urethra is brought up to 0° (level). With the sutures held in this position, a similar procedure is carried out on the opposite side. The bladder is filled to 250 ml and, with the urethra at 0°, pressure on the bladder is firmly and sharply produced while the urethral meatus is observed for leakage. If there is leakage, the sutures are brought up until it stops, and goniometer measurement of the urethral axis is taken. Usually, the urethral axis is deviated less than 15° from the horizontal when continence is achieved.

The sutures anchored through Cooper's ligament are now tied. Almost invariably there is a distance between the Cooper's ligament and the vaginal wall, so that there is a "bow-string" effect on the sutures. (The sutures are *not* tied tightly.) Removing the fatty tissue in this area earlier in the procedure allows approximation of the tissues and subsequent adherence. Obstruction of the ureter occurs in approximately 1% of patients having anterior urethropexies.[40] Therefore, on ascertaining

that the patient is continent, indigo carmine is given intravenously. The bladder is either opened in the midline a distance of 3 to 4 cm and narrow retractors are placed, or suprapubic cystoscopy is used, passing the scope through the bladder fundus. The bladder walls are carefully visualized to ensure that the sutures are safely placed and the ureters are functioning bilaterally. The bladder incision is then closed in a two-layer technique using 3-0 chromic suture in a running continuous manner with the second layer inverting the first layer. If only suprapubic cystoscopy is performed, the opening is closed in a single purse-string absorbable suture. A suprapubic catheter is placed before the closure is completed. The suprapubic catheter remains postoperatively until the patient is voiding consistently with low residual urine (less than 100 cc).

Associated pelvic floor defects must be preoperatively recognized and simultaneously corrected, because after abdominal urethropexy, anterior fixation of pelvic floor structures leads to increased stresses on the middle and posterior compartments.

The question of whether coincident hysterectomy is necessary frequently arises. As a policy, a hysterectomy is not performed for the surgical treatment of genuine stress urinary incontinence unless there is a gynecologic reason. Posterior deficit or tendency toward enterocele is considered a gynecologic indication for pelvic floor restorative surgery, which often includes hysterectomy.

Anterior Colporrhaphy

Anterior colporrhaphy is no longer used in our institution as surgical management of genuine stress urinary incontinence. The technique is still employed, however, to reduce funnelling of the proximal urethra when it exists. In these cases, a standard Kelly-Kennedy plication maneuver is performed in conjunction with standard anterior colporrhaphy. Correction of a cystocele involves correcting lateral defects as well as central defects and is discussed in Chapter 12.

Transvaginal Cystourethropexies

Although compared to abdominal urethropexy, vaginal procedures have higher failure rates, vaginal urethrovesical suspension procedures are quicker than conventional abdominal retropubic procedures and may have somewhat reduced operative and postoperative morbidity. It is certainly the procedure of choice when revising previous urethropexy. The vaginal approach is easier and ultimately has less morbidity than an abdominal approach through the space of Retzius in patients previously operated in this area, because of the remarkable fibrosis that occurs. In conjunction with other pelvic floor procedures, the vaginal approach may be well chosen. In particular, the vaginal needle procedures are valuable for prophylaxis against urinary incontinence. Patients with vault prolapses, and others whose urodynamic evaluations reveal decreased pressure transference or positive standing stress test, with the viscera elevated to the desired postoperative state, are excellent candidates for vaginal urethropexy to prevent the occurrence of "hidden" stress incontinence, which may develop following a pelvic floor restorative surgery.

The vaginal urethropexy operation of choice at our institution is modification of the Pereyra procedure. The patient is placed in lithotomy position with proper leg placement. Marking sutures are placed at least 2 cm lateral to the urethra at the urethrovesical junction, as determined by the bulb of a Foley catheter. Following this, an inverted "U" (Fig. 11D2-15) is drawn on the vagina to mark the lines of incision. (Current neurologic studies are underway to see if this type of vaginal incision produces more neuropathy than separate lateral incisions.) The apex of the inverted U is approximately halfway between the identified urethrovesical junction and the urethral meatus. The limbs of the U extend at least 4 cm. The tissue is injected with saline and the incision made. At this point there is a spreading

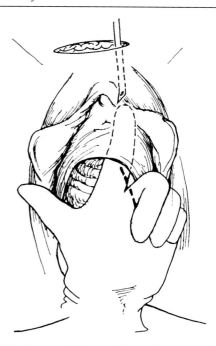

Fig. 11D2-16   Surgeon's finger guiding a Pereyra needle from the suprapubic to the vaginal location during a modified Pereyra procedure.

Fig. 11D2-15   Inverted "U" incision in the vaginal wall during a vaginal urethropexy operation.

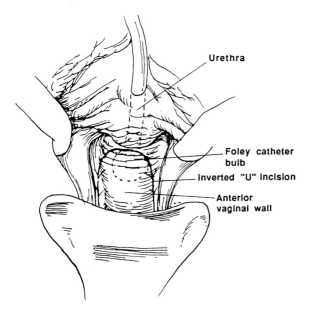

Urethra

Foley catheter bulb

Inverted "U" incision

Anterior vaginal wall

of this tissue, which is actually the muscularis of the vagina. It is identified by shininess and a relative lack of hemorrhage. Scissor dissection is used to extend this tissue, and on each side of the urethra, retropubically using either blunt or sharp dissection, the tissue in this area is penetrated staying close to the symphysis so that the finger enters the space of Retzius. The finger never goes medially, overlying the area of the urethra, but instead moves laterally to the lateral urethral support area. An abdominal incision is made transversely, approximately two finger widths above the symphysis, and passage with a Pereyra needle is made from the suprapubic to the vaginal position with the fingertip held against and guiding the needle (Fig. 11D2-16). A suture of 0 polypropylene that has been sewn in a helical fashion into the submucosa of the vagina, the muscularis of the vagina, and the urethral support tissue, is then brought by the needle to the abdominal location. The same procedure is carried out on the opposite side. The operating table is then placed perfectly level and a goniometer with a level at the lower end is used to determine the degree of angulation of the urethra. A Q-Tip is placed in the urethra for this purpose. The sutures are then elevated to a point bringing the urethral axis to 0°. (Fig. 11D2-17). The bladder is filled with 250 ml of sterile saline and a thrusting maneuver is exerted

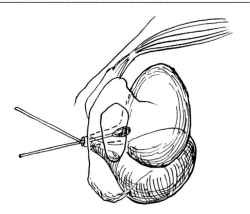

Fig. 11D2-17 Cotton tip in urethra. Deflection from the horizontal may be measured with goniometry.

to the abdominal wall overlying the bladder to test for continence. Thorough urethrocystoscopy is carried out with 0° and 70° cystourethroscopes prior to tying the sutures and testing the bladder for continence. Indigo carmine is given to the patient intravenously, and after tying the sutures both ureters are visualized with the 70° scope to ensure bilateral functioning. The vaginal incision is closed with a running 00 polyglactin suture. The 0° scope ensures that the elevation of the sutures closes the urethrovesical junction and that the sutures are placed neither too far proximal nor distal to that junction. A suprapubic catheter is then placed.

The Gittes procedure can be used alone as a relatively minor surgical procedure or it can be used as an adjunct to other pelvic floor surgery, which is the more common usage. A number 11 knife blade is used to make two stab incisions approximately 4 cm lateral to the midline overlying the symphysis. The Pereyra needle is placed through the rectus fascia in opposition to the posterior aspect of the pubic symphysis and, with a Foley catheter in place and the urethrovesical junction identified by the vaginal fingers, the urethrovesical junction is elevated and the Pereyra needle passed through the vaginal mucosa. A helical stitch is taken through the entire thickness of the vaginal wall in mattress fashion and delivered abdominally with the needle passage. The Pereyra needle is again introduced through the same stab wound abdominally, and after it is through the skin, it is moved at least 2 cm laterally, passed again through the rectus fascia, and delivered to the vagina at the area of the helical stitch. The other end of the helical stitch is then delivered abdominally. The procedure is repeated on the opposite side. Examination with a 0° cystourethroscope is performed to check that there are

no sutures in the urethra or bladder, then elevation of the urethral axis to 0° is carried out while the patient is tested for continence. A 70° scope is used to ensure ureteral function. The sutures are then tied at the abdominal location and the skin pulled up over the tie. All polypropylene sutures are secured with liga clips to prevent the knot's untieing. Long-term results with this procedure, very similar to the original Pereyra procedure, may result in unacceptably high failure rates because suture-tissue surface scarring is the underlying mechanism.

Sling Procedure

The use of abdominal rectus fascia, fascia lata, dura, and synthetic materials each have many advocates. Our preference for sling material is abdominal rectus fascia if healthy tissue is available and no previous surgery was performed at the site. Otherwise, fascia lata is used, or Gortex may be chosen if the patient has had no previous surgery at the urethral-vesical location. Frequently, the strip of fascia is cut in the midline to within 2 cm of the end of the strip, resulting in two limbs with the junction of the two ends used for the urethral location (Fig. 11D2-18). Operating vaginally, the urethrovesical junction is opened as in the vaginal urethropexy procedure, and the space of Retzius is entered.

Fig. 11D2-18 Method of elongating the fascial strip for the pubovaginal sling. **A**, The fascial strip is split through most of its length. **B**, The unsplit portion is anchored beneath the urethra.

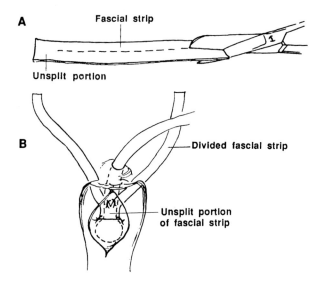

sewn over the rectus fascia with several interrupted permanent sutures.

All patients having sling procedures are taught self-catheterization prior to the surgery, as prolonged time to satisfactory bladder emptying is common.

Vaginal Sling

The vaginal sling as suggested by Raz has been used successfully. This procedure is similar to the above described vaginal urethropexy except that a strip of vagina is left intact (Fig. 11D2-20). This vaginal strip is located just beneath the urethrovesical junction and extends distally over the proximal urethra for a distance of at least 2 cm. The four corners of the vaginal strip are sewn with permanent polypropylene sutures which are then delivered abdominally, elevating the vaginal bridge of tissue in a sling-like manner. The vagina is closed over this bridge of vaginal tissue, thus creating a sling or "patch" composed of full thickness vaginal wall which is not disrupted from its normal anatomic relationship to the urethra.

Vaginal urethropexy procedures produce an anterior focus to the pelvic floor, just as abdominal urethropexy procedures do. Unrecognized or minimal posterior compartment deficits can become exaggerated if not treated simultaneously. Again, the need for careful consideration of the entire pelvic floor when doing reconstructive surgery of any one component is emphasized.

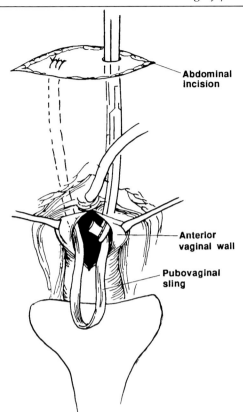

Fig. 11D2-19 Delivery of the pubovaginal sling to retropubic position.

An abdominal incision is made and a long Kelly-type clamp is passed. The sling is then delivered abdominally (Fig. 11D2-19) on both sides going through the rectus fascia. It is sewn beneath the urethra at the urethrovesical junction to include the proximal urethra for at least 2 cm and sewn in place with absorbable suture. The bladder is then examined with a 0° cystourethroscope to verify bladder integrity, the table is leveled and the sling is elevated to approximate a 0° urethral axis. A lower elevation is used if continence is obtained on testing with suprapubic thrust to the bladder filled with 300 ml of fluid. It is important not to elevate beyond 0° with a sling procedure. The abdominal ends of the sling are anchored to the rectus fascia with permanent sutures. Unlike a urethropexy, when the patient increases intraabdominal pressure, there is a direct "pull" which elevates the urethrovesical junction. Thus, elevating beyond 0° is not necessary for relief of stress incontinence and may cause obstruction. Direct visualization of the urethrovesical junction is done at this elevation. Examination with a 70° scope is then carried out to check ureteral function, and the fascial graft is

Fig. 11D2-20 The Raz vaginal sling procedure. The inverted "U" incision is transected at *A-A*, submerged and used as the sling, and overcovered by approximating *A-B*. The vaginal portion is used for the vaginal pubovaginal sling.

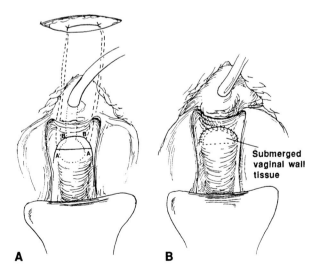

SUMMARY

Anti-incontinence surgical procedures have provided relief to many, but should not be considered the only method of therapy. Cure rates for anti-incontinence procedures tend to give an overly optimistic picture of efficacy because they focus on the symptom of stress incontinence and frequently are subjective in nature. Long-term objective follow-up studies show that only about one half of women operated on are completely dry and without complication at 5 years,[41] with decreased bladder capacity and flow rates and increased urethral resistance and flow times being significant urodynamic parameters changed by the surgery. Most lower urinary tract abnormalities leading to incontinence have a demonstrable neurogenic component (see Chapter 9) and this component is not corrected by surgery. Knowledge of various types of surgery is required so that the patient is not "tailored" to the surgeon's procedure. Other existing defects in the pelvic floor should be recognized and repaired simultaneously to prevent future development of symptoms in the other pelvic floor areas.

REFERENCES

1. Burch JC. Cooper's ligament urethrovesical suspension for stress incontinence. *Am J Obstet Gynecol.* 1968;100:764.
2. Baden WE, Walker T. Urinary stress incontinence: evolution of paravaginal repair. *Female Patient.* 1987;12(2):89–105.
3. Speert H. *Obstetric and Gynecologic Milestones.* New York: MacMillan Co; 1958:446.
4. Watkins TJ. The treatment of cystocele and uterine prolapse after the menopause. *Am J Obstet Gynec.* 1899;15:420.
5. Donald A. A history of the operation of colporrhaphy with remarks on the technic. *J Obstet Gynecol Br Emp.* 1921;28:256.
6. Goebell R. Zur operativen beseitigung der angeborenen incontinentia vesicae. *Ztschr Gynak Urol.* 1910;2:187.
7. Kelly HA. Incontinence of urine in women. *Urol Cutan Rev.* 1913;17:291–293.
8. Stoeckel W. Uber die vermendung der muculi pyramidales bei der operativen behandlung der incontinentia urinae. *Zentrabl Gynak.* 1917;41:11.
9. Price PB. Plastic operations for incontinence of urine and of feces. *Arcl Surg.* 1933;26:1043.
10. Aldridge AH. Transplantation of fascia for relief of urinary stress incontinence. *Am J Obstet Gynecol.* 1942;44:398.
11. Marshall VF, Marchetti AA, Krantz KE. The correction of stress incontinence by simple vesicourethral suspension. *Surg Gynecol Obstet.* 1949;88:509–518.
12. Hodgkinson CP. Relationships of the female urethra and bladder in urinary stress incontinence. *Am J Obstet Gynecol.* 1953;65:560.
13. Green TH Jr. Development of a plan for the diagnosis and treatment of urinary stress incontinence. *Am J Obstet Gynecol.* 1962; 83:632.
14. Burch JC. Urethrovaginal fixation to Cooper's ligament for the correction of stress incontinence, cystocele, rectocele, and prolapse. *Am J Obstet Gynecol.* 1961;81:281–290.
15. Tanagho EA. Colpocystourethropexy: the way we do it. *J Urol.* 1976;116:751–752.
16. Enhorning G. Simultaneous recording of intravesical and intraurethral pressure. A study of urethral closure in normal and stress incontinent women. *Acta Chir Scand.* 1961;270 (suppl):1–68.
17. Pereyra AJ. A simplified surgical procedure for the correction of stress incontinence in women. *West J Surg.* 1959;67:223–226.
18. Pereyra AJ, Lebherz TB. Combined urethral vesical suspension vaginal urethroplasty for correction of urinary stress incontinence. *Obstet Gynecol.* 1967;30:537–546.
19. Pereyra AJ, Lebherz TB. The revised Pereyra procedure. In: Buchsbaum H, Schmidt JD, eds. *Gynecologic and Obstetric Urology.* Philadelphia: WB Saunders Co; 1978:208–222.
20. Pereyra AJ. Revised Pereyra procedure using colligated pubourethral supports. In: Slate EG, ed. *Disorders of the Female Urethra and Urinary Incontinence.* Baltimore: Williams & Wilkins Co; 1978:143–159.
21. Stamey TA. Endoscopic suspension of vesical neck for urinary incontinence. *Surg Gynecol Obstet.* 1973;136:547–554.
22. Raz S. Modified bladder neck suspension for female stress incontinence. *Urology.* 1981;17:82–84.
23. Delancey JOL. Correlative study of paraurethral anatomy. *Obstet Gynecol.* 1986;68:91–97.
24. Gittes RF, Loughlin KR. No-incision pubovaginal suspension for stress incontinence. *J Urol.* 1987;138:568–570.
25. Benson JT, Agosta A, McClellan E. Evaluation of a minimal incision pubovaginal suspension as an adjunct to other pelvic floor surgery. *Obstet Gynecol.* 1990;75:844.
26. Karram MM, Bhatia NN. Patch procedure: modified transvaginal fascia lata sling for recurrent severe stress urinary incontinence. Presented at Eighth Annual Meeting of the American Uro-Gynecologic Society; September 9–11, 1987; San Francisco, Calif.
27. Krantz KE. The anatomy of the urethra and anterior vaginal wall. *Am J Obstet Gynecol.* 1951;62:374–386.
28. Milley PS, Nichols DH. The relationship between the pubourethral ligaments and the urogenital diaphragm in the human female. *Anat Rec.* 1971;170:281–283.
29. DeLancey JOL. Correlative study of paraurethral anatomy. *Obstet Gynecol.* 1986;68:96.
30. DeLancey JOL. Constructional aspects of the extrinsic continence mechanism. *Obstet Gynecol.* 1988;72:296.
31. Ingleman-Sundberg, A. Surgical denervation as therapy for the unstable bladder and urethra. In: Ostergard DR, ed. *Gynecologic Urology and Urodynamics.* 2nd ed. Baltimore: Williams & Wilkins Co; 1985:379.
32. Bergman A, Ballard CA, Koonings PP. Comparison of three different surgical procedures for genuine stress incontinence: perspective randomized study. *Am J Obstet Gynecol.* 1989;160:1102–1106.
33. Beck RP, McCormick S, Nordstrom L. Intraurethral intravesical cough pressure spike difference in 267 patients surgically cured of genuine stress incontinence of urine. *Obstet Gynecol.* 1988;72:302.
34. Bump RC, Copeland WE Jr., Hurt WG, et al. Dynamic urethral pressure profilometry pressure transmission ratio determination in stress incontinence and stress incontinence subjects. *Am J Obstet Gynecol.* 1988;159:749–755.
35. McGuire JE, Lytton B, Kohorn EI, et al. The value of urodynamics in testing in stress urinary incontinence. *J Urol.* 1980;124:256.
36. Bergman A, Koonings PP, Ballard CA. Detrusor instability. Is the bladder the cause or the effect? *J Reprod Med.* 1989;34(10):834–838.
37. McGuire JE. Analysis of failed surgery. *Prog Clin Biol Res.* 1981; 78:351.
38. Sand P, Bowen LW, Panganiban R, et al. The low pressure urethra as a factor in failed retropubic urethropexy. *Obstet Gynecol.* 1987;69:399.

39. Horbach NS, Blanco JS, Ostergard DR, et al. A suburethral sling procedure with polytetra fluorethylene for the treatment of genuine stress urinary incontinence in patients with low urethral closure pressure. *Obstet Gynecol.* 1988;71:648.

40. Eriksen BC. Electrostimulation of the pelvic floor in female urinary incontinence. *Tapir.* (University of Trondheim, Norway) 1989:39.

41. Eriksen BC, Hagen B. Eik-Nes SH, et al. Long-term effectiveness of the Burch colposuspension in female urinary stress incontinence. *Acta Obstet Gynecol Scand.* 1990;69:45.

Urinary Incontinence

11D Surgical Therapies

11D3 Neurostimulation

Emil A. Tanagho

INTRODUCTION

Electrical stimulation to control bladder function has been the subject of extensive research for several decades. Only recently, however, has it reached the phase where it can be applied clinically for the management of a variety of voiding dysfunctions, most importantly urinary incontinence. Our own laboratory has been involved in this work for the last 20 years. In the earliest phase, we attempted to stimulate the spinal cord at the level of the micturition center in the sacral segment to induce bladder evacuation. However, this failed to initiate selective detrusor activity, and we then explored the possibility of stimulating the sacral roots, in the hope that a degree of selectivity would be present among the three pairs of roots to allow separate control of sphincteric function and the detrusor muscle.

After extensive studies and many experimental models, it became clear that sacral root stimulation could provide a means to drive the pelvic floor musculature or induce the external urinary sphincter or urinary bladder to contract. Refinements in technique made it possible not only to stimulate the detrusor to achieve bladder evacuation and the sphincter to maintain an adequate closure mechanism, but also to inhibit the detrusor or sphincteric instability that might be responsible for voiding dysfunction. At the University of California, San Francisco, more than 250 patients have been treated by neurostimulation. They represent a broad spectrum

from complete cord transection, quadriplegia or suprasegmental lesions, to less severe neuropathies and functional disorders, including incontinence, whether owing to sphincteric weakness, an unstable bladder, or unstable pelvic floor.

In our experimental studies,[1-7] we noted that chronic electrostimulation of the sacral roots induced and increased urethral resistance through activation of the muscle fibers of the striated urinary sphincter. Not only was this observed functionally[8,9] but, interestingly, histochemically[10]; that is, the striated urinary sphincter showed evidence of hypertrophy and increased efficiency and a change in characteristics to make it more fatigue-resistant and capable of sustaining an adequate closure pressure.

RATIONALE OF NEURAL STIMULATION

When electrostimulation was applied on the sacral nerve roots in the dog, the closure pressure of the urinary sphincter increased; in addition, with prolonged neurostimulation we detected hypertrophy of the striated muscle fibers of both the urethra and the anal sphincter on the stimulated side. In both the intact and spinalized animal, the stimulated muscle fibers showed a higher overall oxidative activity than did the control muscles.[10] Glycolytic activity also increased, which might be a factor in increasing the fatigue resistance of these hypertrophied striated muscle fibers. With the combination of muscular hypertrophy and increased glycolytic and oxidative activity, chronic neurostimulation raises the hope that it can be used to achieve a well-sustained urethral closure pressure to guard against urinary incontinence.

Aside from the direct effect of neurostimulation on the striated muscles, we noticed an inhibitory response on detrusor activity.[11,12] Neurostimulation can play a major role in the management of urinary incontinence owing to sphincteric weakness and detrusor and sphincteric instability.[13]

Sphincteric Weakness

Neurostimulation to improve the tonus of the striated sphincter has been tried by a variety of techniques. However, the major concern was always striated muscle fatigue. Our own study showed that urinary sphincteric contraction is highly dependent on the frequency of stimulation: a low frequency results in fused weak pressure responses; higher frequencies cause a more appreciable increase in urethral pressure. Frequencies more than 35 Hz induce early fatigue, the rapidity of which is even more precipitous with greater increases in frequency and is almost instantaneous with frequencies over 100 Hz. It was also noted that, with continuous stimulation, the induced sphincteric response would fade away in a short period of time. However, in interrupted stimulation with an on/off ratio of 1 to 2, strong sphincteric contractions were reproducible after each rest interval and could be sustained for an indefinite period of time. What is more interesting is that when the stimulation burst was shortened to a very brief period of time—30 to 60 msec—interrupted by an off-time of twice that duration, unfused sphincteric contractions were induced that resulted in a sinusoidal oscillating closure pressure adequately above the prestimulation baseline and an adequate closure effect on the urethra that could be maintained. With this technique in the experimental model, it was possible to sustain a sufficient sphincteric closure pressure for variable periods of time, extending to several hours.

A major difference between other attempts and that described above is our pulse width of about 200 msec (most other investigators have tried 1 to 1.5 msec). The good sphincteric response obtained with our short pulse width is probably related to the mode of direct nerve stimulation. The charge per phase is reduced, as is the risk of nerve damage. It is known that it is not possible

to eliminate muscular fatigue completely by adjustment of stimulation parameters alone. However, with a greater understanding of the fatigue characteristics of the striated musculature, it is possible that a compromise between sphincteric contractions of short-term and peak tension and those that are long-lasting and of low tension might achieve that goal.

The striated muscle has three main components: fast twitch, slow twitch, and intermediate twitch fibers. The fast twitch fibers generate a high force but fatigue rapidly, whereas the slow twitch fibers are capable of more tonic activity at low levels of force with minimal fatigue. Intermediate fibers (which are essentially fast twitch fibers) are more fatigue-resistant, but generate a lower contraction force. It is clear that neurostimulation, if delivered as a combination of low frequency, wide pulse width, and intermittent pulsing, can sustain an adequate contraction for a long period of time and that this phenomenon has a beneficial effect on the muscular structure. The striated muscles can accommodate overwork, whether in the form of exercise or of chronic electrical stimulation. This adaptation involves changes in the histochemical composition of the muscle fibers and consequently their physiologic characteristics. In accordance with others' findings, we found that chronically stimulated muscles develop more resistance to fatigue than control muscle fibers. Fast twitch glycolytic fibers are converted into fast twitch oxidative glycolytic fibers without any change in the number of slow twitch fibers. These changes take about 8 weeks to develop to the maximum and revert to prestimulation levels between 4 and 8 weeks after stimulation is withdrawn. Restimulation, however, restores the beneficial effect of the previous chronic stimulation in a much shorter period of time.

These studies demonstrated that chronic neurostimulation and activation of the urethral striated muscle through stimulation of the pudendal nerve or sacral root can increase the urethral resistance and its closure efficiency, and can be considered as a possible treatment for urinary incontinence, especially when caused by sphincteric muscle weakness.

Detrusor and Sphincteric or Pelvic Floor Instability

Neurostimulation of the pudendal nerve or the sacral root has been noted to inhibit detrusor contraction. We were convinced that activation of the external sphincter would inhibit or abort detrusor activity as a normal reflex phenomenon, thus minimizing detrusor instability. Increasing the tone within the urinary external sphincter exerts a suppressive effect on detrusor activity. Many patients with voiding dysfunctions in the form of marked urgency or frequency and urge incontinence can benefit from the inhibitory effect of neurostimulation on detrusor hyperreflexia.[14–15]

During our clinical studies, in evaluating patients with a variety of voiding dysfunctions, we tested the integrity of their sacral roots by percutaneous stimulation of S2, S3, and S4. We noted that in those patients with unstable bladders in whom a small volume would trigger a detrusor contraction, stimulation could suppress the detrusor activity and increase the functional bladder capacity.

All patients are tested first by recording responses to stimulation of S2 to S4, first on one side and then on the other. While obtaining urodynamic measurements, we induce the stimulation to see its effect on the pelvic floor muscles (as witnessed clinically by contraction of the levator ani and the anal sphincter) and the region of the external urinary sphincter.

Under local anesthesia, the S3 foramen can be easily found by inserting a spinal needle about one fingerbreadth off the midline at the level of the greater sciatic notch. Once the foramen is identified, an insulated needle is placed and stimulation is initiated from the outside. After the surgeon is satisfied with a good response, the sacral root that gave the most favorable response is stimulated temporarily by a fine wire introduced via the sheath insulating the spinal needle used for testing. This fine wire (itself insulated except for its tip) is taped to the patient's back with Tegaderm and attached to an external receiver unit that is stimulated and adjusted by the patient. The patient is usually asked to adjust his own parameters within his range of tolerance and to report in 3 to 5 days any beneficial effect from this temporary stimulation. If it is shown to have alleviated symptoms by more than 50%, the patient becomes a good candidate for a permanent implant.

Stimulation Parameters

We noted in our patients that sphincteric activity can be recruited by a stimulus of 15 to 20 Hz. This is within the range of maximum comfort, and chronic stimulation at this level has led to no deterioration in sphincteric response. Indeed, some of our patients have received up to 30,000 hours of accumulated stimulation over several years—the longest being more than 9 years. There is, of course, a concern about the optimal frequency parameter because this affects the integrity of the stimulated nerve, and we have noted no damage in chronically stimulated nerves below 20 Hz. We usually use a pulse width of 200 msec with an on-time of 50 msec and off-time of 100 msec. An amplitude of 1 to 4 milliamps seems to be adequate for our purposes and is within the safety margins for preserving neural integrity. These parameters let us sustain adequate urethral closure without evidence of fatigue.

CONCLUSION

Extensive work has been done in the past exploring the potential of neural stimulation in the management of neurogenic bladder.[16–24] Recent attempts have been more successful.[25–32]

Our clinical experience in more than 250 patients treated with neurostimulation supports experimental evidence of the potential value of neurostimulation in the management of urinary incontinence. We were able to predict with a reasonable degree of certainty, through the temporary wire trial, the potential benefit of this technology. The ability to test for responsiveness preoperatively by the simple percutaneous technique avoids unnecessary surgery and saves unnecessary expense. With proper patient selection, including complete urologic and endourologic evaluation, we obtain a success rate ranging between 70% and 75%, with improvement in symptoms in excess of 50%. This approach was especially effective in detrusor hyperreflexia or the unstable bladder with urge incontinence, as well as in patients with moderate pelvic floor and sphincteric weakness. It has the advantage of using a physiologic mechanism that does not jeopardize future management. Activation of the normal reflex responses among the pelvic floor, the external sphincter, and the detrusor muscle is extremely helpful in restoring the stability of the voiding reflex.

In patients with severe intrinsic damage of the external sphincter, neurostimulation is not effective because there is not enough striated muscle tissue to recruit; however, in patients with mild to moderate degrees of pelvic floor and sphincteric weakness, neurostimulation improves the tonus of both (in some cases the anal sphincteric tonus as well) to overcome the minimal weakness and restore continence. Stimulation both increases the closure efficiency and improves the histochemical structure of the striated urinary sphincter to maintain this closure efficiency. With long-term neurostimulation we have not witnessed any evidence of neural deterioration or change in response. After an initial period of adjustment of 2 to 3 months, the parameters remain the same for the duration of stimulation (close to 9 years in one of our patients). Although total experience in this field is rather limited, it is highly encouraging.

SUMMARY

Electrostimulation to control bladder function has been the subject of extensive research for many years. It has reached the phase where it can be applied clinically for the management of a variety of voiding dysfunctions, most importantly for urinary incontinence. Extensive study in many experimental models has made it clear that sacral root stimulation can provide the means to drive the pelvic floor musculature, induce contraction of the external sphincter and, with proper preparation, induce contraction of the urinary bladder.

Besides being able to stimulate the bladder to achieve voiding, one can stimulate the external sphincter to enhance its activity and improve its closure efficiency, thus helping to regain adequate sphincteric control. In our studies, prolonged electrostimulation of the sacral root induced and increased urethral resistance through activation of the striated urinary sphincter and the rest of the pelvic floor. This happened not only functionally but histochemically: the striated urinary sphincter showed evidence not only of hypertrophy and increased efficiency but of a change in its histochemical characteristics to make it more fatigue-resistant and capable of sustaining adequate closure pressure.

In addition to this direct effect on the striated urinary sphincter, neurostimulation of the sacral roots had an inhibitory effect on detrusor activity. We noted that activation of the external sphincter by neurostimulation inhibited or aborted detrusor activity as a normal reflex phenomenon; as such, this could be used to minimize detrusor instability.

All patients are initially tested urodynamically, with responses recorded to stimulation of S2, S3, and S4, unilaterally and then bilaterally. If the desired responses are noted, a wire is left in place for temporary percutaneous stimulation over a few days so that the patient can assess the potential benefits of neurostimulation on symptoms and the degree of urinary incontinence. If the improvement is considered to be more than 50%, the patient is considered for a permanent electrode implant.

Patients with neuropathy as a result of a suprasegmental lesion, traumatic or otherwise, can also benefit from the same technology, not only by achieving urinary control but also by being able to evacuate the bladder and control voiding by neurostimulation of the ventral components of the selected sacral roots.

REFERENCES

1. Heine JP, Schmidt RA, Tanagho EA. Intraspinal sacral root stimulation for controlled micturition. *Invest Urol.* 1977;15:78–82.
2. Jonas U, Jones LW, Tanagho EA. Spinal cord versus detrusor stimulation. A comparative study in six acute dogs. *Invest Urol.* 1975;13:171–174.
3. Jonas U, Heine JP, Tanagho EA. Studies on the feasibility of urinary bladder evacuation by direct spinal cord stimulation. I. Parameters of most effective stimulation. *Invest Urol.* 1975;13: 142–150.
4. Jonas U, Tanagho EA. Studies on the feasibility of urinary bladder evacuation by direct spinal cord stimulation. II. Post-stimulus voiding: a way to overcome outflow resistance. *Invest Urol.* 1975; 13:151–153.
5. Schmidt RA, Bruschini H, Tanagho EA. Urinary bladder and sphincter responses to stimulation of dorsal and ventral sacral roots. *Invest Urol.* 1979;16:300–304.
6. Schmidt RA, Bruschini H, Tanagho EA. Sacral root stimulation in controlled micturition: peripheral somatic neurotomy and stimulated voiding. *Invest Urol.* 1979;17:130–134.
7. Schmidt RA, Tanagho EA. Feasibility of controlled micturition through electrical stimulation. *Urol Internat.* (Basel) 1979;34:199–230.
8. Thuroff JW, Bazeed MA, Schmidt RA, Wiggin DM, Tanagho EA. Functional pattern of sacral root stimulation in dogs. I. Micturition. *J Urol.* 1982;127:1031–1033.
9. Thuroff JW, Bazeed MA, Schmidt RA, Wiggin DM, Tanagho EA. Functional pattern of sacral root stimulation in dogs. II. Urethral closure. *J Urol.* 1983;127:1034–1038.
10. Bazeed MA, Thuroff JW, Schmidt RA, Wiggin DM, Tanagho EA. Effect of chronic electrostimulation of the sacral roots on the striated urethral sphincter. *J Urol.* 1982;128:1357–1362.
11. Tanagho EA. Principles and indications of electrical stimulation of the bladder [in German]. *Urologe.* [A] 1990;29:185–190.
12. Schmidt RA, Tanagho EA. Clinical applications of neurostimulation. *Urologe.* [A] 1990;29:191–195.
13. Tanagho EA. Electrical stimulation. (NIH Health Consensus Development Conference on Urinary Incontinence in Adults). *J Am Geriatr Soc.* 1990;38:352–355.
14. Tanagho EA, Schmidt RA. Electrical stimulation in the clinical management of the neurogenic bladder. *J Urol.* 1988;140:1331–1339.
15. Tanagho EA. Neural stimulation for bladder control. *Sem Neurol.* 1988;8:170–173.
16. Schauman M, Kantrowitz A. Management of neurogenic urinary bladder in paraplegic dogs by direct electric stimulation of the detrusor. *Surgery.* 1963;54:640–650.
17. Nashold BS, Friedman H, Glenn JF, Grimes JH, Barry WF, Avery R. Electromicturition in paraplegia. Implantation of a spinal neuroprosthesis. *Arch Surg.* 1972;104:195–202.
18. Boyce WH, Lathem JE, Hunt LD. Research related to the development of an artificial stimulator for the paralyzed human bladder. *J Urol.* 1964;91:41–51.
19. Caldwell KPS, Flack FC, Broad AF. Urinary incontinence following spinal injury treated by electronic implant. *Lancet.* 1965;1: 846–847.
20. Habib HN. Experience and recent contributions in sacral nerve stimulation for voiding in both human and animal. *Br J Urol.* 1967;39:73–83.
21. Hald T. Neurogenic dysfunction of the urinary bladder. An experimental and clinical study with special reference to the ability of electrical stimulation to establish voluntary micturition. *Dan Med Bull.* (suppl 5) (Copenhagen) 1969;16:1–156.
22. Hald T, Agrawal G, Kantrowitz A. Studies in stimulation of the bladder and its motor nerves. *Surgery.* 1966;60:848–856.

23. Hald T, Meier W, Khalili A, Agrawal G, Benton JG, Kantrowitz A. Clinical experience with a radio-linked bladder stimulator. *J Urol.* 1967;97:73–78.
24. Bradley WE, Timm GW, Chou SN. A decade of experience with electronic stimulation of the micturition reflex. *Urol Internat.* (Basel) 1971;26:283–302.
25. Brindley GS. An implant to empty the bladder or close the urethra. *J Neurol Neurosurg Psych.* 1977;40:358.
26. Brindley GS, Polkey CE, Rushton DN. Sacral anterior root stimulators for bladder control in paraplegia. *Paraplegia.* 1986; 20:365–381.
27. Brindley GS, Polkey CE, Rushton DN, Cardozo L. Sacral anterior root stimulators for bladder control in paraplegia: the first 50 cases. *J Neurol Neurosurg Psych.* 1982;49:1104.

28. Holmquist B. Electromicturition by pelvic nerve stimulation in dogs. *Scand J Urol Nephrol.* (Stockholm) 1968;2(suppl 2):1–27.
29. Stenberg CC, Burnette HW, Bunts RC. Electrical stimulation of human neurogenic bladders: experience with 4 patients. *J Urol.* 1967;97:79–84.
30. Talalla A, Bloom JW, Nguyen Q. Successful intraspinal extradural sacral nerve stimulation for bladder emptying in a victim of traumatic spinal cord transection. *Neurosurg.* 1986;19:955.
31. Tanagho EA. Induced micturition via intraspinal sacral root stimulation. Clinical implications. In: Hambrecht FT, Reswick JB, eds. *Functional Electrical Stimulation.* New York: Marcel Dekker, Inc; 1977:157.
32. Tanagho EA, Schmidt RA. Bladder pacemaker: scientific basis and clinical future. *Urology.* 1982;20:614–619.

Urinary Incontinence

11D Surgical Therapies

11D4 Artificial Sphincter and Periurethral Injections

Rodney A. Appell

INTRODUCTION

Understanding the failure to store urine may be simplified by considering the problem to be located either at the level of the bladder or the level of the urethra. If the incontinence is at the bladder level due to detrusor instability, then the obvious treatment is to decrease the hyperreflexia. If, on the other hand, the problem is caused by urethral sphincteric incompetence, then the treatment involves increasing outflow resistance. Nearly all procedures developed to restore urinary control in this type of outflow disorder are based on the principle of enhancing urethral resistance to the flow of urine. Treatment modalities involve surgical augmentation of intraurethral pressures, and the primary procedures in females are the varying types of slings discussed in Chapter 11D2.

The purpose of this chapter is to discuss additional techniques involving the implantation of an artificial urinary sphincter and the injection of bulk-enhancing agents into the periurethral tissues. Although sling procedures are very successful in handling this type of urinary incontinence in the female, there are certain complications of slings that must be considered. These include possible erosion into the urethra, prolonged or permanent urinary retention, injury to either the bladder or ureters during the surgery, or detrusor instability following surgery. For this reason, techniques for the enhancement of outflow resistance that are an alternative to the usual sling procedures in females will be presented with a discussion of the advantages and disadvantages of each technique.

BLADDER OUTLET INCOMPETENCE

Good candidates for slings, artificial sphincters, and injectable agents are women with low urethral closing pressure in the most proximal portion of the urethra, or bladder outlet incompetence. This decreased urethral resistance may be due to a problem with anatomic support or from a deficit in the intrinsic urethral closure mechanism, so-called Type III stress urinary incontinence.[1] Other causes for this type of urethral failure include myelodysplasia, sympathetic neural injury, and surgical injury or trauma. Characteristically there is total urinary incontinence in any position.

Obviously, urodynamic evaluation to ascertain the etiology of incontinence is mandatory in order to demonstrate poor or absent urethral function. In these cases, the bladder neck and proximal urethra are open at rest in the absence of a detrusor contraction. If the proximal portion of the urethra fails to close, the patient is a suitable candidate—conversely a good closure of the urethra at rest suggests the patient would benefit from a standard resuspension procedure. The combination of fluoroscopy and urethral pressures is a very accurate way to diagnosis proximal urethral sphincter failure. Techniques for combined cystourethrography with measurement of urethral/vesical pressures have been presented elsewhere[2] (see chapters 7 and 8).

More simply, the idea of urodynamics is to classify the disproportion between the bladder and urethral pressures. This volume tolerance equals the leak point, the intravesical volume at which urine leaks through the continence mechanism. The detrusor pressure at the leak point is the leak point pressure (LPP), which may be passive or active. In a patient with absolutely no outflow competence, the leak point pressure is passive and therefore there is no difference between intravesical pressure and subtracted detrusor pressure. The active leak point pressure test which is performed during a Valsalva maneuver with the bladder full is a superb manner in which to judge the success of treatment to increase outflow resistance.

Studies of incontinent women monitored constantly for both urinary leakage and intravesical pressure demonstrate that the intravesical pressure at which leakage is detected is often lower than the recorded urethral pressure performed on the same individual.[3] Thus, the leak point is defined by discovering the intravesical volume at which urine leaks through the continence mechanism, and the LPP is a simple measurement of the intravesical pressure at which the fluid instilled passes through the urethra.[4] From a practical point of view this corresponds to the urethral opening pressure and enables the extent of urethral dysfunction resulting in incontinence to be determined. Urethral failure will be evidenced by a very low or absent leak point pressure, usually below 20 cm/H_2O.

In summary, if the function of the urethral mechanism is grossly impaired, repositioning does not restore its competence, as it is functional urethral length (not anatomic length) and its effective closure pressure that are important. When the patient has a fixed, open bladder outlet (incompetent urethra), then treatment must be designed to increase outflow resistance.

ARTIFICIAL URINARY SPHINCTER

Patient Evaluation and Selection

As discussed above, incontinence may be caused by congenital or acquired disorders that result in an absence or ablation of the urinary sphincters, and correction of this incontinence must be accomplished by increasing bladder outlet resistance.

The artificial urinary sphincter (AUS) is most suitable for patients with pure sphincter incompetency and normal detrusor function. However, even patients with

decreased detrusor contractility may be candidates for AUS if intermittent catheterization can be used also. Again, the diagnosis of urethral incompetence and the status of the detrusor are determined urodynamically and/or fluoroscopically. The success of the artificial urinary sphincter in effecting continence is definitely influenced by the presence of any bladder pathology. The patient with a normal bladder or poor detrusor contractility with unaltered compliance usually benefits from an AUS. Detrusor hyperreflexia, if found urodynamically, must be controlled prior to implantation of the AUS. Adequate bladder capacity is essential (> 125 ml), but residual urine is not a factor. Endoscopic evaluation to determine that viable tissue is present at the prospective cuff site is mandatory and also helpful in determining the proximity of the ureteral orifices to the bladder neck and posterior urethra. As mentioned, careful urodynamic evaluation is essential to establish the bladder response to filling and the combination of LPP and voiding pressure help to determine the pressure-regulating balloon used for an individual patient. This balloon determines the closing pressure with the cuff inflated and deflated. A pressure difference of 40 cm/H_2O usually achieves continence. This endoscopic and urodynamic evaluation of the lower urinary tract is important in assuring an optimal outcome. The only pure contraindications to implanting the AUS are uncontrolled detrusor hyperreflexia and high-grade vesicoureteral reflux.

It is not sufficient to state that patients who have an incompetent urethra are therefore natural candidates for the AUS. They must also have adequate manual dexterity, mental capacity, and motivation to work the pump mechanism each time they need to urinate.

Preoperative Preparation

Preoperative preparation includes prevention of infection. Because the AUS is inserted into a closed space, the procedure can carry organisms into the body. If there is infection postoperatively, the device may have to be removed. Due to tissue viability, the operative site may not be as accessible to natural defense mechanisms and circulating antimicrobials. Therefore, the AUS and the operative instruments are soaked in antimicrobial agents, the wound is sprayed with them, and the proper antimicrobial level is achieved in all tissues before surgery. Also, since a foreign body is being implanted, the urine must be sterile at the time of surgery.

The drug, the route of administration, and the length of coverage are a matter of individual choice although both aerobic and anaerobic coverage is important.

Preoperative shaving and preparation are performed at the time of surgery rather than the previous night to reduce the build-up of surface microbes.

Finally, it is advantageous to know whether the patient is right- or left-handed because it is much easier for the patient to operate a pump if it is placed according to her handedness.

Surgical Technique

Significant advances have been made in both the design and reliability of the AUS. Faulty patient selection and/or surgical technique are now the most common causes of device failure. The American Medical Systems' Sphincter #800™ consists of four components: a pump mechanism, a cuff that encircles the bladder neck and/or urethra, a pressure regulating balloon, and tubing connectors (Fig. 11D4-1). Few devices have been implanted because many surgeons fear the difficulty of placing the cuff around the bladder neck. The so-called urethrovaginal septum is not a true surgical plane, and this is especially challenging in women with Type III stress urinary incontinence, because their urethral incompetence may follow multiple surgical repairs for genuine stress urinary incontinence (Fig. 11D4-2). Even partial injury to these tissues can lead to failure with infection and/or erosion of the cuff into the urethra or vagina.

Cuff placement can be approached via the abdomen or transvaginally. Before describing the two approaches it is important to recognize a few general precautions that are important regardless of approach. Excessive handling of the device components should be avoided.

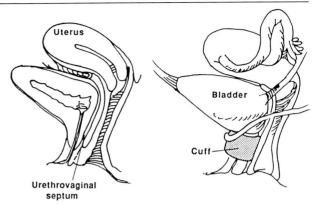

Fig. 11D4-2 Sagittal view of cuff site in urethrovaginal septum. (Reprinted with permission from American Medical Systems, Inc., Minnetonka, MN.)

Silicone-shod hemostats are used for cross-clamping of the tubing. This prevents damage to the tubing that can cause a leak. The entrance of blood into the tubing must be avoided, because this blocks the one-way valves in the pump assembly and results in device malfunction. Liberal irrigation is performed during all connections to prevent this problem. Lastly, to reiterate, antibiotic spray is used liberally throughout the procedure.

After a general or epidural anesthetic the patient is placed in a modified dorsal lithotomy position with the thighs of the patient abducted but minimally flexed toward the abdomen, since the surgical approach for both abdominal and transvaginal procedures requires the ability for intraoperative cystourethroscopy.

Abdominal Approach

A low transverse incision in which the rectus muscles are transected at their insertion (Cherney incision) is important for good exposure of the retropubic space. Palpation of the balloon from a transurethral catheter allows identification of the bladder neck area. After the endopelvic fascia is opened adjacent to the bladder neck on each side, palpation of this catheter helps to localize the area to be dissected (Fig. 11D4-3). One should not hesitate to open the bladder to see the inside as well as the outside of the bladder neck. The proper site for the cuff is inferior to the ureteral orifices and anterior to the vagina. Blunt dissection to expose the lateral margins of the bladder neck and a combination of blunt and sharp dissection to create a posterior passage are performed. The cutter clamp is extremely helpful (Fig. 11D4-4). The value of this clamp is to pinch the tissues that are to be cut. It provides a means of checking placement,

Fig. 11D4-1 The artificial urinary sphincter.

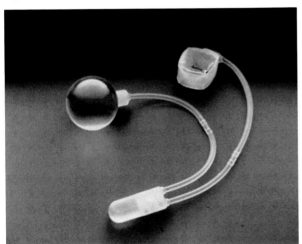

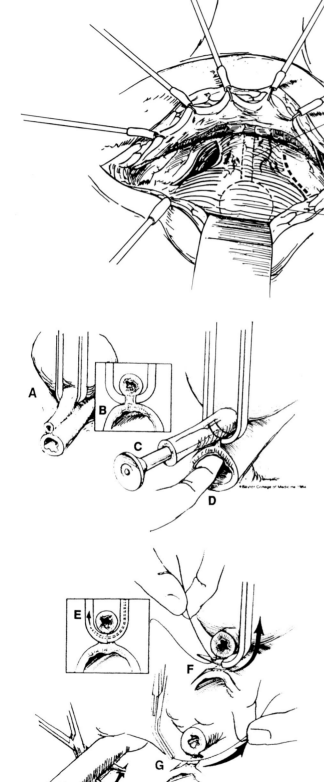

Fig. 11D4-3 Anatomy of the retropubic space demonstrating the location of the Foley catheter balloon, bladder neck, and incision of the endopelvic fascia (bold dashed line) with exposure obtained by Cherney incision. (Reprinted from *Neurourol Urodyn* 1988;7:606, with permission.)

Bladder neck

Foley balloon

cutting the tissue, and providing the passage of a suture to guide instruments for dilation and creation of the passage around the bladder neck. A large right-angled clamp is then placed through this tunnel and spread to accommodate the 2 cm-wide cuff. Injury to the urethra, bladder, or vagina is determined by filling the wound with antibiotic solution and filling the urethra and bladder with air through the urethral catheter, looking for bubbles. Should injury inadvertently occur, the perforation should be repaired before continuing.

The flexible cuff-sizer is then placed around the bladder neck to measure its circumference (Fig. 11D4-5). The cuff should be snug, touching the surface of the bladder neck, but not obstructive. The adult female bladder neck generally requires a 7 to 9 cm cuff. Once the cuff size is selected, slide the end of a clamp through the passage created for the cuff and pull the cuff into position (Fig. 11D4-6A). Finally, thread the tubing through the adaptor hole and snap it over the retaining button to close the cuff in position (Fig. 11D4-6B). An area is then bluntly dissected on one side of the prevesi-

Fig. 11D4-4 "The Cutter Clamp" pinches and holds secure the tissues for identification before it cuts *(A,B)*. Cystoscopy then shows that the urethra is clear *(C,D)*. The cutting blade is advanced into the opposite limb of the device *(E)*. The instrument is dismantled to expose the cutting blade that contains an eye for receiving a suture *(F)*. The instrument is withdrawn with the suture remaining in place for guidance of a large right angle clamp to dilate the passage 2 cm, sufficient for cuff placement *(G,H)*. (Reprinted from *Urol Clin N Amer* 1985;12:311, with permission.)

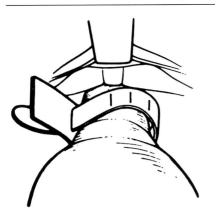

Fig. 11D4-5 Flexible cuff-sizer placed around bladder neck to measure its circumference. (Reprinted with permission from American Medical Systems, Inc., Minnetonka, MN.)

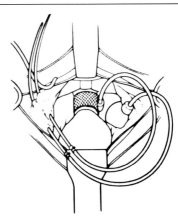

Fig. 11D4-7 Positioning of pressure-regulating balloon and transfer of tubing to subcutaneous portion of abdominal incision. (Reprinted with permission from American Medical Systems, Inc., Minnetonka, MN.)

Fig. 11D4-6 **A**, Positioning the cuff. **B**, Closure of cuff. (Reprinted with permission from American Medical Systems, Inc., Minnetonka, MN.)

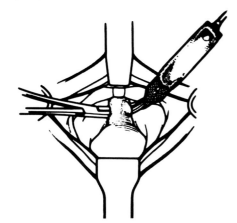

A

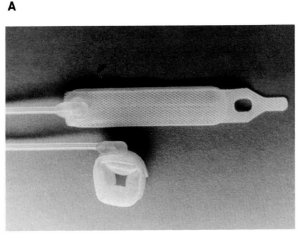

B

cal space for placement of the pressure-regulating balloon (Fig. 11D4-7). This balloon should lie in the submuscular extraperitoneal space. A choice of balloon pressures is available ranging from 51 to 90 cm/H_2O and the closing pressure of the cuff is dependent on this balloon pressure. A pressure just surpassing the active leak point pressure is useful in determining which pressure-regulating balloon to use, as one wishes to use the least amount of pressure that is capable of preventing leakage in the individual patient. In addition, it is important to recognize that erosion will occur if the cuff pressure exceeds the diastolic blood pressure. Once the balloon is selected, it is filled with 22 ml of the recommended fluid and positioned. It is essential that the fluid be isotonic as the silicone acts as a semipermeable membrane. Radiopaque contrast is frequently added for convenience to visualize the components in the postoperative period. Information regarding the make-up of this contrast fluid is provided by the manufacturer. A temporary connection is made between the pressure-regulating balloon and the cuff, allowing the cuff to "charge," that is, to be pressurized to its equilibrium state. This connection is then removed and the balloon aspirated and refilled with 20 ml of the recommended fluid. A tunnel is next created into the labia for insertion of the pump mechanism into a superficial, yet dependent position (Fig. 11D4-8*A*). All tubing is routed from the cuff and balloon to a subcutaneous inguinal position and checked to confirm that there are no kinks present. Connections are then completed between the pump and the cuff and between the pump and the pressure-regulating balloon (Fig. 11D4-8*B*). A functional check of the

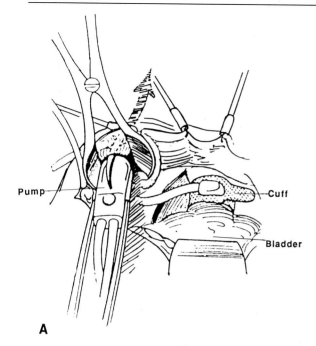

A

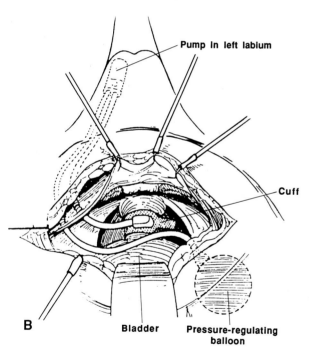

B

Fig. 11D4-8 **A,** Implantation of pump into labia. **B,** Completely connected artificial urinary sphincter in position. (Reprinted from *Neurourol Urodyn* 1988;7:608, with permission.)

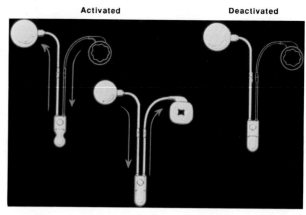

Fig. 11D4-9 Primary deactivation to check functioning of artificial urinary sphincter. (Reprinted with permission from American Medical Systems, Inc., Minnetonka, MN.)

pletely deflate the cuff, then allowing the pump to partially refill for 10 seconds before pressing the deactivation button (Fig. 11D4-9). A 14 French urethral catheter is inserted and the wound is closed, being sure to visualize the prosthetic components during the first layer of closure to prevent inadvertent puncture. Hemostasis is very important because no drains are utilized.

Transvaginal Approach

Due to difficulties in preventing injury to the urethra and bladder neck by the above technique and recognizing that alternative procedures such as the pubovaginal sling are successful even when the sling is made of synthetic material and placed via a combined abdominal/vaginal approach, a vaginal approach to cuff placement may also be considered for implantation of the AUS. The patient is positioned as previously described. A posterior-weighted vaginal retractor is inserted and the labia minora are sutured with silk to the skin laterally for additional retraction to expose the anterior vaginal wall. The urethral catheter is placed and an inverted "U" incision (Fig. 11D4-10A) through the anterior vaginal wall allows the vaginal dissection to be lateral to the urethra and bladder neck. The retropubic space is entered between the pubic bone and the endopelvic fascia to mobilize the urethra and bladder neck sharply and bluntly. The endopelvic fascia is freed from its lateral attachments to the pubic bone and, in this way, bleeding is minimized and bladder or ureteral injury very unlikely. Mobilization is extended down to the level of the ischial tuberosity by sharply dissecting the periurethral scar tissue from any previous surgeries.

prosthesis is determined by cycling the device under cystoscopic control. When finished, the prosthesis is deactivated by squeezing the control pump to com-

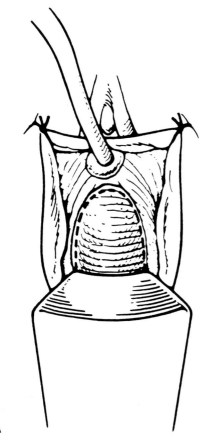

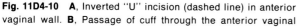

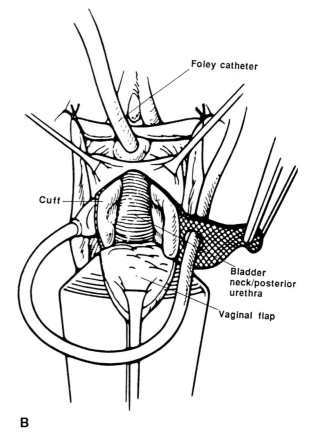

Fig. 11D4-10 A, Inverted "U" incision (dashed line) in anterior vaginal wall. **B**, Passage of cuff through the anterior vaginal incision circumferentially around the bladder neck/posterior urethra. (Reprinted from Appell[6] with permission.)

After the retropubic space is entered, the bladder neck and urethra are mobilized completely from the pubic bone. Once this mobilization is complete the catheter is removed and the calibrated measuring strap is passed around the bladder neck to determine the size of cuff needed, and the cuff is placed into position (Fig. 11D4-10B). Cystourethroscopy is performed to confirm proper placement of the cuff inferior to the ureteral orifices.

At this point attention is paid to the lower abdomen and a small transverse lower abdominal incision is made very close to the pubis. The tubing from the cuff is passed lateral to the bladder into the abdominal incision using either a tonsil clamp or by passing a blunt tubing-transfer needle from the abdominal wound into the vaginal wound, much the same as one would pass the needle carrier in a Pereyra-type bladder suspension. The pressure regulating balloon and pump are implanted through the abdominal wound. All tubing from the 3 components is passed to the subcutaneous inguinal space and filling of the system and connections is accomplished just as described in the abdominal method above. The abdominal incision is closed in the usual fashion, the vaginal incision is closed with 2-0 absorbable suture and a vaginal gauze pack coated with conjugated estrogen cream is left in place for 24 hours.

Postoperative Care

The urethral catheter and vaginal pack are removed on the first postoperative day. The patient is kept on antibiotics for one week and the device is kept deactivated for 6 to 12 weeks. During this period the collateral circulation should be reestablished allowing primary healing of tissues at the cuff site. This has the added benefit of eliminating immediate postoperative pump manipulation, an inherent discomfort for the patient in this early period.

Results and Summary

The results of both the abdominal approach[5] and the transvaginal approach[6] have been excellent with greater than 90% of patients attaining continence. This is not to say that there were no problems requiring surgical revision.[7] However, long-term results were excellent with a minimum of infection and erosion. The success is attributed to appropriate patient selection, judicious use of antibiotics, and primary deactivation. This author feels that the vaginal approach facilitates cuff placement while protecting the urinary organs, and thus far it has demonstrated no increase in infection or erosion compared to the abdominal approach.

The AUS provides continence in patients who fail to store urine secondary to an incompetent bladder outlet, and does so, in most patients, without pressure necrosis or fibrotic contraction of the bladder neck and/or posterior urethra. The AUS is intended to permit intermittent urethral compression, thus allowing the patient to reduce urethral resistance voluntarily during voiding, as opposed to other compressive procedures where the patient is voiding against a relative obstruction. The small number of AUSs implanted is due to surgeons' concerns about technical difficulties encountered during the crucial part of the operation—namely, creating the space for the cuff between the bladder neck and the vagina.

The results with transvaginal placement of the cuff have been most gratifying because they have been more successful than other series where the entire procedure was approached retropubically. The AUS offers a viable option in the management of women with bladder outlet incompetence as it is safe and effective. Best results are obtained in women with total urinary incontinence and no prolapse of the bladder base.

PERIURETHRAL INJECTIONS

Historical Review

Attempts to treat urinary incontinence by the use of injectable agents have been considered and attempted for decades. Sporadic reports[8,9,10] using both sclerosing agents and bulk-enhancing agents have appeared over the years; however, complications and unsatisfactory patient selection delayed acceptance of these techniques. Despite the multitude of positive results using the bulk-enhancing agent polytetrafluoroethylene (Polytef™) over the last two decades,[11–14] this substance has not attained universal acceptance. The reasons for this, as well as the multicenter investigative experience with collagen as a bulk-enhancing agent, will be discussed below.

Patient Evaluation and Selection

Candidates for periurethral injections to augment bladder outlet pressure are, again, patients with either a primary incompetent proximal urethra or those whose disorder of sphincteric function is secondary to either surgery or trauma. Bulk-enhancing agents increase pressure on the urethra and reduce urethral lumenal size, thus establishing additional urethral resistance to the flow of urine. Therefore, patient evaluation and selection as well as the diagnosis of bladder outlet incompetence are no different for patients considering periurethral injection than they are for pubovaginal slings or artificial urinary sphincters, as was discussed in depth earlier in this chapter. However, because this treatment may be performed under local anesthesia (repeatedly, if necessary), significant numbers of elderly and debilitated women have an alternative to catheters and diapers when they are not candidates for surgical repairs such as slings or artificial sphincters. Also, because this technique is an outpatient procedure it should reduce the overall costs of managing incontinence due to bladder outflow incompetence. Any patient undergoing periurethral injections for incontinence should be aware of the fact that the possibility of urinary retention requiring self-catheterization may occur, as well as the need for multiple treatment sessions as the surgeon titrates the amount of material for injection. The major drawback of this technique is the difficulty in ascertaining the quantity of injectable agent required to attain continence.

Polytef™: Technique and Results

Polytef™ is an extremely thick paste that is a sterile mixture of polytetrafluoroethylene micropolymer particles (ranging in size from 4 to 100 µm), glycerin, and polysorbate and must be injected under pressure. Although there are devices to do this endoscopically (Fig. 11D4-11), this author prefers to use the Bruning's otolaryngeal injection (ENT) device (Fig. 11D4-12) which looks like a caulking gun used by otolaryngologists to inject substances in the vocal cords. This has a 16-gauge, 9-cm length needle attached. This technique works exceedingly well and may be used under local anesthesia in some women, but it does require two

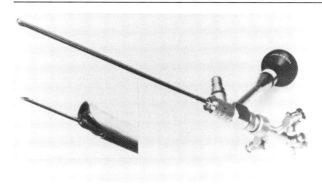

Fig. 11D4-11 Transurethral device for injection of Polytef®. Inset shows needle within sheath.

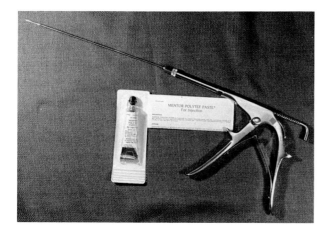

Fig. 11D4-12 Polytef® paste and Bruning's otolaryngeal injection device.

people to do the procedure. The surgeon, while holding the cystoscope in one hand, aims the needle with the other hand into the correct position. The bevel of the needle is directed medially (i.e., toward the lumen) and is slowly advanced while the surgeon looks through the cystoscope to note the bulging of the tip of the needle against the lining of the urethra to ascertain the proper position of the needle prior to actual injection. At this point the surgeon stabilizes the needle periurethrally and the assistant "pulls the trigger" on the device to inject the paste. Although the transurethral method may appear to be more accurate in placement, it is difficult to prevent the paste from coming back into the lumen of the urinary tract via the puncture site and the material is difficult to wash out of the bladder. Additionally, the idea of violating the urinary tract in this manner is worrisome as a cause of bleeding and/or urinary extravasation. One can actually see the material

layering up outside the lining of the urethra, gradually pressing the lumen closed. Ultimately, the cystoscopic view of the posterior urethra from the mid-urethra reveals what appears to be two lateral lobes of a prostate "kissing" in the mid-line. As the injection progresses, resistance develops to the movement of the cystoscope in the urethra.

In my series[15] in which 41 women were treated, 26 patients (63%) were voiding normally and were continent after a single treatment. Two patients (5%), however, experienced permanent urinary retention requiring intermittent self-catheterization. Complications included minor urinary tract infections from the instrumentation and fever of unknown origin lasting for several days without evidence of infection. This questionable allergic response, as well as the well-known risk of particle migration[16] explains the U.S. Food and Drug Administration's hesitancy to fully approve this material.

Contigen®: Technique and Results

Contigen® is a sterile, nonpyrogenic material composed of highly purified bovine dermal collagen that is cross-linked with glutaraldehyde and dispersed in phosphate-buffered physiological saline.

The Contigen® can be injected transurethrally or periurethrally. The transurethral delivery system is designed to be advanced through the working channel of the cystoscope. The needle is advanced into the urethral wall to facilitate injection of the Contigen® into the submucosal tissues of the urethra and periurethra. The delivery system consists of a beveled 20-gauge needle of approximately 1.5 cm attached to a 5 F thermoplastic catheter. The Contigen® itself is provided in a 3 ml luer-lock syringe that easily attaches to the long needle. Each syringe contains 2.5 ml of Contigen®. In this manner, under direct vision, the Contigen® is delivered suburothelially and one can observe the bulking of the surrounding mucosa on either side until it nearly closes in the mid-line.

The possible complications of urethral bleeding and extrusion of the injectable substance are eliminated by using a periurethral rather than a transurethral approach. The vulva is coated with 2% lidocaine jelly and then periurethrally, at the 3 and 9 o'clock positions, 1% plain lidocaine is injected for a total of approximately 2 ml on either side of the urethra. A 20-gauge spinal needle is then placed periurethrally at approximately the 4 o'clock position with the bevel of the needle directed medially (i.e., toward the lumen). The needle is

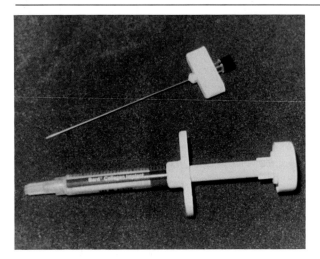

Fig. 11D4-13   Spinal needle and syringe for periurethral Contigen⊤ᴹ injection.

slowly advanced while looking through the cystoscope to notice the bulging of the tip of the needle against the lining of the urethra to ascertain proper positioning of the needle prior to actual injection of the Contigen⊤ᴹ. When this point is reached the 3 ml syringe (Fig. 11D4-13) is attached to the spinal needle and, with one hand stabilizing the cystoscope for direct vision, the second hand injects the Contigen⊤ᴹ. Once the bulge is approximately to the mid-line the needle is removed and placed on the opposite side at approximately the 8 o'clock position and more material is injected. The stopping

point is as described under the section on Polytef⊤ᴹ injection. Fig. 11D4-14 shows the appearance of the bladder neck before and after the Contigen⊤ᴹ injection. One of the great advantages to local anesthesia is having the patient stand and perform a few provocative maneuvers in an attempt to cause urinary leakage. When both the patient and the physician are satisfied, the procedure is terminated.

This summary of results (Table 11D4-1) is based on the first 146 women receiving Contigen⊤ᴹ for urinary incontinence. These 146 patients had a negative immune response to collagen skin test. The cumulative mean volume of Contigen⊤ᴹ required to attain continence in 93% of the patients was 16 ml. Of these patients, 81% were rendered continent within two treatments. These patients were followed more than one year and their leak point pressures rose an average of 41 cm/H²O, indicating that the Contigen⊤ᴹ was successful in increasing urethral outlet resistance. Results of the prospective, open, multicenter investigation demonstrated that Contigen⊤ᴹ can be injected into and around the proximal urethral sphincteric mechanism safely and effectively to treat urinary incontinence.[17] The etiology of the defect, tissue condition at the injection site, and plane of placement of the Contigen⊤ᴹ affects the degree of correction. In general, it can be stated that a given patient is likely to require more than one treatment with Contigen⊤ᴹ to achieve the desired clinical result. The important feature is that once continence is accomplished, patients do not regress. Contigen⊤ᴹ is biocom-

Fig. 11D4-14   **A**, Cystoscopic appearance of bladder neck before, and **B**, after periurethral Contigen⊤ᴹ injection.

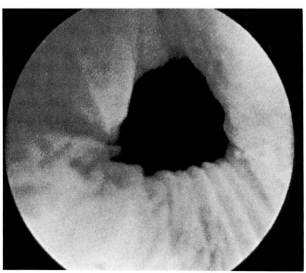

A

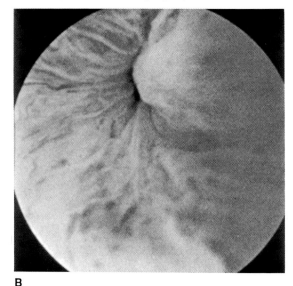

B

Table 11D4-1

Multicenter Results in First 146 Women Receiving Contigen™ Followed for More Than One Year.

Age: 7–85 years
Continence achieved: 93%
Volume injected: 16 ml
Number of injections: 1.7
Leak point pressure: Increase by 41 cm/H_2O

patible and does not begin to degrade for approximately 12 weeks after the injection. By this time the collagen elicits a minimal inflammatory response that enables eventual successful replacement of the bovine collagen with the patient's own collagen,[18] as there is a transformation of the injected collagen into living connective tissue with neovascularization.[19]

SUMMARY

The best results with periurethral injections are in those women who do not have detrusor problems, have adequate bladder capacity, and have no anatomic abnormality. Of the alternative treatments available to patients with severe urinary incontinence due to outlet incompetence, periurethral injections must be compared to the implantation of the artificial urinary sphincter and sling procedures. Many of the patients for whom the above alternative treatments are indicated are unsuitable surgical candidates. Since therapy with injectable agents is less invasive than an open surgical procedure, a significant number of patients who have no options available for resolution of their incontinent state would benefit from periurethral injection therapy.

With respect to the different compounds available, the injection procedure using Contigen™ has been easy to perform under local anesthesia and, thus far, appears free of significant complications. Polytef™, recently renamed Urethrin™ for usage in the urinary tract, has now obtained approval by the U.S. Food and Drug Administration for postprostatectomy urinary incontinence only, as well as its long-standing approval for otolaryngological work. This restricted approval is due to the known migration of Polytef™ particles.[16] Although there were no clinical reports of complications secondary to migration of particles, there is concern because granuloma formation may occur.

As a substance for injection into humans, Contigen™ has the advantage of not eliciting a foreign-body reaction. A minimal inflammatory response results from this noncytotoxic material and there is no evidence for particle migration. The injected collagen seems to be colonized progressively by the host cells and neovessels.[20] Injectable collagen as a biological implant seems to be an attractive alternative to Polytef™ since it is a component of the extracellular protein matrix. However, as with any device, chemical, or compound used in the treatment of medical problems, one should continue to search for improved methods and substances for all purposes. It is clear, however, that injectable techniques in the treatment of urinary incontinence should be pursued, as the procedure is well tolerated by patients of all ages, reduces the need for major surgery, and may enhance the activity of certain other pharmacologic agents. Physicians treating women with urinary incontinence should be prepared to add this treatment modality to his or her armamentarium when readily available.

REFERENCES

1. Blaivas JG. Classification of stress urinary incontinence. *Neurourol Urodyn.* 1984;2:103.
2. Kohorn EI. Role of imaging studies in urinary incontinence in the female. *Obstet/Gynec Rep.* 1989;1:380.
3. James ED. Continuous monitoring. *Urol Clin N Am.* 1979;6:125.
4. McGuire EJ, Woodside JR, Borden TA, et al. The prognostic value of urodynamic testing in myelodysplastic patients. *J Urol.* 1981;126:205.
5. Light JK, Scott FB. Management of urinary incontinence in women with the artificial urinary sphincter. *J Urol.* 1985;134:476.
6. Appell RA. Techniques and results in the implantation of the artificial urinary sphincter in women with type III stress urinary incontinence by a vaginal approach. *Neurourol Urodyn.* 1988;7:613.
7. Donovan MG, Barrett DM, Furlow WL. Use of the artificial urinary sphincter in the management of severe incontinence in females. *Surg Gynecol Obstet.* 1985;161:17.
8. Murless BC. The injection treatment of stress incontinence. *J Obstet Gynaec Br Emp.* 1938;45:67.
9. Sachse H. Treatment of urinary incontinence with sclerosing solutions: indications, results, complications. *Urol Int.* 1963;15:225.
10. Quackels R. Deux incontinences apres adenonectomic queries par injection de paraffine dans de perinee. *Acta Urol Bel.* 1955;23:259.
11. Berg S. Polytef™ augmentation urethroplasty: correction of surgically incurable incontinence by injection technique. *Arch Surg.* 1973;107:379.
12. Politano VA. Periurethral teflon injection for urinary incontinence. *Urol Clin N Am.* 1978;5:415.
13. Schulman CC, Simon J, Wespas E, Germeau F. Endoscopic injection of teflon for female urinary incontinence. *Eur Urol.* 1983;9:246.
14. Deane AM, English P, Hehir M, et al. Teflon injection in stress incontinence. *Br J Urol.* 1985;57:78.
15. Appell RA. Commentary: periurethral polytetrafluoroethylene (Polytef™) injection. In: Whitehead ED, ed. *Current Operative Urology 1990.* Philadelphia: JB Lippincott; 1990:63–65.
16. Malizia AA Jr, Reiman JM, Meyers RP, et al. Migration and granulomatous reaction after periurethral injection of Polytef™ (Teflon). *JAMA.* 1984;251:3277.

17. Appell RA. New developments: injectables for urethral incompetence in women. *Int Urogynecol J.* 1990;1:117.
18. Ford CN, Martin DW, Warner TF. Injectable collagen in laryngeal rehabilitation. *Laryngoscope.* 1984;95:513.
19. Remacle JM, Marbaix E, Bertrand BMG. The value of injectable collagen in vocal and glottic rehabilitation. *Arch Otorhinolaryngol.* 1986;243:233.
20. Remacle M, Marbaix E. Collagen implants in the human larynx. *Arch Otorhinolaryngol.* 1988;245:203.

Urinary Incontinence

11D   Surgical Therapies

11D5   Surgeries for Extrinsic Causes of Incontinence

11D5a   Vesical Vaginal Fistula

Jack R. Robertson

INTRODUCTION

Marion Sims devised and published his technique of closing vesical vaginal fistulae in 1852, whereby he cured 230 of 312 patients at a time prior to the availability of anesthesia and antiseptics. His success was due to exposure of the operative field with his speculum, wide denudation of the edges of the fistula, the use of silver wire sutures, and the constant drainage of the bladder by a catheter tied in the urethra. This pioneering work earned him the title, "father of modern gynecology."[1]

Nearly 50 years later, in 1889, Howard A. Kelly organized and became the first chairman of the Department of Obstetrics and Gynecology at Johns Hopkins University Medical School. He believed that obstetrics and gynecology were each too broad a field and too time-consuming to be combined. He divided the department, appointing John W. Williams to be professor of obstetrics, and making himself professor of gynecology. Kelly's residents were taught to manage the entire pelvic floor, anything in the abdomen, and the entire urinary tract.[2] Because of the prevalence of poorly assisted births at that time, they operated on many vesical vaginal fistulae.

The greatest percentage of vesical vaginal fistulae are now found in third-world countries and are obstetrical in origin. In the United States, where they are now uncommon, vesical vaginal fistulae are usually secondary to hysterectomy and the cure rate is almost 100%.

Vesical vaginal fistulae are easy to detect unless they are tiny and must be differentiated from ureteral vaginal fistulae. Remember that more than one fistula may be present, as this author has seen as many as five fistulae in one patient.

Etiology

The incidence of vesical vaginal fistula, secondary to obstetrics, has decreased in the industrialized countries of the world because of medical access. In third-world countries, however, lack of medical access for obstetric care is the leading etiology of fistulae.

The sources of vesical vaginal fistulae are many. The most common causes in the industrialized world are discussed here.

Surgery

Iatrogenic fistulae usually appear after hysterectomy or anterior colporrhaphy. The mechanism sequence is oozing, hematoma, infection, necrosis, and fistula.

Radiation

Irradiation fistulae may develop in a few months or many years after exposure. The majority occur within three years. It is more difficult to repair fistulae resulting primarily or secondarily from irradiation than are those caused by trauma. The Martius fat pad is especially useful for providing a good blood supply.

Carcinoma

Cancer may contribute to fistula formation in two ways. First, the lesion itself may become infected and erode into the bladder. Second, the fistula may form as a complication of the irradiation or surgery for treatment of the carcinoma.

Infection

Infection may be a cause of the fistula. It results from postoperative abscess of the vaginal vault.

Prevention of Vesical Vaginal Fistula

Most ureteral and vesical injuries occur after abdominal hysterectomy. Visualization of the ureters and clean dissection of the bladder wall from the anterior aspect of the uterus and vagina are essential.[3] These principles provide preparation for more difficult surgeries.

Complex Problems

A variety of procedures are employed if the fistula occurs secondary to hysterectomy. A longer delay before surgery may be necessary. However, the best indication for proper timing is evaluation with the endoscope to see that the edges of the fistula are free of infection.

The transabdominal approach may be indicated with mobilization of the vagina and bladder, excision of the fistula tract, and interposition of a flap of viable omentum between the vagina and bladder closures.[4]

Patients with a small, contracted bladder or a very large fistula may require bladder patching or augmentation with bowel. Fistulae requiring ureteral transplantation or those with poor vascularization, such as occurs with irradiation or diabetes, require the abdominal approach. The goal is to reestablish vascularization in the area of the fistula. This may be accomplished with omental or perineal flaps or with muscle flaps.

The Martius flap is easily available from the bulbocavernosis muscle. The limitation is its length. It is excellent for fistulae of the lower anterior vaginal wall. A useful transplant for the large vesical vaginal fistula is the gracilis muscle.[5] It is mobilized with a skin incision, extending from the pubic tubercle in the inner aspect of the thigh down to the medical aspect of the knee. The vascular pedicle is preserved, and the distal end is pulled through the obturator foramen and fixed under the fistulous closure. The vagina is closed over the gracilis transplant.

Diagnostic Aids and Evaluation of Fistulae

The best chance for a cure is with the first surgical attempt. Chances of a successful repair decrease with each attempt. A tiny vesical vaginal fistula must always be considered if the patient has had previous irradiation, because the fistula may occur years later. Careful work-up of patients with vesical vaginal fistulae is important. The following are recognized methods of evaluation:

1. Instillation of methylene blue, sterile milk, or water in the vagina, and carbon dioxide in the bladder (flat tire test).
2. Indigo carmine test
3. Pyridium test
4. Endoscopic evaluation
5. Intravenous pyelogram
6. Retrograde pyelogram

With the patient in the knee-chest position and using a Sims' speculum, a fistula hidden by the vaginal rugae may be visualized. The vagina is filled with water, and the bladder insufflated with gas. The resulting bubbles of gas entering into the vagina reveal the opening.

The bladder can be filled with methylene blue dye and cotton balls placed in the vagina. The patient is then ambulated, and the cotton balls are later removed. Urine stains indicate a ureteral vaginal fistula; if they are dye-stained, it is a vesical vaginal fistula. Sterile milk can be used instead and does not cause stains. Indigo carmine injected intravenously stains the cotton balls in the case of a ureteral vaginal fistula.

We prefer to give the patient two Pyridium tablets and to insert a vaginal tampon. The patient is ambulated and if dye is present on the tampon, a vesical vaginal fistula or a ureteral vaginal fistula is diagnosed. An intravenous pyelogram would rule out a ureteral vaginal fistula.

Endoscopy is essential in evaluating patients with vesical vaginal fistulae. The patient is placed in the knee-chest position. A Sims' speculum is placed into the vagina for retraction and a rigid or flexible endoscope is introduced through the urethra into the bladder. Carbon dioxide is used for insufflation.[6] The fistula is observed just above the interureteric ridge and the location and function of the ureteral orifices are observed. By manipulating the vaginal aspect of the fistulous tract, the pliability of the bladder wall is observed.

The endoscope is then removed and inserted into the vagina to observe the vaginal aspect of the fistula. A flexible endoscope can usually be maneuvered through the fistulous tract to view the edges of the fistula. Since 1975 we have coupled a television camera to the endoscope, which allows an evaluation of the readiness of the fistula for closure. The fistula is closed whenever the endoscopic view shows it to be clean. No two fistulae are the same.

Preoperative Management

Suprapubic catheter drainage is the most comfortable for the patient if the fistula is small. A menstrual cup with an inserted urethral catheter draining into a leg bag can be used for a large fistula.

The urine should be acidified with an acid ash diet. Any urinary infection must be cultured to determine treatment with the appropriate antibiotic.

One of the problems in vesical vaginal fistula repair is the patient and her family pressuring the physician into premature repair and subsequent failure. A forewarned surgeon will not allow this to interfere with his considered judgment.

General Principles of Fistula Repair

1. If the patient is postmenopausal, estrogen should be given prior to surgery as soon as the diagnosis is made.
2. The catheter is removed one week prior to repair to allow free drainage from the fistula.
3. Either the surgeon must reach the fistula, or the fistula must be brought down to the surgeon. For success a combination of both may be necessary. A large episiotomy or Schuchardt's incision may be necessary for adequate exposure. This is especially true for surgical fistulae, which are always found at the apex of the vaginal vault.
4. The area should be widely mobilized, as it would be for repair of a large cystocele. This is often not done.
5. Do not trim off the scar tissue. Simply fold it in. Trimming may cause bleeding and break down the repair.
6. After the wide mobilization, closure may be accomplished without tension. Two rows of sutures are placed. The ties should not be too tight. Next, the vaginal epithelium is closed.
7. Suprapubic drainage is essential.
8. Antibiotics are seldom used. Culture and sensitivity tests are obtained just before removing the catheter. If indicated, antibiotics are given at this time.

9. All small acute fistulae should have ten days of catheter drainage with intermittent suction, as they may spontaneously close. Electrocoagulation, under cystoscopic control, is usually unsuccessful.

Techniques of Operative Repair

1. Use interrupted sutures. Do not use a purse-string method of suturing.
2. For obstetrical fistulae, the multiple layer closure is essential.
3. Partial colpocleisis is the procedure of choice for posthysterectomy fistulae.

Partial Colpocleisis (Latzko Procedure)

The Latzko procedure has not been well known among gynecologists, and until recently has been little known to urologists. It is used only after total hysterectomy, as it is based on a different principle for the repair of vesical vaginal fistulae.

Posthysterectomy fistulae are always located on the anterior vaginal wall in front of the hysterectomy scar. On the vesical side the fistula is always located above the interureteric ridge. The vesical edges of the fistula are not denuded. The denuded posterior vaginal wall becomes covered by a layer of urothelium. Because the bladder musculature is not sutured to itself, there is no tension on the suture lines. Polyglycolic acid sutures wedged to a urological or gastrointestinal needle are essential.

Technique

The patient is placed in the lithotomy position, using gynecological stirrups. Do not use knee-rest stirrups; they prevent adequate exposure. A small Foley catheter is inserted through the fistula, as traction on the catheter aids exposure. An area with a radius of 1.5 to 2.0 cm from the edge of the fistula is outlined, which includes the anterior and posterior vaginal walls. This area is infiltrated with normal saline or dilute neosynephrine solution (1:100,000) for hemostasis (Fig. 11D5a-1). The vaginal epithelium is denuded with sharp dissection to the edge of the fistula (Fig. 11D5a-2). The scarred edge of the fistula is not freshened as this creates hematoma.

Closure is accomplished with 3-0 polyglycolic acid sutures wedged on a urological needle. The denuded surfaces of the anterior and posterior vaginal walls are sutured together from above downward, being careful not to enter the bladder. The first row of sutures begins

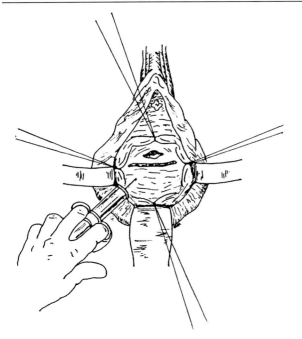

Fig. 11D5a-1 Posthysterectomy fistulae are always located anterior to the scar at the apex of the vaginal vault. Infiltration in four quadrants with a dilute solution of Neo-synephrine® helps make the surgery bloodless.

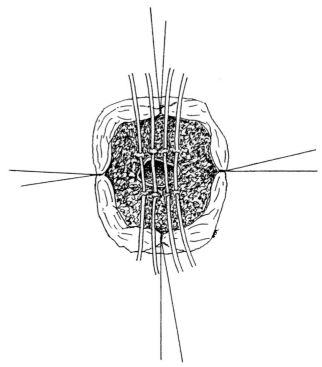

Fig. 11D5a-3 3-0 polyglycolic acid sutures are used for the primary layer. They are tied and the bladder is filled to be sure it is watertight. If so, a suprapubic catheter is placed, deflating the bladder.

Fig. 11D5a-2 The apex of the vagina is denuded anteriorly and posteriorly.

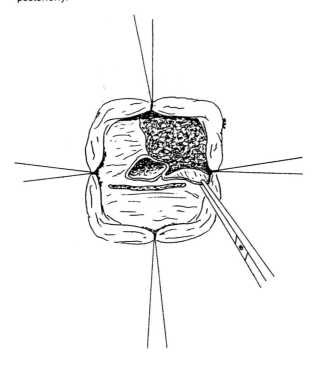

and ends lateral to the fistula's opening (Fig. 11D5a-3). Small bites of tissue are taken, so that tension on the suture line is avoided.

A suprapubic catheter is placed before inserting the second row of sutures. The suture line is checked for water tightness. A second row of sutures approximates the remainder of the raw surface of the anterior and posterior vaginal walls (Fig. 11D5a-4). The vaginal epithelium is approximated (Fig. 11D5a-5).

Postoperative Management of Fistulae

A suprapubic catheter is mandatory as the balloon of the urethral (Foley) catheter lies on the suture line. The catheter may be removed within 24 hours, as there is no tension on the suture line when the bladder distends. However, there is little discomfort with a suprapubic catheter, and the patient can be sent home on the third postoperative day with the catheter to be removed in the office. Catheter irrigation is seldom needed. Antibiotics are rarely given, and if so, only after culture and sensitivity studies.

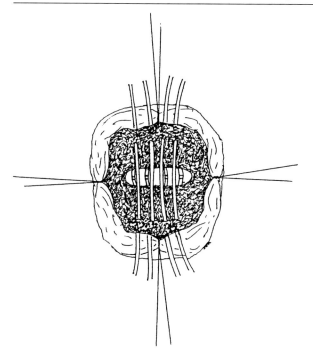

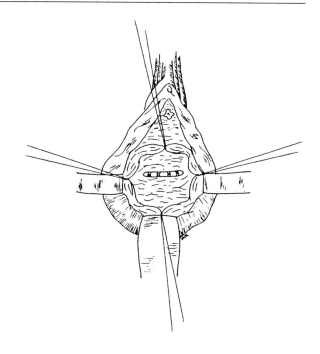

Fig. 11D5a-4 The inverting row of sutures is placed, and the vaginal epithelium is closed with interrupted sutures.

Fig. 11D5a-5 There is little or no shortening of the vaginal vault.

Early ambulation is easy with a suprapubic catheter in place. The patient is given stool softeners and advised not to strain for stool evacuation. Vaginal examination is not done for two months unless urine leakage is obvious. Intercourse should be delayed for four months.

SUMMARY

Vesical vaginal fistulae following gynecologic pelvic surgery are uncommon but still occur. There is a difference of opinion about when to close a vesical vaginal fistula. Because these fistulae have become rare enough that there is no registry, results are controversial.

The artificial compartmentalization of the pelvic floor in the female has created a problem. Many of these patients are now referred by gynecologists to urologists who are also unfamiliar with the vaginal approach for the repair of a vesical vaginal fistula.

Howard Kelly's warning 100 years ago that obstetrics should be separated from gynecology has become a reality; obstetrics is crowding out the surgical training of the gynecologist. However, very few gynecologists are being trained adequately to manage the pelvic floor. Who, then, will be qualified to assume the increasingly complex role of urinary surgeon for women?

REFERENCES

1. Sims JM. On the treatment of vesicovaginal fistula. *Am J Med Sci.* 1852;23:59.
2. Kelly HA. *Bull Johns Hopkins Hosp.* November 1893.
3. Symmonds RE. Incontinence: vesical and urethral fistulas. *Clin Obstet Gynecol.* 1984;27:499.
4. Bender HG, Beck L. Surgery for vesicovaginal fistulas. In: Sanz LE, ed. *Gynecologic Surgery.* Oradell, NJ: Medical Economics Books; 1988:229.
5. Ingelman-Sundberg A. Surgical treatment of urinary fistulae. *Zentralbl Gynakol.* 1978;100:1281.
6. Robertson JR, *Genitourinary Problems in Women.* Springfield, Ill: Charles C Thomas; 1978:5.

CHAPTER 11

Urinary Incontinence

11D   Surgical Therapies

11D5   Surgeries for Extrinsic Causes of Incontinence

11D5b   Urethral Diverticula

Jack R. Robertson

INTRODUCTION

The first successful repair of a urethral diverticulum was described by Hey in 1805.[1] Before 1950 a few more than 100 cases of urethral diverticula were found in the medical records of the Mayo Clinic, Johns Hopkins, and the Cleveland Clinic combined.[2] In 1953 Novak was quoted as saying, "This is a relatively rare condition and no gynecologist will see more than a few in a lifetime."[3] Then Davis developed catheters with double balloons, which effectively isolated the urethra between the intravesical balloon and a sliding or wedge-shaped balloon which tamponaded the external meatus.[4] Using a radiopaque dye for outline, this new technique disproved Novak's prediction, revealing 50 diverticula in 1955, more than the entire previous history of Johns Hopkins Hospital.[5]

The purpose of this chapter is to discuss direct-view urethroscopy, which allows accurate diagnosis as an office procedure. Several different operative approaches are discussed along with the advantage of using urethroscopy at surgery to help lower the complication rate.

Etiology

Huffman in 1948 gave a detailed description of paraurethral ducts and periurethral glands in a classic study.[6] It is postulated that diverticula develop secondary to obstruction of the duct between the urethra and the paraurethral gland, which may lead to abscess formation and rupture back into the urethra. Stones also develop, but carcinoma is infrequent.[7–9]

Incidence

Although the actual incidence of urethral diverticula is unknown, in a study of 300 women who were irradiated for carcinoma of the cervix, Anderson found an incidence of 3%. These patients did not have lower urinary tract symptoms.[10]

Stewart, Bretland and Sidolph[11] evaluated 40 women with persistent lower urinary tract symptoms with positive pressure urethrography and found 16 (40%) with urethral diverticula. The incidence varied between 3% and 4.7%.

Location

The majority of female urethral diverticula are located in the middle or distal third of the urethra. This distribution correlates with the location of the female peri- and paraurethral glands[6] (Fig. 11D5b-1). Occasionally a posterior diverticulum may extend anteriorly and almost encircle the urethra.

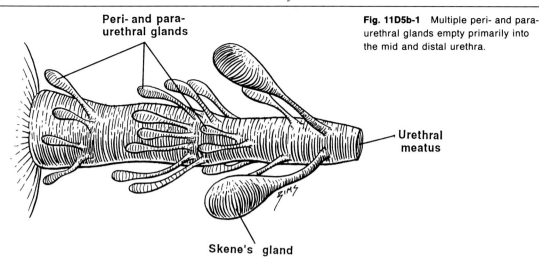

Fig. 11D5b-1 Multiple peri- and para-urethral glands empty primarily into the mid and distal urethra.

Peri- and para-urethral glands

Urethral meatus

Skene's gland

Clinical Symptoms

The symptoms of urethral diverticula are not diagnostic and the classic symptoms of postmicturition dribbling and expression of pus are frequently absent. A great variety of mechanical symptoms are present and may be present for many years without diagnosis.

Urethral diverticulum should be suspected in any patient with chronic lower urinary tract symptoms which are unresponsive to conventional therapy. Although some patients have no symptoms, common complaints are dysuria and difficulty voiding following intercourse. Unless they become infected, wide-mouthed diverticula with good drainage are sometimes asymptomatic. Also, it may be difficult to diagnose a small closed-off diverticulum which produces severe pain.

It should be noted that other maladies of the lower urinary tract mimic the clinical symptoms of urethral diverticula.

Physical Findings

Although physical findings are not always present, a palpable suburethral mass and expression of pus from a tender urethra are classic symptoms. However, urethral palpation in the female is often neglected. As A. Fantl, MD noted during a discussion (September 1988), a report of 100 urological charts found that the male urethra had always been palpated, whereas no mention of urethral palpation was found in 100 gynecological charts.

With the urethroscope acting as a sound in the urethra, a diverticulum may be easily palpated as a soft cushion in 50% of patients. In the author's experience half of diverticula cannot be found by palpation with the examining finger. If pus is expressed, a diverticulum

must be ruled out; however, the pus may be coming from an infected Skene's gland.

Diagnosis

Of patients with urethral diverticula, 50% have more than one and sometimes up to three. A voiding cystometrogram may be used for diagnosis with an accuracy rate of 65%, but urethroscopy frequently reveals two or more diverticula hidden behind the larger diverticulum which is filled with dye.[12]

Positive pressure urethrography, with use of either the Davis or Tratner catheter, is comparable to urethroscopy with an accuracy rate of 90% for either method.

Urethroscopy is essential to diagnose female urethral diverticula because it is an office procedure.[13] The technique begins with instillation of 200 ml of carbon dioxide in the bladder. Two fingers in the vagina push the vesical neck against the symphysis to trap the gas in the urethra (Fig. 11D5b-2). Urethral massage, with direct vision through the 0 degree endoscope, demonstrates the presence of pus or urine exuding from the diverticular orifice.

Preoperative Evaluation

The most important information is the urethral closure pressure profile and its relationship to the diverticular orifice. If urodynamic equipment is not available for the urethral pressure profile, information may be obtained by slowly drawing the urethroscope through the urethra with the gas flowing. If the diverticular orifice is proximal to the area of peak closure pressure, direct dissection with closure of the urethra in layers is

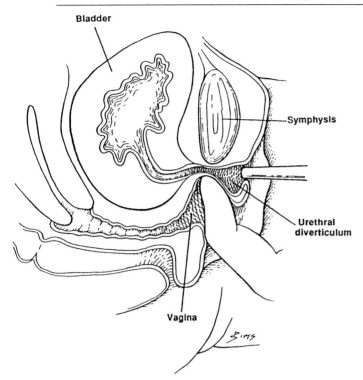

Fig. 11D5b-2 Urethroscopy. The vesical neck is compressed against the symphysis by the surgeon's finger, allowing the urethra to distend with carbon dioxide. The urethra is then massaged to identify the opening into the diverticulum.

required. If the opening of the diverticulum is distal to the peak urethral closure pressure, the Spence procedure is the operation of choice. Genuine stress incontinence will result if a Spence procedure is performed when the urethral diverticular orifice is proximal to peak closure pressure, as the sphincteric mechanism is disrupted.

Again, if urodynamic equipment is not available in the clinician's office, it is essential to use the female urethroscope for preoperative evaluation of the competence and degree of hypermobility of the vesical neck. If the preoperative endoscopic evaluation demonstrates genuine stress incontinence and a poor urethral support, a simultaneous transvaginal needle suspension is the procedure of choice to prevent postoperative incontinence.

Surgical Techniques

Many surgical techniques have been used to identify the boundaries of the the diverticulum transvaginally. Furniss[14] incised the diverticulum and packed the sac with gauze, later excising the resultant urethrovaginal

fistula and granulated sac. Hyams and Hyams[15] also used transurethral gauze packing to facilitate excision.

Young[16] passed a sound through the urethra to stabilize it while the diverticulum was excised transvaginally, and Hunner[17] was the first to create a vaginal flap to cover the incision line so that suture lines were not superimposed. Cook and Pool[18] passed a ureteral catheter transurethrally into the diverticulum, allowing it to coil, which aided the transvaginal excision. Moore[19] exposed the diverticulum transvaginally, incised it and inserted a Foley catheter with the tip removed into the diverticular sac. He inflated the balloon, filling the diverticulum, and then purse-string sutured the opening. This permitted traction as he resected the diverticular sac.

Edwards and Beebe[20] incised the urethral and vaginal wall up to and including the diverticulum, then performed a urethroplasty to repair the incision. Ellik[21] devised a technique for incising diverticula near the bladder neck. He incised the sac transvaginally, packed the cavity with oxycel and oversewed the incision. The surrounding tissues healed by fibrosis. Hirschhorn[22] injected a liquid silastic material into the diverticulum prior to excision. O'Connor and Kropp[23] filled the diverticular sac with a firm fibrin clot formed from human fibrinogen.

Spence and Duckett[24] marsupialized the diverticulum and the distal urethra to the external meatus and lock-stitched the edges to the vaginal mucosa, creating a generous meatotomy. The procedure is analogous to marsupializing a Bartholin's cyst instead of surgically enucleating it. Lichtman and Robertson,[25] the first to report this technique in the gynecological literature, found a low complication rate similar to that of Spence and Duckett.

A recent 10-year report by Roehrborn,[26] on a group of 40 patients who had the Spence marsupialization procedure, also showed a high success rate and low morbidity. The result confirmed the Spence procedure applicability for treatment of most distal urethral diverticula in women.

Surgical Repair

Direct Dissection

As noted, the choice of the surgical method for repair of urethral diverticula depends on the location of the diverticular orifice. If the orifice is proximal to the peak urethral closure pressure site, direct dissection is necessary. This is a difficult procedure for a number of reasons. A normal anatomical fusion of the urethra to the anterior vaginal wall exists, the rate of associated infection is high, and there is a tendency of the diverticulum to partially surround the urethra or extend up under the base of the bladder. Furthermore, no cleavage planes exist, resulting in a tedious, time-consuming operation.

Basic principles of fistula surgery prevail; therefore, adequate dissection and closure in layers with minimal tension follows. For hemostasis normal saline solution is injected submucosally. A half-moon incision is made in the anterior vaginal wall about 0.5 cm below the urethral meatus. A vaginal flap is incised over the diverticulum and reflected inferiorly. A transverse incision is made in the periurethral tissue, which is then reflected superiorly and inferiorly to expose the diverticulum.

Endoscopically the diverticulum is monitored again for size of the orifice, condition of the tissue, and presence of other diverticula. From the vaginal side the diverticulum is opened and the cavity inspected with the endoscope. If peridiverticulitis is confirmed, the friable mucosa is not separated from the vaginal mucosa and fascia, as a partial ablation is indicated. Sharp dissection is required to separate the sac from the vagina and floor of the urethra and preservation of the mucosa of the urethral floor is given utmost care.

Vaginal incision and exposure of the entire area occupied by the diverticulum begins the procedure. At this point it may be helpful to enter the diverticulum and place a Foley catheter for traction. With tedious sharp dissection the entire diverticulum is freed from all surrounding attachments, and the connection to the urethra is definitively identified. The division of the urethral attachment completes the removal of the diverticulum, followed by closure of the urethra.

Interrupted sutures of 3-0 chromic catgut are used to close the urethral defect, inverting the edges, and a second row of mattress sutures approximates the periurethral fascia over the primary sutures. The vaginal flap is then trimmed and approximated with interrupted catgut sutures.

Partial Ablation Technique

With partial ablation the pathology of peridiverticulitis, the site, and the extent of the lesion must be considered (Fig. 11D5b-3A). The vaginal mucosa is dissected free, leaving the diverticulum intact. The sac is entered longitudinally, while the urethral opening is identified. The easily accessible portion of the sac is excised, attempting not to enucleate the sac at its neck (Fig. 11D5b-3B).

The opening is closed side to side with 3-0 chromic catgut. A second layer of sutures is placed, imbricating the previous urethral defect. The remainder of the

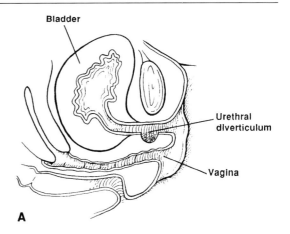

A

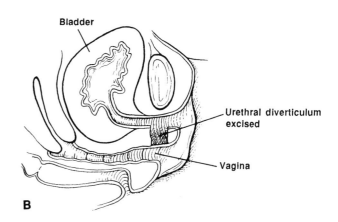

B

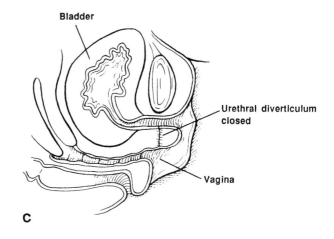

C

Fig. 11D5b-3 Partial ablation technique. **A**, If peridiverticulitis is present, do not dissect out the complete diverticular pocket. **B**, A partial ablation leaves a portion of the sac in situ. **C**, The urethral opening is closed without compromising the urethral floor.

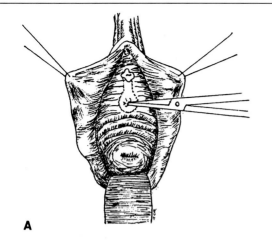

A

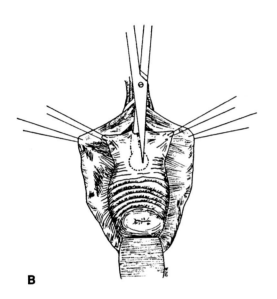

B

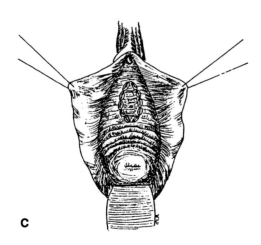

C

Fig. 11D5b-4 The Spence procedure. **A,** If the diverticulum is located distal to the continence zone, a Spence procedure is indicated. **B,** The floor of the urethra is boldly cut through to saucerize the diverticulum. **C,** A running, locking suture is used for hemostasis.

diverticular wall is closed in a double-breasted fashion, and the vaginal mucosa is closed (Fig. 11D5b-3C).

The average hospital stay is six days with this procedure, and in Tancer's series[27] urinary incontinence, fistula formation, or recurrence did not occur. The bladder is filled with 300 ml of saline solution after surgery. A suprapubic catheter is inserted to avoid injury to the suture line from an indwelling urethral catheter, or from complications resulting from intermittent catheterization.

The Spence Procedure

The Spence procedure is designed to marsupialize a urethral diverticulum and is the procedure of choice when the diverticular ostium is distal to the peak urethral closure pressure. The diverticulum is located (Fig. 11D5b-4A) with the 0 degree female endoscope and a Kelly clamp placed on the anterior vaginal wall opposite the diverticular orifice. With one blade of the scissors set in the urethra and the other in the vagina, the intervening septum between the floor of the urethra and the vagina is divided (Fig. 11D5b-4B). After the edges are trimmed, a running, locking suture along the edges assures hemostasis (Fig. 11D5b-4C).

The operation can be performed in 30 minutes in an outpatient facility. There is no need for a vaginal pack, nor is a catheter inserted, and the patient can usually go home a few hours after the procedure. Final healing by granulation results in essentially a large meatotomy.

Complications

Using the standard dissection technique, the complication rate is 17%. Removal of too much urethral mucosa results in urethral strictures; treatment is with gradual dilation. The fistula rate is about 5%, but fistula occurrence can be reduced with antibiotic control.

The Spence procedure can be used for correction if the diverticulum is located distal to the continence zone. This outpatient procedure has a low complication rate.

SUMMARY

Awareness that urethral diverticula are not uncommon is important. Symptoms of urethral diverticula mimic many lower urinary tract abnormalities. Urethroscopy is key to diagnosis and the preoperative work-up may require radiologic as well as urodynamic studies to determine the best surgical procedure.

If the diverticula are distal to the continence zone, the Spence procedure is optimum. If peridiverticulitis is present, the partial ablation procedure is indicated instead of the conventional excision.

The complication rate following the Spence procedure is less than one half of that following the conventional enucleation of the diverticulum. The Spence procedure is an outpatient operation and does not require catheterization.

If catheterization is required with urethral diverticula repair, the suprapubic route is preferred to protect the suture line.

REFERENCES

1. Hey W. *Practical Observations in Surgery*. Philadelphia: J. Humphreys; 1805.
2. Moore TD. Diverticulum of female urethra: an improved technique of surgical excision. *J Urol*. 1952;68:611.
3. Novak E. Editorial comment. *Obstet Gynecol Serv*. 1953;8:423.
4. Davis HJ, Cain LG. Positive pressure urethrography: a new diagnostic method. *J Urol*. 1956;75:753.
5. Wharton LR, TeLinde RW. Urethral diverticulum. *Obstet Gynecol*. 1956;7:503.
6. Huffman JW. Detailed anatomy of the paraurethral ducts in adult human female. *Am J Obstet Gynecol*. 1948;55:86.
7. Davis BL, Robinson DG. Diverticula of the female urethra: assay of 120 cases. *J Urol*. 1970;104:850.
8. Presman D, Rolnick D, Zumercheck J. Calculus formation within a diverticulum of the female urethra. *J Urol*. 1964;91:376.
9. Peters WA, Vaughn ED. Urethral diverticulum in the female: etiological factors and postoperative results. *Obstet Gynecol*. 1976;47:549.
10. Anderson MJF. The incidence of diverticula in the female urethra. *J Urol*. 1967;98:96.
11. Stewart, M, Bretland PM, Stidolph NE. Urethral diverticula in the adult female. *Br J Urol*. 1981;53:353.
12. Robertson JR. Evaluation and management of urethral problems. In: Breen JL, Osofsky HJ, eds. *Current Concepts in Gynecologic Surgery, Advances in Clinical Obsterics and Gynecology*. Baltimore: Williams & Wilkins Co; 1987;3:94.
13. Robertson JR. Endoscopic examination of the urethra and bladder. *Clin Obstet Gynecol*. 1983;26:347.
14. Furniss H. Suburethral abscesses and diverticula in the female urethra. *J Urol*. 1935;33:498.
15. Hyams JA, Hyams NM. New operative procedure for treatment of diverticulum of the female urethra. *Urol Cutan Rev*. 1939;43:573.
16. Young HH. Diverticulum of female urethra. *South Med J*. 1938;31:1043.
17. Hunner GL. Calculus formation in a urethral diverticulum in women: report of three cases. *Urol Cutan Rev*. 1938;42:336.
18. Cook EN, Pool TL. Urethral diverticulum in the female. *J Urol*. 1949;62:495.
19. Moore TD. Diverticulum of the female urethra: improved technique of surgical excision. *J Urol*. 1952;68:611.
20. Edwards EA, Beebe RA. Diverticula of the female urethra. *Obstet Gynecol*. 1955;5:729.
21. Ellik M. Diverticulum of the female urethra: a new method of ablation. *J Urol*. 1957;77:234.
22. Hirschhorn RC. A new surgical technique for removal of urethral diverticula in the female patient. *J Urol*. 1964;92:206.
23. O'Connor VJ Jr, Kropp KA. Surgery of the female urethra. In: Glenn JF, Boyce WH, eds. *Urologic Surgery*. New York: Harper & Row; 1969.
24. Spence HM, Duckett JW. Diverticulum of the female urethra: clinical aspects and presentation of a single operative technique for care. *J Urol*. 1970;104:432.
25. Lichtman AS, Robertson JR. Suburethral diverticula treated by marsupialization. *Obstet Gynecol*. 1976;47:203.
26. Roehrborn, CG. Long-term follow-up study of the marsupialization technique for urethral diverticula in women. *Surg Gynecol Obstet*. 1988;167:191.
27. Tancer ML, Mooppan MMU, Pierre-Louis C, et al. Suburethral diverticulum: treatment by partial ablation. *Obstet Gynecol*. 1983;62:511.

Cystocele

12A   Paravaginal Repair

A. Cullen Richardson

INTRODUCTION

The paravaginal repair yields excellent anatomic and functional results when used to correct the cystourethrocele that results from a separation of the pubocervical fascia from its lateral attachment to the pelvic sidewall. When this defect is accompanied by genuine stress urinary incontinence (SUI), the carefully performed paravaginal repair corrects the SUI almost uniformly. This procedure evolved for the treatment of this one specific anatomic problem.

In this chapter, we will first review the pertinent anatomy. Then we will discuss the rationale for the procedure and the diagnosis of the various anatomic defects that account for cystourethroceles. A detailed description of the operative technique of paravaginal repair will be given. Finally, the history of the evolution of what is now known as the paravaginal repair will be reviewed.

As this procedure requires a detailed understanding of the anatomy of both the pubocervical fascia and pelvic sidewall, we begin by looking at the pelvic floor as a whole and then focus on the areas immediately adjacent to the bladder.

ANATOMY OF BLADDER SUPPORT

Chapter 2 of this book contains a description of the anatomy of genital support. The authors give an over-view of genital support in which the mechanics of support—the interplay between the active striated muscle support and the passive connective-type tissue support—are emphasized. To look more closely at the structural aspect and focus on the supports around the vesical neck, we will approach this somewhat differently. Therefore, let's look at the anatomy again and from a slightly different perspective, giving the big picture and then focusing on those structures adjacent to the vesical neck which are involved in cystocele and/or urethrocele.

The abdominopelvic cavity extends from the diaphragm above to the pelvic floor below, and is the box or house within which reside all of the abdominal and pelvic viscera. Our concerns in gynecology are with the bottom of this box, which becomes the most dependent portion of the cavity when the person assumes erect posture. The bony pelvis surrounds this lower portion of the cavity in a cylindrical fashion. Attached to these bones are various contractile and noncontractile flexible supporting tissues which effectively close this space between the bones, maintaining the viscera inside the cavity. Within this soft tissue closure are openings which, in the female, allow for the passage of the urethra, vagina, and rectum. Collectively, these soft tissue structures are referred to as the *pelvic floor*.

This pelvic floor consists of three layers as listed below. From inside out, they are:

Endopelvic fascia: (See Figs. 12A-1 to 12A-4.) The

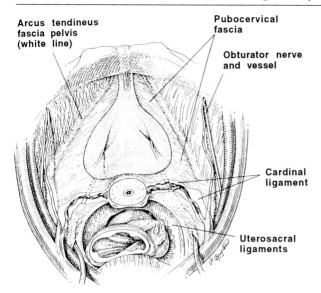

Fig. 12A-1   Endopelvic fascia viewed from above. (Reprinted from *Contemporary OB/GYN* 1990;35,9:100, with permissiom.)

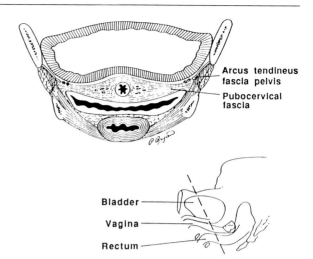

Fig. 12A-3   Diagrammatic cross section at vesical neck. (Reprinted from Skandalakis, et al., *Hernia, Surgical Anatomy and Technique; 1989,* New York: McGraw-Hill, Inc. with permission.)

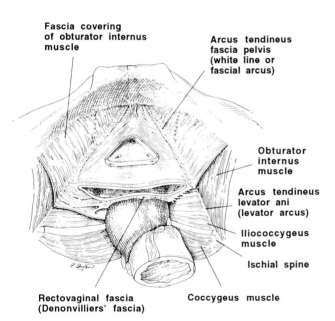

Fig. 12A-2   Relationship of pubocervical fascia and the edge of the vagina to pelvic sidewall. (Reprinted from *Contemporary OB/GYN* 1990;35,9:101, with permission.)

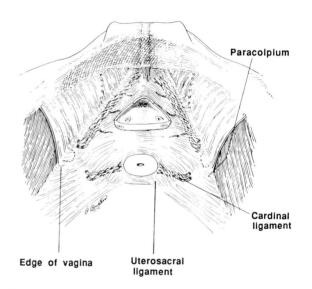

Fig. 12A-4   Pubocervical fascia with bladder removed. (Reprinted from *Contemporary OB/GYN* 1990;35,9:102, with permission.)

network of fibromuscular tissue immediately beneath the peritoneum is usually referred to as the endopelvic fascia. This network surrounds the viscera and fills the space between the peritoneum above and the levatores below. It extends from symphysis to sacrum and ischial spine to ischial spine, yielding a continuity of support from front to back and side to side. In places

it is referred to as ligaments (i.e., uterosacral, cardinal, etc.) though the distinction is a weak one. In other areas it is called *fascia* or covering. Its structure varies from place to place as to density and strength. It is always a mixture of collagen and varying amounts of smooth muscle suspended in a matrix of ground substance. In some areas there are also elastin fibers; these are most abundant in the perivascular area.

Levator muscles: Next, there is the layer of striated muscles of the levator group made up of the pubococcygeus (including the puborectalis), iliococcygeus, and coccygeus muscles. The endopelvic fascia above fuses with and/or merges into the fascial covering of the levator group.

Perineum: The outermost layer is the urogenital diaphragm (urogenital membrane, deep transverse perineii muscle) and its attached underlying intrinsic striated perineal muscles, with their fascial covering.

It is convenient to think of these as three separate layers, but they are intimately connected and each influences the other. The endopelvic fascia is densely connected to the fascial covering of the levatores and contractions of the levatores can alter the contours and position of the endopelvic fascia. Further, the levatores give "backup" support to the fascial support above, just as the perineal structures back up the levatores.

The mechanism of support failure is always from inside out—structures never fall out, they are always pushed out by intraabdominal pressure.

The bladder, uterus with its attached vagina, and rectum are essentially extraperitoneal structures that rest on and are contained within this pelvic floor. When there is a defect in the integrity of the soft tissue closure between the bone, one of these viscera can be pushed outward. The defect is then named according to the displaced viscera, such as urethrocele, cystocele, uterine prolapse, enterocele, and rectocele. This leads to much confusion, because the problem is not with the displaced visceral structure, but with the floor on which the structure is resting or within which it is contained.

For any structure to be pushed out, there must be some break in the continuity of support within the uppermost layer, the endopelvic fascia.

Bladder Support: As shown in Fig. 12A-1, the bladder rests on and is attached to that portion of the endopelvic fascia that we refer to as the pubocervical fascia. This layer of fibromuscular tissue extends from the pericervical tissue in the mid-pelvis ventrally to pass under the symphysis and merge with the urogenital diaphragm. Laterally on each side it fuses into the fascial covering of the muscles of the pelvic sidewall at the arcus tendeneous fascia pelvis (white line). The urethra traverses this layer tangentially, beginning above it at the vesical neck and terminating below it at the external meatus.

Many have tried to subdivide this area into smaller areas, to which various names are given such as pubourethral ligaments, and so on. When dissecting different cadavers, one finds many minor variations, particularly adjacent to the urethra. There are just no consistent structures to which one can assign the term ligament, for clearly it is a continuous hammock-like structure

that blends laterally into the fascia over the muscles of the pelvic sidewall (the obturator internus and levatores) and centrally is continuous with and blends into those fibers that we call bladder pillars and cardinal ligaments. By way of the pericervical tissue it maintains mechanical continuity through the uterosacral fibers all the way to the sacrum.

All operations for cystocele revise the pubocervical fascia. It is either plicated from below (as in the classic anterior vaginal repair and Kelly urethroplasty) or pulled upward and reattached to some structure from above (as in the Marshall-Marchetti-Krantz procedure [MMK] and its many modifications).

Rationale for Paravaginal Repair

What happens to this layer of support under the bladder that allows the bladder to sag, such as in a cystocele? It was traditionally taught that cystoceles result from a generalized stretching or attenuation of the pubocervical fascia, and that this attenuated or stretched fascia was found beneath the vaginal covering of the bulging mass of the cystocele.

A chance observation in a patient more than 20 years ago caused the author to doubt this traditional view. When the patient strained and pushed out a cystourethrocele, she also everted the right superior sulcus of her vagina. When this area alone was supported, the bladder and urethra no longer descended. It was clear that the supporting tissue had broken away from its attachment to the lateral pelvic wall.

This observation was incompatible with the two concepts that had always been taught. First, this was clearly an isolated break in the supports, and second, it was at the pelvic sidewall, not involving the bulging mass that was coming through her vaginal opening.

At the time, the author considered this an unusual aberration, but started questioning just where laterally this tissue attached. He began doing dissections both at autopsy and in fixed cadaver material. He also began to look more closely at all patients with cystourethroceles. It was clear that the original patient was no exception. With careful examination, most patients with cystourethroceles were found to have isolated defects, and often the problem was at the pelvic sidewall.

After one year of autopsy dissections, the author and his partner operated on the first patient, reattaching the fascia to the pelvic sidewall on the right side only. Her cystourethrocele was cured and she was relieved of her symptom of SUI.

After performing about 65 such operations, the con-

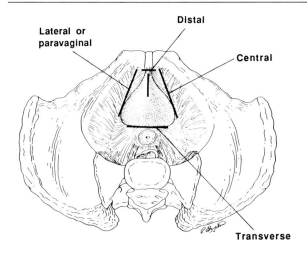

Fig. 12A-5 The four defects: four areas in which pubocervical fascia can break or separate. (Reprinted from *Contemporary OB/ GYN* 1990;35,9:105, with permission.)

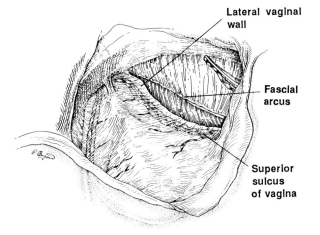

Fig. 12A-6 Paravaginal defect. Note the separation of the lateral attachment of the pubocervical fascia from its attachment to the fascial covering of the obturator internus and levator muscles. (Reprinted from *Contemporary OB/GYN* 1990;35,9:106, with permission.)

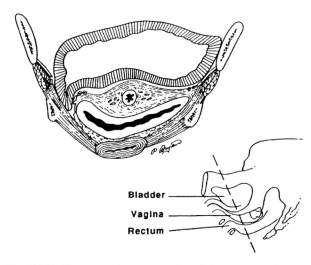

Fig. 12A-7 Diagrammatic cross section of the paravaginal defect. (Reprinted from Skandalakis, et al., *Hernia, Surgical Anatomy and Technique* New York: McGraw-Hill, Inc.; 1989, with permission.)

cept and results were published.[1] This report was designed primarily to document the concept of isolated breaks as opposed to generalized stretching.

With continuing observation, the isolated nature of the defects remained, but clearly the break was not always at the pelvic sidewall. Four areas are now identified in which this continuity can be interrupted, compromising support to the bladder (Fig. 12A-5). They are now referred to as the four "defects" seen with cystocele and/or urethrocele.

Diagnosis

The distinction of the various defects is of paramount importance because each anatomic defect requires a different operative procedure for its correction. They can be distinguished only by careful physical examination performed with a knowledge of normal anatomy. The four defects are: the paravaginal defect, transverse defect, central defect, and distal defect. The findings for each are described as follows:

Paravaginal defect: (See Figs. 12A-6 and 12A-7.) Here the lateral attachment of the pubocervical fascia separates from its attachment to the fascial covering of the obturator internus and levator muscles. This separation may be unilateral or bilateral. It usually yields a combination urethrocystocele. Because the vagina is attached to the pubocervical fascia, when the break is in this area, the lateral superior vaginal sulcus descends, the bladder neck becomes hypermobile, and often there is SUI.

When the superior sulcus is supported on each side,

the cystourethrocele disappears. If the defect is unilateral (more often on the right), then support of the sulcus on that side alone corrects the cystourethrocele. It is in the correction of this defect (and only this defect) that the paravaginal repair is appropriate.

Transverse defect: This defect is named transverse defect because it is a transverse separation of the pubocervical fascia from its attachment to the pericervical ring of fibromuscular tissue, into which not only the pubocervical fascia but also the cardinal and uterosacral ligaments merge. When this defect occurs alone, it yields a large cystocele but the vesical neck remains well supported. The bladder dissects downward, obliterating the anterior vaginal fornix. Support of the lateral sulci of the vagina has little effect.

This separation of the fascia away from the cervix alone does not cause stress urinary incontinence. The usual problem experienced by patients with this anatomic defect is residual urine.

The transverse defect can occur in conjunction with a paravaginal one. This is often the case in patients with total prolapse.

The vaginal approach works well for this problem. It should be emphasized, however, that it is important to close this break in the fascia anteroposteriorly—not side to side.

Central defect: This is any break in the central portion of the hammock between its lateral, dorsal, or ventral attachments. These are surprisingly uncommon in our patient population. On casual inspection, these patients' cystourethroceles look very similar to those accompanying the paravaginal defect. However, with support of the lateral superior sulcus of the vagina on each side, the cystocele will persist.

A central separation can occur secondarily, following high suspension of the lateral portion of the fascia from above as in the Burch modification of the MMK.

In treatment of this defect, a traditional anterior vaginal repair is necessary. After careful reflection of the vaginal mucosa off of the underlying fascia, one can distinguish the edges of the fascial defect, and the job then is to simply reapproximate the broken edges.

Distal defect: This defect is rare but does occur. Here the distal urethra is avulsed or separated from its attachment by way of the urogenital diaphragm (urogenital membrane or deep transversus perineii muscle) from its attachment to the overlying symphysis. This would include those patients who have had an amputation of the distal urethra as part of a radical vulvectomy.

Often these patients have distressing urinary incontinence that is difficult to repair. At present, it is not clear just what the best approach is for these patients. In our experience, one of the sling procedures usually works.

As mentioned above, a combination of two or more defects does occur. Many patients with complete prolapse have both a transverse defect in front of the cervix and a paravaginal one laterally. When this is found, the patient requires both a repair of the transverse defect as well as the paravaginal repair.

In our patient population, about 80% to 85% of those patients we see with cystoceles do have paravagi-

nal defects. Of the patients with cystourethrocele accompanied by stress urinary incontinence, more than 95% have paravaginal defects. Thus the paravaginal repair is the operation of choice in about 95% of our patients with SUI.

TECHNIQUE OF PARAVAGINAL REPAIR

A Pfannensteil incision is made through skin, subcutaneous tissue, and fascia. The peritoneum is freed from the undersurface of the rectus muscles and the recti are retracted. (Better exposure can be obtained by detachment of the rectus muscles from the superior pubic ramus as in the Cherney incision, but once experience is gained, the Pfannensteil will be sufficient.) The retropubic space is entered by incising the transversalis fascia at its attachment to the superior pubic ramus. The transversalis fascia is then "wiped off" of the superior pubic ramus laterally until the obturator notch can be palpated or seen. The bladder is drawn medially away from the sidewall of the pelvis. The left hand of the surgeon is inserted into the vagina. While holding the bladder with a sponge stick (Fig. 12A-8A), the lateral superior sulcus of the vagina is elevated and the prominent veins coursing down the lateral sulcus of the vagina are exposed. The separation of the lateral sulcus (as indicated by the veins in the sulcus) from the pelvic sidewall can be appreciated.

The object of this procedure is to reattach the lateral sulcus of the vagina with its overlying pubocervical fascia to the pelvic sidewall at the level to which it was originally attached. Remember, this is at the level of the arcus tendeneous fascia pelvis (white line) which runs from the back of the lower edge of the symphysis to the ischial spine. It is wise at this point to palpate these two landmarks, for this is the level to which the fascia is to be reattached.

The first stitch placed on each side is the "key suture," for it is the placement of this stitch that determines where along the pelvic sidewall the vagina is reattached.

The vesical neck can be palpated with the vaginal hand. Then, draw in your mind an imaginary arc (convex toward the symphysis) at the level of the vesical neck. The lateral extent of this arc is the location of the vaginal bite of this first stitch.

While elevating the lateral superior sulcus, a full thickness stitch is placed through the lateral sulcus beneath the prominent veins (Fig. 12A-8B). Before releasing the needle, traction is placed on the needle holder

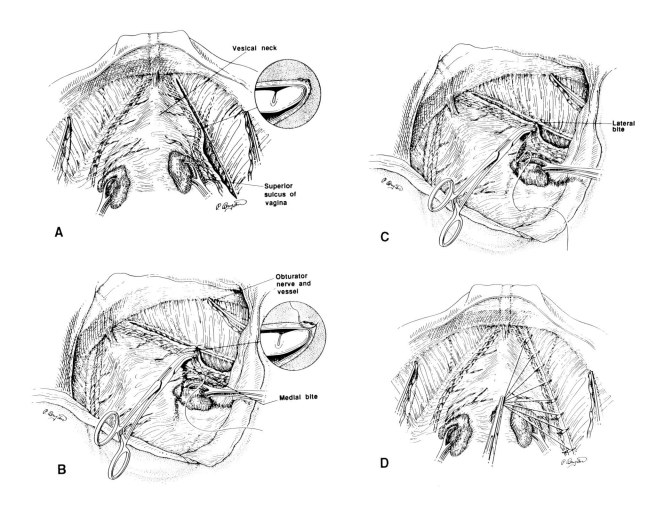

Fig. 12A-8   Paravaginal repair technique. **A**, Elevation of lateral superior sulcus of vagina with vaginal hand. **B**, First medial bite in repair; note stitch is placed through the lateral sulcus *beneath* the prominent veins. The tip of the needle holder is moved toward the ischial spine. **C**, Completed first, or key, suture. The lateral bite is taken through the obturator fascia and around the remnant of the fascial arcus. **D**, Completed procedure. (Reprinted from *Contemporary OB/GYN* 1990;35,9:108–109, with permission.)

moving its tip toward the ischial spine. While palpating with the vaginal hand, this traction is carried backward until the external meatus of the urethra can be felt to be drawn immediately beneath the middle of the lower edge of the symphysis (Fig. 12A-8C). The lateral (pelvic wall) bite is then taken. This suture is held and not tied.

Following the placement of this first stitch, additional sutures are placed through the vaginal sulcus with its overlying fascia and the pelvic sidewall at about 1 cm intervals—both dorsally (toward the ischial spine) and ventrally (toward the pubic ramus). Dorsally, the last stitch should be about 1 cm in front of the ischial spine.

Ventrally, the last stitch should be as close as possible to the pubic ramus. When all sutures are placed, they are then tied (Fig. 12A-8D).

Permanent suture should be used. We have principally used silicon-coated dacron on a medium GI needle (Davis and Geck, 3-0 Tycron, on the T-5 needle.) Because this is a coated and very slick suture, at least 6 throws must be placed for knot security.

The procedure is repeated on the opposite side. Generally, the right side is repaired first because most patients have a defect only on the right (the reason for this is unknown). Even if there is no defect on one side, the junction between the vagina and the pelvic sidewall should be reinforced by placing sutures around the junction of the pubocervical fascia to the fascia over the obturator internus as described above.

The retropubic space is then irrigated with warm Ringer's lactate solution. Hemostasis is checked at this time.

Drains are rarely used in the retropubic space. They are used only when extensive previous surgery has required major dissection.

Many times when the sutures are placed there is some bleeding around the needle puncture sites. This usually stops as soon as the sutures are tied.

Figures 12A-6 and 12A-7 show a defect that has occurred by a separation immediately medial to the arcus. This sometimes occurs, but more commonly the entire arcus is separated from the lateral pelvic wall. Rarely, the separation is down the middle of the arcus and remnants can be identified on both the pelvic and vaginal sides.

When the entire arcus is pulled away, it is necessary to locate the level at which it originally attached as described above. Remember the arcus extends from a point 1 cm up and 1 cm lateral to the midline of the lower edge of the symphysis back to the ischial spine. For the dorsal two thirds of the way, the fascial arcus (white line) overlies the levator arcus (arcus tendineus levator ani) which is the semitendinous origin of the iliococcygeus muscle. Usually when the fascial arcus is torn away, careful palpation locates the levator arcus.

Nevertheless, establish a mental line between the two points referenced above and it is along this line that the vagina is to be reattached. When the fascial arcus is torn away, incorporate the levator arcus in the lateral bite of the stitches in the upper two thirds of the repair, as it is a strong structure and can hold a suture.

An indwelling urethral catheter is not used during or after the procedure. However, until one gains sufficient experience in the procedure, the indwelling Foley catheter helps as a landmark in locating the urethra and bladder neck.

Results

This procedure has been done by the author and his partner, James B. Lyon, M.D., over 800 times, either as a primary operation for cystourethrocele with SUI or as a secondary procedure in those patients who had failed prior surgery for SUI and/or cystourethrocele. We continue to get 95 + % satisfactory results in both groups. We define satisfactory results by the following:

1. Correction of the cystourethrocele
2. Relief of stress urinary incontinence
3. Preservation of normal voiding function
4. No persistent postoperative bladder dysfunction

Similar results have been obtained by others who are employing this approach.[2-4]

One gratifying aspect of our results is that there have been no ongoing voiding difficulties (so common following MMK and its many modifications) in any of the more than 800 patients. All of the patients except one have voided normally within 72 hours of surgery. The one exception voided on the fifth day. Most patients (80%) void immediately after surgery. We use straight catheterization two or three times if necessary, and if the patient is still unable to void, we leave in an indwelling Foley catheter for 24 hours. Less than 5% of patients require the Foley catheter.

Similarly, no patient experienced an unstable bladder postoperatively unless they had evidence of detrusor instability preoperatively.

For emphasis, it should be repeated that this operation is appropriate only for patients whose cystourethrocele (with or without SUI) is the result of a paravaginal defect as described above.

SUMMARY

If defects in pelvic support occur as isolated breaks, it is possible to approach the defect directly, repair it, and restore the normal anatomy. The paravaginal repair is just that: an attempt to restore normal anatomy.

The only alternative to restoration of the normal anatomy is the creation of a compensatory abnormality. The MMK is an example of this—the urethra is reattached in an abnormal location (to the back of the symphysis) in an attempt to stop abnormal urine loss.

Clearly a restoration of normal anatomy has the best chance of restoration of normal function. Although this operation was performed originally in response to a single observation in a single patient, it has evolved into a useful procedure.

Again, the paravaginal repair is not an operation for SUI. It is a procedure designed to correct a cystourethrocele due to a paravaginal defect which may or may not be accompanied by the symptom of SUI. SUI is not a single disease entity, but is a symptom of an underlying anatomic or functional problem.

Why SUI occurs so frequently, but not uniformly, with paravaginal defects is yet to be determined. The mechanism of urinary continence in the female is complex. Urodynamic studies show some sphincteric activity along the entire length of the urethra. Clearly the striated muscles involved in pelvic support are involved as well as the inherent smooth muscle within the urethra and bladder neck.

A point to remember is that the paravaginal repair reattaches the supports lateral to the vesical neck and urethra to the fascia overlying the striated muscles of the pelvic sidewall. There are no rigidities created as is the case when these structures are attached to the pubic bone or Cooper's ligament, as with the MMK or its many modifications. As pointed out in Chapter 2, mechanically there is always a delicate interplay between the passive connective tissue and the striated muscle.

We have found that in a patient with genuine stress incontinence (according to the definition of the International Continence Society) in whom one can demonstrate a paravaginal defect, one can predict with 99% accuracy that if the normal anatomy is restored, the patient will be cured of her SUI.

As to the existence of isolated breaks in the pelvic supporting tissues in support defects other than cystocele, we have continued to study this and are increasingly convinced that they exist. This is particularly true in rectocele where the defect is in the rectovaginal fascia.

In the repair of rectocele, just as with cystocele, the task is to identify the break in the rectovaginal fascia and repair it directly. This can be done almost uniformly. The rectovaginal fascia, when dissected in the autopsy room, is a very strong structure. In its normal state it is almost transparent, but quite strong.

In the future, the primary approach to all patients with support defects will be first to assess where the breaks have occurred. Then determine if it is possible to approach them directly. If so, the operative procedure should be designed to restore normal anatomy. If this is not possible (and only when not possible) then consider those procedures that create a compensatory abnormality.

The remaining enigma is that sometimes the primary problem is with the striated muscle, particularly of the levator sling (puborectalis and pubovaginal portions of the pubococcygeus). In those patients with denervation or abnormal loss of muscle tone and an increase in muscle length, few surgical approaches are successful. (Attempts to address this with levatoplasty are discussed in Chapters 13D, and 16, and a description of the procedure is found in Chapter 14D2.) Clearly, we will make a major breakthrough when we develop a procedure for this problem that is consistently successful.

REFERENCES

1. Richardson AC, Lyon JB, Williams NL. A new look at pelvic relaxation. *Am J Obstet Gynecol.* 1976;126:568.
2. Richardson AC, Edmonds PB, Williams NL. Treatment of stress urinary incontinence due to paravaginal fascial defect. *Obstet Gynecol.* 1981;57:357.
3. Shull BL, Baden WF. A six-year experience with paravaginal defect repair for stress urinary incontinence. *Am J Obstet Gynecol.* 1989;160:1432.
4. Youngblood JP. Paravaginal repair. *Contem OB/GYN.* 1990;35: 28.
5. White GR. An anatomic operation for the cure of cystocele. *Am J Obstet Dis Wom Child.* 1912;65:286.
6. White GR. Cystocele, a radical cure by suturing lateral sulci of vagina to white line of pelvic fascia. *JAMA* 1909;53:1707.
7. Figurnov KM. Surgical treatment of urinary incontinence in women. *Akusherstvo I Ginekologiia* 1948;6.
8. Inman WB. Suspension of the vaginal cuff and posterior repair following vaginal hysterectomy. *Am J Obstet Gynecol.* 1974;120: 977.
9. Durfee RB. Anterior vaginal suspension operation for stress incontinence. *Am J Obstet Gynec.* 1965;92:615.
10. Goff BR. The surgical anatomy of cystocele and urethrocele with special reference to the pubocervical fascia. *Surg Gynecol Obstet.* 1948;87:725.

HISTORICAL APPENDIX

When the paravaginal repair was originally reported in 1974, no claim of originality was made. The paravaginal defect seemed so obvious that certainly someone had suggested this previously. Our literature search at that time, however, was not fruitful. In about 1982, Dr. David Nichols, while reading the book, *Cystocele In America,* by Ricci, saw a synopsis of a paper given in 1911 by a Dr. George R. White,[5] "An Anatomical Operation for the Cure of Cystocele." He pulled this article from the American Journal of Obstetric, Gynecology and Diseases of Children, Vol. 65, p. 286, 1912. Subsequently the other report by Dr. White in the AMA journal of the previous year was found.[6] Dr. Nichols was kind enough to send both reports to me with a note indicating that it sounded similar to what I was describing as the paravaginal repair. In this article, Dr. White clearly expressed most of the concepts which we had been promoting for some 15 years and which we have reiterated in this chapter.

As Dr. White was from Savannah, Ga., an attempt was made to see if there were any further writings by him on this subject. We found only that Dr. White was forced for health reasons to move briefly to Arizona in 1913. He returned to Savannah and died as a young man in 1915, a few short years after this report. I was unable to trace any descendants still in Savannah.

Clearly Dr. White was a man of vision and ahead of his time. His articles were obviously based on careful thought and meticulously done anatomic work. He differed so widely with the accepted teachings of his day that he was simply ignored. When he presented his views to the American Medical Association, his discussants never even referred to anything that he had said; they just proceeded to describe their operation for cystocele. Unfortunately, Dr. White did not live long enough to continue to report on his approach and to convince his peers.

At the time of his second report, Dr. White had performed this procedure vaginally in the living patient but with uniformly satisfactory results. But he described doing the operation abdominally in the autopsy room, and it was this procedure that he envisioned as someday being the "easiest and simplest way to accomplish (the reattachment of the vagina to the pelvic sidewall)." He stated further in this paper in 1912, " . . . I doubt not that the transperitoneal suture of the vagina to the white line of the pelvic fascia will form a part of the ideal operation for procidentia."

In reading these short reports carefully, one is impressed with the wealth of very accurate observations and the careful logic of the descriptions. After working on this for more than twenty years, the author can find nothing in Dr. White's report with which to differ, except that not all cystoceles are the result of the lateral separation of the fascia from the pelvic sidewall, though it is the most common cause.

Dr. K.M. Figurnov[7] described a vaginal operation for urinary incontinence very similar to Dr. White's original procedure. He advocated a resuspension of the anterior vaginal wall to the fascial arcus. He reported doing this more than 200 times with only one surgical failure.

Others have advocated using the white line or other points on the lateral pelvic wall for vaginal suspension. Dr. Byron Inman[8] published a paper suggesting the use of sutures out to the fascia of the pelvic sidewall at the level of the vaginal apex when adequate cardinal and uterosacral ligaments are not available. Durfee[9] recommended placing one suture on each side into the obturator fascia in his modification of the Burch procedure.

In 1976, Drs. Wayne Baden and Tom Walker of Temple, Texas, had developed a vaginal operation for stress incontinence that was designed to reattach the structures lateral to the urethra and bladder neck to the pelvic sidewall in treatment of a syndrome which they referred to as "urethral detachment." They had identified (but not yet reported) a subset of patients in whom they deemed the pathology to be a detachment of the lateral supports of the urethra from the pelvic sidewalls. Subsequently, Dr. Baden suggested the term "paravaginal repair" for the procedure we had been doing. He was a great help in making us classify and accurately describe the procedure in unmistakable language.

In 1948, Dr. Byron Goff[10] reported that in anatomic studies he was unable to find any evidence of attenuation of the pubocervical fascia in cystocele. Surely there were others who focused on either the lack of attenuation of the fascia as a cause of cystocele or the use of the sidewall in repair of cystocele. Once recognized, it seems so simple that it must have occurred to many others during the 150 years of surgery for this condition.

Cystocele

12B Vaginal Approach to Cystocele Repair

J. Thomas Benson

INTRODUCTION

In the previous chapter on paravaginal repair of cystocele, the significant advance of recognizing structural lateral defects as a component of cystocele development was made. Repairing this by the abdominal route was well explained. In this chapter, we will emphasize the recognition of defects leading to the cystocele development and how to repair such defects from the vaginal route. Diagnosis of cystocele by type, location, and grade will be explained. Causes of surgical failure will be enumerated. Then, techniques of anterior colporrhaphy and vaginal paravaginal cystocele repair will be described.

The pathophysiologic development of a cystocele involves anatomic defects of either the vaginal wall, the vaginal supportive structures, or both. Proper surgical repair requires recognition of the underlying defects, a process assisted by identifying the type, location, and grade of the cystocele. *It is uncommon for the anatomic defects to involve only the anterior vaginal wall.* The anterior vaginal wall lies on the posterior vaginal wall, which is in turn supported by the levator plate. Recognition of defects in these structures should lead to simultaneous correction to restore the integrity of the entire pelvic floor.

TYPES OF CYSTOCELE

A cystocele developing from stretching of the anterior vaginal wall past the point of accommodation is termed a *pulsion* or *distention* cystocele. The distention typically occurs with parturition when the lateral attachments of the vaginal wall remain intact and the anterior central portions are stretched. The effects of this distention may become more marked with aging, hormonal deprivation, and, perhaps, neurologic changes. A pulsion or distention cystocele has loss of rugae, especially over the anterior vaginal wall (Fig. 12B-1), unlike the generalized rugae loss seen with atrophy.

A cystocele resulting from loss of the lateral vaginal support is termed a *displacement* or *traction* cystocele. The attachment to the arcus tendineus is lost either

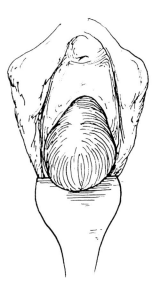

Fig. 12B-1 Pulsion cystocele. Note the absence of rugae, the central location, and the intact lateral supports.

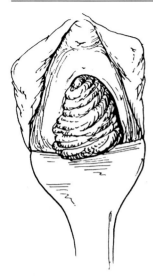

Fig. 12B-2 Traction cystocele. In this type of cystocele, the rugae are often preserved, but there is a loss of lateral attachment.

unilaterally or bilaterally. A cystocele of this type is often characterized by retention of rugae (Fig. 12B-2). The lateral detachment may be appreciated by gently pulling with skin hooks in the region of the lateral vaginal sulci. It may also be demonstrated by noting the patient's lack of ability to elevate the lateral sulci of the anterior vaginal wall when asked to "squeeze."

Most cystoceles involve a combination of distention and displacement elements. The existing defects may be thought of as "lateral" with the displacement type, and "central" with the distention type. Surgical correction requires repairing the appropriate defect.

Location

A cystocele may be defined as anterior or posterior in relationship to the interureteric line. An anterior cystocele involves the trigone and urethrovesical junction and is frequently associated with increased bladder neck mobility, lack of effective transference of intraabdominal to midurethral pressures, and stress incontinence. A posterior cystocele is associated with relative fixation of the urethrovesical junction and prolapsing of the bladder superior to this level. They are generally not associated with stress urinary incontinence and may indeed demonstrate "paradoxical continence." In this condition the "flap" effect of the more acute posterior urethrovesical angle leads to continence, which may be lost when this type of cystocele is repaired. Preoperative recognition of paradoxical continence by manually supporting the cystocele while performing a standing stress test (see Chapter 6) will allow selective surgical support to the urethrovesical junction to prevent loss of continence when the cystocele is repaired.

Combinations of posterior and anterior cystocele commonly occur. Development of relaxation more distally, the so-called "urethrocele," is uncommon. Dissection in the area of the distal urethra is, therefore, not required in most cystocele repairs and, in fact, may add to postoperative voiding dysfunction.

Grades of Cystocele

A cystocele is considered grade one if during the patient's Valsalva maneuver in the upright position the cystocele does not reach the introitus. If the introitus is reached by the anterior vaginal wall during the patient's Valsalva maneuver in the upright position, the cystocele is grade two. If during this same maneuver the cystocele protrudes beyond the introitus, it is grade three, and if it is beyond the introitus at rest it is grade four.

Surgical Failures

The most common cause of surgical failure with cystocele is the inappropriate choice of procedure. The majority of surgeries for cystocele are performed vaginally, assuming only a central defect of a pulsion type cystocele. Cystoceles with lateral defects are not corrected by such an operation; likewise, if only the lateral defects are corrected in a combination cystocele, the remaining pulsion or central cystocele will still be present and the problem will eventually recur.

Failed treatment of genuine stress urinary incontinence associated with cystocele may occur due to incorrect procedural choice. Treatment by anterior colporrhaphy alone has failure rates as high as 40% to 45%.[1,2] If there is associated low urethral pressure, treatment by either anterior colporrhaphy or urethropexy has high failure rates, suggesting that sling procedures may be a better choice (see Chapter 11D1).

Surgical methodology may also lead to failure. In pulsion cystocele it is of utmost importance to enter the vesicovaginal space so that the entire fibromuscular wall of the vagina is utilized in the repair (Fig. 12B-3).

Attempts to correct the lateral defect of traction cystocele by elevation of the lateral anterior vaginal wall and suspension of it to the retropubic space as described in the "four corner technique" have unacceptably high rates of failure. This technique relies entirely on suture integrity and there is no anatomic site for adhesion formation.

Another cause of surgical failure is neglecting to simultaneously correct rectocele defects in Denonvilliers' fasciae or large levator hiatus defects (see Chapter 16). Since the anterior vaginal wall rests on the poste-

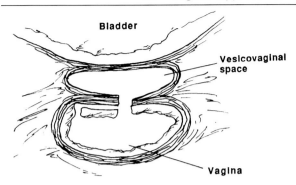

Fig. 12B-3 Vesicovaginal space. Entry into this space allows the full thickness of the fibromuscular vaginal wall to be utilized in repair of pulsion cystocele.

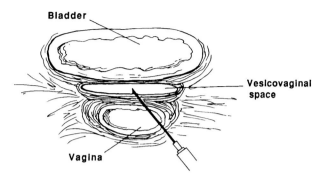

Fig. 12B-4 Penetration into the vesicovaginal space is recognized by diminished resistance after the needle perforates the wall's full thickness.

rior vaginal wall and the posterior wall on the levator plate, proper restoration of Denonvilliers' fasciae and/or levatoplasty may function as an important adjunct to prevent recurrence of the cystocele or any existing vault descent.[3]

Surgical Techniques

Anterior Colporrhaphy for Pulsion Cystocele

The area of the pulsion defect is identified and Allis clamps are placed in the sagittal line at the superior and inferior aspects of the defect. In the combined anterior and posterior pulsion cystocele repair, the incision extends superiorly to halfway between the urethrovesical junction and the external urethral meatus. The entire thickness of the vaginal wall is incised so that the vesicovaginal space is entered. Recognition of the entire vaginal wall may be simplified by injection of saline. Frequently, one may employ a glass barrelled syringe to feel the diminished resistance of the vesicovaginal space when the needle perforates the wall's full thickness (Fig. 12B-4). The fibromuscular bladder capsule is then plicated using 3-0 chromic suture. At this point the full thickness of the anterior vaginal wall is either resected and closed with full thickness sutures or, as in Fig. 12B-5, the patient's right vaginal flap is split, the superficial portion excised, and the remaining left vaginal flap is sewn to the undersurface of the split right flap. Anterior type cystocele repair involves dissecting the urethrovesical junction from the vagina. Preoperatively, if the patient is deemed to have objective genuine stress urinary incontinence with loss of transference of abdominal forces to the urethra, and a normal urethral closing pressure in the upright position with a full blad-

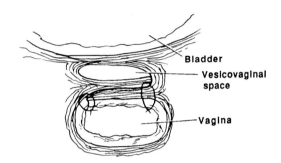

Fig. 12B-5 The overlapping technique for pulsion cystocele. One and one-half thicknesses of anterior vaginal wall are used for support.

der (> 20 cm/H_2O), the modified Pereyra urethropexy is performed and thus the muscularis of the vagina is split (see Chapter 11D2). If the patient has shown significant funneling (vesicalization), then the entire fibromuscular layer of the vagina is incised, the urethrovesical junction freed, and an appropriate number of vertical mattress (Kelly-Kennedy type) sutures are placed to plicate the funnel and restore normal configuration and caliber to the proximal urethra. This area is then supported by full-thickness, interrupted absorbable sutures in the vaginal wall and urethral supports (pubourethral ligaments) (Fig. 12B-6).

Another method of overlap repair using permanent sutures is performed by splitting both sides of the anterior vaginal wall and overlapping the two deeper layers (the so-called "pubovaginal fascia"). Permanent Gortex type sutures may be used, which become incorporated into the tissue's connective substance. These sutures are applied in a "near side one, far side two, near side two, far side one" pattern. The superficial layer may then be trimmed and closed with absorbable suture. This method again uses one and one-half full thickness vaginal wall for support, using permanent suture.

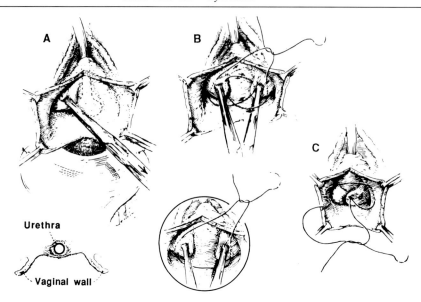

Fig. 12B-6 "Pubourethral ligament" support to proximal urethra in case of vesicalization of urethra. **A**, The vaginal wall is opened beneath the urethra (note inset below). The clamp is grasping the right pubourethral ligament. **B**, Right and left pubourethral ligaments are included in the suture. Circled inset below shows an alternate suture. **C**, The suture is tied. (Reprinted from Nichols DH, Randall CL, *Vaginal Surgery*, 3rd ed, Baltimore: Williams & Wilkins Co; 1989:256, with permission.)

Vaginal Paravaginal Cystocele Repair for Traction Cystocele

The vaginal approach to traction cystocele accomplishes the same anatomic restoration as the abdominal paravaginal cystocele repair (see Chapter 12A). The intent is the same: to reestablish continuity of the vaginal and urethral supports to the arcus tendineus from its point of origin at the inferior pubic symphysis to its attachment at the ischial spine. This procedure was first described by White in 1909.[4,5]

The urethrovesical junction is identified with the bulb of a Foley catheter and bilateral marking sutures are placed 2 to 3 cm lateral to this junction. Subsequent marking sutures are placed on the anterior vaginal wall at areas which, when elevated to the arcus tendineus, correct the traction cystocele. Four or five such sutures are placed progressively along the line of the arcus tendineus toward the ischial spine. If there is sufficiently supportive cardinal-uterosacral ligament complex in this area, it may be utilized. Otherwise, the defect continues to the ischial spine, and an apical vault (or uterine) prolapse is present, which may require correction with a McCall culdoplasty and/or a bilateral sacrospinous suspension approached from the posterior vaginal side (see Chapter 13D3). The marking sutures are placed prior to any surgical incision so that the distor-

tion occurring during the procedure does not lead to improper suture placement. After injecting the muscularis of the vaginal wall with saline, an inverted "U" incision, or bilateral sulci incision is used (Fig. 12B-7A). The fibromuscular layer of the vaginal wall is opened and dissection with scissors is carried out in the avascular space lateral to the proximal urethra and inferior to the bladder (Fig. 12B-7B). Then, using blunt or, when necessary, sharp dissection, the "urethral supports" are traversed so that the operator's finger is now retropubically in the space of Retzius (Fig. 12B-7C). The obturator canal is palpated and dissection is bluntly carried out in a direction along the arcus tendineus toward the ischial spine, being careful to avoid the obturator nerve and vessels by remaining posterior and inferior to them (Fig. 12B-7D).

The bladder is then reflected medially and, with direct visualization, a Deschamps ligature carrier is used to place Gortex sutures in the obturator internus fascia. These sutures are anterior to the internal pudendal vessels and nerves and lateral to the inferior hypogastric nerve plexus overlying the iliococcygeal muscle. At least 4 sutures should be placed, beginning near the ischial spine and extending along the arcus tendineus to the symphysis. They are then sewn into the vaginal wall (Fig. 12B-7E) on the lateral aspect of the U-shaped incision line, a line indicated by the previously placed

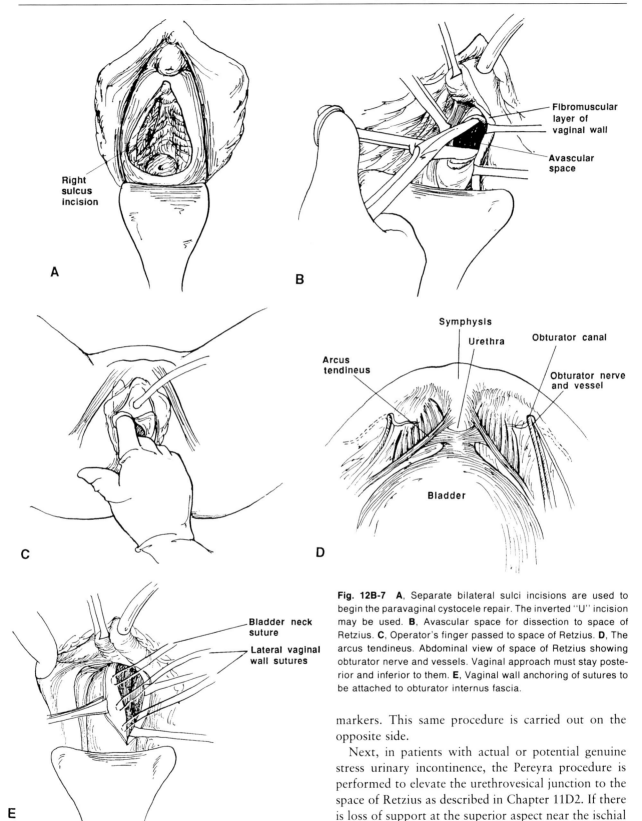

Fig. 12B-7   A, Separate bilateral sulci incisions are used to begin the paravaginal cystocele repair. The inverted "U" incision may be used. **B**, Avascular space for dissection to space of Retzius. **C**, Operator's finger passed to space of Retzius. **D**, The arcus tendineus. Abdominal view of space of Retzius showing obturator nerve and vessels. Vaginal approach must stay posterior and inferior to them. **E**, Vaginal wall anchoring of sutures to be attached to obturator internus fascia.

markers. This same procedure is carried out on the opposite side.

Next, in patients with actual or potential genuine stress urinary incontinence, the Pereyra procedure is performed to elevate the urethrovesical junction to the space of Retzius as described in Chapter 11D2. If there is loss of support at the superior aspect near the ischial spine (i.e., a vaginal vault "inversion" prolapse), a

McCall culdoplasty and/or a bilateral sacrospinous ligament suspension is performed (see Chapter 13D). The
anterior vaginal wall is then closed with running continuous 2-0 polyglactin sutures. The anterior vaginal wall
is supported and the lateral sutures are tied. At this
point the bladder is filled to 300 ml of sterile saline and
the patient is tested for continence by direct application
of force over the suprapubic region. The urethrovesical
(Pereyra) sutures are then elevated until continence is
established. A goniometer is used to measure urethral
axis (see Chapter 6). The sutures are then tied and
treated as with the modified Pereyra or with the Gittes
modification.

During lateral dissection for the vaginal paravaginal
repair the operator may conceptualize the line of the
arcus tendineus as arising from the lower one sixth of
the pubic bone, 1 cm from the midline and extending to
the ischial spine. The fascial attachments of the paraurethral tissues and the anterior vaginal wall are to this
line and muscular attachments to the medial border of
the levator ani muscle occur in essentially the same area
(Fig. 12B-8). It is to this area that the lateral attachments of the anterior vaginal wall will be reestablished
in cases where they are defective. Therefore, lateral
cystocele defect can be completely corrected from the
vaginal route, and remaining central or pulsion type
cystocele defects may be simultaneously corrected with
the anterior colporrhaphy techniques. This type of anatomic repair of lateral vaginal wall defect is much more
successful than attempts to elevate the lateral vaginal
wall to the retropubic location. This may be due to the
presence of an anatomic area of adherence along the
arcus tendineus, whereas suspending the anterior vaginal wall with the same retropubic passage of sutures
used for the urethrovesical junction depends solely on
the integrity of the supporting suture, with no area of
anatomic approximation for adhesion and support.

Learning the surgical anatomy of this area from the
abdominal route is probably preferable. Under guidance from the "abdominal" surgeon, the "vaginal" surgeon can be directed during each case until the anatomy
of the region is sufficiently understood to operate vaginally without guidance.

SUMMARY

Standard anterior colporrhaphy performed as the
only therapy for cystocele has led to very disappointing
results. Recognizing that cystocele can be due to defects
either centrally or laterally has led to improved results
by recognizing and correcting all of the defects present.
The lateral defects leading to traction type cystoceles
can be repaired either abdominally or vaginally. Learning the repair by both routes frees the pelvic floor surgeon from limitation of surgical approach to correct all
the patient's pelvic floor defects.

REFERENCES

1. Baden WD, Walker T. Urinary stress incontinence: evaluation of
   paravaginal repair. *Fem Patient.* 1987;2:89–105.
2. Stanton SL, Tenagho EA. Preface. In: Stanton SL, Tenagho EA,
   eds. *Surgery of Female Incontinence.* New York: Springer–Verlag;
   1980.
3. Lucente V, Benson JT, McClellan E. Restoration of the levator
   ani for the treatment of genital tract prolapse: the retrorectal
   levatoplasty. Presented at AUGS meeting; November 3, 1990;
   Tarpon Springs, Fl.
4. White GR. Cystocele—a radical cure by suturing lateral sulci of
   vagina to the white line of pelvic fascia. *JAMA.* 1909;53:1707–
   1709.
5. White GR. An anatomic operation for the cure of cystocele. *Am
   J Obstet Dis Wom Child.* 1912;65:286.

Fig. 12B-8   The arcus tendineus viewed from above.

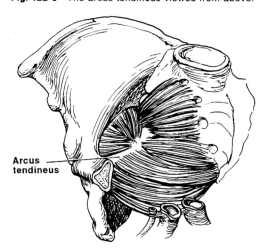

Arcus
tendineus

Vaginal Dysfunction

13A   Sexual Function in the Postmenopausal Female

Barbara B. Sherwin

INTRODUCTION

Although disturbances in aspects of sexual functioning are commonly reported by menopausal women, it is not clear whether they are causally related to the endocrine changes that are a hallmark of this reproductive event. In this chapter, an attempt will be made to assess the impact of the sex steroids on sexual behavior in postmenopausal women by examining both the mechanisms of action of hormones on various tissues and the empirical evidence regarding the consequences of changes in the endocrine milieu that occur at the time of menopause.

Endocrine Changes

It is likely that waning ovarian follicular activity and its eventual cessation are key events in the endocrinologic changes that occur in the perimenopausal period. Several years before the menopause, there is an increase in circulating follicle-stimulating hormone (FSH) and a decrease in estradiol and progesterone.[1] Estrogen production by the postmenopausal ovary is minimal and ovarian removal is not accompanied by any significant further decrease in circulating or excreted estrogens.[2]

In women, both the adrenal gland and the ovary contain the biosynthetic pathways necessary for androgen synthesis and secretion. The ovary produces ap- proximately 25% of plasma testosterone, 60% of androstenedione, and 20% of dehydroepiandrosterone (DHEA), whereas the adrenal gland produces 25% of circulating testosterone, 40% of androstenedione, 50% of DHEA and 90% of dehydroepiandrosterone sulphate (DHEAS). The remainder of circulating androgens in the female are thought to arise through peripheral conversion, which likely accounts for the production rate of 50% of testosterone and 25% of DHEA.[3] About 50% of women produce even greater amounts of androgens after the menopause due to ovarian stromal hyperplasia that occurs under the influence of high luteinizing hormone (LH) levels.[4] However, when it occurs, this increase in ovarian testosterone production is time-limited, so that eventually, testosterone levels decrease in all women.

Aspects of Sexual Behavior

As more research findings on hormones and sexual behavior were accumulating during the 1960s and 1970s, it became clear that the inconsistencies in the literature were largely due to a lack of standard definitions. Sexuality is not a unitary phenomenon but rather is composed of identifiably distinct but interrelated processes. The word "libido," commonly used to describe all aspects of sexual behavior, confused the research effort.

Davidson and colleagues[5] suggested that the components of sexual behavior could be conceptualized under two major headings. The first category subsumes those behaviors associated with libido or sexual motivation, such as sexual desire, sexual fantasies, and satisfaction or pleasure, whereas potency refers to pelvic vasocongestion, orgasmic contractions, and possible extragenital responses. This definition has since served as a useful heuristic tool for defining and investigating sexual dysfunction in both men and women, because it lends itself to an analysis of the component parts of sexuality and their selective regulation by psychosocial and physiologic factors. In females, therefore, we can operationally define and measure sexual motivational factors such as desire and fantasies, as well as potency or sexual response factors such as vaginal lubrication and orgasm. A comprehensive description of sexual behavior, therefore, requires the differential evaluation of these behavioral elements which probably have different physiologic and psychologic bases.

Epidemiology of Sexual Dysfunction after Menopause

Survey data on the frequency and type of sexual problems after menopause generally show a high incidence of problems in postmenopausal women. Percentages of women complaining of specific dysfunctions appear in Table 13A-1. It is important to note that in most of these surveys, subjects were patients at a menopause clinic, so these incidences cannot be generalized to a nonclinical population. Nonetheless they serve to point out that one third to one half of women who seek medical care postmenopausally complain of a problem in sexual function.

The extent to which the husband's diminished libido and/or potency influences the decline in the women's sexual behaviors has also been disputed. Although several authors have concluded that the "husband effect," and not menopausal endocrine changes, was primarily responsible for decrements in sexual activity,[6,7] others have found little evidence in support of this contention.[8,11,13] Although the issue has not been resolved, it does seem clear from hormone replacement studies that are reviewed later in this chapter that decrements in both sexual desire and response may occur in postmenopausal women, independent of any problems in their partners. Moreover, it is of interest that in Hällström's[8] study of 800 perimenopausal Swedish women, declining sexual interest occurred more commonly in lower socioeconomic groups. His interpretation that education leads to greater freedom from cultural inhibi-

Table 13A-1
Epidemiologic Data on Aging and Frequency of Female Sexual Behaviors

Study	Sexual Interest	Coitus	Orgasm
Kinsey and colleagues[6]	?	↓53%	↓48%
Pfeiffer and Davis[7]			
46–50 yrs.	↓7%	?	?
61–65 yrs.	↓51%	?	?
Hällström[8]			
46–54 yrs.	↓52%	↓	↓16%
55–64 yrs.	↓68%	↓	↓24%
McCoy and Davidson[9]	↓85%	↓	NC
Sarrel and Whitehead[10]	↓39%	↓	↓32%
Cutler and colleagues[11]			
44–52 yrs.	↓10%	↓	↓20%
Hunter and Whitehead[12]		?	NC
Hällström and Samuelsson[13]	↓33%	?	?

? = Not assessed; ↓ = Decrease; NC = No change.

tions and sexual stereotypes serves to further underline the myriad determinants of sexual behavior.

Various research paradigms are used to investigate the concomitants and possible etiology in declining sexual function in peri- and postmenopausal women. The three most commonly used strategies are correlational studies, psychophysiologic studies, and hormone replacement therapy studies. Research findings from each of these groupings will be reviewed.

Correlational Studies

Several investigators tested the association between circulating levels of sex steroids and sexual behavior in postmenopausal women. Bachmann and coworkers[14] found that neither estradiol nor testosterone levels differentiated sexually active and inactive untreated postmenopausal women, but that sexually active women had less vaginal atrophy than did inactive women. Interestingly, of the 29 sexually inactive women in their sample, 32% cited their partner's disinterest, whereas 25% cited their own disinterest as reasons for their celibacy. In accordance with Hällström's[8] finding, Bachmann's study also found that sexually inactive women had lower incomes.

In a longitudinal study, cycling perimenopausal women were followed for at least one year beyond the cessation of their menstrual cycles. Compared with their premenopause data, the women had fewer sexual thoughts or fantasies and experienced less vaginal lubrication during sex after menopause. Although estradiol and testosterone levels both showed significant declines from pre- to postmenopause, higher testosterone levels were associated with coital frequency.[15] Since 38% of subjects dropped out of the study before its completion because of the need for estrogen replacement therapy, it is likely that the decline in sexual functioning was underestimated in this biased sample.

Perimenopausal women with irregular menstrual cycles between the ages of 44 to 52 years failed to report significant deficits in sexual desire, response, or satisfaction, although those whose estradiol levels were low did report a decrease in coital activity.[16] The relationship between testosterone levels and sexual behavior was not reported in that study.

Psychophysiologic Studies

The development in the 1970s of the vaginal photoplethysmograph allowed for the objective, physiologic measurement of sexual arousal in women. The vaginal photoplethysmograph is an acrylic probe containing a light-emitting diode and photo-detector for measures of vaginal vasocongestion.[17] The instrument is designed to be inserted into the vagina as a tampon and is used to quantify changes in vaginal pulse amplitude in laboratory settings as a result of exposure to sexual stimuli. Morrell and coworkers[18] tested a group of young, regularly cycling women and groups of premenopausal and postmenopausal women who were exposed to erotic film and fantasy. The vaginal pulse amplitude of the premenopausal subjects did not differ from that of the young cycling women. However, both the young cycling women and the premenopausal subjects had significantly greater responses (more vaginal vasocongestion) than a group of untreated postmenopausal women. The differences in circulating levels of estradiol and testosterone between the groups mimicked their psychophysiologic differences. That is, plasma levels of both estradiol and testosterone were lower in the postmenopausal women compared to those in the other two groups. It should be noted that in the postmenopausal group, 54% complained of inadequate lubrication and 36% experienced dyspareunia. The authors suggested that low estradiol levels may have accounted for the diminished vascular response to erotic stimuli.

In a second psychophysiologic study, premenopausal women and estrogen-treated and untreated postmenopausal women were investigated to determine whether differences in hormone status were associated with differences in physiologic and subjective sexual responses.[19] The three groups did not differ in either average or maximum vaginal pulse amplitude to erotic and neutral videotapes, nor in latency of sexual response. However, the untreated postmenopausal women reported significantly less vaginal lubrication in response to the erotic film compared to the perimenopausal and the estrogen-treated postmenopausal subjects. Because there was no relationship between estradiol levels and vaginal pulse amplitude, the authors concluded that estrogen is important in maintaining vaginal lubrication and the perception of arousal, but not in determining vaginal vasocongestion. Moreover, testosterone levels were associated with higher levels of physical sensations during sexual arousal, although not with genital responses.

In a recent, well-controlled, prospective study, menopausal women were tested before treatment and after random assignment to groups for treatment with either Premarin, 0.625 mg; Premarin, 0.625 mg and Provera, 5 mg; Premarin, 0.625 mg and methyltestosterone, 5 mg; or placebo.[20] All women in the hormone-treated groups had significantly reduced frequency of hot flush compared to the placebo group. Hormone treatment did not significantly alter mood ratings, sexual behaviors, or psychophysiologically measured sexual arousal. However, the combined estrogen-testosterone preparation significantly increased reports of pleasure from autoerotic or self-stimulating behavior.

In summary, two of the three psychophysiologic studies failed to find an effect of estrogen on vasocongestive responses during sexual arousal, but did observe that vaginal lubrication was estrogen dependent. More important perhaps, is the consistent finding in these studies that testosterone contributed to the pleasurable physical sensations associated with sexual arousal, although it was unrelated to actual genital responses.

Hormone Replacement Therapy Studies

The paradigm that is perhaps most powerful for the study of the specificity of the sex steroids on female sexuality involves administering hormone replacement therapy to women who have undergone total abdominal hysterectomy (TAH) and bilateral salpingo-oophorectomy (BSO). When both ovaries are removed from premenopausal women, circulating testosterone levels decrease significantly within the first 24 to 48 hours postoperatively.[21] The fact that women are deprived of ovarian androgen production following this surgical procedure provides a rationale for administering both estrogen and androgen as replacement therapy.

In Great Britain and Australia, subcutaneous implantation of pellets containing estradiol and testosterone has been used as a treatment for menopausal symptoms for several decades. This route of sex-steroid administration results in a slow, constant release of the sex hormones over a period of at least six months.

In a single-blind study, both surgically and naturally menopausal women who complained of loss of libido (undefined) despite therapy with conjugated equine estrogen were implanted subcutaneously with pellets containing estradiol, 40 mg, and testosterone, 100 mg.[22] By the third month after implantation, patients reported a significant increase in libido and enjoyment of sex, as well as in the frequency of orgasm and of initiation of sexual activities. These changes occurred concurrent with a significant increase in plasma testosterone levels.

In another single-blind study, a group of premenopausal women (mean age 44.5 years) and a group of naturally and surgically menopausal women (mean age 53.3 years) were implanted with subcutaneous pellets containing estradiol, 50 mg, and testosterone, 100 mg.[23] Loss of libido was a presenting symptom in more than 80% of patients in both groups, and hormone implant therapy reversed the symptom in two thirds of the patients.

Twenty women who had experienced a severe loss of libido despite treatment with oral estrogens and progestins that adequately relieved other symptoms, such as hot flushes and vaginal dryness, randomly received subcutaneous implants of either estradiol, 40 mg, or of a combined pellet containing estradiol, 40 mg, and testosterone, 50 mg.[24] Self ratings of various aspects of sexual functioning were carried out after implantation. After 6 weeks, the loss of libido in the single implant group remained, while the combined group showed significant symptomatic relief. The mean peak testosterone concentrations after testosterone implantation slightly exceeded the upper limit of the normal female range.

Although these implant studies were single-blind, in two of them patients were preselected on the basis of loss of libido that had been unresponsive to estrogen alone,[22,23] and the third study contained an estrogen-alone control group as a basis for comparison. Despite methodologic flaws, results of these studies strongly suggest that testosterone and not estrogen is primarily critical for libido or sexual desire in women.

During the past decade, several prospective, well-controlled studies of general and sexual effects of combined estrogen-androgen (E-A) parenteral preparations in surgically menopausal women were carried out. In all of them, premenopausal women who needed to undergo TAH and BSO for benign disease were randomly assigned to one of four treatment groups postoperatively. Those who received an E-A preparation or androgen alone (A) intramuscularly following surgery had greater energy level and sense of well-being than those who received estrogen alone (E) or placebo (PL).[25] Administration of the androgen-containing preparations (E-A and A) were also associated with lower somatic and psychologic symptom scores than E or PL.[26] Moreover, all women treated with hormones following surgery had more positive moods than those given PL.[27]

Androgenic effects of sexual behavior were also investigated in these studies of women who had all been happily married for at least 5 years. It was also ascertained that they and their husbands were in good general health. The women monitored several aspects of their sexual behavior daily for a total of 8 months; 1 month preoperatively, and during 2 three-month postoperative treatment phases that were separated by a placebo month. All drugs were given intramuscularly every 28 days. In the E-A combined preparation, 1 ml contains testosterone enanthate, 150 mg; estradiol dienanthate, 7.5 mg; and estradiol benzoate, 1 mg. Women who received either of the androgen-containing drugs reported an enhancement of sexual desire (Fig. 13A-1) and arousal (Fig. 13A-2), and an increase in the number of sexual fantasies compared with those treated with E or PL.[28] Ratings of women treated with androgen did not differ from those of a second control group comprised of women who had undergone TAH but whose ovaries had been retained (CON). This occurred even though patients in the CON group were on average 10 years younger than the oophorectomized women. However, the frequencies of coitus or orgasm did not differ as a response to the various hormonal treatments. Sherwin and Gelfand[29] subsequently confirmed these findings in surgically menopausal women who were treated with the E-A drug on a long-term basis, compared with a group that received long-term E alone, and a third group that remained untreated following their TAH and BSO at least 2 years earlier.

Taken together, the findings from both the subcutaneous implant pellet studies and the controlled studies that used intramuscular hormonal preparations provide compelling evidence that the addition of testosterone to an estrogen replacement regimen is associated with an

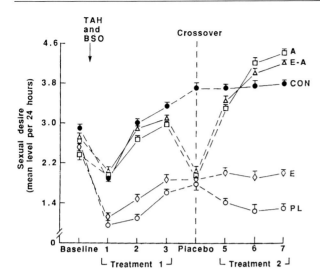

Fig. 13A-1 Mean level of sexual desire plus or minus SEM (standard error of the mean). The treatment groups are combined estrogen-androgen, *E-A* (△), estrogen alone, *E* (◇), androgen alone, *A* (□), placebo, *PL* (○), and hysterectomy, *CON* (●). (Reprinted from Sherwin[28] with permission.)

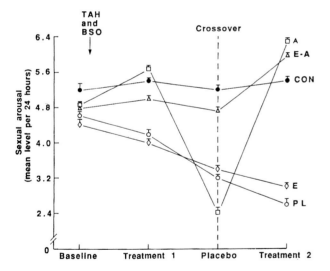

Fig. 13A-2 Mean level of sexual arousal plus or minus SEM (standard error of the mean). The treatment groups are combined estrogen-androgen, *E-A* (△), estrogen alone, *E* (◇), androgen alone, *A* (□), placebo, *PL* (○), and hysterectomy, *CON* (●). (Reprinted from Sherwin[28] with permission.)

enhancement of sexual desire, interest, and enjoyment of sex in postmenopausal women. These findings also allow the conclusion that in women, as well as in men,[30] testosterone has its major effect on the cognitive, moti-

vational, or libidinal aspects of sexual behavior, such as desire and fantasies and not on physiologic responses. Moreover, studies of nonhuman primates strongly suggest that testosterone exerts this effect on sexual desire via mechanisms that impact directly on the brain, rather than by any effect on peripheral tissues.[31]

Side Effects of Estrogen-Androgen Combined Replacement Therapy

In our studies of surgically menopausal women given 1 ml of an injectable E-A preparation every 28 days,[25–29] we observed a 15% to 20% incidence of mild facial hirsutism that recedes when the dose is modified. Other virilizing side effects such as deepening of the voice were not reported with this dose. Recently, after decreasing the dose of the combined drug to 0.5 ml (75 mg of testosterone per month intramuscularly), we noted a reduction in the incidence of hirsutism to less than 5% of patients. Given intramuscularly, the E-A combined drug we use does not adversely affect the lipoprotein lipid profile,[32] a finding that cannot be generalized to other hormonal preparations or to other routes of administration. However, in a recent pilot study we determined that the daily oral administration of 0.625 mg of esterified estrogens, and 1.25 mg of methyltestosterone for at least 6 weeks did not cause any significant change in the lipid profile of postmenopausal women thus treated.[33] Levels of sex hormone binding globulin, a hepatic protein, also remained within the normal range of female values following the long-term intramuscular administration of the combined E-A preparation.[34]

SUMMARY

Epidemiologic studies provide evidence that a considerable number of postmenopausal women complain of disturbances in some aspect of sexual functioning. Given that estrogen is responsible for the integrity of the tissues of the reproductive tract, decreased vaginal lubrication and dyspareunia may be due to estrogen depletion in these women. However, it is clear that sexual dysfunctions, specifically lack of sexual desire and interest, occur in postmenopausal women who are being treated with exogenous estrogen. This is reported more frequently by surgically menopausal women who were deprived of ovarian androgen production than by naturally menopausal women whose ovaries may continue to secrete androgens for some period of time after the menopause. Evidence from well-controlled studies now strongly suggests that the administration of a combined E-A preparation in the postmenopause enhances the motivational or libidinal aspects of sexuality such as desire and interest. When the sexual complaint is associated with a natural or surgical menopause, exogenous testosterone combined with estradiol is frequently effective in reversing the symptom. However, when the sexual dysfunction has been life-long or when its onset predates the menopause considerably, then hormone therapy may not be sufficient to restore levels of sexual desire and psychologic counselling should be sought.

REFERENCES

1. Sherman BW, Korenman SG. Hormonal characteristics of the human menstrual cycle throughout reproductive life. *J Clin Invest.* 1975;55:699.
2. Judd HZ, Lucas WE, Yen SSC. Serum 17β-estradiol and estrone levels in postmenopausal women with and without endometrial cancer. *J Clin Endocrinol Metab.* 1976;43:272.
3. Longcope C. Adrenal and gonadal steroid secretion in normal females. *Cl Endocrinol Metab.* 1986;15:213.
4. Judd HL, Judd GE, Lucas WE, Yen SCC. Endocrine function of the postmenopausal ovary: concentrations of androgens and estrogens in ovarian and peripheral vein blood. *J Clin Endocrinol Metab.* 1974;39:1020.
5. Davidson JM, Gray GD, Smith ER. The sexual psychoendocrinology of aging. In: Meites J, ed. *Neuroendocrinology of Aging.* New York: Plenum Press; 1983;221–258.
6. Kinsey AC, Pomeroy WB, Martin CE, Gebhard PH. *Sexual Behavior in the Human Female.* Philadelphia: WB Saunders; 1953.
7. Pfeiffer E, Davis GC. Determinants of sexual behavior in middle and old age. *J Am Geriat Soc.* 1972;4:151.
8. Hällström T. Sexuality in the climacteric. *Clin Obstet Gynecol.* 1977;4:227.
9. McCoy NL, Davidson JM. A longitudinal study of the effects of menopause on sexuality. *Maturitas.* 1985;7:203.
10. Sarrel PM, Whitehead MI. Sex and menopause: defining the issues. *Maturitas.* 1985;7:217.
11. Cutler WB, Garcia CR, McCoy N. Perimenopausal sexuality. *Arch Sex Behav.* 1987;16:225.
12. Hunter MS, Whitehead MI. Psychological experience of the climacteric. *Menopause: Evaluation, Treatment and Health Concerns.* New York: Alan R. Liss Inc; 1989:211–224.
13. Hällström T, Samuelsson S. Changes in women's sexual desire in middle life: the longitudinal study of women in Gothenberg. *Arch Sex Behav.* 1990;19:259.
14. Bachmann G, Leiblum SR, Kemmann E, Colburn DW, Swartzman L, Shelden R. Sexual expression and its determinants in the postmenopausal woman. *Maturitas.* 1984;6:19.

15. McCoy N, Davidson JM. A longitudinal study of the effects of menopause on sexuality. *Maturitas.* 1985;7:203.
16. Cutler WB, Garcia CR, McCoy N. Perimenopausal sexuality. *Arch Sex Behav.* 1987;16:225.
17. Tahmousch AJ, Jennings JR, Lee AL, Camp S, Weber F. Characteristics of a light-emitting diode-transistor photoplethysmograph. *Psychophysiology.* 1976;13:357.
18. Morrell MJ, Dixen JM, Carter S, Davidson JM. The influence of age and cycling status on sexual arousability in women. *Am J Obstet Gynecol.* 1984;148:66.
19. Myers LS, Morokoff PJ. Physiological and subjective sexual arousal in pre- and postmenopausal women taking replacement therapy. *Psychophysiology.* 1986;23:283.
20. Myers LS, Dixen J, Morrissette D, Carmichael M, Davidson JM. Effects of estrogen, androgen, and progestin on sexual psychophysiology and behavior in postmenopausal women. *J Clin Endocrinol Metab.* 1990;70:1124.
21. Vermeulen A. The hormonal activity of the postmenopausal ovary. *J Clin Endocrinol Metab.* 1976;42:247.
22. Burger HG, Hailes J, Menelaus M, Nelson J, Hudson B, Balazs N. The management of persistent menopausal symptoms with estradiol-testosterone implants: clinical, lipid and hormonal results. *Maturitas.* 1984;6:351.
23. Cardozo L, Gibb DMF, Tuck SM, Thom MH, Studd JWW, Cooper DJ. The effects of subcutaneous hormone implants during the climacteric. *Maturitas.* 1984;5:177.
24. Burger H, Hailes J, Nelson J, Menelaus M. Effect of combined implants of estradiol and testosterone on libido in postmenopausal women. *Lancet.* 1987;294:936.
25. Sherwin BB, Gelfand MM. Effects of parenteral administration of estrogen and androgen on plasma hormone levels and hot flushes in surgical menopause. *Am J Obstet Gynecol.* 1984;148:552.
26. Sherwin BB, Gelfand MM. Differential symptom response to parenteral estrogen and/or androgen administration in the surgical menopause. *Am J Obstet Gynecol.* 1985;151:153.
27. Sherwin BB, Gelfand MM. Sex steroids and affect in the surgical menopause: a double-blind cross-over study. *Psychoneuroendocrinology.* 1985;10:325.
28. Sherwin BB, Gelfand MM, Brender W. Androgen enhances sexual motivation in females: a prospective cross-over study of sex steroid administration in the surgical menopause. *Psychosom Med.* 1985;47:339–351.
29. Sherwin BB, Gelfand MM. The role of androgen in the maintenance of sexual functioning in oophorectomized women. *Psychosom Med.* 1987;49:397.
30. Bancroft J, Wu FCW. Changes in erectile responsiveness during androgen replacement therapy. *Arch Sex Behav.* 1983;12:59.
31. Everitt BJ, Herbert J. The effects of implanting testosterone propionate in the central nervous system on the sexual behavior of the female rhesus monkeys. *Brain Res.* 1975;86:109.
32. Sherwin BB, Gelfand MM, Schucher R, Gabor J. Postmenopausal estrogen and androgen replacement and lipoprotein lipid concentrations. *Am J Obstet Gynecol.* 1987;156:414.
33. Sherwin BB, Youngs DD. Effects of oral estrogen-androgen preparation on lipid metabolism in postmenopausal women. Abstracts of the Workshop Conference on Androgen Therapy: Biologic and Clinical Consequences; Marco Island, FL. Jan, 1990.
34. Sherwin BB, Gelfand MM. Individual differences in mood with menopausal replacement therapy: possible role of sex hormone-binding globulin. *J Psychosom Obstet Gynecol.* 1987;6:121.

Acknowledgments: The preparation of this manuscript was supported by Grant #MA-8707 from the Medical Research Council of Canada awarded to B.B. Sherwin.

CHAPTER 13

Vaginal Dysfunction

13B Pathogenesis

J. Thomas Benson

INTRODUCTION

Vaginal dysfunction can be defined both obstetrically and gynecologically. Obstetric vaginal dysfunction refers to the failure of the vagina to accommodate the vast requirements of parturition. This frequently relates to the configuration and size of the bony structure, the most nonyielding pelvic floor component. The subsequent muscular, fascial, vascular, and neurologic damage comprises many of the underlying etiologies of female pelvic floor disorders.

Vaginal dysfunction from a gynecologic viewpoint encompasses the functions of fertilization and sexual response. Both of these functions involve a partner. Unlike other systems, then, the pathogenesis of vaginal dysfunction is not limited to consideration of just the patient.

As with other pelvic floor disorders, vaginal dysfunctions do increase with advancing age[1] so that more than one quarter of postmenopausal women describe sexual problems. Many older women are sexually inactive because they lack a partner. Currently, in the United States there are only 69 men for every 100 women age 65 and older.[2] Response to this cultural phenomenon is an apparent change in the expectation that wives should be younger than husbands. In 1983, the woman was at least five years older than the man in 6.2% of all U.S. marriages, a 67% increase compared to the 1970 statistics.[3]

Vaginal dysfunction as it relates to infertility refers to failure of seminal reception, pooling, and capacitation, whether caused by structural or chemical factors. Vaginal dysfunction in sexual response may be classified chiefly into problems of dyspareunia or laxity. Increased understanding of vaginal physiology promotes improved therapeutic techniques for restoration when the vagina is a component of pelvic floor disorder, as it is so often.

VAGINAL PHYSIOLOGY

Compared to the male, the presence of the reproductive tract in the woman constitutes a focal weakness in the pelvic floor and explains the increased frequency of its disorders in women. As the weakest portion of the pelvic floor, the vagina is subjected to all the vectors of force caused by gravity, damaged by the trauma of childbirth, and finally insulted by hormonal deprivation. The focus of pelvic floor disorders is therefore on the vagina.

For the various portions of the vagina to act synchronously in sexual response, proper anatomic relationship to other pelvic floor viscera and supports must be present. The horizontal alignment of the upper portion of the vagina in a posterior direction overlying an intact levator plate with a competent levator hiatus, allowing all the pelvic floor viscera to function in a unified manner, is necessary. Mobility of the upper vagina so that its attachment to supporting structures allows forward and upward expansion while synchronously acting with perineal musculature for sphincteric effect, in unison with the urinary and colorectal system, must be achieved.

Studies of pelvic floor disorders as outlined in this book, encompassing the clinical, radiologic, ultrasound, manometric, electrodiagnostic, and histopathologic investigations all have reference to the vaginal attachments and relationships. For discussion purposes, vaginal function can be divided into introital and apical considerations.

Introital Physiology

Much of our understanding of vaginal physiology stems from the epochical work of Masters and Johnson.[4,5] Introital muscular activity involves the transverse perineal, bulbocavernosus, and external anal sphincter muscles of the perineum, and the compressor urethra and urethrovaginal sphincter of the urogenital diaphragm. Configurations of this musculature in living subjects are found by 360 degree radial ultrasound and magnetic resonant imaging to be somewhat different than anatomic studies based on cadaver material. For instance, the anal sphincter musculature has a substantial anterior component, unlike that depicted in the anatomic literature.[6] This musculature works in coordinated fashion, principally served neurologically by branches of the pudendal nerve. Autonomic nervous control through the pelvic plexus has profound effects on sphincteric smooth musculature in the urinary, vaginal, and colorectal systems as well as vascular effects (see Chapter 9A).

The vestibular, urethrovesical, and external rectal vasculature are involved to a marked degree in introital sexual response. The phenomenon of lubrication is a somewhat generalized response depending on initial dilation of the perivaginal veins, including those of the bulbous vestibule, pudendal, urethrovaginal, vesical, and external rectal plexuses. Associated with the vascular events are color and rugal changes in the vaginal mucosa, with flattening and darkening of color as the excitement stage evolves. The transverse rugal corrugations are more marked in the anterior wall, especially in the nullipara, and become notably less distinct secondary to the vascular swelling as the excitement stage continues. During the plateau stage of sexual response the basal congestion becomes even more pronounced causing the central lumen of the outer one third of the vagina to be reduced to one third of its previous size.

This congested area, in addition to the engorged labia minora, forms the "orgasmic platform" that aids in seminal fluid retention by the high, firm, perineal support. The "gripping" effect thus created also functions in penile containment. The platform release occurs rapidly after orgasm, but may take up to 30 minutes to dissipate if no orgasm occurs.

After initial relaxation during the excitement stage, the muscular component of the orgasmic platform becomes most pronounced during the orgasmic phase. At this time there are regular, strong contractions in the outer one third of the vagina. The contractions are usually three to six in number occurring in intervals of about 0.8 seconds initially, then increasing intervals occur for a total of ten to fifteen contractions.

Apical Physiology

Changes in the vaginal apex occur during sexual response. The inner two thirds of the vagina undergo lengthening and distention beginning in the excitement stage, with the uterus elevating out of the true pelvis. This phenomenon is dependent on anterior location of the uterine fundus and support of the round ligament area, as the retroverted uterus will not undergo such elevation. Partially, as influenced by the levator attachment (see Chapter 2), the transverse vagina anterior to the cervix undergoes widening and the vagina lengthens (see Chapter 4). In the resolution phase, zonal relaxation of the upper two thirds of the vagina occurs, principally involving the lateral and posterior walls, and the cervix returns to the preexcitement location in about 3 to 4 minutes, somewhat more rapidly than the posterior and lateral vaginal wall return. Realization of the increased width of the vagina in the apical portion is important in planning surgical restoration in pelvic floor defect surgery.

Introital Dysfunction

Introital dysfunction may become pronounced when neurogenic, vascular, or muscular elements, or any combination of these, have functional derangement. The symptomatology of introital dysfunction is chiefly dyspareunia or laxity.

Dyspareunia

Dyspareunia as a symptom of vaginal introital dysfunction is inseparable from the pathophysiology involved in vaginismus.[7] Etymologically, "dyspareunia" means "bad or difficult mating." Current concepts that consider dyspareunia to be pain during intercourse have narrowed the focus into artificially compartmentalized, antagonistic viewpoints regarding organic features on one hand, and psychologic features on the other hand. As considered by psychiatrists, dyspareunia is defined in women as the occurrence of pain in the absence of organic disease, localized to the vagina and/or lower pelvic area from penetration or thrusting of the penis in the vagina. And, as listed under the classification of psychosexual disorders in *The Diagnostic and Statistical Manual of Mental Disorders* (DSM III),[8] vaginismus has traditionally been diagnosed in the psychiatric literature only when the spasm is sufficient to prevent vaginal penetration. This viewpoint promotes the impression that intromission is virtually impossible in women with vaginismus because of the involuntary muscle contraction, and that if vaginismus is present, concurrent dyspareunia is invariable. Therefore, if vaginismus is the cause of the dyspareunia, the primary diagnosis is vaginismus.[9]

In actuality, dyspareunia and vaginismus are undeniably linked. Repeated dyspareunia is likely to result in vaginismus, and vaginismus may be the causative factor in dyspareunia. Also considered are aspects of sexual dysfunction thought to involve learning theory.[10] Either lack of learning or faulty learning may cause expectations leading to a learned dysfunction or pain.

The most successful and logical explanation of pathogenesis of dyspareunia with introital vaginal dysfunction postulates the causality to be a continuum of both physical and psychogenic factors with a potential for both to be equal contributors.[11] Vaginismus is not an all-or-nothing phenomenon. It occurs in varying degrees and can occur at varying times. It has, in fact, been classified[12] into four degrees: the first degree is characterized by perineal and levator spasm which is relieved with reassurance; the second degree with perineal spasm maintained throughout pelvic examination; the third degree with levator spasm and elevation of the buttocks; and the fourth degree with levator and perineal spasm leading to adduction and retreat. Any painful condition of the vaginal introitus invokes psychologic responses associated with anxiety and intrapsychic conflict leading to vaginismus, which further increases the introital dyspareunia to make a classic "vicious cycle." The therapy[7] of the introital dysmenorrhea must combine any organic factor with treatment of the vaginismus, which is so well managed during the examination by teaching the patient that she can be in control of the vaginal introital musculature and describing and legitimizing a plan for employing these principles in her relationship with her partner.

In ascertaining organic cause of introital dyspareunia, there is probably no place in medicine where history is of more importance. Careful search for the chronology of the painful events is probably the most valuable diagnostic tool.

Organic Lesions

Organic lesions are present in approximately one third of cases of introital dyspareunia.[13] Embryologically, the urethra above the mesonephric duct and the anterior vaginal wall below it both take origin from the urogenital sinus. The posterior ends of the Müllerian ducts contact the epithelium of the urogenital sinus at the level where the Wolffian ducts open into the sinus, the Müllerian tubercle. The junction of the epithelium of the Müllerian ducts in the urogenital sinus epithelium is debatable. Some observers consider the junction to be at the squamocolumnar junction of the endocervix,[14] whereas some believe it to be in the upper one third of the vagina,[15] and still others feel it is at the junction of the endocervix at the endometrium.[16] Nevertheless, all are in agreement that tissues derived from the urogenital sinus constitute the most sensitive tissues to steroid sex hormones, such sensitivity affecting the urethra as well as the vagina.

Excessive secretion of androgenic steroid during embryonic life can lead to defective development of the introitus to the point that satisfactory coitus is impossible. Operation for ambiguous genitalia prior to menarche, an important point psychologically, frequently results in a small vaginal orifice that requires further surgery to achieve satisfactory coitus.

A congenital anomaly of congenital shortening between the fourchette and urethra accompanied by a firm perineum, a thick hymen, and a small introitus is a common congenital cause of introital dyspareunia.[17] In this condition the dyspareunia is partially caused by pressure on the external urethral meatus, always a consideration because of the sensitivity of the urethra.

Other congenital anomalies such as transverse septae require surgical removal. Longitudinal septae as a rule do not cause dyspareunia. Vagina agenesis (Mayer, Rokitansky, Kuster, Hauser syndrome) of course is an easily recognizable congenital defect leading to dyspareunia.

Organic causes of introital dyspareunia can usually be diagnosed by careful examination. Vulvar episiotomy scars are commonly associated with such dyspareunia. Mediolateral episiotomies tend to produce the problem more than midline ones, although both certainly can. Scars from perineoplasty are common offenders. Bartholin duct dilatation during a sexual response in diseased ducts can be a cause of dyspareunia, as can scars from Bartholin duct excision.

Cystic lesions of the introitus occur, such as mesonephric cysts and paraurethral cysts, or perineal or vaginal endometriosis. Urethral polyps are fairly common also. Urethritis and "urethral syndrome" are commonly associated with dyspareunia, and the association of vaginismus with urethral syndrome is strong. Rigid hymen and hymenitis have long been considered local organic causes. Vulvar disease includes herpetic infection, dystrophy, radiation damage, and allergic reactions to deodorants and restrictive clothing. Vascular defects such as glomus tumors were also described as leading to dyspareunia.[18]

The effects of estrogen deprivation are distinctly apparent in this condition.[19] The vulva loses its thick, adipose layer and the vaginal mucosa becomes pale, friable, and dry. Lubrication is impaired. Infrequent coitus leads to loss of elasticity and as many as 30% of postmenopausal patients complain of dyspareunia.

Vaginal bands which are described as occurring between portions of the hymen and only becoming obvious at the time of sexual arousal,[20] and conditions postulated to be due to inadequate rupture of the hymen[21] may cause dyspareunia. One of the most distressing and common forms of dyspareunia is iatrogenically caused by improperly performed posterior colporrhaphies where the levator ani is brought together in a nonanatomic position between the vagina and rectum. The creation of transverse tender bands leading to dyspareunia in this classic Halban-Hegar posterior colporrhaphy resulted in virtual disuse of the posterior colporrhaphy in many localities. Properly performed levatoplasties utilizing anatomic correction (see Chapter 16) should not have this associated sequela.

Apical Dysfunction

Apical dysfunction has profound relevance to anatomic supporting structures of the pelvic floor. It is now realized that there is a 35% to 40% increase in apical vaginal length and upper end vaginal expansion to as much as 6 cm during sexual excitation. Such changes in position and length are dependent on proper maintenance of the anterior vaginal lateral supports to the arcus tendineus and levator attachments in the absence of the uterus. When the uterus is present, the same structures in addition to anterior uterine supports with round ligament are functional. Any pathologic process which may limit this elevation or increase tissue sensitivity may lead to the development of deep dyspareunia.

Dyspareunia

Just as with introital dyspareunia there is unavoidable overlapping of the organic symptomatology with psychologic input. Just as introital dyspareunia and vaginismus are coexistent with introital dysfunction, deep dyspareunia is associated with pelvic floor musculature disorders and significant psychologic input, because the patient senses loss of control with decreased sexual response, thereby increased anxiety again causing a vicious cycle. The associated pelvic floor dysfunctions that are present when the vaginal apical supporting structures are lost may be in urinary and anorectal realms. The urinary and anal dysfunction further heightens the anxiety associated with the sexual dysfunction, to add to both the organic and psychologic distresses.

The pathologic processes limiting the elevation and expansion of the upper vagina may be extrinsic and may not be a primary disorder of support mechanisms. Any process leading to inflammation such as endometriosis or pelvic inflammation may contribute to dyspareunia. The support loss processes change the upper vaginal elevation and expansion and, in addition, have vascular effects. Tourniquet-type effect on venous pelvic vasculature is considered to lead to the development of deep dyspareunia in the "pelvic congestion syndrome."[22] Disputes over the psychologic versus organic factors in this condition have been ongoing since its description in 1952, but as already emphasized, both components should be considered, because both are invariably present. The vascular effects in the pathogenesis of apical or deep dyspareunia can explain why the pain is occasionally perceived as being unilateral. Vascular disturbance following tubal ligation have been found to cause unilateral pain.[23]

An all too common cause of apical dyspareunia is iatrogenic shortening of the vaginal vault in association with hysterectomy. The cervix does constitute a portion of the anterior vaginal wall and removing that compromises the length of the anterior vaginal wall, especially if closed transversely. Excessive apical vaginal removal is commonly performed with hysterectomy for benign disease, resulting in shortened vaginal length. This has a particularly profound effect if shortened to the point that the vagina cannot occupy a horizontal position to rest on the levator plate. If either increased levator hiatus, shortened vagina, or both factors are present, vaginal inversion can occur and lead to vault prolapse. Shortened vaginal length can affect the elevation and widening of the apex so that a sexual dysfunction develops. It is an unfortunate situation because it is difficult to remedy surgically. Perineorrhaphy does add some vaginal length at the distal portion, but restoring vaginal length at the apical portion is not easily achieved, short of grafting procedures.

Laxity

Vaginal dysfunction may be secondary to laxity and not actually produce symptomatology of either introital or deep dyspareunia.

Introital Laxity

The symptomatology of introital laxity has its pathogenesis in disturbance of formation of the orgasmic platform. The orgasmic platform is important in both penile containment and gripping and in seminal pooling. Thus its disturbance may lead to sexual dysfunction or even problems associated with infertility.

The pathogenesis of introital laxity is generally obstetric in origin, having to do with actual architectural disturbance of the perineal musculature. Combined with this we are recognizing more and more the significance of neurogenic disturbance, particularly in damage of the pudendal nerve (see Chapter 9). The cloacal sphincter musculature giving rise to the perineal muscles, as well as the external anal sphincter and urethral sphincteric apparatus, are primarily supplied by the pudendal nerve. Typical lower motor neuron defects can occur, adding to the problem of disturbed architecture of the musculature by leading to laxity within the muscles on a lower motor neuron disease basis. The recognition of the neurogenic component leads to changes in therapy so that not only is the muscular architecture restoration important, but also attempts are made to prevent further damage of the pudendal nerve. Thus, if it is recognized that the pudendal nerve can be damaged by stretching of it by excessive movement of the perineum, then properly performed restorative surgery will diminish the perineal excursion. Therefore, continued trauma to the pudendal nerve by straining the perineum during defecation can be prevented.

Apical Laxity

Apical laxity is, of course, associated with structural defects and support defects that allow for the development of vaginal vault inversion, as described above. In addition, neurogenic components may also exist. The levator musculature adjunctive supports rely on neurogenic supply not only from the pudendal nerve, but also through other branches of the pelvic plexus supplying the levator musculature from above. Disorders of pelvic plexus innervation do arise commonly from disorders of lumbosacral vertebra and cord and cauda equina disorders, and disorders of the pelvic floor plexuses themselves. Thus, diseases involving the lumbosacral spine or even conditions involving the pelvic plexus, such as surgery, may affect levator supporting systems. Within these areas are multitudes of interactive reflexes having to do with bladder detrusor and external urethral sphincter interaction, as well as rectal and anal canal interaction. Thus, a neurogenic component to apical laxity problems is as important as the structural defects. Support losses are related to neuropathy, as indicated in Chapter 9, and in fact localized neuropathies may be related to the presence or absence of associated urinary incontinence and anal incontinence.

Vascular changes are associated with apical defects as well as muscular and neurologic changes. With the defect there is a diminution in the vesical, external rectal, pudendal, and vascular responses which play such a profound role in sexual physiology.

SUMMARY

The pathogenesis of vaginal dysfunction in pelvic floor defects is complex, multifactorial, and interrelated to other components of pelvic floor dysfunction. It is difficult to evaluate the sexual dysfunction because controlled empirical studies with populations selected by appropriate statistical methods do not exist. However, increased understanding of the pathogenesis of vaginal dysfunction with pelvic floor difficulties combined with appreciation of the fact that sexual function is a component of the healthy, elderly woman, should allow the pelvic floor surgeon to approach the subject in a comprehensive manner.

REFERENCES

1. Bachman GA, Leiblum SR, Grill J. Brief sexual inquiry in gynecologic practice. *Obstet Gynecol.* 1989;73:425.
2. *Projection of Population of the United States: 1982 to 2050.* Washington, DC: Bureau of the Census; October 1982. 922-P-25.
3. Klinger M, Vartabedian L, Wispe L. Age difference in marriage and female longevity. *J Mar Family.* 1989;51:195.
4. Masters WH, Johnson VE. *Human Sexual Response.* New York: Bantam; 1981.
5. Masters WH, Johnson VE. *Human Sexual Response.* New York: Little, Brown and Co; 1966.
6. Aronson MP. In vivo study of the anatomy of anal continence

using magnetic resonance imaging: Implications for surgical repair of lacerations and anal incontinence. Presented at Society of Gynecologic Surgeons, XVI Annual Meeting; March 7, 1990; New Orleans.

7. Steege JF. Dyspareunia and vaginismus. *Clin Obstet Gynecol.* 1984;27(3):750–759.

8. *Diagnostic and Statistical Manual of Mental Disorder,* 3rd ed. Washington DC: American Psychiatric Association; 1980.

9. Levay A, Sharpe L. Sexual dysfunction: diagnosis and treatment. In: Lief H, ed. *Sex and Problems in Medical Practice.* Monroe, Wis: American Medical Association; 1981.

10. Sotile W, Kilmann P. Treatment of psychogenic female's sexual dysfunction. *Psychol Bull.* 1977;84:619.

11. Sanderg G, Quecillon RP. Dyspareunia: an integrated approach to assessment and diagnosis. *J Fam Pract.* 1987;24;1:66–69.

12. Lamont O. Vaginismus. *Am J Obstet Gynecol.* 1978;131:632.

13. Fink P. Dyspareunia: current concepts. *Med Asp Hum Sex.* 1972; 6:28.

14. Vilas E. Uber der entwicklung der menschlichen scheide. *Z Anat Entwicklungsqesh.* 1932;98:263.

15. Koff AK. Development of the vagina in the human fetus. *Contrib Embryol.* 1953;24:59.

16. Fluhmann CF. The developmental anatomy of the cervix uteri. *Obstet Gynecol.* 1960;15:62.

17. Huffman JW. Dyspareunia of vulvovaginal origin. *Postgrad Med.* 1983;73(2):287–296.

18. Kohorn EI, Merino MJ, Goldenhersh M. Vulvar pain and dyspareunia due to glomus tumor. *Obstet Gynecol.* 1986;67:415.

19. Bachman GA, Leiblum ST, Sandler B, et al. Correlates of sexual desire in postmenopausal women. *Maturitas.* 1985;7:211.

20. Sarrell OM, Steege JF, Maltzer M, et al. Pain during sex response due to occlusion of the Bantholine gland duct. *Obstet Gynecol.* 1983;62:261.

21. O'Donnell RP. Chronic honeymoon cystitis. Correction by Surgery Part I. *Br J Sexual Med.* 1978;2:20.

22. Duncan EH, Taylor HC. A psychosomatic study of pelvic correction. *Am J Obstet Gynecol.* 1952;64:1.

23. El-Minawa MF, Mashhor N, Relia MS. Pelvic venous changes after tubal sterilization. *J Reprod Med.* 1983;28:641.

Vaginal Dysfunction

13C   Nonsurgical Therapies

Jerry S. Benzl

INTRODUCTION

Pelvic relaxation syndrome, as manifested by genuine stress incontinence, cystocele, rectocele, uterine prolapse, and certain types of female sexual dysfunction, is almost always associated with either dysfunction of the pelvic floor muscles, pathologic stretching of the paravaginal connective tissues, and/or disruption of the lateral fasciae attachments of the vagina.

Connective tissue and fasciae defects are not addressed here because they are a surgical problem when grossly disrupted. Instead, we will focus on the functional importance of the pubococcygeus muscle and the use of pelvic muscle physiotherapy for the nonsurgical treatment of pelvic relaxation syndrome.

THE PUBOCOCCYGEUS MUSCLE

Within the muscular pelvic floor the pubococcygeus muscle, which originates in the os pubis and inserts in the coccyx, is a principal part of the physiologic complex of muscles which close the pelvic outlet. It contributes to the support and sphincteric control of the urethra, vagina, and rectum, and is essential for maintaining the tone of other pelvic muscles, both striated and smooth.[1] Urinary continence is promoted by pubococcygeus muscle contraction in response to increased intraabdominal pressure. Such contractions have been shown to functionally lengthen and compress the urethra, and to elevate the urethrovesical junction into an area of transmitted abdominal pressure.[2]

Initial damage to the pubococcygeus muscle occurs primarily during childbirth. Over time, associated factors such as muscle debility due to disuse or aging, atrophy due to inadequate postmenopausal estrogen levels, hereditary tissue weakness, or chronic increases in intraabdominal pressure (i.e., chronic cough, obesity, or occupations that require repeated heavy lifting), compound the damage. Eventually, progressive pelvic descent leads to pudendal nerve neuropathy and severe pubococcygeus neuromuscular dysfunction.[3] Fortunately, much of this neuromuscular dysfunction can be prevented or reversed utilizing the techniques of therapeutic exercise and electrical stimulation of the pubococcygeus muscle.

ACTIVE VS PASSIVE PHYSIOTHERAPY

Physiotherapy of the pubococcygeus muscle can be divided into two phases: active and passive. Active physiotherapy requires the patient to have voluntary control of her pubococcygeus muscle in order for her to participate in the neuromuscular reeducation and training process. The patient is made aware of correct pubococcygeus muscle function, learns to contract this muscle properly, and therapeutically exercises her pelvic floor to achieve the desired results. Passive physiotherapy is recommended for those patients who do not have voluntary control of their pubococcygeus muscle and cannot learn to contract this muscle despite extensive neuromuscular retraining efforts. Their pubococcygeus muscle has usually atrophied to such a severe degree that voluntary cortical control is absent and little muscular function remains. To effectively reverse pubococcygeus muscle atrophy, direct electrical stimulation is applied to produce "passive" muscle contractions. After muscle strength and awareness of pubococcygeus muscle function have been restored by electrical stimulation therapy, active physiotherapy can be prescribed to more fully develop pelvic floor neuromuscular reflexes.

ACTIVE PHYSIOTHERAPY

Many patients demonstrate awareness of function and have good voluntary control of the pubococcygeus muscle. These patients can be easily identified during vaginal palpation and only need to perform therapeutic gynecologic exercises (TGEs) to improve neuromuscular function. Patients with poor pubococcygeus function need additional instruction. The utilization of vaginal manometry or other biofeedback techniques are useful when teaching these patients to correctly exercise their pubococcygeus muscle (see Chapter 4B). Once awareness of function has been established, a therapeutic gynecologic exercise program can be started.

Although protocols may vary, most gynecologic exercise programs apply the following basic principles of muscle exercise physiology: (1) initial effort is concentrated on isolation of the specific muscle or muscle group, (2) after several weeks of training, when the muscles have adapted and the correct contraction movements are learned, the number of repetitions is gradually increased, and (3) each time a new target number of repetitions is reached, the muscles are contracted a little harder to increase contraction strength. It is important that both the strength and number of the contraction exercises are increased gradually so that optimum results are obtained without causing unnecessary muscle discomfort. Some researchers therefore advocate the use of a written exercise plan to help avoid exercise-induced muscle soreness.[4-6]

There is a great variation from study to study in the number of daily contraction exercises that are suggested. Recommendations range from 50 to 100 exercises or more per day, usually in divided sessions.[7-9] To treat urinary incontinence, Kegel recommended 300 contraction exercises per day.[10] This amount of exercise may seem excessive and time consuming, but once the patient becomes proficient these exercises can be completed in less than 10 minutes per day. It is important to understand that skipping daily repetitions is second only to improper contraction technique as a cause for failure of this treatment modality.

THERAPEUTIC GYNECOLOGIC EXERCISES

There are four different gynecologic contraction exercises your patient should practice to help regenerate her pubococcygeus muscle strength and restore reflex function: the flick contraction exercise, the hold contraction exercise, the pull-up contraction exercise, and the reflex contraction exercise.

The *flick contraction exercise* is performed by contracting and relaxing the pubococcygeus muscle in rapid one second bursts, each time contracting the muscle as tightly as possible. This exercise is the easiest to learn and helps develop the maximum contraction strength.

The *hold contraction exercise* is performed by holding the contraction at maximum strength for approximately four seconds. Initially most patients cannot maintain these contractions and may lose 50% or more of the maximum recorded pressure change. As control improves and the maximum contraction strength is maintained, the total contraction time should be increased and maintained, for ten seconds or more. This exercise is particularly useful for patients with urinary incontinence because prolonged pubococcygeus muscle contractions are usually required to help them stay dry during times of urge or stress.

The *pull-up contraction exercise* is performed by dividing the pubococcygeus muscle contraction into four parts, contracting the muscle in controlled increments to the point of maximum tension, and then releasing the contraction in an equally controlled manner. This contraction exercise has benefits in certain types of sexual dysfunction. In women with perceived "vaginal looseness" this exercise can bring added satisfaction to both partners when performed during coitus. Also, learning to relax the pubococcygeus muscle may help patients with vaginismus.[11]

The *reflex contraction exercise* is the most important of the four exercises, particularly in the treatment of women with urinary incontinence. Only training the pubococcygeus muscle to contract strongly does not necessarily mean that function is improved. To improve specific functions, the strengthened pubococcygeus muscle must be trained to respond to sudden increases in intraabdominal pressure. By consciously practicing pubococcygeus muscle exercises during activities that produce incontinence, the patient is gradually conditioned to automatically use this muscle. The ultimate goal of gynecologic exercises is not raw muscle strength or contraction ability alone, but the development of an intact contraction reflex that functions when needed in a spontaneous way.

PASSIVE PHYSIOTHERAPY

Electrical stimulation therapy of the neuromuscular structures of the pelvic floor has been in clinical use for more than two decades and is advocated for the treatment of a wide variety of urogynecologic disorders. Suggested indications include dysmenorrhea, vaginismus, dyspareunia, interstitial cystitis, stress incontinence, urge incontinence, and hyperreflexic bladder.[12–16] Studies have shown that the electrical stimulus can be successfully delivered by numerous modalities, including direct bladder stimulation, stimulation of the spinal sacral nerve, and stimulation of the pudendal nerve via anal or vaginal devices.[13,16,17] Because of psychologic, aesthetic, and general comfort considerations, transvaginal electrical stimulation has become the most commonly employed method of electrical stimulation therapy in women.

ELECTRICAL STIMULATION: MODES OF ACTION

The pubococcygeus muscle and the striated muscle component of the urethra are innervated by S4 (partially by S3 and S5) through the somatic pudendal plexus. The smooth muscles of the urinary bladder and urethra receive motor innervation from the parasympathetic pelvic nerves and the sympathetic hypogastric plexus.

Animal and clinical research indicates that the effect of transvaginal electrical stimulation is mediated via both the afferent and efferent segments of the pudendal nerve.[18] Stimulation of the efferent branch of the pudendal nerve with a weak alternating electric current causes the pubococcygeus and periurethral striated muscles to contract, increasing urethral closure pressure. Bladder inhibition during electrical stimulation occurs via two reflex arcs. The afferent limb of the pudendal nerve

initiates both reflex arcs and then the parasympathetic pelvic nerves and the sympathetic hypogastric nerves mediate the bladder inhibition.

Transvaginal electrical stimulation is best tolerated at an electrical current strength of less than 10 V set at a frequency of 10 to 50 Hz. Studies have demonstrated that a stimulation frequency of 50 Hz on a pulse duration of 1 to 2 msec is the most effective setting to stimulate striated muscle contraction and urethral closure. For bladder inhibition a stimulation frequency of 10 Hz on a pulse duration of 2 msec produces the best results.[18–20] By programming different electrical parameters such as pulse patterns, current intensity, and tissue impedance, intermediary degrees of both increased urethral pressure and bladder inhibition can be attained.

ELECTRICAL STIMULATION METHODS

Three different methods of electrical stimulation are currently employed for the treatment of urinary incontinence and pelvic muscle relaxation and are classified according to the time of application: (1) acute-maximal electrical stimulation, (2) chronic electrical stimulation, and (3) intermittent electrical stimulation.

Acute-maximal electrical stimulation consists of 15 to 20 minute applications of electrical stimulation via anal plug or vaginal pessary electrodes. The intensity of stimulation is maintained just below the patient's discomfort or pain threshold. As accommodation to the stimulus occurs, the intensity is gradually increased. Positive effects of this therapy may last from several days to several months with initial urodynamic cures observed in 50% of the patients.[21]

Chronic electrical stimulation is delivered via an anal plug or vaginal pessary which is maintained in place for 8 to 12 hours per day. The intensity of stimulus is adjusted by the patient to her individual comfort level. Patient acceptance and the ability to wear the device are major limiting factors of this modality. For some women, such as those who have failed multiple treatment regimens, chronic electrical stimulation is an acceptable option.

To date, the most clinically useful method of electrical stimulation has been the intermittent form. Intermittent transvaginal electrical stimulation has been shown to significantly improve the subjective symptoms in 87% of patients with genuine stress incontinence and in 69% of patients with detrusor instability.[22] This method is particularly useful when combined with active pelvic floor exercises in those patients with severe muscle atrophy and/or the inability to perform pubo-

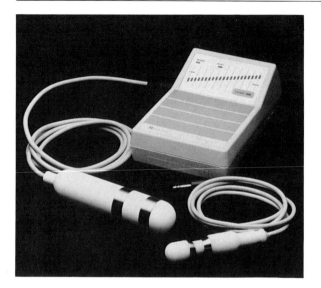

Fig. 13C-1 The Microgyn II transvaginal electrical stimulation device. (Manufactured by InCare Medical Products, Libertyville, Illinois.)

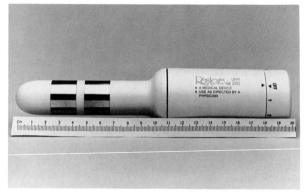

Fig. 13C-2 The Restore Unit transvaginal electrical stimulation device. (Manufactured by Interactive Medical Technologies, Inc., Ventura, California.)

coccygeus contraction exercises on their own. A vaginal pessary electrode (Fig. 13C-1) or a vaginal probe (Fig. 13C-2) is used by the patient to stimulate pubococcygeus muscle contractions, and passively exercise this muscle for 15 to 20 minutes per day. This passive exercise helps to regenerate atrophic muscle tissue, improve muscle contraction strength, establish awareness of pubococcygeus function, and allows the patient to advance to therapeutic gynecologic exercises more rapidly.

Patient Selection

Before receiving electrical stimulation therapy the patient should undergo careful urogynecologic, urodynamic, and neurologic evaluation to obtain a precise diagnosis of the type and degree of incontinence. General measures such as treating urinary or vaginal infections, prescribing adequate estrogen replacement therapy, and pubococcygeus muscle contraction exercise training should be tried before electrical stimulation treatments are started.

Each patient should undergo a trial of in-office electrical stimulation to assess her tolerance and acceptance prior to prescribing an electrical stimulation device for home use. There must be a strong understanding on the patient's part that physiotherapy, be it active or passive, is not a cure but an ongoing treatment that helps her control the condition. The patient will need to make a commitment to long-term therapy because, as in any muscle exercise program, if the exercises are not continued on a regular basis, any symptomatic improvement in her condition would be gradually lost. On the other hand, once the restoration of pubococcygeus muscle function has been achieved (usually within 12 to 14 weeks), many patients can maintain the positive results without electrical stimulation therapy by adhering to a routine of 10 minutes of therapeutic gynecologic exercise per day.

SUMMARY

Careful evaluation of patients and the proper application of active and passive physiotherapy provides a safe, effective means of treatment for many urogynecologic disorders. There is ample clinical evidence to indicate that restoring pubococcygeus muscle tone and function can, in many cases, alleviate the symptoms of pelvic relaxation syndrome.

The preventive aspects of pelvic muscle physiotherapy are also important. Success is directly related to patient compliance, and optimum results are achieved when the patient is reevaluated periodically. An assessment of pubococcygeus muscle function and patient education should be a routine part of every pelvic examination.

REFERENCES

1. Kegel A. Stress incontinence and genital relaxation. *Ciba Clinical Symposium.* 1952;4:35–51.
2. DeLancey JOL. *Anatomy of the Extrinsic Continence Mechanism.* Proceedings of the International Continence Society (Boston);1986:22–24.

3. Snooks SJ, Badenoch DF, Tiptaft RC, Swash M. Perineal nerve damage in genuine stress incontinence: an electrophysiological study. *Br J Urol.* 1985;57:422–426.

4. Henderson J. A pubococcygeal exercise program for simple urinary incontinence: applicability to the female client with multiple sclerosis. *J Neurosc Nurs.* 1988;20(3):185–188.

5. Dougherty M, Bishop K, Abrams R, Batich C, Gimotty P. The effect of exercise in the circumvaginal muscles in postpartum women. *J Nurs Midwif.* 1989;34(1):8–14.

6. Taylor K, Henderson J. Effects of biofeedback and urinary stress incontinence in older women. *J Gerontol Nurs.* 1986;12(9):25–30.

7. Burgio K, Whitehead W, Engel B. Urinary incontinence in the elderly. *Ann Intern Med.* 1985;104:507–515.

8. Baigis-Smith J, Smith D, Rose M, Newman D. Managing urinary incontinence in community-residing elderly persons. *Gerontologist.* 1989;29(2):229–223.

9. Norton C. Female incontinence. In: *Nursing for Continence.* Beaconsfield, NY: Beaconsfield Publishers; 1986:109–127.

10. Kegel A. Physiologic therapy for urinary stress incontinence. *JAMA.* 1951;146(10):915–916.

11. Lamont J. Vaginismus. *Am J Obstet Gynecol.* 1978;131(6):632–636.

12. Mannheimer L, Whalen E. The efficacy of transcutaneous electrical nerve stimulation in dysmenorrhea. *Clin J Pain.* 1985;2:75–83.

13. Scott R, Hsueh G. A clinical study of the effects of galvanic vaginal muscle stimulation in urinary stress incontinence and sexual dysfunction. *Am J Obstet Gynecol.* 1979;135:663.

14. Fall M, Carlsson C, Erlandson B. Electrical stimulation in interstitial cystitis. *J Urol.* 1980;123:192.

15. Sotiropoulos A. Management with electronic stimulation of muscles of pelvic floor. *Urology.* 1975;6(3):312–318.

16. Grimes J, Nashold B, Currie D. Chronic electrical stimulation of the paraplegic bladder. *J Urol.* 1973;109:242–245.

17. Krauss D, Lilien O. Transcutaneous electrical nerve stimulator for stress incontinence. *J Urol.* 1981;125:790–793.

18. Erlandson B, Fall M, Carlsson C. The effect of intravaginal electrical stimulation on the feline urethra and urinary bladder. *Scand J Urol Nephrol Suppl.* 1978;44:19–30.

19. Godec C, Cass A, Ayala G. Bladder inhibition with functional electrical stimulation. *Urology.* 1975;6(6):663.

20. Fall M. Does electrostimulation cure urinary incontinence? *J Urol.* 1984;131(4):664–667.

21. Eriksen B, Bergmann S, Eik-Nes S. Maximal electrostimulation of the pelvic floor in female idiopathic detrusor instability and urge incontinence. *Neurourol Urodynam.* 1989;8:219.

22. Bent A, Richardson D, Ostergard D. Transvaginal electrical stimulation in the treatment of genuine stress incontinence and detrusor instability. *Neurourol Urodynam.* 1989;8:363.

CHAPTER 13

Vaginal Dysfunction

13D   Surgical Therapies

J. Thomas Benson

INTRODUCTION

The vaginal dysfunctions which can be surgically addressed are those characterized by dyspareunia, vaginal laxity, and vaginal prolapse.

As outlined in Chapter 13B, dyspareunia is a chief manifestation and one which, on carefully chosen occasions, can be improved surgically. Dyspareunia will be considered chiefly from the viewpoint of introital problems, with the surgical correction of contracture following perineorrhaphy and contracture secondary to dystrophy. Surgical correction of vaginal laxity will be outlined. Both vaginal and abdominal approaches to surgical correction of vaginal prolapse with emphasis on levator plate restoration will be described.

Apical Dyspareunia

Apical vaginal dysfunction leading to dyspareunia may be due to extensive adjacent disease or to support tissue disease. The presence of disease external to the vaginal apical tissue and supporting structures requires diagnosis by careful physical examination and frequently visualization either endoscopically or with laparotomy. Correction of extensive disease follows standard gynecologic surgical principles.

Correction of apical vaginal function leading to dyspareunia caused by lack of support is as outlined in therapy for anterior support problems (Chapter 12) or

posterior support problems (Chapter 16) or vaginal prolapse later in this chapter.

Introital Dyspareunia

As outlined in Chapter 13B, the pathogenesis of introital dyspareunia is varied. Nowhere can a preoperative evaluation be more important than with introital dyspareunia. As indicated, the organic features and the psychologic features of vaginismus are virtually always concomitant and must be carefully evaluated. The therapy for vaginismus relies on retraining the patient for control of the voluntary musculature, and surgical intervention should be postponed until full benefits of correction of the vaginismus are obtained. The concept of the vaginal orifice being contracted to the point requiring surgery requires preoperative demonstration of (1) the anatomic defect, (2) the evidence that vaginal dilatation alone is not effective, and (3) the coital relationship to the defect must be present.

The dyspareunia may be secondary to actual introital contraction, or may be related to hymenal or vestibular chronic inflammatory processes, or to the lower urinary tract with the urethral-meatus being the focal point of the dyspareunia.

Urethral Meatal Surgery

In 1959 O'Donnell[1] described "relative hypospadias" that he associated with an inadequate rupture of the hymenal ring causing lower urinary tract inflammation and dyspareunia. A surgical procedure for relief of these symptoms was described.

There are varied opinions regarding the validity of this entity. Careful evaluation of patients with recurrent lower urinary tract inflammation reveals very few who have difficulty on an anatomic, surgically correctable basis. The comparison of female lower urinary tract function with the male's urinary tract function has led to many years of improper consideration of increased resistance being a factor leading to lower urinary tract infection. For that reason the female urethra has been subjected to dilatations and other procedures to overcome this "resistance," which is rarely found in carefully defined urodynamic studies. Furthermore, the concept that the female bladder is completely sterile and that the proximal urethra has no bacterial invasion is erroneous. The true situation is that bacteria are frequently introduced into the female bladder. The bladder has adequate expulsive properties that promptly rid it of the intruding pathogens. Other than obstruction of the outflow with such things as diaphragms, tampons, or surgical procedures, the obstructed flow rate is usually caused by expulsive problems relating to poor detrusor function. Such diminished expulsive power of the detrusor can occur in various conditions, many of which stem from deficiencies in the cauda equina and are related to neurologic dysfunctions in the lower spinal column (see Chapter 9A). Attention must be paid to all these elements of lower urinary tract function before one takes the step of surgical correction of urinary meatal difficulties to either relieve dyspareunia or symptoms of recurrent cystitis.

In carefully selected patients, some have hymenal attachment to the urethral meatus such that eversion of the meatus occurs readily with introital penile intromission, and relief may be obtained by a modified O'Donnell procedure. As indicated in Fig. 13D-1A, the hymenal attachment lateral to the urethral meatus is incised. We frequently use a straight hemostat to incise a pie-shaped area of hymenal tissue (see Fig. 13D-1B). After excising the triangular-shaped piece of tissue, hemostasis is secured with a Heaney type suture utilizing 3-0 polyglactin suture material. In these procedures we try to avoid glycerol impregnated chromic catgut, which has been shown to be associated with increased dyspareunia when used with perineal repair.[2]

Some patients with urinary meatal coital pain are helped by transportation of bulbocavernosus pads to the area beneath the urethra (Martius procedure). This may be performed as a unilateral or bilateral procedure

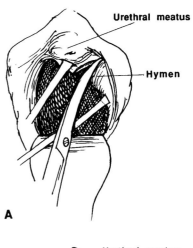

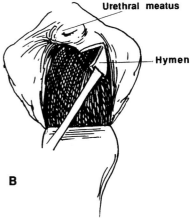

Fig. 13D-1 **A**, Incision of hymen lateral to urethral meatus. **B**, Removal of pie-shaped section of hymenal meatal attachment.

and has applicability for many other urethrovaginal disorders, such as fistulas.

Vestibulitis

In 1983, the International Society for the Study of Vulvar Disease Congress[3] named the symptom complex of chronic burning vulvar discomfort *vulvodynia*. The term *vulvar vestibulitis syndrome* was coined[4] to describe pain on vestibular touch with point tenderness and physical findings confined to the vestibular erythema. A surgical procedure for correcting introital dyspareunia ascribed to infection of the minor vestibular gland was adopted.[5] The cure rate with the surgical therapy, however, has been disappointing, with some series showing only 59% cure rate.[6] Patients with diffuse acetyl white areas involving the skin and mucous membrane have better response with low-dose topical 5-fluorouracil, whereas CO_2 laser vaporization and argon laser photocoagulation are somewhat effective in those patients with painful vestibular erythema. Many of these patients, even with negative histologic examination, demonstrate human papilloma virus with DNA hybridization techniques.[7]

Introital Contracture

Generally speaking, there are two types of contraction of the vaginal introitus necessitating surgical relief; one is contraction that is iatrogenic following a perineorrhaphy, and the second is the contraction resulting from chronic vulvar dystrophy.

It is important to recognize the fundamental differences between the two because repair involves completely different surgical principles. The contraction following a perineorrhaphy generally results from an excessive perineal skin excision with distortion of the perineal musculature, which pulls medially and fibroses. With this type there is adequate loose posterior vaginal wall skin just above the contracted introitus. In patients with chronic vulvar dystrophy the skin is inelastic, thin, and atrophic. The labia are largely effaced and the posterior vaginal wall skin is not adequate and loose, but instead is atrophic and fibrous. Frequently, the urethral orifice may be almost covered by the more anterior location of the thinned posterior commissure.

Correction of Contracture Following Perineorrhaphy

In this condition there is no actual shortage of vaginal skin. Simply making a vertical incision and closing it horizontally will not be adequate in these conditions except when the condition is due entirely to skin contracture. Most cases involve more than just skin contracture and include the musculature of the perineal body, which generally is fibrosed and adhered medially. The operation must repair this musculature to separate it so that it falls laterally, and to accomplish this the fibrotic tissue must be excised. The skin incision (Fig. 13D-2A) is not made vertically, but instead is made horizontally along the line of the posterior commissure.

The skin flaps are elevated by undermining and freeing, generally with Dean scissors. At this point one sees that the musculature is adhered together with fibrotic bands. With finger in the rectum, the external anal sphincter can be identified and protected and the large amount of fibrous tissues removed. Usually, a considerable amount of tissue must be removed to completely excise all the fibrous tissue present. Following this, the perineal musculature is separated laterally and, after ascertaining that the small but adequate perineal body is present, closure is made in a transverse fashion (Figs. 13D-2B–D). In completing the transverse closure there is usually a "dog-eared" effect laterally, and this tissue is simply excised. Thus, the loose vaginal skin is brought down in a transverse fashion over the perineum, reconstituting an adequate vaginal introitus. Careful examination at the time of surgery identifies any remaining bands of introital tissue, which should certainly be treated prior to completing the surgical procedure.

Vaginoplasty for Contracture Secondary to Dystrophy

Because there is inadequate tissue available in this area for reconstruction, a grafting with healthy, unaffected full-thickness skin is required. The posterior vaginal wall is split in the posterior longitudinal axis and undermined until the introitus and lumen are of adequate size, and then the graft is placed to make up the posterior defect. The graft is obtained from the immediate adjacent tissue and is triangular in shape with the point of triangle distally so that good blood supply remains present. As indicated in Fig. 13D-3A, an incision to the right of the midline in the posterior vaginal wall and perineum is made, and, with the Dean dissecting scissors, the edges are undermined. The same procedure is performed on the opposite side until an adequate introitus is created. The raw posterior area is ready to receive the graft (Fig. 13D-3B). The graft is created, as indicated in Fig. 13D-3C, from the left labium majora and thigh and remains attached to the base. The second incision of the graft, as indicated in Fig. 13D-3D, is made and forms the other side of the triangle. The skin graft is dissected free from the underlying fat and is the same general shape as the recipient area, with the donor area being larger. The apex and skin fat is transfixed to the apex of the recipient area and with 3-0 polyglycolic suture the graft is sewn into place on the receiving bed. The donor side then has the skin edges undermined and it is closed with 2-0 polyglycolic sutures to the middle of it, starting from the superior aspect and then, starting at the inferior aspect, the second suture closes to the middle to avoid puckering posteriorly near the anus. The final figure (Fig. 13D-3E) shows the lower poste-

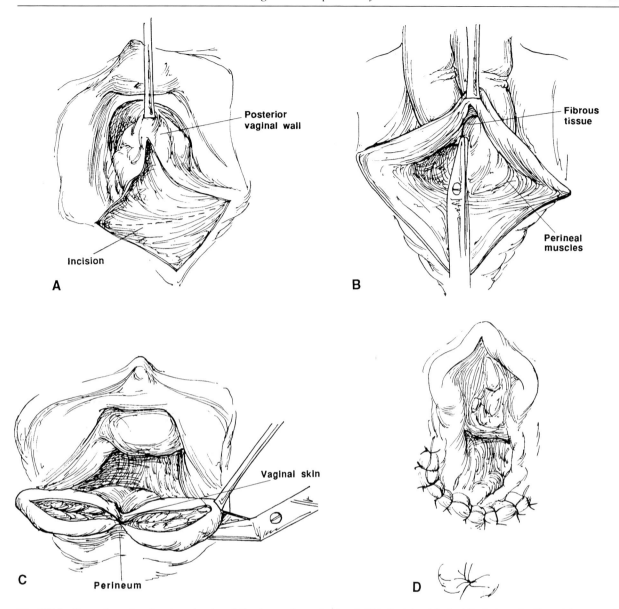

Fig. 13D-2 Correction of perineal contracture following perineorrhaphy. **A**, Skin incision (*dashed line*) along the line of the posterior commissure. **B**, Excision of fibrous tissue and lateral separation of perineal musculature. **C**, Closure in transverse fashion and excursion of "dog ears." **D**, Vaginal skin is brought transversely over the perineum to complete the closure.

rior vaginal wall with adequate introitus and the closed donor site.

Operations for Vaginal Laxity

Preoperative considerations again are paramount in preparing to operate on a patient for vaginal laxity. Following the same principles as outlined for surgery for dyspareunia, the psychologic evaluation must be thorough, and anatomic defect must be present and conservative attempts to improve function with exercise regimens should be tried before resorting to surgical repair.

The condition with the most obvious anatomic defects are chronic complete perineal tears. Many of these defects involve the anal sphincters, both external and internal. They are by nature located more anteriorly, but careful preoperative evaluation will reveal a surpris-

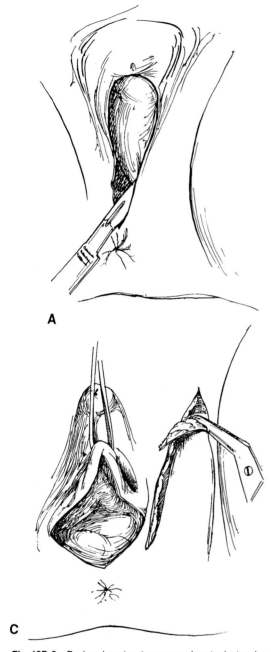

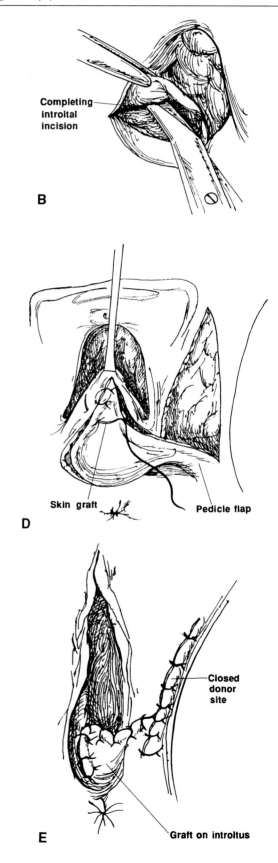

Fig. 13D-3 Perineal contracture secondary to dystrophy. **A,** Incision is made in vagina and perineum. **B,** Preparation of raw posterior area to receive graft. **C,** Creation of graft from left labium majora and thigh. **D,** Transfixion of graft. **E,** Completed procedure.

ing loss of muscular activity. Such preoperative evaluation can delineate the area of scar and fibrosis which is not useful in the repair, and can indicate the area of viable muscle tissue that can be used. Preoperative evaluation with needle electromyography is one way to

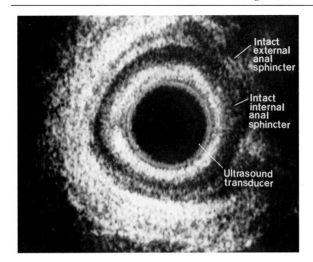

Fig. 13D-4 Concentric ultrasound showing a normal internal and external anal sphincter. (Courtesy of C. Bartram, St. Mark's Hospital, London.)

ascertain the location of functioning tissue (see Chapter 9C). Also extremely helpful is preoperative evaluation with concentric radial ultrasound. Fig. 13D-4 shows concentric ultrasound study of the external anal sphincter with normal sphincter, and Fig. 13D-5 shows a patient with torn sphincter musculature.

Operating for vaginal laxity, especially when it involves chronic third-degree or fourth-degree perineal tear, is not to be confused with operating for anal incontinence. Repairing the sphincter alone in a patient complaining of incontinence to solids leads to frustrating results. If the patient has anal incontinence, then factors outlined in Chapter 14 should be considered. In operating for vaginal laxity the anal sphincter defect is

Fig. 13D-5 Concentric ultrasound showing laceration of the anal sphincter.

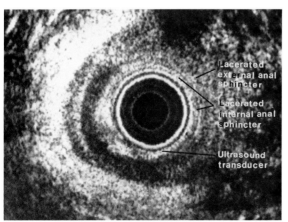

repaired as a concomitant to the repair of the laxity. Restoration of the superficial transverse perineal and bulbocavernosus muscle, in addition to restoration of the muscles of the urogenital diaphragm (urethrovaginal sphincter) gives the desired result. To be avoided is bringing the levator musculature (pubococcygeus) together overlying the rectum and posterior to the vagina in a nonanatomic location. This can lead to dyspareunia, as so often occurs with rectocele repair incorporating this type of approximation. If the levator plate is judged to be inadequate, then attention and repair to that should be a separate surgery through a different surgical site (see Chapter 14D2).

Excess vaginal and perineal skin is present in this condition and surgery for reconstruction involves removal of the excess skin. An inverted "V" incision is made with the apex of the V just above the area of the urethral vaginal sphincter, and the extensions of the V going lateral to the anal sphincter. The ends of the limbs should be approximated before making the incision to ensure that the introitus is adequate at the completion of the procedure when these two ends are approximated. A transverse line connects the two limbs of the V, and the vaginal tissues present in the now defined triangle are excised. Again, the principle of excision of scarred tissue is adhered to. If a chronic fourth-degree defect exists, the rectal wall edges are sutured, inverting the mucosal edge after excising the scarred portion. The cut ends of the external anal sphincter are identified. The external sphincters are reapproximated. For this, at least three 0 polyglycolic sutures are used, usually in mattress fashion, to incorporate the external sphincter. The musculature of the urethrovaginal sphincter and then the bulbocavernosus and superficial transverse perineal muscles are approximated. Subcutaneous tissue is closed and, finally, the vaginal skin edges and perineal skin edges are approximated. When the external anal sphincter has to be re-united, sphincterotomy at 5 o'clock is performed to prevent postoperative gas "buildup" by temporarily relaxing the sphincter.

Preoperative bowel preparation is advisable in these situations, as is a high fiber diet and early ambulation.

Points of Emphasis

In closing the rectal defect after trimming the edges and removing fibrotic tissue, the first layer of sutures inverts the mucosal edge. The second layer of sutures is placed in a Lembert fashion to invert the first layer. It is surprising how much retraction can occur at the external anal sphincter when it is chronically torn. If not recognized preoperatively by electromyography or ul-

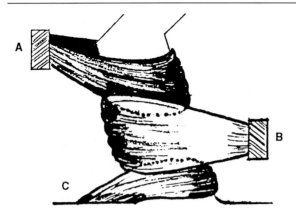

Fig. 13D-6 Vectors of force in the external anal sphincter. *A,* Anterior directed puborectalis. *B,* Posterior attachments of the external anal sphincter to coccyx. *C,* Anteriorly directed superficial external sphincter attachment to the perineal body. (Reprinted from *Invest Urol* 1975;12:412, with permission.)

trasound or other study, it must be searched for by passing Allis or tissue forceps in the direction of the retracted muscle mass until it can be clamped and pulled medially. Next, in placing the interrupted sutures in the external anal sphincter, each of the three sutures should be placed as much as possible in a plane at right angles to the previous suture. Vectors of force in the external anal sphincter are actually in three planes, as depicted in Fig. 13D-6. The sutures placed should recapitulate these force directions by anterior attachment of superior (puborectalis) and inferior (perineal) sutures and posterior (coccygeal) attachment of middle. Oversewing the prerectal fascia over the approximated external sphincter musculature gives added support.

Vaginal Prolapse

Vaginal prolapse, of course, refers to failure of attachment of the vagina. The same pathophysiology is involved with uterine prolapse and, in advanced degrees, the therapy after removing the uterus is essentially the same for vaginal vault prolapse as it is for uterine procidentia.

The basic anatomic principles remain: (1) The support of the uterosacral and cardinal complexes act to retain the posterior, horizontal alignment of the upper vagina, and (2) the upper vagina and rectum then are supported by the levator plate, so that forces acting on the pelvic floor tend to cause posterior and not inferior displacement of the upper vagina. In vaginal prolapse, these principles are violated.

Degrees of vaginal vault descent are somewhat difficult to standardize. The prolapse of the vagina may be thought of as an "inversion" process when there is a loss of superior attachments with telescoping of the apical portion, or as an "eversion" process involving the more introital parts of the vagina. Estimation of the amount of prolapse may be done by reference to the ischial spine or reference to the perineum. As with procidentia, when the vagina is completely inverted in the resting state it may be referred to as grade four vaginal vault prolapse. With the vaginal apex at the introitus at rest and exiting the introitus with the Valsalva maneuver is comparable to a grade three prolapse. Lesser degrees are more aptly divided into percentiles. The vagina, generally having a length of 6 to 7.5 cm along the ventral wall and 9 cm along the dorsal wall, may be thought of as being prolapsed 50% of its length when it reaches within four cm of the introitus.

Vaginal prolapse is rarely an isolated event. Anteriorly, there is usually associated cystocele and, posteriorly, there is frequently associated rectocele or enterocele.

The anterior defects leading to cystocele constitute an important part of the surgical repair of vaginal prolapse. For that reason the area of defect must be recognized for proper anterior vaginal wall repair to be a component of the surgery for vaginal prolapse (see Chapter 12).

The posterior component or rectocele-enterocele likewise must be identified. Defecography is sometimes helpful to delineate the relationship of rectocele to the vault prolapse. In many cases of vault prolapse there is retention of the rectum in a more anatomically normal position (Fig. 13D-7). This occurs when the urogenital prolapse is "sliding" down the anterior surface of the rectovaginal septum. Frequently, however, rectocele is an associated component of the vaginal vault prolapse and must be identified and repaired (see Chapter 16). Enterocele is very commonly associated with vaginal prolapse and may frequently be appreciated preoperatively. Intraoperative identification is sometimes the first time it is possible to diagnose, and repair of the enterocele is a concomitant part of the repair of the vaginal prolapse. Diagnosis by defecography is now possible (Chapter 7A).

The method of repair for vaginal prolapse generally falls into three types. The actual removal of the vagina with total colpectomy or colpocleises is a definitive method of repair which closes the levator hiatus virtually completely, but, of course, leads to inability for proper vaginal sexual function. This point deserves serious consideration. Many patients in the age group com-

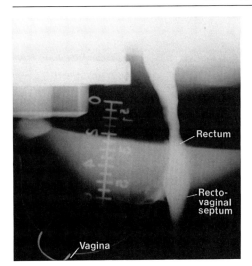

Fig. 13D-7 Defecography (voiding proctogram) showing the rectum in a normal anatomic relationship while the vagina is completely prolapsed, "sliding" down the rectovaginal septum.

monly associated with vaginal prolapse tell the attending physician that loss of vaginal function is unimportant. However, this answer is frequently given because they feel they are not supposed to be having sexual activity or that their situation is such that they will not have opportunity for sexual activity in the future. With the changing life expectancy and social mores, many patients, even in markedly older age groups, establish new relationships for which retention of sexual function becomes important. Furthermore, even if sexual functioning is not resumed, the psychological self-image associated with sexuality can be affected by the thought that introital sexual functioning is no longer possible. For these reasons this method of surgical repair for vaginal prolapse is decidedly inferior to one preserving vaginal functioning.

Methods of vaginal prolapse repair that retain vaginal function are methods of pelvic floor reconstruction which can be performed either vaginally or abdominally. Debates as to which approach is best do not overcome the fact that for every pelvic floor surgeon, there are patients for whom an abdominal approach is best because of associated intraabdominal pathology, and there are patients for whom the vaginal approach is preferable with the concomitant vaginal procedures. Therefore, it behooves the pelvic floor surgeon to maintain expertise in both surgical methods.

To evaluate the merits of each approach we are conducting a prospective, completely randomized study in which all patients with 50% or greater vaginal vault

prolapses are operated by either the abdominal or the vaginal approach. The abdominal approach involves the correction of lateral anterior wall defects (abdominal paravaginal cystocele repair); the closure of the posterior cul-de-sac (anterior posterior directed sutures as a modification of the Moschcowitz procedure); abdominal colposacral suspension using Gortex material; and, when indicated, anterior and posterior colporrhaphy and levatoplasty performed from the vaginal approach. The other part of the study encompasses the vaginal approach, using a vaginal paravaginal cystocele repair when there are lateral defects; central cystocele repair when defect is present in this area; bilateral sacrospinous vaginal vault suspension using Gortex; McCall type culdoplasty for superior defects; posterior colporrhaphy when indicated for rectocele repair; excision of enterocele sac when present; and levatoplasty when indicated. In both parts of the study, if the patient has genuine stress urinary incontinence, she also has urethropexy performed using the Burch modification (see Chapter 11D2) for the abdominal group, or the Pereyra modification (see Chapter 11D2) for the vaginal group.

Preliminary results on the prospective randomized series with 92 patients followed for 2 to 25 months show recurrence rates of 4.7% for the abdominal group and 9% for the vaginal group. The overall morbidity is < 10%. The time to resume normal voiding was significantly different between the two groups, with the abdominal group resuming normal voiding in an average of 4 days while the vaginal group averaged approximately 11 days. The hospitalization length, although expected to be lower in the vaginal group, has not been statistically different.

Preliminary nerve studies were performed on the two groups, evaluating the pudendal nerve, the perineal nerve, the cauda equina, the pelvic plexus, and proximal S2, S3, and S4 roots. These studies are conducted on patients pre- and postoperatively to determine if there is a significant difference with the two routes of surgery as far as possible damage to the pelvic nerves. Preliminary data suggest more nerve damage with the vaginal route.

Levator Plate

Vaginal prolapse is frequently related to levator plate deficiencies. Most patients that have vaginal vault prolapse have a markedly widened levator hiatus. Therefore, suspension of the vaginal vault by either method is more apt to fail if there is no levator plate intact posterior to the vagina, where it can act as a buttress under the posteriorly directed, horizontal upper vagina. Evaluation of the levator plate may be clinical, radiologic, or with ultrasound (Chapter 7).

Clinical evaluation with the patient in the upright position, or in a lateral Sims' position straining reveals perineal descent if the levator plate is inadequate. In this condition the anal verge leads the descent of the pelvic floor. Measurement of the ischial tuberosities and concomitant measurement of the anal verge reveal that the deficient levator plate can move the anal verge more than 2 cm. The anal verge then occupies a position which is below the ischial tuberosities. If the movement is less than 2 cm and/or the final location with a strong Valsalva maneuver is above the ischial tuberosities, then levator plate insufficiency is unlikely. For this purpose a clinical perineometer (Fig. 13D-8) may be used.

Performance of the levatoplasty is outlined in Chapter 14D2, as this procedure was originally outlined for surgical therapy of fecal incontinence. Its use as an adjunctive surgery for vaginal prolapse in pelvic floor defect is independent of its function in surgery for fecal incontinence. The procedure is a valuable adjunct in our surgical therapy and is especially helpful in cases that had failed surgery for vault prolapse. In our series of 36 patients so treated, evaluated with a follow-up time from 6 months to 2 years, 32 retained good vault support, 4 had 50% descensus recur, and none had recurrent vault inversion. This series includes patients who failed previous surgery for vault suspension in 18 (50%) instances.

PRINCIPLES

As with most pelvic floor surgeries, understanding and operating in natural spaces markedly reduces blood loss and facilitates anatomic correction.

Sutures used for vaginal vault prolapse are a combination of polyglycolic absorbable sutures and permanent sutures. Permanent sutures used may be Gortex or monofilament polypropyline. Permanent braided sutures are avoided because if infection occurs, their mechanical structure has areas where antibiotics cannot reach bacterial reservoirs. Infection may then require

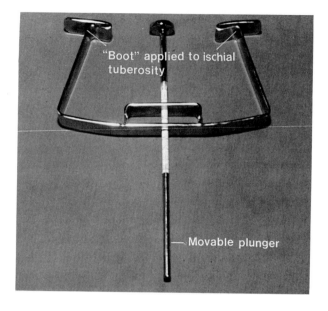

Fig. 13D-8 The clinical perineometer is an instrument used to measure descent of the perineum.

suture removal, whereas monofilament sutures do not have this propensity. The monofilament polypropyline sutures do have memory, and small ligaclips are frequently used after tying the knots to prevent that memory from causing the suture to untie. A headlight seems essential in this type of surgery because so many of the spaces being operated are not accessible to good illumination by operating room lights. We use a very helpful tool, the Vital-Vue© 7120 (Fig. 13D-9), which is a sterile, disposable surgical instrument with an obturator that combines suction, illumination, and irrigation system (manufactured for Davis & Geck, Danbury, CT 06810, USA). When prosthetic tissue such as Gortex is used, the irrigant solution used with the Vital-Vue instrument contains 50,000 U bactiracin and 70 mg gentamicin in 100 cc normal saline.

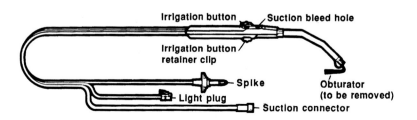

Fig. 13D-9 The Vital-Vue© is an instrument used during vaginal vault surgery.

PROCEDURES

Total Colpectomy

This procedure removes all of the vaginal wall and associated enterocele, then uses the pubococcygeal muscle and completely closes the levator hiatus.

Because of the nature of the healing with this procedure, pulling of the urethra into a more inferior location commonly occurs. Therefore, prophylaxis against the development of stress urinary incontinence must be considered. If preoperatively the patient already has a condition of decreased transference of abdominal pressures to the midurethra, then vaginal urethropexy may be employed concomitantly with the procedure (see Chapter 11D2). With the inverted apex of the vagina securely held, a transverse incision is made at the prolapsed apical portion (Fig. 13D-10A). An incision is made to the introitus on the anterior vaginal wall going through the complete thickness of the anterior vaginal wall in the vesical vaginal space (Fig. 13D-10B). The bladder is separated from its vaginal attachment and, if it is deemed unnecessary to do needle urethropexy, then Kelly-Kennedy plication sutures are placed at the vesical neck. The prolapsed apical portion or the vagina is then elevated, and beginning at the fourchette (Fig. 13D-10C) transverse incision is made. Entering the rectovaginal space the vaginal wall is incised sagittally and dissected free from the rectum. Lateral incisions are then made (Fig. 13D-10D) and the anterior lateral walls of the vagina are dissected from the underlying peritoneal covering and the entire vaginal wall excised at the introitus (Fig. 13D-10E). The peritoneum remaining represents the hernial sac of the enterocele, which is excised and then closed. The edge of the pubococcygeus muscle is identified and separated so that medial mobilization can occur, and with 0 polyglycolic suture, a series of interrupted sutures are placed in the levator ani, closing the levator hiatus (Fig. 13D-10F). After ensuring complete hemostasis, the remaining vaginal wall is closed in running suture, a suprapubic catheter is placed, and the procedure is completed.

Abdominal Colposacral Suspension

The patient is positioned on the operating table in universal stirrups or with pillows beneath each knee so that the surgeon's nondominant hand has access to the vagina. A Pfannenstiel incision is generally used, al-

though a midline incision may be used. The abdominal cavity is entered, any necessary lysis of adhesions performed, and the pelvis visualized. The initial step of the procedure is closure of the cul-de-sac. Because of the propensity of circular purse-string sutures to relax and allow small bowel herniation, purse-string sutures in the Moschcowitz fashion are no longer employed. Instead, interrupted anterior posterior sutures using Gortex suture are used. The ureters are carefully visualized. Closure is usually with two layers of interrupted sutures. At this point the retroperitoneum overlying the sacral promontory is opened in the midline. Stay sutures are placed on each side of the opening as the incision is continued down overlying the closed cul-de-sac and extending to the vaginal apex, which has been previously located and held by Kocher clamps (Fig. 13D-11). A Gortex patch is sewn to at least one-half of the posterior vaginal wall, after opening the peritoneum overlying the wall. Six to eight interrupted sutures are used. The anchoring is done with Gortex sutures and goes through the complete muscular wall of the vagina. The Gortex is thus placed retroperitoneally. With care not to exert any tension, the graft is anchored to the cul-de-sac closure sutures, and finally is approximated to the second or third sacral vertebra where it attaches to the anterior longitudinal ligament overlying the sacrum. The attachment at this point assists in maintaining horizontal alignment of the upper vagina and is made with at least four Gortex sutures. The needle used for the placement of these sutures is a number five curved Mayo needle which is strong, so that needle breakage is not apt to occur. The arc of the needle must be carefully followed. Hemostasis can occasionally be difficult in the presacral area due to retraction of the vessels into the sacral foramina. Liga clips are frequently effective, as is pressure. Should these methods prove ineffective, stainless steel sterile thumbtacks can be used to press immediately over the vessel, should all other attempts fail to achieve satisfactory hemostasis. The middle sacral vessels should be sought by palpation prior to placing the sutures in the anterior longitudinal ligament. In some patients the anterior longitudinal ligament is very poorly formed and attenuated. The retroperitoneum is then closed over the Gortex prosthesis in a running 2-0 polyglycolic suture. At this point the visceral peritoneum is closed and attention is turned to the space of Retzius. There are lateral cystocele defects in all cases of vault prolapse, which are now corrected by the abdominal paravaginal cystocele repair as described in Chapter 12A. Inspection of the interior of the bladder to ascertain that the permanent sutures are not through the vagina and to ascertain proper ureteral function is imperative. This can be done at this juncture

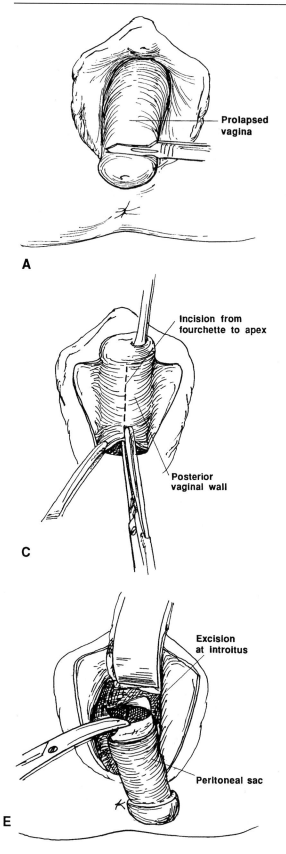

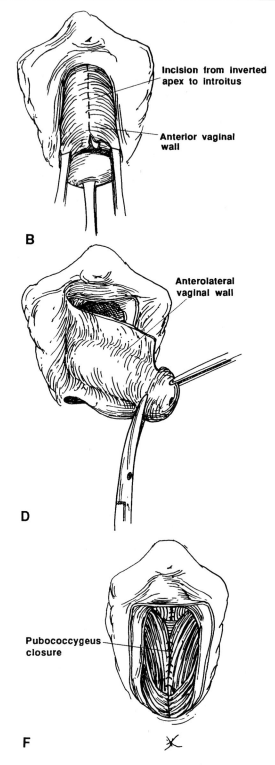

Fig. 13D-10   Total colpectomy. **A**, The initial incision. **B** The posterior incision at the perineum *(dashed line)*. **C** The transverse incision from the fourchette to apex *(dashed line)*. **D**, The dissection of the anterolateral walls from the peritoneal sac. **E**, The excision of the peritoneal sac. **F**, The closing levators.

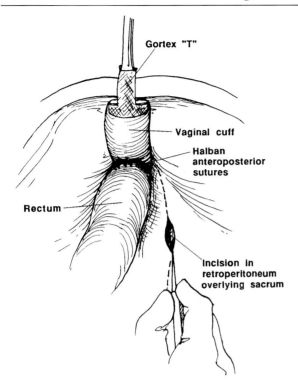

Fig. 13D-11 The abdominal colposacral suspension. Halban anteroposterior stitches are used to close the cul-de-sac. The Gortex is sutured to the vaginal cuff.

through cystotomy incision or through a smaller incision with a cystoscope. This can be deferred to the vaginal portion of the procedure where cystourethroscopy may be utilized. Indigo carmine is given to evaluate ureteral function. After closure of the fascia and skin the patient is placed in the lithotomy position and posterior colporrhaphy is performed as for rectocele repair (see Chapter 16). If a levatoplasty is deemed necessary it is performed as the final step in the operation.

Vaginal Approach

The anterior wall defect in the vaginal prolapse is operated on as the first portion of the procedure. This is accomplished by the vaginal paravaginal cystocele repair as described in Chapter 12B. Concomitant use of Pereyra modification of urethropexy is performed again in those patients showing decreased abdominal to midurethral pressure transmission on preoperative urodynamic testing with the vaginal vault supported. If urethropexy is deemed necessary, needle urethropexy is performed as described in Chapter 11D2.

Following the anterior and superior wall reattachment, attention is turned to the posterior wall. A transverse incision is made at the introitus marking the lateral extremes of the transverse incision and bringing them together as they will be when the procedure is completed to make sure the introitus has adequate size. A "V"-shaped incision is made in the perineal skin, and with the surgeon's finger in the rectum the retrovaginal space is identified and entered. The posterior vaginal wall is opened utilizing the full thickness of the vaginal wall with the opening going to the rectovaginal space. Near the vaginal apex any enterocele will be encountered. If enterocele is encountered, the peritoneum is opened, the bowel content displaced into the abdominal cavity, and a permanent purse-string suture is placed to close the peritoneal sac and the excess hernial sac is removed. Placing the cuff on traction defines the uterosacral ligaments that can now be approximated.

Superior (apical) defects are managed by such uterosacral approximation. Permanent sutures are placed through the entire thickness of vaginal wall excluding the mucosa, to the uterosacral ligament, to anterior rectal wall (and posterior cul-de-sac), to opposite uterosacral ligament and through the vaginal wall again. Two to four such sutures are usually required and tying of the sutures is delayed until all are in place (Fig. 13D-12).

Some patients have adequate reconstruction at this point. Many, however, still need more support of the posterior apical tissues. These need bilateral sacrospinous attachment. Following the apical defect closure, the patient's right rectal pillar overlying the ischial spine is identified and is gently opened with a right angle clamp. A Breisky Navratil retractor is placed through

Fig. 13D-12 Uterosacral cuff approximation.

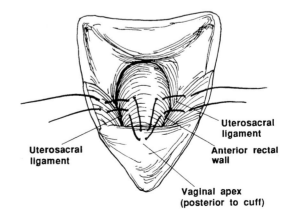

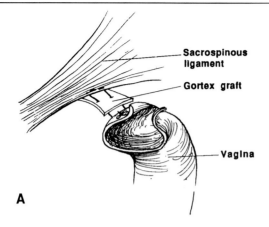

A

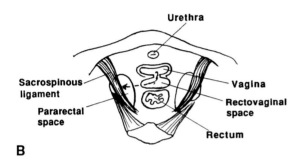

B

Fig. 13D-13 A, The sacrospinous suspension utilizing a Gortex graft placement on the right side. Procedure would be repeated on the left side for a bilateral suspension. **B**, Approach to the sacrospinous ligament through the rectovaginal and then pararectal spaces (indicated by *arrow*).

the defect in the rectal pillar, holding the rectum medially. A second curved retractor is placed with traction exerted anteriorly, and a third laterally (the three retractors are approximately at 12, 4, and 8 o'clock) and, thus, visualization of the sacrospinous ligament (coccygeus muscle) can be carried out (Figs. 13D-13*A*, *B*). At a distance of at least 2 cm medial to the ischial spine a Babcock clamp is placed on the ligament. With Deschamps ligature carrier a suture of 0 proline, 60 inches in length, is placed into the ligament *under direct observation*. It is placed into the ligament and brought out so that it does not go behind the ligament, avoiding the pudendal vessels or the nearby sciatic nerve roots. This suture is then brought out so that the insertion through the sacrospinous ligament represents the midpoint of the doubly folded suture. The suture can then be cut and in this manner there are now two sutures going through the sacrospinous ligament. Careful evaluation to determine that the suture is placed at least 2 to 4 cm medial to the ischial spine is carried out and rectal examination is performed to determine that there is no perforation of the rectal wall. If the vagina is too small to easily reach both sacrospinous ligaments, a Gortex patch may be used. These sutures are then placed through a patch of Gortex which is 1 mm in thickness and rectangular in shape with approximately 4 cm by 3 cm. At the other end of the Gortex are two more sutures or proline. The Gortex is anchored to the

Fig. 13D-14 MRI study of nulliparous female subject. **A**, Line of cut (solid dark diagonal line) for view shown in **B**. Note "H" configuration produced by lateral vessels in **B**.

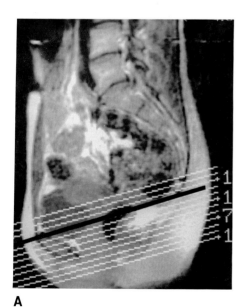

A

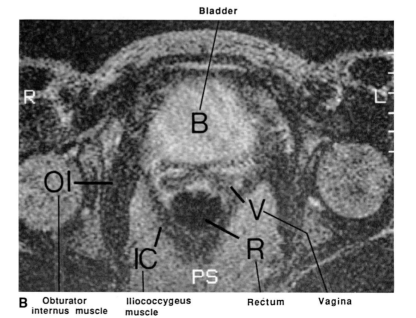

B Obturator internus muscle   Iliococcygeus muscle   Rectum   Vagina

sacrospinous ligament and the two sutures at the other end of the Gortex are anchored to the vaginal cuff going through the full thickness of the muscularis. They are held at this point and not tied down because this would elevate the vaginal cuff to a point making it difficult to close the sagittal incision in the vaginal wall. The same procedure is carried out on the left side and a Gortex patch placed to the left sacrospinous ligament if necessary. The bilaterally placed Gortex patches now substitute for the patient's cardinal ligament and uterosacral ligament complex. The correction of any rectocele is carried out at this point as described (see Chapter 16) and the vaginal wall is closed halfway to the introitus. At this point, the four sutures placed into the vaginal cuff, two going to each sacrospinous ligament, are then tied elevating the vaginal apex. The Gortex extensions prevent the bilaterally elevated vaginal support from compressing the rectum. Any necessary perineorrhaphy is completed and the vagina is thus anatomically restored to its proper horizontal axis with repair of the lateral and apical defects. In those patients in whom a deficient levator plate is present, levatoplasty is carried out as a final part of the restorative surgery.

With both the abdominal and the vaginal routes of vaginal prolapse repair, the vagina should be supported in the anatomically correct posterior inclination. Magnetic resonance imaging studies on living, nulliparous subjects (Figs. 13D-14A, B) depict vaginal support to the area of iliococcygeus muscle originating from the obturator internus fascia, a support satisfactorily accomplished with the described procedures.

REFERENCES

1. O'Donnell RN. Relative hypospadias potentiated by inadequate rupture of the hymen: a cause of chronic inflammation of the lower part of female urinary tract. *J Int Coll Surg.* 1959;32:374.
2. Spencer JAD, Grant A, Elbourne D, et al. A randomized comparison of glycerol-impregnated chromic catgut with untreated chromic catgut for the repair of perineal trauma. *Br J Obstet Gynaecol.* 1986;93:426–430.
3. Burning vulva syndrome: report of the ISSVD task force. *J Reprod Med.* 1984;29:459.
4. Friedrich EB Jr. Vulvar vestibulitis syndrome. *J Reprod Urol.* 1987;32:110.
5. Woodruff JD, Parmley TH. Infection of the minor vestibular glands. *Gynecology.* 1983;62:609.
6. Reid R, Greenburg MD, Daoud Y, et al. Colposcopic findings in women with vulvar pain syndromes. *J Reprod Med.* 1988;33(6):523.
7. Turner MLC, Marinoff SC. Assertion of human papillomavirus with vulvodynia and the vulvar vestibulitis syndrome. *J Reprod Med.* 1988;33(6):533.

Fecal Incontinence

14A   Social and Economic Factors

Elizabeth McClellan

INTRODUCTION

Fecal incontinence is underreported, underrecognized, and poorly understood. Even the definition of fecal incontinence lacks standardization. A suggested definition for purposes of discussion is "involuntary excretion or leakage of feces in inappropriate places or at inappropriate times twice or more in the past month."[1] This lack of ability to retain rectal contents may be further classified as temporary, occasional, uncontrolled, or contained.[2] Involuntary release of flatus or partial fecal soiling is categorized as minor fecal incontinence. Major fecal incontinence refers to deficient control of stools of normal consistency.[2] Double incontinence refers to fecal incontinence accompanied by urinary incontinence.

Little is known about the incidence and prevalence of fecal incontinence and its effect on those who suffer from it. An extensive literature review conducted with the assistance of the British based Incontinence Advisory Service revealed fewer than 30 journal articles and book references directly addressing fecal incontinence in a comprehensive fashion. Fecal incontinence appears to have only recently received significant medical attention, as virtually none of the publications were written prior to the mid-1970s and most were written in the late 1980s.

The Incontinence Action Group established by the King's Fund Centre reported in 1983 that the bulk of incontinence teaching is done in geriatric medicine courses in undergraduate medical school. Less than half of British medical schools even provide a geriatric medicine course. Of these courses, an average of 21 minutes was spent on the subject of fecal incontinence. The Incontinence Action Group found that urology and gynecology department teaching in the area of incontinence was "very sparse." Twelve schools and teaching hospitals in Great Britain spent an average of 23 and 21 minutes, respectively, discussing fecal incontinence.[3] No comparable studies have been conducted in the United States.

In this chapter, a review of published information is presented as well as new data on the prevalence, economic impact, and psychologic impact of fecal incontinence. Clinical applications are discussed, and future direction in the areas of education, diagnosis and management, and research is suggested.

PREVALENCE

Fecal incontinence prevalence rates (the percentage of a population affected at a given time) vary within the literature. The Incontinence Action Group reported a British fecal incontinence prevalence rate of 0.5% in adults ages 15 and older. Approximately one half of those afflicted have not sought treatment for their incontinence.[3] Another British study found the prevalence rate of fecal or double incontinence among patients known to London health agencies was 0.4 per 1000 females ages 65 or older. This figure is roughly double that of men of the same age group. In the community, the prevalence of fecal or double incontinence was greater. A prevalence rate of 1.7 per 1000 females ages 15 to 64 was noted. Again, the rate rose among females 65 or older to 13.3 per 1000 females. Among those surveyed from the community, fecal or double incontinence was more common among males in the younger age group than females but more common in females than males in the older age group.[1]

Among the hospitalized elderly in the United Kingdom, fecal incontinence prevalence rates of 13% to 66% have been reported.[4,5] A 1985 study of the elderly in private British nursing homes found a 33% prevalence rate for fecal incontinence.[5] In Manchester, England, a 10% prevalence rate was determined after surveying 30 residential homes for the elderly.[6]

Double incontinence has been shown to be twelve times as likely as isolated fecal incontinence.[1] Ten to 25% of those with urinary incontinence are also afflicted with fecal incontinence.[7] The prevalence of bowel and bladder problems in extended care facility residents was reported by the United States National Center for Health Statistics to be 34% among those 65 to 74 years of age and 48% among those 85 or older.[8] In a British study of 1559 female patients presenting for urodynamic investigation, 3% reported fecal soiling. In females diagnosed with detrusor instability and neurologic conditions, 48% and 39% respectively experienced fecal incontinence.[9]

Between February 1988 and February 1989, we conducted a study at our referral based, tertiary care urogynecology practice in Indianapolis evaluating 171 females for the presence of urinary and fecal incontinence. The females presented with symptoms or established diagnoses of bladder dysfunction including dysuria, incontinence, recurrent urinary tract infections, cystocele, painful bladder syndrome, diminished urinary flow, urethral syndrome, and fistulae. The females ranged in age from 13 to 89 and all resided in the community. Of these, 82% ($n = 141$) suffered with urinary incontinence. A surprising 41% ($n = 58$) of those with urinary incontinence had accompanying fecal incontinence! Of the total population, 35% ($n = 60$) experienced fecal incontinence. Double incontinence was present in 34% of the total population ($n = 58$). Isolated fecal incontinence was present in only 1% ($n = 2$). Of those who experienced fecal incontinence, 40% ($n = 24$) had major incontinence and the remaining 60% ($n = 36$) had minor incontinence. In this

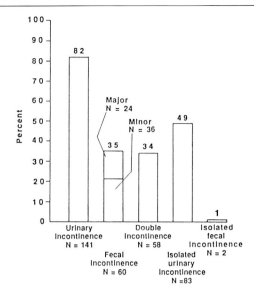

Fig. 14A-1 Prevalence of incontinence among all females presenting to our urodynamic center between February 1988 and February 1989 with complaints of bladder dysfunction.

study, patients complaining only of inability to control flatus were not classified as fecally incontinent (Fig. 14A-1). Of note, constipation, defined as straining greater than 25% of time spent defecating, less than two bowel movements per week, or feeling that the bowel was never completely evacuated, was experienced by 59% ($n = 100$) of these females.

Three extended care facilities in the Indianapolis area were surveyed to establish a fecal incontinence prevalence rate among this population. An inner city extended care facility, a suburban extended care facility, and a surrounding community extended care facility were studied. The majority of the residents required heavy or total care, although a handful of residents were able to do some or all activities of daily living independently. The total sample population was comprised of 249 females and 64 males ages 19 to 103. Of the females, 62% ($n = 154$) were incontinent of urine, 51% ($n = 127$) were incontinent of stool, and 50% ($n = 125$) were doubly incontinent. These figures were greater than those of the male residents. Of the males, 53% ($n = 34$) were incontinent of urine, 45% ($n = 29$) were incontinent of stool, and 44% ($n = 28$) were doubly incontinent (Fig. 14A-2 and Table 14A-1).

The mean number of urine incontinent episodes per incontinent resident each 8 hour shift was 2.1; the mean number of stool incontinent episodes per incontinent resident each 8 hour shift was 0.9.

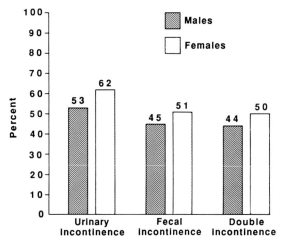

Fig. 14A-2 Prevalence of urinary and fecal incontinence among sample of extended care facility residents in Indianapolis.

Several factors may account for the variability among reported prevalence rates. Differing patient populations, selection bias, differing survey techniques, and differing definitions of incontinence are such factors. Patient denial and reluctance to disclose incontinence are additional factors. One study demonstrated that 10% of urine incontinent persons initially denied having incontinent episodes until further follow-up questions were asked by medical personnel.[10] It may be postulated that persons are more hesitant to discuss fecal incontinence due to its more private nature.

ECONOMIC IMPACT

Management of incontinence is a tremendous economic burden for those affected and their caregivers. Consider the previously described sample of extended care facilities. The three facilities averaged 23.67 minutes per episode of incontinence for cleaning the resident and changing linens. Based on the mean daily urinary incontinent episodes per entire sample population, a total of 467.25 hours are spent cleaning and changing the 188 incontinent residents for urine loss each day. If stool incontinent episodes occurred separately from urine incontinent episodes, an additional 166.16 hours per day would be spent cleaning and changing the 156 incontinent residents for fecal soiling (Table 14A-2). The above examples demonstrate only part of the economic burden of urinary and fecal incontinence in extended care facilities. An indirect cost of urinary and fecal incontinence is that personnel are obligated to spend so much time cleaning and changing the incontinent that they may be able to give only cursory attention to other resident needs.[11,12] On the other hand, when caregivers are repeatedly confronted with the disagreeable chore of cleaning up incontinent episodes, they may tend to avoid the incontinent person, further confounding difficulties in the management of these people.[11] Other indirect costs are those associated with prevention and management of skin breakdown secondary to the caustic effect of feces on the skin. In a study by Brocklehurst,[13] fecal incontinence was found to be a positive correlate of bacteriuria in patients in geri-

Table 14A-1
Incontinence Prevalence Rates Among Individual Extended Care Facilities

	Inner City	Suburban	Surrounding Community
Males	23	28	13
Females	106	86	57
Urinary incontinence			
Males	22%($n=5$)	64%($n=18$)	85%($n=11$)
Females	55%($n=58$)	63%($n=54$)	74%($n=42$)
Double incontinence			
Males	17%($n=4$)	54%($n=15$)	69%($n=9$)
Females	42%($n=44$)	59%($n=51$)	53%($n=30$)
Incontinent episodes/ Incontinent resident/ 8 hours			
Urine	2.5	2.4	1.5
Stool	1.5	0.6	0.5

Table 14A-2
Time Spent Cleaning Incontinent Residents Among
Individual Extended Care Facilities

	Mean Minutes Cleaning per Incontinent Episode	Mean Hours Cleaning per 24 Hours	
		Urine	Stool
Inner city	22	173.25	80.85
Suburban	36.5	315.36	74.46
Surrounding community	12.5	49.69	8.13

atric wards. Frequent exposure of stool to female genitalia has been implicated in increased risk of infection.[2]

Laundry and disposable undergarment charges must also be considered a significant direct cost to the institutionalized, hospitalized, and community-dwelling incontinent population. In the United States more than $400,000,000 are spent annually on adult undergarments for urinary and anal incontinence.[14]

In the community-dwelling population, the cost of diagnostic testing, a cost often borne by third-party payors, comprises a part of the economic impact of fecal incontinence. In a study including 29 patients reporting chronic diarrhea, most were extensively investigated for diarrhea when, on closer scrutiny, it was discovered that the major, previously unreported and unrecognized problem was incontinence to liquid feces.[15]

Society as a whole is financially impacted by fecal incontinence. Incontinence is the second most common impetus behind institutionalization of the elderly, ranking above even mental incompetence.[14] Fecal incontinence may be secondary to urinary incontinence in the decision to institutionalize because it is less common, but it is generally thought to be more unpleasant for the caregiver.[13] Institutional care of the elderly, at present an enormous challenge, is expected over the next few decades to become an even larger problem.[5]

PSYCHOLOGICAL IMPACT

It is difficult to determine the full psychological impact of fecal incontinence on the sufferer. Very little is known about the psychological aspects of fecal incontinence because no large scale scientific studies have been conducted in this arena. It is known that defecation is a profoundly private function[2] and that bowel dysfunc-

tion is the most fundamental of all personal problems, even surpassing sex in priority.[16] Fecal incontinence is embarrassing to discuss primarily for the afflicted but also for many caregivers. The sense of isolation and alienation that may accompany fecal incontinence can be reinforced by medical personnel who are unwilling or unable to openly discuss fecal incontinence.[10] In one British poll, 55% of fecally incontinent persons had not verbalized their problem to their family physician.[1]

Because bladder and bowel control are learned in early childhood, loss of control often signifies a loss of adulthood and independence and produces an identification with the negative aspects of aging. A decrease in feelings of well-being may result.[17] Various authors have associated fecal incontinence with feelings of anxiety, frustration, helplessness, depression, moodiness, sadness, pessimism, and decreased self-esteem. The assumption that these relationships are causal is simply hypothetical at present because no scientific study has explored these relationships in depth. In studies of the effect of urinary incontinence on psychological well-being, continent women reported statistically higher emotional well-being and greater life satisfaction than did incontinent women in the same age category. In those with increasing severity of urinary incontinence, feelings of well-being were proportionally decreased.[18] This observation may be partially related to the overall health of the women and not due simply to the presence or absence of urinary incontinence. The psychosocial impact of incontinence on the individual has not been found to be directly proportional to the severity of incontinence as demonstrated by objective means.[10,17,19,20] The perception of severity is unique to the individual.

Incontinent women report more sexual dysfunction than continent controls.[21] In separate studies of females with urinary incontinence, women demonstrating both genuine stress urinary incontinence and detrusor instability reported that urinary problems had negatively affected their sexual relationships.[21,22] Five mechanisms may be responsible for sexual dysfunction in the incontinent female.[22,23] Dyspareunia resulting from tissues irritated by leakage or from anatomic changes caused by previous pelvic floor surgery has been reported. Depression and decreased libido presumably arising from decreased feelings of self-worth may be causes of sexual dysfunction. Embarrassment about odor or coital incontinence may be another reason for sexual difficulties. Lastly, incontinence can be used as a means for avoiding intercourse when more deep-rooted problems exist in a sexual relationship. It is presently unknown whether the relationship between sexual dysfunction and urinary incontinence would also be found in a group of women with isolated fecal incontinence or if the presence of double incontinence would exaggerate sexual dysfunction.

Two studies reported an association between urinary incontinence and alteration in daily activities and social contacts.[18,19] Situations in which accessibility to the toilet was either unknown or not available resulted in avoidance of that situation or activity. This observation can presumably be inferred of fecal incontinence as well. In a study at an American Veteran's hospital, the unpredictability of fecal incontinent episodes created more distress for the caregivers than did the actual episodes themselves.[11] Anecdotally, our patients with fecal incontinence collaborate this observation, admitting that unpredictability of accidents is the reason they often become essentially homebound.

CLINICAL APPLICATIONS

An awareness of the prevalence of fecal incontinence dictates that direct and specific questions must be incorporated into history taking, especially among patients with urinary incontinence. Simply asking if one is incontinent is inadequate.[7] One study found that questions about urinary loss were readily understood whereas questions regarding fecal incontinence were often misunderstood.[1] Multiple questions may be required to assess for the presence of a problem with fecal incontinence. For example, fewer than half of patients suffering from fecal incontinent episodes ranging in frequency from less than once per month to daily volunteered this information on their presentation to a gastrointestinal clinic. Their incontinence was revealed only after closer questioning.[24]

Asking questions regarding the sensitive topic of fecal incontinence requires that permission to verbalize be given. Active listening skills and patience are necessary for effective communication. An awareness of one's own attitudes regarding feces and fecal incontinence must be examined.[16] Intolerance and disgust on the part of the physician or caregiver are readily perceived by patients.

After identifying a problem with fecal incontinence, a positive attitude toward treatment should be conveyed. Often, a nonhelpful defeatist attitude prevails, as demonstrated by a study of British nursing home residents. Only 4% of fecally incontinent residents were referred for care of their incontinence, even though 75% were fecally incontinent for longer than one year. Sixty days following treatment for fecal incontinence, 66% were no longer incontinent.[6]

SUMMARY

The ability to clinically recognize and manage fecal incontinence lags far behind the extent and implications of the problem. Fecal incontinence prevalence rates of 41% in community-dwelling females with urinary incontinence and 51% in extended care facility female residents demand advancement in our understanding of fecal incontinence. Improvement in the areas of education, diagnosis and management, and research is desperately needed to prevent a situation where desire for treatment is met by medical personnel without the knowledge or skills to respond.[3]

Education of both the medical and public sectors must be expanded. Undergraduate medical and nursing curricula should include a comprehensive discussion of fecal incontinence with supporting detailed coverage in textbooks. Postgraduate education could be enhanced by incorporating fecal incontinence into gynecology, geriatric, urology, surgery, gastroenterology, and medicine department teachings. Continuing medical education lectures and conferences would also be beneficial. Teaching programs for extended care facility administrators and caregivers would greatly aid the fecally incontinent institutionalized population. Education of the public might best begin by introducing the subject of fecal incontinence in the news media and lay publications. Individual patient teaching could occur in clinical practice by early identification and discussion of risk factors.

An improved ability to diagnose fecal incontinence and initiate management is needed. Education of medical personnel plays a critical role in achieving this goal. In addition, tertiary level continence centers within referral zones could serve as resources for evaluation and treatment of fecal incontinence.

Perhaps most importantly, further research into the prevalence, economic impact, and social implications of fecal incontinence is needed. Using meaningful, standardized definitions, U.S. fecal incontinence prevalence rates should be established. Accurate estimates of the costs of fecal incontinence should be determined. Psychological health, including sexuality, and its association with fecal incontinence need scientific exploration. An important area for study involves examining potential etiologic factors in the development of fecal incontinence. Only when the causes of fecal incontinence are well understood can consistently effective medical and surgical management be achieved. We are all pioneers in this exciting, if unglamorous, field of fecal incontinence.

REFERENCES

1. Thomas TM, Egan M, Walgrove A, et al. The prevalence of fecal and double incontinence. *Commun Med.* 1984;6:216.
2. Mowlam V, North K, Myers C. Managing fecal incontinence. *Nurs Times.* 1986;82:55.
3. Kings Fund Centre. Action on incontinence: report of a working group. *Project Paper 43.* 1983;1.
4. Brocklehurst JC. The problems in old age. *Proc Roy Soc Med.* 1972;65:66.
5. Clarke M, Hughes AO, Dodd KJ, et al. The elderly in residential care: patterns of disability. *Health Trends.* 1979;11:17.
6. Irvine RE. Fecal incontinence is not inevitable. *Br Med J.* 1986; 292:1618.
7. Jeter KF. The patient with urinary incontinence. *Home Health Care Pract.* Palo Alto, California: Health Market Research; 1986; 169.
8. Wells T. Conquering incontinence. *Geriatr Nurs.* 1990;11:133.
9. Lewis P, Abrams P, Shepherd A. The incidence of bowel symptoms in urodynamic patients. *Neurourol Urodyn.* 1990;9:357.
10. Herzog AR, Fultz NH. Prevalence and incidence of urinary incontinence in community-dwelling populations. *J Am Geriatr Soc.* 1990;38:273.
11. Habeeb MC, Kallstrom MD. Bowel program for institutionalized adults. *Am J Nsq.* 1976;76:606.
12. Henry M. Fecal incontinence. *Nurs Times.* 1983;79:61.
13. Brocklehurst JC, ed. *Textbook of Geriatric Medicine and Gerontology.* 3rd ed. Edinburgh: Churchill Livingstone; 1985.
14. Lahr CJ. Evaluation and treatment of incontinence. *Sunburst Biomedical Corporation: Incontinence.* 1987;1.
15. Read NW, Harford WV, Schmulen AC, et al. A clinical study of patients with fecal incontinence and diarrhea. *Gastroenterology.* 1979;76:747.
16. Stewart M. Constipation and fecal incontinence in the elderly. *Med Wom Fed.* 1971;53:25.
17. Norton PA. Prevalence and social impact of urinary incontinence in women. *Clin Obstet Gynecol.* 1990;33:295.
18. Herzog AR, Fultz NH, Brock BM, et al. Urinary incontinence and psychological distress among older adults. *Psychol Aging.* 1988; 3:115.
19. Wyman JF, Harkins SW, Choi SC, et al. Psychosocial impact of urinary incontinence in women. *Obstet Gynecol.* 1987;70:378.
20. Norton C. The effects of urinary incontinence in women. *Int Rehab Med.* 1982;4:9.
21. Walters MD, Taylor S, Schoenfeld LS. Psychosexual study of women with detrusor instability. *Obstet Gynecol.* 1989;75:22.
22. Hilton P. Urinary incontinence during sexual intercourse: a common, but rarely volunteered symptom. *Br J Obstet Gynaecol.* 1988;95:377.
23. Sutherst JR. Sexual dysfunction and urinary incontinence. *Br J Obstet Gynaecol.* 1979;86:387.
24. Leigh RJ, Turnberg LA. Fecal incontinence: the unvoiced symptom. *Lancet.* 1982;1:1349.

CHAPTER 14

Fecal Incontinence

14B Pathogenesis

M. M. Henry

INTRODUCTION

It is probable that an unrepresentative sample of the fecally incontinent patient population is referred to surgeons for treatment. Usually the patient is female in middle age; it is unusual for elderly patients with dementia (possibly the most common cause in the West) to be referred to a surgeon for treatment of anal incontinence. In the experience of the surgical unit at St. Mark's Hospital, London, incontinence occurs in women and men in a ratio of 8:1, although in the elderly the sex incidence is probably more equal. For the individual affected the consequences may be devastating, leading to a loss of self-esteem and a sense of social alienation.

When considering possible causative factors it is important to begin by differentiating between minor and major functional impairment because the etiology is likely to differ and treatment options differ markedly.

MINOR ANAL INCONTINENCE

Minor anal incontinence is defined as the occasional minor staining of underwear and/or loss of control to flatus. At this level the degree of social disability is likely to be minimal and rarely indicates severe underlying disease or disorder.

Simple anal pathology such as third degree hemor-

rhoids, prolapsing anal polyp, or anal fissure causing failure of normal local hygiene may cause minor soiling, which can be rapidly diagnosed on simple anal examination, including proctoscopy. Persistent symptoms may be indicative of loss of internal anal sphincter control. This may in turn be the consequence of previous anal surgery (e.g., anal dilatation, hemorrhoidectomy, sphincterotomy, or anal fistula surgery) or of a complete rectal prolapse. In the latter, the internal sphincter damage is probably the result of trauma caused by the frequent prolapse of four layers of edematous rectal wall giving rise to a "self-dilatation." Under certain circumstances the internal sphincter is noted to be deficient where there was no history of prior trauma. Why this should develop spontaneously is not known and is the subject of current research.

Less commonly, patients with damage to the striated component of the anal sphincter mechanism develop major degrees of anal incontinence, and these are discussed in detail below.

MAJOR ANAL INCONTINENCE

Major incontinence is defined as the frequent and uncontrollable passage of formed stool and therefore is of sufficient severity to represent a significant degree of disability to the individual concerned. Severe gastrointestinal infections (e.g., cholera, shigella, salmonella, amebiasis) and severe inflammatory bowel disease may lead to anal incontinence in spite of normal sphincter and pelvic floor function. With infective disease the normal control mechanisms are "swamped" by the presence of copious quantities of liquid stool, such that their capacity to cope is exceeded. In the presence of inflammatory bowel disease a similar mechanism may occur, but in addition the capacity of the rectum as a reservoir organ is reduced by fibrous tissue.[1]

Other patients to be considered with major incontinence usually are shown to have a significant deficit of their external anal sphincter and/or pelvic floor muscles, sometimes seen in addition to a weak internal sphincter as well. In our experience at St. Mark's Hospital, London, the majority of such patients were shown to have histologic evidence of severe denervation of the striated musculature.[2,3] The histologic findings were later confirmed by sophisticated neurophysiologic studies,[4] and nerve conduction studies demonstrated that in the majority the denervation was secondary to damage to the pudendal nerves.[5] In a small proportion of patients a mixed central (cauda equina) and peripheral nerve lesion can be demonstrated.[6] This evidence strongly suggests that anal incontinence is usually neurogenic in origin, the latter arising from injury to the distal part of the innervation of the pelvic floor muscles.

THE CAUSES OF PELVIC FLOOR DENERVATION

Childbirth

About 40% to 60% of women with anal incontinence report a difficult childbirth[2] and the hypothesis that childbirth might be a major factor in initiating denervation injury was investigated by Snooks and colleagues[7] in a study from St. Bartholomew's Hospital, London. It was found that the innervation to the external anal sphincter muscle was damaged during vaginal delivery, but did not occur following cesarean section. The abnormalities found were most marked in multiparous women and correlated most strongly with a prolonged second stage of labor, application of obstetric forceps, and with a large fetus. Substantial recovery from nerve damage as determined by measurement of the pudendal nerve latency occurred within the first 2 months after delivery, but recovery was least complete in the multiparous woman delivered with forceps assistance. It seems probable that a difficult vaginal delivery may result in distal nerve damage as a consequence of stretching of the pelvic floor (and its nerve supply) and

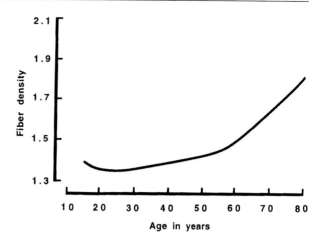

Fig. 14B-1 Fiber density of external anal sphincter muscle in normal population showing the relationship to age. With increasing age there is an increase in fiber density, particularly after 60 years, indicating that muscles normally denervate with advancing age.

probably also from direct compression by the fetal head of the nerves which lie in the sidewall of the pelvis.

In the study outlined above, four patients were incontinent immediately following delivery and they remained incontinent 2 months after delivery. Not all patients with traumatic childbirth present with incontinence immediately after childbirth, but instead the symptoms may appear several years later. Under these circumstances, additional denervation takes place as a response to aging, since it is well recognized that all skeletal muscle denervates as a normal physiologic response to the aging process (Fig. 14B-1). If the muscle is already partially denervated, then age denervation may be sufficient to cause a functional disability several years after the initial trauma.

Constipation and Defecation Disorders

Denervation was also demonstrated in the pelvic floor muscles of patients who have constipation and defecation disorders such that they strain excessively.[8,9] Such patients are often observed to display the physical sign of perineal descent. On examination of a normal, healthy individual in the left lateral position, during a straining effort the perineum descends approximately 2 cm but remains above the plane of the bony outlet of the pelvis. In patients with abnormal descent, however, the perineum descends well below the bony outlet during a straining effort.[8] The terminal portion of the pudendal nerve in the adult is approximately 9 cm; in patients with abnormal descent of 2 cm to 3 cm, a stretching force to the distal portion of the pudendal nerve of 20% to 30% is exerted. Since irreversible nerve damage was shown to develop when nerves are stretched by as little as 12%,[10] it is possible that stretching of these nerves (during straining) leads to secondary neuropathic damage. Studies of patients show a linear, quantifiable relationship between the degree of nerve damage and the degree of perineal descent,[11] lending support to this hypothesis. In addition, it was shown that short periods of straining induce temporary prolongation of the pudendal nerve latency.[12]

Other Causes

Denervation may less commonly be associated with diabetes mellitus[13] or other lower motor neuron lesions such as cauda equina, tumor, or trauma. Anal incontinence may be a feature in disseminated neurologic disorders such as multiple sclerosis, in which denervation may be a feature.[14]

Traumatic damage to the pelvic floor leading to disruption of the anorectal angle may cause significant incontinence. Such injury is occasionally seen after major pelvic injuries where there is fracture across the bony ring of the pelvis or rarely after impalement injury. Damage to the external sphincter can occur with anal fistula surgery or following a third degree perineal tear associated with traumatic vaginal delivery. In both circumstances incontinence may develop, particularly if there was synchronous traumatic damage to the innervation of the sphincter. This has important therapeutic implications because simple anal sphincter repair in patients who have denervation damage usually is associated with a poor clinical outcome.[15]

Suprasegmental factors contribute to normal bowel control, and when these are deficient, such as in spinal cord injury, stroke, and dementia, these patients are frequently incontinent. Deficient cortical awareness of rectal filling and poor cortical control of neuromuscular function are presumably part of the explanation of the prevalence of incontinence in the elderly.[16] In addition, such patients develop fecal impaction, which in turn causes reflex relaxation of the internal sphincter, so permitting leakage of liquid stool and severe soiling.

SUMMARY

Minor incontinence is usually the result of local anal disease and can be readily diagnosed on simple anal examination and proctoscopy. Severe anal incontinence is due either to severe trauma of the anal sphincter muscles or to denervaton of the striated musculature. The latter is most commonly caused by obstetric damage (e.g., traumatic childbirth) and less frequently may be associated with tumors or traumatic lesions affecting the cauda equina.

REFERENCES

1. Farthing MJG, Lennard-Jones JE. Sensibility of the rectum to distention and the anorectal distention reflex in ulcerative colitis. *Gut.* 1978;19:64–69.
2. Parks AG, Swash M, Urich H. Sphincter denervation in anorectal incontinence and rectal prolapse. *Gut.* 1977;18:656–665.
3. Beersiek F, Parks AG, Swash M. Pathogenesis of anorectal incontinence: a histometric study of the anal musculature. *J Neurol Sci.* 1979;42:111–127.
4. Neill ME, Parks AG, Swash M. Physiological studies of the pelvic floor in idiopathic fecal incontinence and rectal prolapse. *Br J Surg.* 1981;68:531–536.
5. Kiff ES, Swash M. Slowed conduction in the pudendal nerves in idiopathic (neurogenic) fecal incontinence. *Br J Surg.* 1984;71:614–616.
6. Snooks SJ, Henry MM, Swash M. Abnormalities in central and peripheral nerve conduction in anorectal incontinence. *J Roy Soc Med.* 1985;78:294–300.
7. Snooks SJ, Swash M, Henry MM, Setchell ME. Injury to innervation of the pelvic floor sphincter musculature in childbirth. *Lancet.* 1984;ii:546–550.
8. Henry MM, Parks AG, Swash M. The pelvic floor musculature in the descending perineum syndrome. *Br J Surg.* 1982;69:470–472.
9. Snooks SJ, Barnes PRH, Swash M, Henry MM. Damage to the innervation of the pelvic floor musculature in chronic constipation. *Gastroenterology.* 1985;89:977–981.
10. Sunderland S. *Nerves and Nerve Injuries.* 2nd ed. Edinburgh: Churchill Livingstone; 1978;62–66.
11. Jones PN, Lubowski DZ, Swash M, Henry MM. Relation between perineal descent and pudendal nerve damage in idiopathic fecal incontinence. *Int J Colorect Dis.* 1987;2:93–95.
12. Lubowski DZ, Swash M, Nicholls RJ, Henry MM. Increase in pudendal nerve terminal motor latency with defecation straining. *Br J Surg.* 1988;75:1095–1097.
13. Rogers J, Levy DM, Henry MM, Misiewicz JJ. Pelvic floor neuropathy: a comparative study of diabetes mellitus and idiopathic fecal incontinence. *Gut.* 1988;29:756–761.
14. Hinds JP, Eidelman BH, Wald A. Prevalence of bowel dysfunction in multiple sclerosis. A population survey. *Gastroenterology.* 1990;98:1538–1542.
15. Laurberg S, Swash M, Henry MM. Delayed external sphincter repair for obstetric tear. *Br J Surg.* 1988;75:786–788.
16. Brocklehurst JC. Management of anal incontinence. *Clin Gastroenterol.* 1975;4:479–487.

CHAPTER 14

Fecal Incontinence

14C   Nonsurgical Therapies

James H. MacLeod

INTRODUCTION

Most presentations on fecal incontinence dwell on its surgical aspects, while paying only lip service to its conservative management. Yet, there are a great many incontinent patients in whom surgery is not indicated; and many patients with chronic, severe fecal incontinence can now be helped considerably with conservative measures.

The purpose of this chapter is to indicate the many areas in which nonoperative methods may alleviate fecal incontinence and, not infrequently, eliminate it; sometimes nonoperative methods are the sole procedure, sometimes they are a supplement to corrective surgery. This chapter describes those procedures.

The currently available nonoperative procedures for incontinence involve (1) biofeedback, and (2) pharmacologic and behavioral methods of treatment. In recent years, biofeedback has become a valid form of treatment, and many advances have evolved in the pharmacologic and behavioral areas.

INDICATIONS FOR CONSERVATIVE TREATMENT

The form of conservative treatment depends on the type and severity of the patient's incontinence. A classification is presented in Table 14C-1.

Indications for surgery are limited to cases of traumatic origin, if the sphincter muscle and innervation remain intact and the patient has had a trial of biofeedback, and to some cases of pudendal neuropathy, also after a trial of biofeedback. Rectal prolapse should be corrected surgically whenever feasible and as soon as possible, because it causes continuing nerve injury.[1] Rarely, incontinence of neurologic or congenital origin may benefit from sphincter supplementation with a nearby muscle,[2] or with a silastic sling.[3]

Operative repair is not indicated for incontinence caused by other causes. Surgery does not correct incontinence caused by loss of sphincter innervation, nor will it correct that due to a sensory or a reservoir deficit.

Candidates for conservative treatment of fecal incontinence may, therefore, exhibit any of the following indications:

1. loss of innervation of the anorectal musculature
2. traumatic origin, except as noted above
3. perineal descent, in most cases
4. sensory deficits
5. reservoir deficits
6. previously failed surgery
7. refused surgery
8. health too poor to undergo surgery
9. chronic diarrhea or dementia, which can negatively affect surgical outcome

Table 14C-1
Classification of Incontinence

Component	Category
Motor	
Innervated	Anorectal surgical laceration
	Obstetrical laceration
	Penetrating wound
Noninnervated	Upper motor neuron
	Cerebral—dementia, cerebrovascular accident, multiple sclerosis
	Spinal cord—trauma, tumor, herniated disc, multiple sclerosis
	Lower motor neuron
	Conus—ischemia, multiple sclerosis
	Cauda—trauma
	Peripheral—stretch injury with pudendal neuropathy—obstetric injury, chronic constipation, rectal prolapse
Sensory	
Decreased coordination of sphincter contraction with rectal distention	
Increased rectal sensory threshold	
Neurologic disease	
Diabetes	
Reservoir	
Colon capacity and motility—inflammatory bowel disease	
Rectal capacity and compliance	
Rectal resection—anterior resection, ileoanal anastomosis "c" or "s" pouch	
Rectal ischemia	
Radiation proctitis	
Inflammatory bowel disease	
Mixed	
Motor and sensory—neurologic, diabetes	
Motor, sensory and reservoir—impaction, postoperative repair of imperforate anus	

SELECTION OF TREATMENT

Selection of treatment is influenced by several factors. These include the cause and severity of incontinence,[9,10] its impact on the patient's life, and the level of comprehension and motivation the patient possesses for solving the problem.

Minor degrees of incontinence frequently respond to sphincter exercises or to antidiarrheal medication, whereas more severe incontinence may require biofeedback, surgical correction, or behavioral management.

The effect of incontinence on the quality of the patient's life determines, in large part, the nature and intensity of treatment. Leakage of flatus or an occasional smear on the clothing is quite a different matter from the loss of a formed bolus of stool.

Finally, motivation and comprehension are important to all forms of treatment, but are especially necessary to biofeedback.

Components of Continence

Although choice of treatment for incontinence involves the factors mentioned above, the very basis of the choice stems from determining which of three components that govern fecal continence is or are affected, as therapies are specific and vary accordingly. These three components are the motor, sensory, and reservoir functions (Table 14C-2).

Continence at rest is maintained by tonic contraction of all of the sphincter muscles: the internal sphincter

Table 14C-2
Physiology of Continence

Component	Innervation	Role
Motor		
External sphincter (& perineal body)	Somatic	Lateral closure
Puborectalis (anorectal angle)	Somatic	Lateral closure flap-valve closure
Internal sphincter	Autonomic	Relaxation on rectal distention, contracted at rest; "fine tuning" of continence
Sensory		
Rectal sensation	Autonomic	Warns of rectal filling
Anal sensation	Somatic	Sampling of rectal contents; discrimination of gas, liquid & solid; warns of breach of continence mechanism
Reservoir		
Rectal capacity & compliance	Autonomic	Retention of adequate volume; distensibility without increase in pressure
Colon motility	Autonomic	Volume and consistency of stool and rate of delivery to rectum

Reprinted from *Endoscopy Rev* Nov/Dec 1988:47 with permission.

Table 14C-3
Mechanisms of Continence

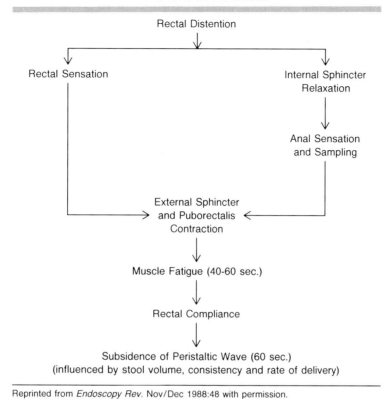

Reprinted from *Endoscopy Rev.* Nov/Dec 1988:48 with permission.

maximally, and the external sphincter and puborectalis minimally. The voluntary muscles contract further in response to perianal stimulation, postural changes, and to increases in intraabdominal pressure; but the mechanisms of continence are set in action fully by rectal distention (Table 14C-3).

A sense of rectal fullness, mediated by nerve endings outside the rectum, probably in the levator muscles,[4,5,6] leads to reflex internal sphincter relaxation, allowing rectal contents to come in momentary contact with the lining of the upper anal canal, thus enabling "anal sampling" (i.e., discrimination between gas, liquid, and solid) to take place, with warning of an impending breach of the continence mechanism.[7]

A voluntary contraction of the external sphincter and puborectalis muscles occurs in response to rectal distention and to anal sampling, closing the anal canal by lateral compression. In addition, puborectalis contraction renders the anorectal angle more acute, creating a flap-valve effect.[8]

However, these muscles can contract maximally for only 40 to 60 seconds; continence beyond that time depends on the reservoir function of the rectum which includes both an adequate capacity (300 to 500 cc) and compliance (the ability to distend to accommodate oncoming stool without a corresponding increase in intrarectal pressure) until subsidence of the peristaltic wave.

Rectal accommodation is further dependent on the volume and consistency of the stool and the rate at which it is delivered to the rectum. This is in turn dependent on the activity of the distal colon.

These multiple components of continence are, to some extent, redundant so that there is some compensation by the others when one is lost. Although all three are necessary to fecal continence, some components are more important than others; most critical are the external sphincter and puborectalis muscles.

Evaluation of Continence

All of these factors can be evaluated by a thorough history and anorectal examination (Tables 14C-4 and

Table 14C-4
History

Name	Sex	Age

Duration of i/c

Degree of i/c
Discharge   Soiling   Urgency   Gas   Liquid   Solid

Bowel Habit
BM's/day

stool consistency: watery   loose   formed   hard

Frequency of i/c
episodes/da.   # day/wk   time of day   night

Relevant Medical History

Grav/para status	Traumatic delivery?
Hx a/r surgery	GI Surgery
Trauma to perineum	
To spinal cord (level)	
Neurologic disease	Diabetes Radiation
Urinary incontinence	Impotence
Medication for diarrhea	Other illnesses
Other medications	

Reprinted from *Endoscopy Rev* Nov/Dec 1988:52 with permission.

Table 14C-5
Examination

Inspection

Perianal soiling	Excoriations	Scarring
Patulousness	Keyhole deformity	Wink
	sphincter defect:	
Straining:		site:
perineal descent		
prolapse		

Digital Exam

Sphincter:		Sphincter defect:
resting tone	max squeeze	site:
Accessory muscle contraction		
Anorectal angle:		
at rest	contraction	straining
Patulousness	Closing reflex	
Posttraction	Bidigital	Impaction

Anoscopy
Scarring
Prolapse of mucosa or hemorrhoids

Sigmoidoscopy
Stool consistency
Escape of insufflated air
Internal intussusception or prolapse

Reprinted from *Endoscopy Rev* Nov/Dec 1988:52 with permission.

14C-5).[11,12] A neurologic examination or an investigation of chronic diarrhea may be indicated as well.

In recent years several centers established laboratories for the study of manometry, electromyography, and defecography, both for research purposes and as methods of clinical evaluation. These studies have contributed greatly to our understanding of the pathophysiology of incontinence, but they remain cumbersome to perform, difficult to interpret, and are not generally available to the average practitioner.

The history and physical examination remain the most important part of evaluation.[13] Clinical examination can provide a simplistic but adequate appraisal of all the components of continence. Evaluation should include assessment of sensory, motor, and reservoir functions with identification of the deficient component.

Although the strength of sphincter tone and contraction can be estimated by anorectal digital examination, opinion is divided as to its accuracy.[14,15,16] At any rate, the devices used in biofeedback give a reasonably accurate indication of the strength of external sphincter contraction.

An intrarectal balloon is used to measure the rectal sensory threshold and to evaluate rectal capacity and compliance.[17] In its simplest form, the balloon is a condom, a finger cot, or the finger of a surgical glove. It is tied securely around the tip of a length of polyethylene tubing that is inserted into the rectal ampulla, then gently inflated.

Two volumes are determined, the sensory threshold and the maximum tolerated volume. The former is the volume at which the first sensation of rectal distention occurs (normal value 15 ml); the latter is the maximum volume of rectal distention which the patient will tolerate. It measures rectal capacity (normally 400 to 500 ml) and gives an indication of compliance.

The degree of incontinence can be quantified roughly by the history and examination, and more precisely by means of the saline continence test, where the patient is placed on a commode under which is placed a funnel and a graduated cylinder. Saline is run into the rectum through a polyethylene tube at the rate of 60 ml/min for 25 minutes.

The first leak (over 10 ml) and the total amount retained are measured. A 1500 ml volume is generally tolerated by normally continent patients. However, almost invariably, incontinent patients leak when about 500 ml are instilled.[16] This is an excellent overall measure of susceptibility to incontinence.

MANAGEMENT OF INCONTINENCE ACCORDING TO THE COMPONENT AFFECTED

Biofeedback

Biofeedback is based on the premise that if the patient can see the result of his efforts, those efforts will become more efficient and effective.[11,20,32,33] It enhances muscle rehabilitation success by increasing awareness of the weakened muscles and improving motivation through a more personal interaction between patient and caregiver, thus promoting a more conscientious adherence to the exercise program. The latter benefit was remarked on by several authors.[19,20,22–30]

As it applies to fecal incontinence, biofeedback facilitates anal sphincter exercises and coordination of sphincter activity with rectal distention by providing immediate visual documentation of the effectiveness of sphincter contractions.

A form of biofeedback is available for each component of continence—the motor component being treated most commonly and successfully, the sensory one less so, and the reservoir function infrequently and with the least success.

External sphincter contraction is not a reflex, but a learned response.[18,35] The objective of motor biofeedback is to relearn that specific motor response. According to Bennett and coworkers, every muscle has latent motor units which can become activated with exercise.[35]

Biofeedback improves sensory function as well, perhaps by recruiting adjacent neurons.[36,37] The patient who can perceive rectal distention can be trained to increase that perception and to intensify and coordinate the strength of external sphincter contraction in response to it.[38]

Biofeedback is less successful in improving the reservoir component. It may be enhanced by feedback from a modification of the saline continence test. Schiller and colleagues,[39] in one case, placed the infusion bottle where the patient could observe it and gave verbal encouragement while the saline was instilled during several training sessions. A sevenfold increase in retention of the saline was achieved and maintained, as was continence. Improvement of the motor and sensory functions by biofeedback may, to some extent, compensate for a diminished reservoir function.

Each component of biofeedback may be effective for some patients. External sphincter injury may respond to sphincter training, and those with increased sensory threshold to rectal distention may learn to recognize smaller volumes with sensory biofeedback. Still others with adequate sensation and muscle strength may benefit from synchronized treatment with sensory and motor biofeedback.[40]

Because it is harmless and painless, there are no absolute contraindications to biofeedback. It is, therefore, the treatment of choice for sensory or motor incontinence,[30,32] and is often helpful in retraining the patient after sphincter repair.[32] Biofeedback is less effective, however, in reservoir cases and those with loss of innervation. Its value is also less certain in patients with diarrhea.[25,32,37]

The requirements for successful biofeedback are: (1) a comprehending and motivated patient, (2) the ability to sense rectal distention, and (3) the ability to contract the external sphincter.

Therefore, biofeedback is of value in improving puborectalis and external sphincter tone, in sensitizing patients with sensory deficit, and in coordinating muscular contraction in response to rectal distention.[21]

A trial of this painless, inexpensive, and risk-free treatment modality is worthwhile in any case in which there is detectable sphincter muscle activity in a motivated and comprehending patient.

Motor Deficits

The value of sphincter exercises alone in sphincter muscle rehabilitation has been substantiated by the test of time. Although the exercises alone frequently restore continence, instruction in their execution is difficult to communicate. Because biofeedback is not present during ordinary sphincter exercises, the immediate reinforcement and the ability to correct improper technique is not available to these patients. Therefore, results are frequently poor.[21]

Hopkinson and Lightwood[31] described a method of anal sphincter stimulation in 1966 involving the use of a dumbbell-shaped plug containing two electrodes connected to a portable tetanizing current generator. Although they and a few others reported satisfactory results,[10,32] most reports were not encouraging.[21,32–34]

Motor Biofeedback

There are four phases of motor biofeedback training, as follows:

1. With the intraanal electrode or balloon in place, patients are instructed in external sphincter con-

traction. While viewing the display, they experiment with different maneuvers until the proper response is produced repeatedly. Extraneous muscle contraction (of the buttock, abdomen, thigh, back, and even neck) are discouraged, because they dissipate the force of contraction and lead to early fatigue.[20,34,41] It should be noted, however, that in some neurologic cases contractions of the buttocks must be accepted as a necessary substitute for sphincter contraction.

2. The external sphincter contraction is synchronized with distention of the intrarectal balloon.
3. The display is removed from the patient's view and contractions are practiced without it.
4. Patients are encouraged to regularly perform sphincter exercises, using the same maneuvers, during the intervals between sessions.

Treatment is continued until continence is satisfactory or until it is determined that no improvement can be achieved (Table 14C-6).

THE THREE BALLOON METHOD

The three balloon system developed by Schuster and associates[42-44] is the most widely used method of motor biofeedback. The equipment consists of a probe with three balloons—an intrarectal one, which can be inflated to distend the rectum, and two intraanal balloons, the proximal one which records internal sphincter contraction and relaxation, the distal one recording external sphincter contraction. All of the balloons are connected to a recorder by way of pressure transducers which record all pressure measurements simultaneously (Fig. 14C-1).

Fig. 14C-1 Coronal section through the anus and rectum. The anorectal musculature is labeled at left. Note the three-balloon system located in the ampulla, the region of the internal sphincter, and the external sphincter, respectively. The tracings indicate the pressure changes for each balloon after distention of the balloon in the ampulla.

Table 14C-6
Biofeedback Protocol

Have the patient keep an incontinence diary and bring it at each visit for review.

After inserting the apparatus, instill 60–150 ml of air, so as to enable the patient to distinguish the nature of the stimulus. Then instill 5 ml at 2–3 second intervals until the change in rectal sensation is felt; time the interval from instillation to verbal response.

The normal patient should respond to 15 ml of air or less. If the volume is not recognized, or the response is delayed beyond 2 seconds, rechallenge with the same volume, telling the patient when the volume is injected.

When the volume is recognized, concentrate on eliminating the delay and on reducing the volume necessary to stimulate recognition, by 5 ml decrements.

Instruct the patient to squeeze the anus and, while watching the display, try to get as high a reading as possible; maintain the contraction for as long as possible. Discourage extraneous muscle contractions. Allow short rest intervals of 15 to 30 seconds, as required.

Record the highest reading reached and maintained for 3 seconds and record the longest duration achieved. It's best to do this early in the session, before fatigue develops.

Once the patient is performing well, move the meter out of sight and observe the performance.

The average session should last about 30 minutes. Coach the patient in proper contraction, with plenty of verbal encouragement.

Instruct the patient in sphincter exercises to be performed between sessions: sphincter contractions of 20–30 seconds each, 30 times twice daily.

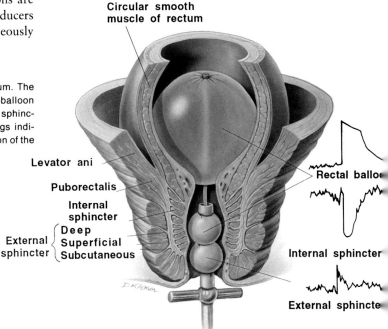

Engel, Nikoomanesh and Schuster, in 1974, were the first to report this technique. Of eight patients, four became fully continent and two were improved.[43]

In 1979, Cerulli, Nikoomanesh and Schuster reported on the use of biofeedback in 50 incontinent patients. Success was defined as "complete disappearance of incontinence or at least a 90% decrease in the frequency of incontinence; therefore, a patient with daily incontinence could have no more than one episode every ten days."[44] Their success rate was 71%. Results were best in patients with incontinence caused by anorectal surgery (92%) and worst in cases caused by neurologic condition (45%). Subsequently, several investigators reported similar success rates.[25,28,39,45,46]

ELECTROMYOMETRIC METHOD

In 1967, Haskell and Rovner[47] reported a 71% success rate using electromyography with needle electrodes to train patients in sphincter contraction. However, the procedure involved too many needle insertions to be generally acceptable. The electromyometric method substitutes an intraanal plug for the needle electrode and an electromyometer for the electromyograph.[11,20,34,41] It displays external sphincter contraction only, by means of an intraanal plug containing two electrodes which may be either concentric or linear (Fig. 14C-2). The plug is adapted to an electromyometer in such a way that the electric impulses generated by the contracting sphincter are audibly and visibly conveyed to the patient as a guide in these exercises.

In my last reported series,[20] 113 patients with anal incontinence in whom conventional sphincter exercises were ineffective were treated by this method—89 in the

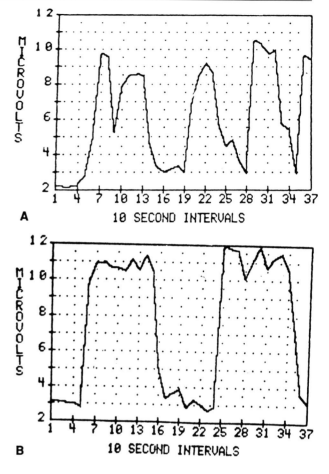

A

B

Fig. 14C-3   Data printout of the signal produced by muscle contraction, showing the peak value before **A**, and after **B**, biofeedback therapy with the Biocomp 2001 (scale 8μV). (Reprinted from *Gastroenterology* 1987;93:292, with permission.)

Fig. 14C-2   Anal plug that is adapted to an electromyometer. (Reprinted from *Gastroenterology* 1987;93:292, with permission.)

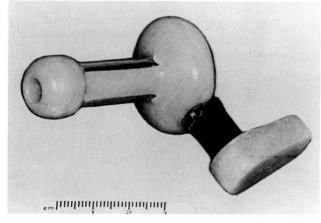

office and 24 in the hospital rehabilitation department. Various electromyometers were used*; in the last 16 cases the Biocomp 2001™ electromyometer (Biofeedback Research Institute, Wilshire Blvd., Los Angeles) was used in conjunction with an Apple computer (Fig. 14C-3). With the plug in place and the electromyometer (EMM) or computer screen in view, patients were instructed in sphincter contraction during an average of 3.34 one-hour sessions.

---

*The actual value of the signal is not as important as an increase in the value from session to session; neither is it as important as actual restoration of continence. Several patients achieved continence with no measured increase in performance. Thus, a change in instrument should not bias results and adaptation of the anal plug to any electromyometer should be just as effective.

Table 14C-7

Results of Biofeedback According to Cause of Anal Incontinence

Cause	Total	Satisfactory	
		No.	Percent
Traumatic			
Obstetric	16	10	63
Postoperative			
Hemorrhoidectomy	19	16	84
Fistulectomy	21	19	90
Keyhole deformity	13	0	0
Excision carcinoma	2	1	50
Lateral sphincterotomy	3	2	67
Anterior resection	3	0	0
Multiple operations	2	1	50
Subtotal	79	49	62
Nontraumatic			
Radiation	3	3	100
Neurologic	3	1	33
Idiopathic	25	17	68
Rectal prolapse (postrepair)	3	1	33
Subtotal	34	22	65
Total	113	71	63

Reprinted from *Gastroenterology* 1987;93:293 with permission.

cess rate with hospital treatment was only 46% as compared with a 67% rate in the office. This difference is attributable to the fact that hospital patients were treated by technicians, although well-trained ones, rather than by the doctor, which emphasizes again the importance of personal interaction between patient and physician in patient motivation.[22]

SWAN ATTIKA METHOD

The Swan Attika apparatus (Swan Attika (Europe) Ltd, 9, Kapetan Stamati Street, GR-83100 Samos. Greece), with a latex rubber probe and a battery-powered control and display unit (Fig. 14C-4) combines many of the best features of both of the foregoing methods.[48] It is just as inexpensive as the electromyometric method and is easier to use than either of the other methods described.

To date, the author has used this equipment in 47 patients with a 70% success rate.

Sensory Deficits

Testing for sensitivity to rectal distention is easily performed and should be carried out in all incontinent

The success rate, as determined using Cerulli's criteria,[44] was 63% (Table 14C-7). As in Cerulli's series, biofeedback was most successful in those patients who were incontinent after anorectal surgery and least successful in those of neurologic origin.

Although a success rate of 63% is certainly acceptable in patients who would otherwise have remained incontinent or have undergone surgery, it is less than Cerulli's success rate of 71% and is substantially less than that of 74% achieved in my previous series.[82]

The difference can be attributed to two factors. The first is *case selection,* whereby cases are included or excluded on the basis of how they directly affect the outcome of the study. For example, in the present series there were 13 cases of keyhole deformity,** all of which were treatment failures. When these cases were excluded from the series the success rate rose to 71%. There were no such cases in my previous series.[34]

Location of treatment is the second factor. The suc-

**Keyhole deformity is a condition occurring after partial division of the sphincter complex posteriorly during either fissurectomy or fistulectomy, whereby a small gutter is formed resulting in chronic seepage of mucus, stool, or both.

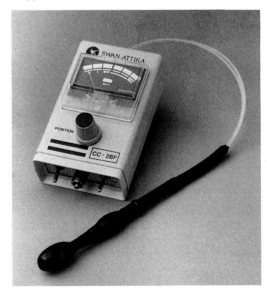

Fig. 14C-4 The Swan Attika apparatus has a detachable rectal balloon; below this is a squeeze-sensitive anal chamber, which senses the activities of the internal and external sphincters and the puborectalis. The handheld display incorporates a pressure transducer as well as an amplifier and sensitivity controls. Pressure changes are displayed on an analog meter. (Reprinted from *Endoscopy Rev* Nov/Dec 1988:55, with permission.)

patients before commencing treatment, especially if surgery is contemplated. Impairment of rectal sensitivity may well doom any proposed operation to failure.[25] One should suspect a sensory deficit if an incontinent patient displays normal sphincter contraction.

Sensory biofeedback is indicated in those patients who (1) have a normal sensory threshold, but fail to coordinate external sphincter contraction with rectal distention, or (2) have an elevated sensory threshold to rectal distention which may be due to a neurologic deficit, increased rectal compliance, or diabetic neuropathy.

A small number of patients have been found to have abnormalities of rectal sensation, and in some cases this is combined with a motor deficit.[49] They may be able to contract the external sphincter when instructed to do so, but are unable to perceive rectal distention and are thus deprived of the appropriate warning signal.

All of the methods of biofeedback described here, in addition to recording external sphincter contraction, allow sensory testing with an intrarectal balloon and coordination of external sphincter contraction with rectal distention (the electromyometric method does so only if the plug has a central channel). The Schuster 2-balloon manometric method records relaxation of the internal sphincter as well.

Patients with neurologic impairment, but with some innervation intact, may benefit from both motor and sensory biofeedback, although most require behavioral measures as well.[37,50,51]

A raised rectal threshold of sensitivity occurs in children with encopresis and in adults with recurrent fecal impaction.[80] These patients usually require behavioral and pharmacologic measures, but may derive some benefit from sensory biofeedback.[28]

Up to 20% of diabetics develop both a peripheral and autonomic neuropathy with an increased threshold of conscious rectal sensation and impaired external sphincter contraction in response to rectal distention.[36] Many also have chronic diarrhea caused by autonomic neuropathy.[26,39,52] Treatment consists of control of the diabetes[39] and sensory biofeedback.

Buser and Miner[53] found that a few patients have a delayed response to rectal distention because they respond to the wrong stimulus. That is, they take no action until they feel the sphincter being stretched by the full rectum. These patients were able, with sensory retraining by intrarectal balloon distention, to correct the sensory delay, improve the sensory threshold, and eliminate incontinence in 10 of 13 cases.

Sensory Biofeedback

The purpose of sensory biofeedback, therefore, is to decrease the threshold of awareness to rectal distention and to eliminate any delay in response. It is performed as follows:

1. Determine the smallest volume of rectal distention sensed and time the verbal response to it (normally less than 2 seconds.
2. Repeat the process until the patient can reliably detect distention to the threshold without delay.
3. Administer progressively smaller volumes in decrements of 5 ml of air.
4. Each time a smaller volume is sensed consistently, without delay, decrease the volume further.
5. Repeat the procedure until a normal level is reached or no further improvement can be attained.
6. Coordinate sensation and sphincter contraction, if necessary.[25,36,53]

Reservoir Deficits

Reservoir disorders, fortunately, are few in number, because they are difficult to treat. They fall into two main categories: disorders of the colon, and disorders of the rectum.

Colonic Disorders

Diseases of the colon range from irritable bowel syndrome to inflammatory bowel disease, with shortened transit time, rapid delivery of the stool to the rectum, and a more liquid stool. The major factor in the rapidity and forcefulness of entry of stool into the rectum is the motility of the left colon.

Many incontinent patients have a history of episodic diarrhea with urgency incontinence, most frequently caused by underlying irritable bowel syndrome,[54] which may be difficult to manage. Approximately one fourth of patients with irritable bowel syndrome are occasionally incontinent even if they have a strong sphincter.[55] On the other hand, control of diarrhea with constipating agents may improve symptoms to the extent that a proposed operation becomes unnecessary.[56]

It is equally important to realize that incontinence is a common but frequently unvoiced symptom in patients with diarrhea and may be the real reason the patient is seeking help. Of 76 patients with diarrhea reported by

Leigh and Turnberg,[57] half were incontinent, but only half of these volunteered that information. The rest admitted to incontinence only on direct questioning.

Other studies report similar findings.[10,16,58] Apparently diarrhea is a more socially acceptable symptom than incontinence. Conversely, doctors may interpret incontinence in the patient with diarrhea as a manifestation of severe diarrhea.

Rectal Disorders

Disorders of the rectum with decreased capacity and compliance consist of two types.[2,65] The first type occurs after resection of the rectum and pulling down of colon or small bowel into the pelvis to replace the rectum. This type results from anterior resection of the rectum, ileoanal anastomosis, with or without an ileal pouch, and surgical correction of imperforate anus. The colon is very different from the rectum in terms of structure and function, and the small bowel is even more markedly different due to its thicker, more muscular wall and lowered compliance.[59] Normal bowel function and continence are usually recovered by 6 months to 1 year,[60,61] but results will be poor if there has been an anastomotic leak or pelvic sepsis. The resulting edema and scarring produces an unyielding rectum with a markedly diminished capacity.[60,62,63]

In the case of a surgically repaired imperforate anus, especially where the defect was high, all three components of continence may be affected. Allen and coworkers[64] and Arnbjornsson and colleagues[65] both found that both maximum sphincter contraction and the critical threshold for rectal distention were improved.

Scarring and inflammation of the rectum, the second disorder type, is caused by inflammatory bowel disease, such as chronic ulcerative colitis,[66] Crohn's disease of the colon,[67] rectal ischemia,[26] and radiation proctitis.[68] In such cases there is rapid, forceful passage of stool through the rectum and anal canal; occasionally, rectal distention is so painful that there is voluntary inhibition of the external sphincter.

With inflammatory bowel disease the maximum tolerable volume is less than in normal subjects, and correlates with the activity of the disease.[66,67]

There is no specific treatment for reservoir deficits. Biofeedback by saline retention may be attempted,[39] but in most cases, behavioral and pharmacologic measures, such as the use of steroid enemas, loperamide, and bulk agents, must be taken to improve stool consistency, decrease colonic motility, and alleviate urgency incontinence.

MANAGEMENT OF INCONTINENCE BY PHARMACOLOGIC AND BEHAVIORAL MEASURES

Indications and Goals

Although applicable to any incontinent patient, pharmacologic and behavioral measures are most often applied as a supplement to biofeedback or operative repair, for many patients with deficient reservoir function, in most patients with neurologic disorders, and for those with recurrent fecal impaction.

The aims of bowel management programs are to achieve optimal fecal consistency, control the time of evacuation, and to provide satisfactory skin care.

Control of Fecal Consistency

Converting a patient's stool from loose to solid may actually render the patient with borderline sphincter function continent. This can be done by treating a specific illness like inflammatory bowel disease, which may be causing the loose stools, with steroids.

Increasing fecal bulk with agents such as psyllium seed or methylcellulose to bind water in the stool and decrease pressure in the sigmoid colon[69] can also have this effect (although in some cases it is necessary to restrict dietary fiber in order to decrease the fecal volume).

Lastly, slowing of the intestinal transit by use of opiate derivatives, allowing water absorption from the stool, can produce continence. Loperamide is more effective than diphenoxylate, without the latter's frequent side effects which include the potential addictiveness of codeine.[70] Loperamide also increases the resting pressure of the internal sphincter,[71–74] and enhances rectal compliance.[25,37]

Encouragement of Regular Evacuation

This is a sine qua non of incontinence management. Granted, not all patients need a daily bowel movement, but continence is more readily maintained if the entire sigmoid colon is evacuated completely at regular interval.[75]

This may be accomplished by the following measures:

1. The patient should have regular meals and a well-

balanced diet which provides adequate hydration and roughage, including bulk agents if necessary.

2. The gastrocolic reflex can be promoted. Increased colonic activity with mass movement of the contents peaks about 30 minutes after meals, most markedly in the morning. Capitalizing on this event by sitting on the commode for 10 to 15 minutes after breakfast each day may be enough to establish regularity and restore continence.

3. Suppositories and or enemas can be used, if necessary, at the same time each day, usually in the morning. If the incontinence-free time between enemas is too short, a constipating drug may be administered.

4. Finally, for those patients who cannot retain an enema, the following measures may be of help.

Often only small amounts of water (50 ml) are necessary to irrigate the rectum successfully.[32] For these patients a soft-tipped, water-filled bulb syringe may suffice to stimulate rectal contractions and empty the rectum. The syringe is inserted well into the anal canal, so that the bulb is pressed firmly against the perineum and the water is expressed into the rectum.

By using a latex cone and disposable irrigating equipment, some incontinent patients can become regular, like the ostomate. The lubricated cone tip is inserted firmly into the rectum and tap water is allowed to flow by gravity from a bag at shoulder level, the volume being adjusted to each patient's needs. This method was judged successful by Nicosia and Becker[77] in 12 of 17 patients (all of whose incontinence was of neurogenic origin) and was a complete failure in none.

Schandling and Gilmour[78] devised a special enema continence catheter with an inflatable intrarectal balloon and an exterior baffle which prevents displacement of the balloon. All of 112 incontinent children with spina bifida were rendered continent, in the sense that they acquired the ability to expel the bowel contents at a chosen time and in a designated place with no more than three inadvertent minor escapes of fecal material during one month.

The emphasis of all these habit-training programs is on the prevention of constipation by regular elimination.[30] Some common complaints of patients listed by Dietrich and Okamoto[79] were that the process takes too long, that it is difficult to incorporate into the home life, and that there are too many economic deterrents.

On the basis of these complaints, Alterescu[80] suggests that dietary modifications be realistic and that any recommendations be simple and introduced one at a time. If the demands of the regime are too great, failure will result.

Perianal Skin Care

The bed-confined, incontinent patient requires especially diligent nursing care of the perianal skin.

Control of stool consistency by the measures previously described is the most important measure, as liquid stool can break down the skin barrier and produce a raw perineum in a matter of hours.

Lessening the contact time of stool with the skin is vitally important for the same reason. The skin should be cleansed gently with warm water immediately after each bowel movement.

Protection of the skin requires augmentation of the normal skin barrier. The best skin protectants are ointments with a petrolatum base that create a water-impermeable film. When the skin is macerated, these ointments are less helpful. Instead, and particularly if there is continuous mucous leakage, powders containing talc, zinc oxide, or cornstarch which have a drying effect can be used, as can lotions and exposure to air. Water-soluble creams may soothe the irritated skin, but have little barrier effect.[11]

The Hollister Fecal Incontinence Collector (Hollister Inc., 2000 Hollister Drive, Libertyville, Illinois 60048) consists of a drainable pouch like a stoma bag, and a skin protective barrier which adheres to the perineum, anal cleft, and inner surfaces of the buttocks, thus holding the collector firmly in place while protecting the perianum. Although this appliance is rarely necessary, in the presence of severe, intractable, and uncontrollable diarrhea, such as that occasionally seen in Crohn's disease, it may well prevent severe skin damage and eliminate the need for endless turning and changing of the patient.

Dodge and coworkers[81] described and classified various external products, including disposable pads and diapers, and if the patient is confined to bed, reusable or disposable underpads. The choice depends on the severity of the incontinence, the degree of dependence, the patient's eyesight, dexterity, and personal preference.

Moisture and prolonged contact with feces leads to maceration, ulceration, and to superficial fungus and yeast infections. Aluminum sulfate and calcium acetate (Domeboro's solution(TM)) is useful as an irrigant for cleansing macerated skin. If the skin is superficially ulcerated, hydrocortisone, 1% cream may be helpful. A cholestyramine ointment has been suggested for the treatment of perianal ulcerations secondary to ileoanal anastomosis or to severe diarrhea (in which the effluent may be ileal in nature). Antifungals such as 3% iodochlorhydroxyquine (Vioform™) or antimonilials such as Nystatin™ are occasionally useful.

SPECIAL SITUATIONS

Care of Institutionalized Patients

Fecal incontinence in the elderly is a leading cause of nursing home placement.[99,100] The patient should be helped to be socially acceptable even if he or she is bedridden. Tobin and Brocklehurst[96] treated 82 elderly institutionalized patients, three quarters of whom were mentally impaired, by behavioral methods. At two months, two thirds of the patients were no longer incontinent.

Neurologic Conditions

In both cerebral cortical and spinal cord conditions, the power to inhibit intrinsic rectal contractions by external sphincter contraction is lost. The spinal cord patient also has lost the ability to sense rectal distention. In both cases, spontaneous reflex evacuation occurs and defecation is fairly complete. Typically, a formed stool is passed in the early morning, usually after food intake. So, it makes sense to arrange for the patient to be on the commode at that time.[74,82,83]

Particularly in the case of spinal cord lesions, the aim is to regulate reflex evacuation (with or without the use of laxatives and enemas). Evacuation may be triggered 15 to 20 minutes after a meal, or after insertion of a suppository, by some or all of the following measures: (1) skin stimulation of the inner surface of the thigh and perianum; (2) digital stimulation with downward traction on the puborectalis; (3) abdominal massage along the course of the colon, especially on the left side; (4) leaning forward and straining, if any of the abdominal musculature innervation is intact.

In the cases of cauda equina lesions, not only is rectal sensation lost, but activity in the descending colon is often impaired[75] so that bowel evacuation is mechanically more difficult and impaction more frequent. Defecation is accomplished in response to vague stimuli such as sweating and abdominal discomfort, possibly perceived via the sacral sympathetic plexus. Habit training is imperative to regulate evacuation, and suppositories, enemas, and even manual removal may be necessary.

Lesser degrees of innervation loss, as in partial paraplegia, myelomeningocele, and multiple sclerosis may benefit from motor or sensory biofeedback alone or in combination with behavioral and pharmaceutical measures. Those patients suffering from dementia do better with behavior modification.

Fecal Impaction

This disorder involves all three major components of continence. It is a common cause of soiling in the elderly, especially in the immobilized or senile patient. The impacted stool blunts rectal sensation, creates excessive rectal compliance, and chronically inhibits sphincter tone. As a result there is leakage of liquid feces around the impacted stool with overflow incontinence.[96]

The seepage and soiling are constant, unlike the situation in neurologic disorders, and may give the mistaken impression of diarrhea. *It is important to rule out impaction by digital examination before treating incontinence or diarrhea in the elderly or debilitated patient.*

There are two aspects of treatment: immediate relief of the impaction, and prevention of recurrence.

Immediate treatment involves one or two enemas given daily until there is no fecal return and the rectum is empty on digital examination. If the stool is hard, an oil retention enema may be administered. Manual removal is unpleasant for the examiner, unpleasant and painful for the patient, and usually unnecessary. On the rare occasion when relief is urgent, only a portion of the main bolus need be extracted, following which enemas can be given until the bowel is empty.

Usually in these cases most or all of the colon is full of stool, and frequently enemas must be given for several days until there is no fecal return, abdominal palpation reveals no stool, and the rectum is empty on digital examination. Failure is usually due to inadequate emptying of the bowel.[25]

Prevention of recurrence requires keeping the bowel empty; therefore, habit training is begun with regular visits to the toilet after meals. If necessary, a suppository is inserted once daily (against the rectal wall, not into the fecal mass).[80] Glycerin suppositories may be adequate, although bisacodyl suppositories are necessary more frequently than they are in neurologic patients. If these measures are unsuccessful after three days, an enema is given.[25]

Other general measures include avoidance of constipating drugs and increasing the patient's activity and mobility when possible.

Relapse is frequent unless the cause is eliminated and regular evacuation established. Biofeedback, both motor and sensory, may be of help in restoring rectal sensibility and sphincter tone.[38]

Encopresis

This is a form of recurrent impaction with overflow incontinence which occurs in children. It consists of diminished ability to detect stool in the rectum related to a markedly increased threshold of rectal sensation to distention.[96]

Psychologic factors undoubtedly play a role, but psychiatric therapy is long and difficult with relatively meager results. On the other hand, pediatricians and surgeons have had considerable success with management programs.[28,97,98]

Certain features are common to all programs:

1. A complete examination is performed.
2. The parents and child are interviewed; any serious emotional disturbance is ruled out and the mechanism of the condition is explained to the parents. It is made clear that the child is not willfully soiling, and attempts are made to motivate the child.
3. The bowel is evacuated completely (1 to 2 enemas usually are sufficient).
4. Behavioral treatment is begun with bowel training.
5. Laxatives are administered regularly. Among those favored are lactulose, mineral oil, and Senokot.(TM)
6. A daily record is kept and submitted to the physician regularly.
7. A system of rewards (praise, candy, or special privileges) and punishments (ranging from nonchalance, through disapproval and loss of privileges, to cleaning up after his own incontinence episodes) is carefully planned and instituted (there is controversy on the use of punishments).

Biofeedback has also been used successfully in the management of this condition.[28]

Myelomeningocele

This condition occurs in 0.1% of births.[84,85] With aggressive medical and surgical treatment, 80% to 90% now survive, and of these, 90% suffer from fecal incontinence.[86] So rehabilitation has become increasingly important in the management of this disease.

There is significantly increased threshold to rectal distention as compared to controls,[87] and the external sphincter cannot be squeezed voluntarily.[43,44,88–90]

Several investigators found biofeedback efficacious.[44,90–95] However, Whitehead and coworkers[90] concluded that biofeedback is beneficial only in those with lesions below L2, and then only if combined with behavioral therapy.

Wald[92,93] reported that response to biofeedback correlates most strongly with rectal sensory thresholds and that impaired sensation is associated with a poor response to biofeedback. In his series, all those with normal rectal sensation had neuromotor deficits of L5, S1, or lower.

The initial evaluation should include testing for perianal sensation, voluntary contraction of the external sphincter, fecal impaction with overflow incontinence, and the minimum volume of rectal distention that will produce rectal sensation.[89]

The requirements for successful biofeedback treatment of myelomeningocele are patient motivation, control of sphincter or gluteals, and the ability to sense rectal distention (to a maximum of 60 ml).[93]

Rectal distention is begun with large volumes. The patient is trained to recognize progressively smaller volumes and to synchronize voluntary external sphincter or gluteal contractions with the distention. Many more sessions (6 to 12) than usual are necessary; however, there should be some indication of improvement after 2 to 3 sessions. If not, attempts should be discontinued and behavioral measures instituted.[81]

SUMMARY

Behavioral medicine has had a considerable impact on the management of fecal incontinence. Habit training and biofeedback are the treatments of choice in many types of incontinence and are successful in a high percentage of appropriately selected cases.

Results vary depending on the component of continence affected. Results are best in those cases in which the affected component is motor, and poorest in those patients with disorders of rectal compliance, as well as in demented patients.

The management of fecal incontinence also requires considerable sensitivity on the part of the physician, because many of these patients are understandably anxious.

REFERENCES

1. Yoshioka K, Hyland G, Keighley MRB. Critical assessment of the quality of continence after postanal repair for fecal incontinence. *Br J Surg.* 1989;76:64–68.
2. Corman ML. Gracilis muscle transposition for anal incontinence: late results. *Br J Surg.* 1985; 72(suppl):S21–S22.

3. Labow SB, Hoexter B, Moseson MD, et al. Modification of silastic sling repair for rectal procidentia and anal incontinence. *Dis Colon Rectum.* 1985;28:684–685.
4. Scharli AF, Kiesewetter WB. Defecation and continence: some new concepts. *Dis Colon Rectum.* 1970;13:81–107.
5. Williams NS, Price R, Johnston D. The long-term effects of sphincter preserving operations for rectal carcinoma on function of the anal sphincter in man. *Br J Surg.* 1980;67:203–208.
6. Lane RH, Parks AG. Function of the anal sphincters following coloanal anastomosis. *Br J Surg.* 1977;64:596–599.
7. Bennett RC, Duthie HL. The functional importance of the internal anal sphincter. *Br J Surg.* 1964;51:355–357.
8. Parks AG. Anorectal incontinence. *Proc R Soc Med.* 1975;68:681–690.
9. Miller R, Bartolo DCC, Roe A, Cervero F, Mortensen NJMcC. Anal sensation and the continence mechanism. *Dis Colon Rectum.* 1988;31:433–438.
10. Keighley MRB, Fielding JWL. Management of fecal incontinence and results of surgical treatment. *Br J Surg.* 1980;67:757.
11. MacLeod JH. Fecal incontinence: a practical program of management. *Endoscopy Rev.* 1988:45–56.
12. Rosen L, Khubchandani IT, Sheets J, Stasik JJ, Riether RD. Management of anal incontinence. *Am Fam Phys.* 1986;33:129–137.
13. Corman ML. *Colon and Rectal Surgery.* 2nd ed. Philadelphia: JB Lippincott; 1989:182.
14. Hallan RI, Marzouk DEMM, Waldron DJ, Womack NR, Williams NS. Comparison of digital and manometric assessment of anal sphincter function. *Br J Surg.* 1989;76:973–975.
15. Henry MM, Parks AG, Swash M. The pelvic floor musculature in the descending perineum syndrome. *Br J Surg.* 1982;69:470–472.
16. Read NW, Harford WV, Schmulen AC, Read MG, Santa Ana CA, Fordtran JS. A clinical study of patients with fecal incontinence and diarrhea. *Gastroenterology.* 1979;76:747–756.
17. Devroede G. Anal incontinence. *Dis Colon Rectum.* 1982;25:90–95.
18. Whitehead WE, Orr WC, Engel BT, Schuster MM. External anal sphincter response to rectal distention: learned response or reflex. *Psychophysiology.* 1982;19:57–61.
19. Burgio, KL, Robinson JC, Engel BT. The role of biofeedback in Kegel exercise training for stress urinary incontinence. *Am J Obstet Gynecol.* 1986;154:58–64.
20. MacLeod, JH. Management of anal incontinence by biofeedback. *Gastroenterol.* 1987;93:291–294.
21. Tuckson WB, Fazio VW. Anal incontinence. In: Fazio VW, ed. *Current Therapy in Colon and Rectal Surgery.* Philadelphia: BC Decker; 1990.
22. Devroede G, Duguay-Perron C. Biofeedback: the light at the end of the tunnel? Maybe for constipation (lett) *Gastroenterology.* 1981;80:1089–1090.
23. Wald A. Use of biofeedback in treatment of fecal incontinence in patients with myelomeningocele. *Pediatrics.* 1981;68:45–49.
24. Orne MT. The efficacy of biofeedback therapy. *Annu Rev Med.* 1979;30:489–503.
25. Wald, A. Fecal incontinence: effective nonsurgical treatments. *Postgrad Med.* 1986;80:123–129.
26. Devroede G. Ischemic fecal incontinence and rectal angina. *Gastroenterol.* 1982;83:970–980.
27. Devroede G, Arhan P, Schang JC, Heppell J. Orderly and disorderly fecal continence. In: Kodner, ID, Roe JP, eds. *Colon, Rectal and Anal Surgery: Current Techniques and Controversies.* St. Louis: CV Mosby; 1985:40–62.
28. Olness K, McParland FA, Piper J. Biofeedback: a new modality in the management of children with fecal soiling. *J Pediatr.* 1980;96:505–509.
29. Gaarder KR. *Clinical Biofeedback: a Procedural Manual.* Williams & Wilkins Co; 1977:91.
30. Whitehead WE, Schuster MM. *Gastrointestinal Disorders: Behavioral and Physiological Basis for Treatment.* Orlando, Fla: Academic Press; 1985:29–275.
31. Hopkinson BR, Lightwood R. Electrical treatment of anal incontinence. *Lancet.* 1966;1:297–298.
32. Penninckx FM, Elliot MS, Hancke E, et al. Symposium: fecal incontinence. *Int J Colorect Dis.* 1987;2:173–186.
33. Collins CD, Brown BH, Duthie HO. An assessment of intraluminal electrical stimulation for anal incontinence. *Br J Surg.* 1969;54:542–546.
34. MacLeod JH. Biofeedback in the management of partial anal incontinence. *Dis Colon Rectum.* 1983;26:244–246.
35. Bennett RC. A review of the results of orthodox treatment for anal fistulae. *Proc R Soc Med.* 1962;55:756–757.
36. Wald A, Tunuguntla AK. Anorectal sensorimotor dysfunction in fecal incontinence and diabetes mellitus: modification with biofeedback therapy. *N Engl J Med.* 1984;310:1282–1287.
37. Wald A. Disorders of defecation and fecal continence. *Cleveland Clin J Med.* 1989;56:491–501.
38. Marzuk PM. Biofeedback for gastrointestinal disorders: a review of the literature. *Ann Int Med.* 1985;103:240–244.
39. Schiller LR, Santa Ana C, Davis GR, Fordtran JS. Fecal incontinence in chronic diarrhea: report of a case with improvement after training with rectally infused saline. *Gastroenterology.* 1979;77:751–753.
40. Latimer PR, Campbell D, Kasperski J. A components analysis of biofeedback in the treatment of fecal incontinence. *Biofeedback Self-Regul.* 1984;9:311–324.
41. MacLeod JH. Biofeedback in the management of partial anal incontinence: a preliminary report. *Dis Colon Rectum.* 1979;22:169–171.
42. Schuster MM. Behavioral approaches to the treatment of gastrointestinal motility disorders. *Med Clin North Am.* 1981;65:1397–1411.
43. Engel BT, Nikoomanesh P, Schuster MM. Operant conditioning of rectosphincteric responses in the treatment of fecal incontinence. *New Engl J Med.* 1974;290:646–649.
44. Cerulli MA, Nikoomanesh P, Schuster MM. Progress in biofeedback conditioning for fecal incontinence. *Gastroenterol.* 1979;76:742–746.
45. Goldenberg DA, et al. Biofeedback therapy for fecal incontinence. *Am J Gastroenterol.* 1980;74:342–345.
46. Riboli EB, Frascio M, Pitto G, Reboa G. Biofeedback conditioning for fecal incontinence. *Arch Phys Med Rehabil.* 1988;69:29–31.
47. Haskell B, Rovner H. Electromyography in the management of the incompetent anal sphincter. *Dis Colon Rectum.* 1967;10:81–84.
48. Constantinides CG, Cywes S. Fecal incontinence: a simple pneumatic device for home biofeedback training. *J Ped Surg.* 1983;18:276–277.
49. Lubowski DZ, Nicholls RJ. Fecal incontinence associated with reduced pelvic sensation. *Br J Surg.* 1988;75:1086–1088.
50. Kiff E, Swash M. Slowed conduction in the pudendal nerves in idiopathic (neurogenic) fecal incontinence. *Br J Surg.* 1984;71:614–616.
51. Kiff ES, Swash M. Normal proximal and delayed distal conduction in the pudendal nerves of patients with idiopathic fecal incontinence. *J Neurol Neurosurg Psych.* 1984;47:820–823.
52. Feldman M, Schiller LR. Disorders of gastrointestinal motility associated with diabetes mellitus. *Ann Int Med.* 1983;98:378–384.
53. Buser WD, Miner PB. Delayed rectal sensation with fecal incontinence: successful treatment using anorectal manometry. *Gastroenterology.* 1986;91:1186–1191.
54. Read NW, Bartolo DCC, Read MG. Differences in anal function in patients with incontinence to solids and in patients with incontinence to liquids. *Br J Surg.* 1984;71:39–42.

55. Siegel D, Tucker H, Enck P, Whitehead W, Schuster MM. Symptoms differentiating irritable bowel syndrome (IBS) from other G.I. disorders. *Gastroenterology.* 1984;86:1251. Abstract.

56. Keighley MRB, Fielding JWL. Management of fecal incontinence and results of surgical treatment. *Br J Surg.* 1983;70:463–468.

57. Leigh RJ, Turnberg LA. Fecal incontinence: the unvoiced symptom. *Lancet.* 1982;1:1349–1351.

58. Cann PA, Read NW, Holdsworth CD. Irritable bowel syndrome: relationship of disorders in the transit of a single solid meal to symptom patterns. *Gut.* 1983;24:405–411.

59. Heppell J, et al. Physiologic aspects of continence after colectomy, mucosal proctectomy and ileoanal anastomosis. *Ann Surg.* 1982;195:435–443.

60. Pedersen IK, Christiansen J, Hint K, Jensen P, Olsen J, Mortensen PE. Anorectal function after low anterior resection for carcinoma. *Ann Surg.* 1986;204:133–135.

61. Suzuki H, Matsumoto K, Amano S, Fujioka M, Honzumi M. Anorectal pressure and rectal compliance after low anterior resection. *Br J Surg.* 1980;67:655–657.

62. Lane RHS, Parks AG. Function of the anal sphincters following coloanal anastomosis. *Br J Surg.* 1977;64:596–599.

63. Cohen M, Rosen L, Khubchandani I, Sheets J, Stasik J, Riether R. Rationale for medical or surgical therapy in anal incontinence. *Dis Colon Rectum.* 1986;29:120–122.

64. Allen MC, Orr WC, Robinson MG. Anorectal functioning in fecal incontinence. *Dig Dis Sci.* 1988;33:36–40.

65. Arnbjornsson E, Breland U, Kullendorff CM, Mikaelsson C, Okmian L. Physiotherapy to improve fecal control after Stephens' rectoplasty in high imperforate anus. *Z Kinderchir.* 1986;41:101–103.

66. Farthing MJG, Lennard-Jones JE. Sensibility of the rectum to distention and the anorectal distention reflex in ulcerative colitis. *Gut.* 1978;19:64–69.

67. Buchmann P, Mogg GAG, Alexander-Williams J, Allan RN, Keighley MRB. Relationship of proctitis and rectal capacity in Crohn's disease. *Gut.* 1980;21:137–140.

68. Varma JS, Smith AN, Busuttil A. Correlation of clinical and manometric abnormalities of rectal function following chronic radiation injury. *Br J Surg.* 1985;72:875–878.

69. Connell AM. Dietary fiber and diverticular disease. *Hosp Prac.* 1976;11:119–124.

70. Palmer KR, Corbett CL, Holdsworth CD. Double-blind crossover study comparing loperamide codeine and diphenoxylate in the treatment of chronic diarrhea. *Gastroenterology.* 1980;79:1272–1275.

71. Bannister JJ, Read NW, Donnelly TC, Sun WM. External and internal sphincter responses to rectal distention in normal subjects and in patients with idiopathic fecal incontinence. *Br J Surg.* 1989;76:617–621.

72. Read M, Read NW, Barber DC, Duthie HL. Effects of loperamide on anal sphincter function in patients complaining of chronic diarrhea with fecal incontinence and urgency. *Dig Dis & Sci.* 1982;27:807–814.

73. Rattan S, Culver PJ. Influence of loperamide on the internal anal sphincter of the opossum. *Gastroenterology.* 1987;93:121–126.

74. McKirdy HC. Effect of loperamide on human isolated internal sphincter. *Proc Physiol Soc.* 1981;C16:20–21.

75. Longo WW, Ballantyne GH, Modlin IM. The colon, rectum, and spinal cord patient; a review of the functional alterations of the denervated hindgut. *Dis Colon Rectum.* 1989;32:261–267.

76. Nicosia JF, Becker C. Bowel management of anal incontinence. *Am Soc Col Rect Surg.* Annual Meeting. 1985.

77. Shandling B, Gilmour RF. The enema continence catheter in spina bifida: successful bowel management. *J Ped Surg.* 1987;22:271–273.

78. Dietrich S. Okamoto G. Bowel training for children with neurogenic dysfunction: a follow-up. *Arch Phys Med Rehabil.* 1982;63:166–170.

79. Alterescu V. Fecal incontinence. *J Enterostom Ther.* 1986;13:44–48.

80. Dodge J, Bachman C, Silverman H. Fecal incontinence in elderly patients. *Postgrad Med.* 1988;83:258–270.

81. Brocklehurst JC. Bowel management in the neurologically disabled: the problems in old age. *Proc Roy Soc Med.* 1972;65:66–69.

82. Brocklehurst JC. Management of anal incontinence. *Clin Gastroenterol.* 1975;4:479–487.

83. Freeman JM. Neural tube defects: risks of occurrence and recurrence. In: Freeman JM, ed. *Practical Management of Myelomeningocele.* Baltimore: University Park Press; 1974:4–7.

84. Elwood JH, Elwood JM. *Epidemiology of Anencephalus and Spina Bifida.* London: Oxford University Press; 1980.

85. Brocklehurst G, Forrest D, Sharrard WJW, Stark G. Spina bifida for the clinician. *Clin Dev Med.* London: S.I.M.P. with Heinemann Medical; 1976.

86. Loening-Baucke V. Factors determining outcome in children with chronic constipation and fecal soiling. *Gut.* 1989;30:999–1006.

87. Whitehead WE et al. Biofeedback treatment of fecal incontinence in patients with meningomyelocele. *Dev Med Child Neurol.* 1981;23:313–322.

88. Wald A. Biofeedback for neurogenic fecal incontinence: rectal sensation is a determinant of outcome. *J Ped Gastroenterol & Nutrit.* 1983;2:302–306.

89. Whitehead WE, Parker L, Bosmajian L, et al. Treatment of fecal incontinence in children with spina bifida: comparison of biofeedback and behavior modification. *Arch Phys Med Rehabil.* 1986;67:218–223.

90. Loening-Baucke V, Desch L, Wolraich M. Biofeedback training for patients with myelomeningocele and fecal incontinence. *Dev Med Child Neurol.* 1988;30:761–790.

91. Wald A. Biofeedback therapy for fecal incontinence. *Ann Int Med.* 1981;95:146–149.

92. Wald A. Biofeedback for neurogenic rectal incontinence: rectal sensation is determinant in outcome. *J Pediatr Gastroenterol Nutr.* 1983;2:302–306.

93. Wald A, Chandra R, Chiponis D, Gabel S. Anorectal function and continence mechanisms in childhood encopresis. *J Pediatr Gastroenterol Nutr.* 1987;6:554–558.

94. Whitehead WE, Parker LH, Masek BJ, Cataldo MF, Freeman JM. Biofeedback treatment of fecal incontinence in patients with myelomeningocele. *Dev Med Child Neurol.* 1981;23:313–322.

95. Tobin GW, Brocklehurst JC. Fecal incontinence in residential homes for the elderly: prevalence, etiology, and management. *Age Ageing.* 1986;15:41–46.

96. Meunier P, Mollard P, Marechal JM. Physiopathology of megarectum: the association of megarectum with encopresis. *Gut.* 1976;17:224–227.

97. Wright L, Walker CE. Treatment of the child with psychogenic encopresis. *Clin Pediatr.* 1977;16:1042–1045.

98. Young GC. The treatment of childhood encopresis by conditioned gastroileal reflex training. *Behav Res Ther.* 1973;11:499–503.

99. Williams FC. Introductory remarks. NIH Conference on Incontinence in the Elderly. National Institute on Aging, Bethesda, MD. 1982.

Fecal Incontinence

14D   Surgical Therapies

14D1   Indications and Methodologies of Anal Sphincter Repair

John J. Murray and Malcolm C. Veidenheimer

INTRODUCTION

The psychologic and social consequences of fecal incontinence are profound. Afflicted individuals suffer greatly from the desperate anxiety and self-imposed social isolation that frequently accompany the disorder. The various operative and nonoperative measures proposed for the treatment of fecal incontinence reflect the multiple anatomic, neurologic, and physiologic derangements that can give rise to the problem. Direct repair of acquired anal sphincter injuries provides the most satisfactory outcome of any treatment for fecal incontinence. Accurate selection of patients for sphincter repair and close attention to the technical details of the procedure should maximize the chances for success.

ETIOLOGY OF ACQUIRED ANAL SPHINCTER INJURIES

Problems related to childbirth are the most common cause of anal sphincter dysfunction. Tearing and stretching of levator and sphincter muscles may occur with any delivery but are most commonly seen as a sequel to precipitate delivery or as a result of prolonged labor. In many instances an episiotomy was performed and subsequently enlarged as a result of a tear. Obstetric lacerations that involve the rectum and anus are usually repaired at the time of injury. In some instances the primary repair may not accurately appose the muscle layers of the levator and sphincter region, and in other instances hemorrhage or infection may supervene, leading to dehiscence of the repair. Incomplete healing of tears and repaired episiotomies may result in development of rectovaginal fistulas. In other circumstances, the rectovaginal septum may harbor indolent infection resulting in a septal abscess that drains spontaneously into the rectum or vagina, producing a rectovaginal fistula. Such an event may occur months or years after the original injury.

Anal sphincter injury may result from prior anorectal operation, most commonly as a complication of the management of complex abscess or fistula. Attempts at draining the abscess or performing fistulotomy may result in division of excess musculature, especially when the rectovaginal septum is involved. Large abscesses involving the ischiorectal fossa may result from more proximal penetration of the anorectal wall. The subsequent fistulous tract may encompass the puborectalis muscle. In reality, most extrasphincteric fistulas have an iatrogenic origin. In attempting to identify the internal opening of the fistula, false passages that transgress the levator muscles and enter the rectum above the level of the puborectalis muscle may be created inadvertently. Should a fistulotomy then be performed, the entire sphincter complex must be sacrificed. Less commonly, excision of an anal fissure performed with undue enthusiasm may result in injury to the sphincter muscle mechanism. Indeed, the simple operation of anal sphincterotomy, designed to divide only the distal portion of the internal anal sphincter, may result in trouble with control if incorrectly performed. Extensive hemorrhoid resection that inadvertently injures the sphincter muscle or puborectalis muscle may also cause incontinence. Anal dilation, performed in some centers as the operation of choice for hemorrhoids and anal fissure, may be complicated by fecal incontinence. Vigorous four-finger dilation, especially in elderly patients, may result in irreparable damage to the sphincter muscles or to their nerve supply, resulting in prolonged and sometimes permanent incontinence.

Prolapse of the rectum may also lead to fecal incontinence. Although this may reflect an associated traction injury to the pudendal nerves, recurring intrusion of the rectum through the anal canal may cause stretching of the anal levatores and sphincters to such a degree that normal muscle tone is lost. When the rectum is reduced, the sphincter mechanism is unable to close the anal canal completely, and the anal orifice becomes patulous, allowing mucus and fecal material to escape from the rectum and appear at the perineal region (Fig. 14D1-1). Although this represents an acquired injury to the anal sphincter, no anatomic defect in the sphincter muscle is present.

Impalement injuries to the perineum produce traumatic disruption of the rectum, anus, and surrounding musculature and lead to varying degrees of fecal incontinence. Trauma to the anal area may also result from insertion or extraction of foreign bodies. Anal sexual activity may traumatize the sphincter mechanism to such a degree that the anus takes on the patulous appearance seen in the patient with chronic rectal prolapse. Fractures of the pelvis may cause nerve injuries that interfere with the function of the levator and sphincter muscles. Incontinence in this circumstance is not the result of direct injury to the anal sphincter.

EVALUATION OF PATIENTS

History

Successful treatment of patients with fecal incontinence begins with a comprehensive evaluation to determine the cause for incontinence as well as any complicating factors. Nearly all patients with anal incontinence have some historical basis for the condition. Therefore, detailed inquiries should be made regarding obstetric delivery, past history of perineal trauma, and previous operations in the region. It is also important to make inquiries about the presence of protrusions such as rectal prolapse. A detailed sexual history should also be obtained. Specifically, the physician should determine whether anal intercourse or the insertion of various objects into the anal canal is a habit of the patient.

The decision to proceed with repair of anal sphincter injuries is in large measure determined by the extent of disability experienced by the patient. True fecal incontinence should be distinguished from urgency and seepage. Is the patient able to differentiate flatus from stool? Does the patient have incontinence of flatus only or of stool and flatus? Does all stool escape from the anal canal or does seepage occur only at the time of a bout of diarrhea? Is the material that escapes from the anus truly feces or mucus secretion? Inquiries should be made about sensation in the area. Does the patient feel there is a numbness? Is the patient aware when stool escapes from the anal canal or does the presence of the stool go unnoticed for long periods of time? Does the patient have an urgency to evacuate and, if so, how long can the patient wait once the urge appears before the actual need to reach the bathroom? How much staining does the patient experience? Is it enough to require the use of a pad or does the patient have to wear some sort of absorbent underwear? It is also important to determine whether there is escape of fecal material and flatus through the vagina as well as through the anus, suggesting a concomitant rectovaginal fistula. Major problems with excoriation of the perianal skin should be investi-

Fig. 14D1-1 Patulous anal orifice in patient with rectal procidentia.

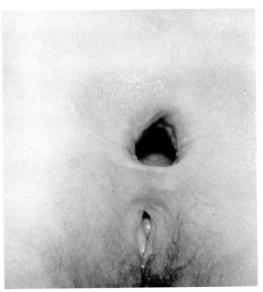

gated, and it should be noted whether certain skin applications relieve skin irritation.

Physical Examination

Physical examination should confirm the presence of a segmental defect in the sphincter muscle complex and permit identification of associated problems that may complicate sphincter repair. When the patient is properly positioned on the examining table, either in stirrups or in the prone jackknife position, the physician should be able to examine the perineum and note whether a cloacal deformity at the anovaginal region exists from previous obstetric trauma. The presence of a rectovaginal fistula or fistula in ano may also be identifiable by inspection. The presence of prolapsing mucous membrane or a true rectal prolapse should readily be apparent at the time of inspection, especially if the patient is asked to strain while assuming a squatting position over the commode. The degree of effacement and thinning of the rectovaginal septum should be apparent on visual examination, and any scars from previous trauma or surgical repair should be assessed at the time of inspection. When the patient is asked to strain, the physician should be able to note the presence of perineal descent, reflecting neurogenic injury to the muscles of the pelvic floor.

Careful digital examination of the anus and vagina permits an assessment of much of the detail needed to make decisions regarding the repair of anal sphincter injuries. The resting tone of the anal musculature as well as the extent of any palpable muscle defect should be noted. When the patient is asked to tighten the sphincter muscles, the force of contraction can be assessed and the integrity of sphincter innervation confirmed. During the same maneuver, it should be determined whether the puborectalis muscle is intact. The examiner can hook the index finger over the upper edge of this muscle and, by sweeping along its surface, identify any defects in the muscle body. When the anus is examined, the patient should be asked to strain down, simulating defecation, to determine the presence of an internal rectal prolapse. Any fistula identified should be cannulated with a probe to determine the course of the fistula. For rectovaginal fistulas, the level of the communication between the rectum and the vagina should be determined. Perianal sensation should also be assessed by pinprick or scratching. The anocutaneous reflex, or contraction of the external anal sphincter in response to stimulation of the perianal skin, can be identified visually and confirmed with electromyography. Absence of

the reflex or prolonged latency of the reaction can be caused by a lesion in the conus medullaris or a neuropathy involving the afferent or efferent limbs of the reflex arc. Absence of the reflex in elderly patients should be confirmed with electromyography because eliciting the reflex with mechanical stimulation in this group can be difficult.[1]

Endoscopic examination of the distal colon should minimally include a screening for signs of inflammatory bowel disease. Evidence of active inflammatory bowel disease involving the anus and rectum would generally preclude repair of anal sphincter injuries. Both anal manometry and electromyography in the sphincter and levator regions may have a role in the assessment of patients with fecal incontinence. Details of these examinations are noted elsewhere in this book. Despite the scientific usefulness of electromyography and anorectal manometry, the final judgment must be based on the history and physical examination. Much of the decision making can be based on the strength of those two assessments, even in the absence of manometry and myography.

ANAL SPHINCTER REPAIR

Not all individuals who sustain a focal injury to the anal sphincter require operative repair. Patients experiencing minor seepage or occasional urgency incontinence with liquid bowel movements may benefit from a trial with diet modification and antimotility agents. Biofeedback programs and physical therapy regimens to enhance the performance of the residual sphincter mechanism may also prove helpful. Patients experiencing excessive seepage or frank fecal incontinence are unlikely to benefit from these nonoperative measures. Direct repair of the anal sphincter injury is most likely to be successful when neuromuscular function is preserved and at least one half of the circumference of the external sphincter remains intact. These criteria for successful repair can be confirmed preoperatively with electromyography.

The appropriate time for repair of anal sphincter injuries is determined by the nature and extent of the original injury. Initial management of traumatic perineal injuries that involve the anal sphincter should be limited to wound debridement to remove foreign material, fecal debris, and devitalized tissue. Further wound contamination is minimized by proceeding with proximal fecal diversion and irrigation of the distal colonic segment. It is unlikely that the severed muscle of the anal sphincter can be approximated without tension. To avoid further tissue destruction from uncontrolled wound sepsis, uncontaminated tissue planes should be left intact. Dissection and mobilization of severed ends of sphincter muscle to attempt approximation and primary repair should scrupulously be avoided. However, an attempt at repair of third-degree perineal lacerations resulting from obstetric trauma should be undertaken at the time of injury. Layered closure of the wound with approximation of the transected sphincter muscle generally produces a good functional result. The successful outcome following immediate repair of obstetric injury to the anal sphincter stands in contrast to the outcome following immediate repair of anal sphincter injury from other causes. This difference may be attributable to the coexistent laxity of the pelvic floor and perineal muscles in women with obstetric trauma, which permits apposition of the divided sphincter muscle without tension.[2] In all other circumstances, including cases of wound dehiscence following immediate repair of obstetric lacerations, definitive repair of injuries to the anal sphincter should be postponed for 3 to 6 months. This interval permits resolution of inflammation and edema. Delay also promotes contracture and closure of soft tissue defects. Postponing repair for 3 to 6 months permits mature scar tissue to develop at the severed ends of sphincter muscle, which facilitates secure suture placement at the time of repair. Repair of iatrogenic anal sphincter injury arising as a complication of fistula operation may be undertaken in 3 to 6 months if the suppurative process is controlled.

Preoperative preparations should include mechanical cleansing of the colon followed by the administration of oral antibiotics, as would be given before elective colonic resection. Broad-spectrum parenteral antibiotics should also be administered perioperatively as prophylaxis against wound infection. To avoid the consequences of postoperative urinary retention, a Foley catheter is inserted at operation. Operative identification of the residual sphincter muscle in patients who have undergone previous unsuccessful attempts at repair or in whom injury is associated with extensive soft tissue loss may be facilitated by the use of a nerve stimulator. In this circumstance, it is preferable to perform operation with the patient under general anesthesia and to avoid the use of muscle relaxants. Otherwise, general or regional anesthesia may be used. The location of the sphincter injury determines the position of the patient on the operating table. The lithotomy position is used for repair of defects confined to the anterior midline of the anal circumference. The prone jackknife

position is preferred for repair of all other injuries.

For repair of injuries involving the posterior or lateral quadrants of the anal sphincter, the overlying scar is excised and the skin incision extended in a curvilinear direction along the anal margin. The extent of the incision varies according to the size of the original wound and the degree to which the ends of divided muscle have retracted. The incision frequently involves more than half the circumference of the anus (Fig. 14D1-2*A*). Subcutaneous scar tissue is excised, and the ends of the divided external sphincter are identified. Care is taken to preserve a rim of fibrous scar tissue at the edge of the divided muscle (Fig. 14D1-2*B*). The sphincter muscle is dissected from the adjacent anoderm and ischiorectal fat for a distance of 1 to 2 cm to achieve the necessary mobility to permit repair without tension. Injury to the supporting neurovascular bundles that enter the body of the muscle in the posterolateral quadrants should be avoided. The plane of dissection should extend to the depth of the anorectal ring to restore adequate length to the anal canal. When defects in the posterior or lateral quadrants of the anal sphincter are being repaired, additional mobility in the remnants of sphincter muscle can be obtained by dividing the anococcygeal ligament.[3]

Reconstruction begins with repair of defects in the anal mucosa resulting from excision of scar or residual fistula. If adequate mobility of the free edges of the sphincter muscle can be obtained, the ends of muscle are overlapped for 1 to 2 cm and secured with one or two rows of synthetic absorbable mattress sutures (Fig. 14D1-2*C*). The sutures should encompass the rim of scar tissue preserved at the free edge of divided muscle to provide a more secure repair. An overlapping repair is preferable to simple apposition of the muscle ends. Sutured apposition of the ends of the divided sphincter muscle has been associated with a higher rate of treatment failure.[4] By increasing the surface area in contact between the muscle ends, the overlapping repair provides a more secure union to overcome the tendency for retraction of the muscle ends on active contraction. The distinct substantial muscle bundles envisioned with this technique and depicted in medical illustrations represent the ideal but, frequently, not the actual circumstance. The quality of the repair is influenced by previous attempts at repair, the extent of tissue destruction, and the quality of the residual muscle. Occasionally, repair is limited to simple plication of attenuated muscle and scar. In this setting any attendant functional improvement probably results from narrowing and elongation of the anal canal rather than from improved function of the reconstructed anal sphincter.

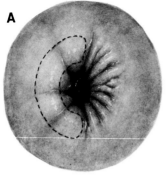

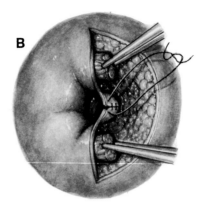

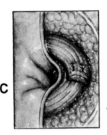

Fig. 14D1-2 Repair of posterior or lateral sphincter injuries. **A,** Retraction of divided sphincter muscle. **B,** Identification and mobilization of divided sphincter muscle following excision of skin and subcutaneous scar. **C,** Completed overlapping repair. (Reprinted from *Surg Clin North Am* 1980;60:459, with permission.)

Soft tissue coverage of the repaired sphincter muscle protects the repair and promotes more rapid healing. This is usually accomplished by primary closure of the incision. When this is not possible, an advancement flap or rotation flap consisting of skin and subcutaneous tissue from the adjacent buttock can be used to cover the repair and to restore the circumference of the anal margin.

Although the same principles apply to the repair of midline anal sphincter injuries resulting from obstetric trauma, successful repair must include reconstruction of the perineal body to correct the ectopic displacement of the anus that frequently accompanies these injuries. Repair begins with a cruciate skin incision centered over the remnant of the rectovaginal septum (Fig. 14D1-3). V-shaped flaps of skin and subcutaneous tissue are developed laterally. Dissection in the rectovaginal septum can be facilitated by the infiltration of a mixture of saline with epinephrine (1:200,000) to separate the tissue planes and aid in hemostasis. Dissection proceeds in this plane to the level of the puborectalis muscle, which is plicated in the anterior midline with several interrupted sutures (Fig. 14D1-4). The ends of the divided external sphincter are identified and dissected from adjacent scar tissue. Again, care is taken to preserve a rim of scar tissue at the edge of the divided muscle bundles. The muscle ends are overlapped or approximated and secured with a series of interrupted synthetic absorbable sutures. The remnants of the su-

perficial transverse perineal muscle are also approximated. The vaginal and rectal mucosa are trimmed to excise any associated fistula. The skin flaps are advanced medially and secured with subcuticular synthetic absorbable sutures to restore the skin bridge between the anus and vagina (Fig. 14D1-5). If necessary, a closed suction drain is placed in the subcutaneous space to obliterate a residual cavity.

Fig. 14D1-3 Cruciate skin incision overlying attenuated perineal body. (Reprinted from *Surg Clin North Am* 1985;65:41, with permission.)

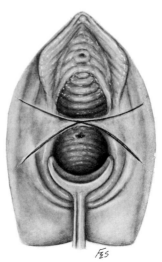

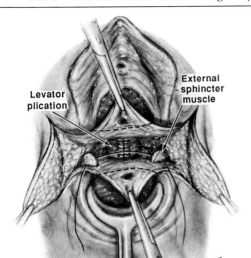

Fig. 14D1-4   Anterior plication of puborectalis muscle and identification of remnants of external sphincter. (Reprinted from *Surg Clin North Am* 1985;65:41, with permission.)

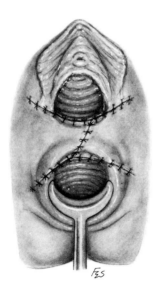

Fig. 14D1-5   Advancement flap anoplasty to reconstruct perineal body. (Reprinted from *Surg Clin North Am* 1985;65:41, with permission.)

Concomitant fecal diversion at the time of sphincter repair has been recommended in some reports, particularly for the treatment of patients who have large sphincter defects or who have undergone previous unsuccessful repair.[3,5] Other surgeons have successfully repaired all types of anal sphincter injury without reliance on a complementary diverting colostomy.[6,7] Excluding cases of traumatic injury where a colostomy is required for initial management of the perineal wound, current experience indicates that a diverting colostomy is unnecessary for the successful repair of most anal sphincter injuries. However, postoperative care requires close attention to bowel management to avoid the potential for wound contamination and disruption of sphincter repair that can result after spontaneous defecation in the immediate postoperative period. Preoperative mechanical cleansing of the colon and postoperative restriction to a clear liquid diet for 3 to 5 days usually ensure that spontaneous defecation does not occur in the immediate postoperative period. The duration of bowel confinement may be extended by adding codeine, diphenoxylate hydrochloride (Lomotil), or deodorized tincture of opium to the postoperative regimen. However, use of these medications by a patient whose diet is unrestricted may precipitate fecal impaction, a potentially disastrous complication. When normal bowel function returns, the patient may resume a regular diet supplemented with a psyllium-seed bulk laxative to optimize stool consistency and avoid constipation. The Foley catheter may be removed when perineal spasm and discomfort subside, which usually occurs by the third postoperative day.

RESULTS

The reported complication rate after repair of anal sphincter injuries ranges from 13% to 27% (Table 14D1-1).[3,5-7] Wound infection is common to all of the series listed. Despite the findings of Pezim and colleagues,[7] who reported no correlation between postoperative wound sepsis and poor functional outcome, most investigators have identified an increased risk for dehiscence of sphincter repair in the presence of infection.[3,5,6,8] Wound infection may also result in fistula in ano. Management of the fistula may jeopardize whatever portion of the repair remains intact. Symptomatic anal stenosis has been reported as a complication of sphincter repair by investigators who rely more frequently on a concomitant colostomy.[3,5] The problem of delayed wound healing is not confined to patients whose wounds are allowed to heal by secondary intention. Corman[2] reported a mean duration of 7 weeks to achieve wound healing in 28 patients who underwent rectovaginal reconstruction and advancement flap anoplasty for repair of obstetric injuries to the anal sphincter. Delay in wound healing resulted from separation of the skin flaps used to reconstruct the perineal body.

Table 14D1-1

Postoperative Morbidity After Anal Sphincter Repair.

Study	No. of Patients	No. With Colostomy	Operative Morbidity	Complications					
				Wound Sepsis	Hematoma	Dehiscence	Fistula	Stricture	Delayed Healing
Stricker et al.[8]	47	7	—	4	2	1	—	—	—
Fang et al.[6]	79	5	16%	2	3	—	—	—	—
Browning and Motson[3]	97	93	27%	2	—	4	7	16	25
Yoshioka and Keighley[5]	27	10	22%	5	—	—	—	1	—
Pezim et al.[7]	40	—	13%	5	—	—	—	—	—

Table 14D1-2

Functional Results After Anal Sphincter Repair.

Study	No. of Patients	Percent Continent for Liquid and Solid Stool	Percent with Improved Functional Status
Browning and Motson[3]	97	78	91
Stricker et al.[8]	20	—	80
Fang et al.[6]	79	58	95
Yoshioka and Keighley[5]	27	33	81
Miller et al.[9]	14	71	
Laurberg et al.[10]	18	50	83
Pezim et al.[7]	33	—	76

Analysis of functional results achieved with direct repair of anal sphincter injuries reveals substantial variation in the reported ability to render patients continent for liquid and solid stool (Table 14D1-2). This discrepancy may reflect differences in criteria used to assess outcome as well as variations in patient population. Correlation of the mechanism of sphincter injury with the functional outcome after repair reveals a diminished likelihood for rendering patients continent for liquid and solid stool after operative injury to the anal sphincter. In some series, these patients constitute the majority of those treated for anal sphincter injury.[3,5] Laurberg and colleagues[10] and Roberts and coworkers[11] demonstrated that a proportion of patients with fecal incontinence after obstetric injury have an associated neurogenic injury to the external sphincter and muscles of the pelvic floor. As a result of this progressive neuropathic damage to the pelvic floor, repair of the anal sphincter defect may be associated with a less successful outcome.[10] Associated pudendal nerve injury is the most likely cause for treatment failure in patients undergoing repair of obstetric injuries to the anal sphincter.[3,5] The inconsistent presence of this neuropathy in patients with obstetric injury to the anal sphincter, as well as the variable time course required for its clinical expression, may contribute to the variation in reported continence for liquid and solid fecal material after sphincter repair. As a group, however, 80% to 90% of patients undergoing repair of anal sphincter injuries report improvement in their functional status.

SILASTIC ANAL SLING

For the patient whose sphincter injury is not amenable to repair or whose repair has failed, alternate treatment options are limited. Anal encirclement procedures using fascia lata femoris, gracilis muscle, or Silastic sheeting have been used to alleviate incontinence by increasing the passive resistance of the anal canal to spontaneous defecation. Labow and others[12] originally described the use of a band of Dacron-impregnated Silastic as a modification of the Thiersch procedure for treating rectal prolapse. Larach and Vasquez[13] subsequently reported a successful outcome in two of four patients in whom the Silastic sling was implanted for treatment of incontinence.

The procedure is performed with the patient under general or regional anesthesia after mechanical cleansing of the colon. Antibiotics are administered orally the day before operation to provide prophylaxis against wound infection. Parenteral antibiotics may be used in the perioperative period for the same purpose. With the patient in the prone jackknife position, curvilinear incisions overlying the ischiorectal fossa are made (Fig. 14D1-6A). The incisions are placed lateral to whatever sphincter muscle remains and extend to a sufficient depth to accommodate a 1.5- to 2.0-cm band of Silastic sheet. Subcutaneous tunnels are created anteriorly and posteriorly to connect these incisions (Fig. 14D1-6B). The anococcygeal ligament is divided when the posterior tunnel is developed. In women, great care must be taken in making the anterior tunnel because the plane between the rectum and vagina may be thin (Fig. 14D1-6C). A 1.5- to 2.0-cm band of Dacron-impregnated Silastic is tunneled circumferentially to encompass the remaining sphincter muscle and perianal soft tissue (Fig. 14D1-6D). The ends of the band are overlapped and secured with nonabsorbable monofilament sutures or a linear stapling device (Fig. 14D1-6E). The Silastic band should be sufficiently lax to permit insertion of the distal interphalangeal joint of the index finger into the

Fig. 14D1-6   Silastic anal sling procedure. **A**, Bilateral skin incisions are placed lateral to residual sphincter muscle. **B**, Kelly clamps are used to develop perianal tunnels. **C**, Subcutaneous tunnels are completed. **D**, Silastic sheet is tunneled around the anus. **E**, Silastic sling is tightened and secured with a linear stapler. (Reprinted from *Surg Clin North Am* 1985;65:44–45, with permission.)

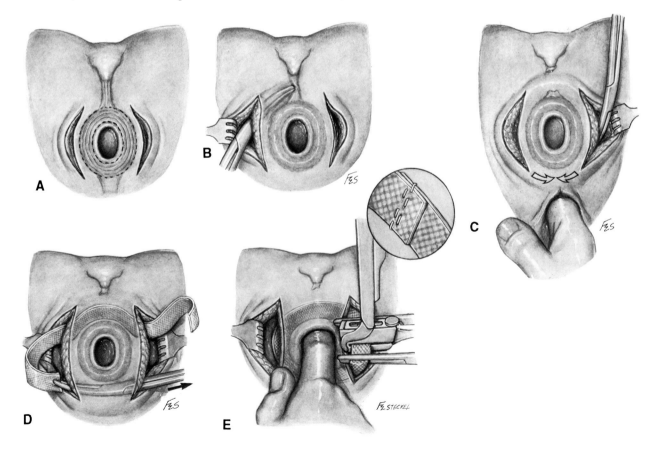

anus. The Dacron-impregnated Silastic material has enough elasticity along its longitudinal axis to permit passage of a fecal bolus through the anus. The incisions are irrigated and closed in layers with absorbable suture material. Postoperative care requires close attention to bowel management to ensure success with this procedure. Patients are advised to follow a high-residue diet supplemented with a psyllium-seed bulk laxative. Judicious use of antimotility agents or cathartics may be necessary to improve the functional result and minimize the potential for fecal impaction. Infection is the most serious complication after placement of a Silastic perianal sling. Successful management of wound sepsis usually requires removal of the sling. Infection occurring in the immediate postoperative period usually results from wound contamination during operation. Wound infection presenting as a late complication usually results from erosion of the sling through the perianal skin or into the rectum or vagina. To diminish the likelihood for skin erosion, the sling should be placed deep enough to ensure a margin of 1 to 2 cm between the outer edge of the sling and the perianal skin.

Stricker and colleagues[8] reviewed the results in 14 patients after placement of a Dacron-Silastic sling to treat incontinence. Follow-up at 1 year revealed improved control in seven patients. The symptoms of incontinence were unchanged in two patients. Five patients required removal of the sling because of a poor result (one patient) or perineal erosion or infection (four patients). With prolonged follow-up ranging from 2 to 10 years, improved control persisted in six patients. As the final alternative before a permanent colostomy for treating incontinence, the functional outcome afforded with a Silastic perianal sling is reasonable.

SUMMARY

Operative repair of acquired anal sphincter injuries provides the best opportunity for successful treatment of fecal incontinence. Unfortunately, candidates for sphincter repair comprise only a portion of the population afflicted with incontinence. Successful repair of anal sphincter injuries must begin with careful preoperative patient evaluation to select those individuals who are most likely to benefit from surgery. Comprehensive historical review and physical examination augmented by anal manometry and electromyography will identify patients with focal sphincter injuries and preserved neuromuscular function.

The timing for sphincter repair depends on the nature of the injury and the presence of associated infection or soft tissue loss. Preoperative mechanical cleansing of the colon and judicious use of perioperative antibiotics will minimize the potential for postoperative wound infection. The technique for repair is determined by the type and location of the sphincter injury. Crucial principles of repair include the careful dissection of the sphincter muscle to protect its neurovascular supply, preservation of a rim of fibrous scar tissue at the edge of the severed muscle, and sufficient mobilization of the transected sphincter muscle to permit approximation without tension. The treatment of obstetric injuries to the anal sphincter must also incorporate anterior plication of the puborectalis muscle and reconstruction of the perineal body. Adherence to these guidelines for patient selection and operative technique should result in a substantial improvement in the functional status of the majority of patients treated.

REFERENCES

1. Pedersen E. The anal reflex. In: Henry MM, Swash M, eds. *Coloproctology and the Pelvic Floor. Pathophysiology and Management.* London: Butterworths; 1985:104–111.
2. Corman ML. Anal incontinence following obstetrical injury. *Dis Colon Rectum.* 1985;28:86.
3. Browning GGP, Motson RW. Anal sphincter injury: management and results of Parks sphincter repair. *Ann Surg.* 1984;199:351.
4. Blaisdell PC. Repair of the incontinent sphincter ani. *Surg Gynecol Obstet.* 1940;70:692.
5. Yoshioka K, Keighley MS. Sphincter repair for fecal incontinence. *Dis Colon Rectum.* 1989;32:39.
6. Fang DT, Nivatvongs S, Vermeulen FD, Herman FN, Goldberg SM, Rothenberger DA. Overlapping sphincteroplasty for acquired anal incontinence. *Dis Colon Rectum.* 1984;27:720.
7. Pezim ME, Spencer RJ, Stanhope CR, Beart RW Jr, Ready RL, Ilstrup DM. Sphincter repair for fecal incontinence after obstetrical or iatrogenic injury. *Dis Colon Rectum.* 1987;30:521.
8. Stricker JW, Schoetz DJ Jr, Coller JA, Veidenheimer MC. Surgical correction of anal incontinence. *Dis Colon Rectum.* 1988;31:533.
9. Miller R, Orrom WJ, Cornes H, Duthie G, Bartolo DCC. Anterior sphincter plication and levatorplasty in the treatment of faecal incontinence. *Br J Surg.* 1989;76:1058.
10. Laurberg S, Swash M, Henry MM. Delayed external sphincter repair for obstetric tear. *Br J Surg.* 1988;75:786.
11. Roberts PL, Coller JA, Schoetz DJ Jr, Veidenheimer MC. Manometric assessment of patients with obstetric injuries and fecal incontinence. *Dis Colon Rectum.* 1990;33:16.
12. Labow S, Rubin RJ, Hoexter B, Salvati EP. Perineal repair of rectal procidentia with an elastic fabric sling. *Dis Colon Rectum.* 1980;23:467.
13. Larach SW, Vasquez B. Modified Thiersch procedure with Silastic mesh implant: a simple solution for fecal incontinence and severe prolapse. *South Med J.* 1986;79:307.

CHAPTER 14

Fecal Incontinence

14D   Surgical Therapies

14D2   Postanal Repair

M. M. Henry

INTRODUCTION

The operation of postanal repair was devised by Parks[1] as a means of restoring anal continence principally in patients with neuropathy of the pelvic floor and external anal sphincter musculature (see Chapter 14B). The technique was devised as a response to physiologic and anatomic studies which had identified the important role that an acute anorectal angle played in anal continence in the normal state.[1] In this procedure, access to the pelvic floor musculature is gained posteriorly via the avascular space that exists between the smooth muscle of the internal sphincter and rectum and the striated muscle of the external sphincter and pelvic floor (the intersphincteric space). Once the pelvic floor muscles and external sphincter have been displayed, these are then plicated posterior to the midline using a nonabsorbable suture material. It was originally believed that the procedure was effective because of (a) restoration of the anorectal angle, (b) lengthening of the anal canal, (c) support of the pelvic floor, and (d) improved mechanical advantage caused by shortening the muscle fibers. There is little evidence to support these hypotheses, but there seems to be no doubt that the anal canal is lengthened[2] and that the squeeze pressures are improved by the procedure.[3] Lengthening of the anal canal presumably increases the resistance to the spontaneous evacuation of rectal contents via the anus.

. Indications

As stated above, the principal indication for this procedure is neuropathy of the pelvic floor musculature, usually as a consequence of previous obstetric trauma. Under usual circumstances the decision to proceed to surgery is based on clinical grounds rather than on laboratory results. Hence, a patient who is severely handicapped by a functional disability should be offered postanal repair even if preoperative testing reveals a severe deficit.

Preoperative Preparation

If the rectum is inadvertently opened allowing fecal contamination, severe pelvic sepsis may be the result. For this reason a full mechanical bowel preparation with perioperative antibiotic chemoprophylaxis is recommended.

The Operation

The patient is placed in the lithotomy position and the subcutaneous tissues posterior to the anus are infiltrated with a weak adrenaline solution (1:300,000). A V-shaped incision is made approximately 1 cm posterior to the anus with its apex at the tip of the coccyx (Fig. 14D2-1). A flap of skin contained within the inci-

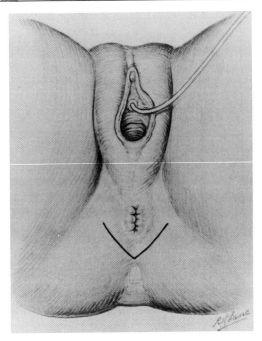

Fig. 14D2-1 Patient who was previously catheterized is placed in the lithotomy position and a V-shaped incision created posterior to the anus with the apex directed toward the coccyx.

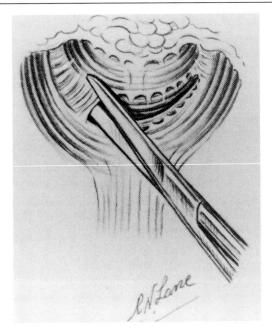

Fig. 14D2-3 The commencement of the dissection of the intersphincteric space using scissors.

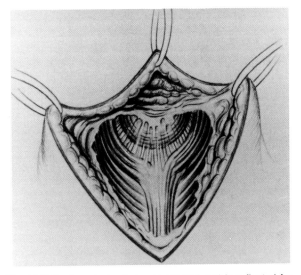

Fig. 14D2-2 An anterior flap was created and is reflected forward to expose the lower borders of the internal and external anal sphincters.

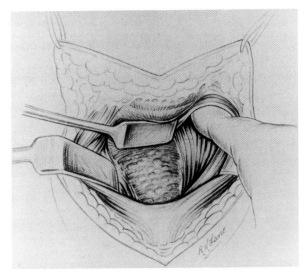

Fig. 14D2-4 The dissection continues using blunt dissection. The internal anal sphincter (anterior) is dissected free from the external anal sphincter (posterior).

sion is lifted forward to expose the inferior borders of the internal and external sphincters (Fig. 14D2-2). The intersphincteric space is identified between the two muscles (Fig. 14D2-3). This step can be difficult and may be facilitated by looking for the longitudinal smooth muscle fibers (the terminal fibers of the taeniae

coli) which course within the intersphincteric space and are eventually inserted into the perianal skin. The plane is then dissected by a combination of sharp and blunt dissection (Fig. 14D2-4). In order to expose the upper surface of the levator ani muscles, Waldeyers fascia needs to be divided by sharp dissection (Fig. 14D2-5).

Once the levator muscle is exposed, suturing can be done. At the highest level, a lattice is constructed across

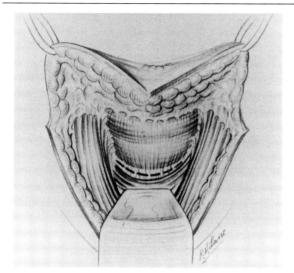

Fig. 14D2-5 At the level of the anorectal junction a dense layer of fascia is encountered within the intersphincteric space (Waldeyers fascia). This must be divided by sharp dissection in order to gain access to the pelvis.

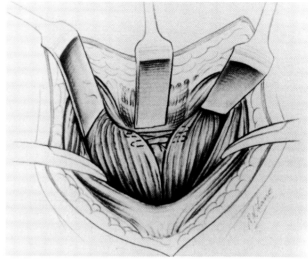

Fig. 14D2-7 The more caudal muscles comprising the levator complex are more mobile and can be plicated and brought into the midline position. These latter two steps are responsible for restoring the posterior levator muscle bulk and hence decreasing the obliquity of the anorectal angle.

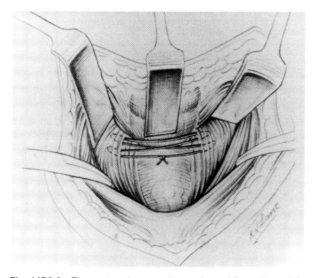

Fig. 14D2-6 The rectum has now been cleared from the pelvic floor and a lattice of sutures (0 prolene) have been inserted into the highest component of the levator muscle complex (ileococcygeus).

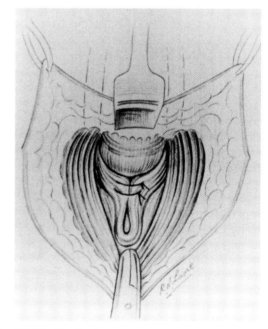

Fig. 14D2-8 Finally the external sphincter muscle fibers are plicated using 2/0 prolene.

the ileococcygeus muscle with O prolene (Fig. 14D2-6). Below this level the puborectalis muscle is approximated, ensuring that the sutures are not subject to undue tension (Fig. 14D2-7). Ideally a small gap in the midline is left to allow for any edema which may develop postoperatively. Finally the fibers of the external sphincter are plicated (Fig. 14D2-8) and the skin partially sutured to avoid secondary sepsis.

Postoperative Care

Excessive straining should be avoided to prevent disruption of the repair. For this reason a regimen of laxatives sufficient to cause stool softening is advisable in the postoperative period. This can later be supplemented by the daily use of an irritant suppository in an attempt to induce effortless rectal emptying and reduce soiling. This can only be employed when the wound is almost healed.

Results

In Parks' original series,[1] 83% of patients reported excellent function postoperatively. In an analysis of the overall St. Mark's experience of the operation, 56% of 129 patients were either fully continent or only incontinent of flatus; a further 14% were incontinent of liquid stool only.[4] Keighley's[5] early results showed that 63% were continent of solid and liquid stool. The later results were less favorable.[6] Of 114 patients, only 32% claimed to have complete continence, and although 62% had an improvement, they did suffer from episodes of incontinence, particularly in the presence of diarrhea.

Morbidity

Problems with the wound occurred in 19% of the total St. Mark's experience of 242 patients.[4] These included ischemia of the skin flap, wound infection, wound breakdown, fistula, and hematoma formation. On the other hand, Miller and coworkers[7] reported a negligible morbidity in 17 patients, although details were not provided. There is only one report of a death: an obese, diabetic patient died from a pulmonary embolus on the seventh postoperative day.[8]

SUMMARY

This technique is an attractive one because it is not technically complex if the operator has become adept at identifying and dissecting out the intersphincteric space. The results compare well with other surgical procedures developed for treating this condition. Where postanal repair fails to restore reasonable anal continence, the creation of a colostomy should be considered. Most patients prefer an abdominal wall stoma to stoma in the perineum.

REFERENCES

1. Parks AG. Anorectal incontinence. *Proc R Soc Med Lond.* 1975; 68:681–690.
2. Womack NR, Morrisson JFB, Williams NS. Prospective study of the effects of postanal repair in neurogenic fecal incontinence. *Br J Surg.* 1988;75:48–52.
3. Browning GGP, Parks AG. Postanal repair for neuropathic fecal incontinence: correlation of clinical result and anal canal pressures. *Br J Surg.* 1988;70:101–104.
4. Henry MM, Simson JNL. The results of postanal repair: a retrospective study. *Br J Surg.* 1985;72 (suppl):17–19.
5. Keighley MRB. Postanal repair for fecal incontinence. *J R Soc Med Lond.* 1984;77:285–288.
6. Keighley MRB. Postanal repair. *Int J Colorect Dis.* 1987;2:236–239.
7. Miller R, Bartolo DCC, Locke-Edmunds JC, Mortensen NJMcC. Prospective study of conservative and operative treatment for fecal incontinence. *Br J Surg.* 1988;75:101–105.
8. Yoshioka K, Keighley MRB. Critical assessment of the quality of continence after postanal repair for fecal incontinence. *Br J Surg.* 1989;76:1054–1057.

CHAPTER 15

Rectal Prolapse: Pathogenesis and Management

Kenneth E. Levin and John H. Pemberton

INTRODUCTION

Rectal prolapse is an uncommon, often disabling condition that has long fascinated surgeons. Although first described in 1500 BC in the Ebers Papyrus,[1] many aspects of its etiology and treatment remain controversial to this day. Few clinical disorders have generated such a large number of surgical procedures with varying degrees of success as has rectal prolapse. Only in the last few decades has our understanding of the pathophysiology, coupled with better surgical techniques, led to improved long-term rates of success. The aims of this chapter are to define the confusing terminology of rectal prolapse, describe its etiology, and outline appropriate steps in the evaluation of patients with rectal prolapse. Surgical procedures will be illustrated with their results and complications along with an outline of our preferred surgical management approaches.

Terminology

Confusing terminology is a major problem in the study of rectal prolapse. The terms that must be distinguished are *mucosal prolapse, internal intussusception* (occult rectal prolapse) and *complete rectal prolapse* (procidentia). *Mucosal prolapse* is caused by a looseness or breaking down of the connective tissue between the submucosa of the rectum and anal canal and the underlying muscle.[2] This usually starts in the anal canal

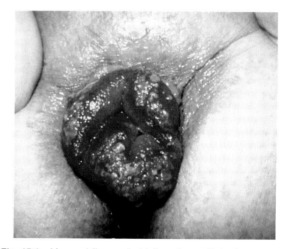

Fig. 15-1 Mucosal (hemorrhoidal) prolapse. Note the presence of linear mucosal folds and erosions. Compare this figure of mucosal prolapse with that of a complete rectal prolapse (Figure 15-3).

and, in its earliest form, is represented by prolapsing hemorrhoids. With progression, more anal canal mucosa (hemorrhoids) and distal rectal mucosa protrudes, leading to the characteristic picture of linear mucosal furrows and absence of the perianal sulcus (Fig. 15-1). Mucosal prolapse does not progress to complete rectal prolapse and is considered part of the spectrum of hemorrhoidal disease.

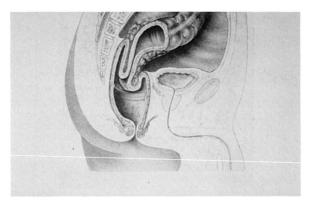

Fig. 15-2 Diagram of internal intussusception (occult rectal prolapse). The rectum folds into itself and is progressively forced caudad until it reaches the top of the anal canal. By definition, an occult prolapse does not protrude through the anus.

Internal intussusception of the rectum (occult rectal prolapse) (Fig. 15-2) is a distinct clinical entity that may represent the precursor of complete rectal prolapse.[2,3] It is probably an early stage in the progression of the disorder, occurring internally before the prolapsed rectum becomes evident externally through the anal orifice. It can only be diagnosed reliably by obtaining a defecating proctogram. *Complete rectal prolapse,* then, is defined as protrusion of the full thickness of the rectal wall through the anal orifice (Fig. 15-3).

ETIOLOGY

The precise cause of rectal prolapse is not completely understood. Many theories have been proposed to explain its etiology, but only two gained widespread popularity. Moschcowitz[4] proposed in 1912 that rectal prolapse was a form of sliding hernia with an abnormally deep pouch of Douglas, forming a hernial sac. As a result of increased intraabdominal pressure, the anterior wall of the rectum would be pressed into the rectal lumen by the hernial sac. Ultimately, the intraabdominal contents overcome the resistance offered by the rectum itself and by the posterior supporting structures of the pelvis, and herniate through the levator musculature, resulting in rectal prolapse. Supporting this theory are specific anatomic features (Box 15-1, Fig. 15-4) usually found in patients with prolapse.[4,6]

The theory of Moschcowitz was refuted by Devadhar in 1965,[5] which was, in turn, substantiated by Broden and Snellman in 1968.[6] These authors theorized that rectal prolapse represented a rectorectal intussusception of the middle rectum and that the common anatomic features were secondary rather than predisposing in nature. Cineradiographic techniques demonstrated that when a patient with rectal prolapse strained at stool, the first thing that happened was intussusception of the rectum. The intussusception originated circumferentially in the rectal wall at the level of the peritoneal reflection in the pelvis (about 6 to 8 cm above the anal

Fig. 15-3 A, Complete rectal prolapse. Note the "concentric ring" appearance of the folds of the rectal wall. **B,** By placing the examining thumb in the centrally located orifice of the prolapse and the index finger near the junction of the skin and mucosa, the thickness of the prolapse is appreciated, as is the sulcus between the prolapse and the perineal skin.

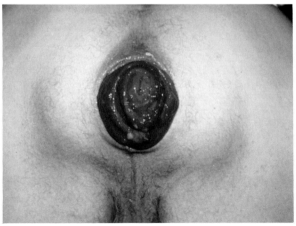

A

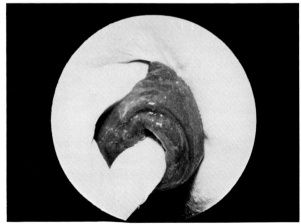

B

Box 15-1
Anatomic Features Associated with Rectal
Prolapse

Abnormally deep rectosigmoid or rectovesical
    pouch
Lax and atonic pelvic floor musculature
Redundant rectosigmoid colon
Lax and atonic anal sphincter
Lack of normal sacral fixation of the rectum

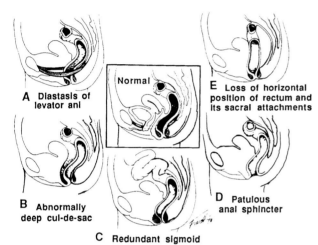

Fig. 15-4 The anatomic features that are associated with complete rectal prolapse but do not cause it. (Reprinted from Henry MM, Swash M, *Coloproctology and the Pelvic Floor: Pathophysiology and Management*, London: Butterworths; 1985, with permission.)

the rectum loosens on its mesentery. As this occurs, the fixed point becomes lower and lower, and the intussusception on subsequent straining is seen to begin just above the new fixed point. When it reaches a point of stronger fascial attachment in the region of the lateral stalks, it hesitates for variable lengths of time. Eventually, repeated pressure from above caused by straining overcomes this barrier and the bowel further protrudes, so that the first observed point of protrusion becomes the mucocutaneous junction. As the bowel rolls from inside out, there is no specific lead point which comes down from above; in other words, the intussusception does not stay at the rectosigmoid junction, but as time progresses it is seen to start in a lower position depending on where the rectum is fixed at that time.

As a consequence of this sequence of events, with rectorectal intussusception, a pseudomesorectum is sometimes formed; the sigmoid mesentery is lengthened, the cul-de-sac is deepened, the supporting elements of the rectum and rectosigmoid are stretched and lengthened and eventually atrophy, and the levators and sphincter musculature are altered from slight weakness and loss of tone to actual atrophy and true patulousness.[7]

Characteristically, the anus of a patient with com-

Fig. 15-5 Etiology of complete rectal prolapse. This is a diagrammatic representation of a radiologic study performed by Theuerkauf et al.[7] **A**, Metal beads were sewn about the orifice of the complete rectal prolapses *(4)* and at defined intervals cephalad *(3,2,1)*. **B**, The prolapse was then reduced. Note now the position of the metal beads. The circle of beads *(4)* is the most cephalad. **C**, As the rectum prolapses again, bead *1* exits first followed by *2*. **D**, Bead at position *3* prolapses next. **E**, The rectum has again prolapsed completely. This experiment confirmed that the pathogenesis of complete rectal prolapse was intussusception. (Reprinted from Theuerkauf[7] with permission.)

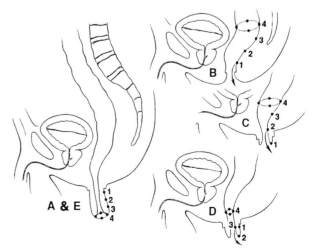

verge). Internal intussusception (occult prolapse) was demonstrated cineradiographically to represent the precursor to complete rectal prolapse. Enterocele, which corresponds to the sliding hernia of Moschcowitz,[4] was a late manifestation of chronic intussusception associated with defecation straining.

Theuerkauf and coworkers[7] noted cineradiographically that the prolapse does not begin originally at 6 to 8 cm inside the rectum, as proposed by Broden and Snellman.[6] Rather, their studies showed that the intussusception begins at the rectosigmoid junction by chance or accidental happening, and not because of any congenital or acquired defect[7] (Fig. 15-5). The intussusception then pulls the rectosigmoid area away from its congenital attachments, and with repeated straining, plete rectal prolapse is patulous and gaping, and fecal incontinence frequently accompanies this condition. It is probable that a gaping anus and compromised sphincter are an effect of the intruded prolapse rather than a cause of the disorder.[2] However, damage to the sphincter from obstetrical trauma or extensive fistulotomy has been implicated as a contributing factor in some patients.[8] The pathogenesis of complete rectal prolapse then is intussusception. The reason for rectal intussusception in the first place is unknown.

Porter[9] performed EMGs in patients with rectal prolapse and found complete and protracted inhibition of the puborectal muscle with straining; this might predispose such patients to formation of a prolapse. Parks, Swash, and Urich[10] proposed that because some patients with rectal prolapse also had descending perineums and fecal incontinence, denervation of the puborectal and external anal sphincter muscles was likely. With prolonged straining at defecation over decades, the pudendal nerves would be progressively stretched until injury occurred. The puborectal muscle and external anal sphincter would therefore be lax and allow a prolapse to progressively form. However, the pelvic floor abnormalities cannot be responsible directly for the rectal intussusception itself, which occurs 6 to 8 cm above the puborectal muscle.

What may occur is that patients have difficulty expelling fecal contents, thus prompting them to strain at stool for prolonged periods of time. This straining sometimes occurs because the puborectal muscle fails to relax appropriately.[11] Solitary rectal ulcers may occur at this stage in the development of prolapse. In response to prolonged increases in intraabdominal pressure, the lax rectum begins to intussuscept into itself. With continued straining over decades, the pelvic floor muscles and external anal sphincter may become partially denervated because the pudendal nerve is stretched; episodes of incontinence may occur. As the rectum descends further, a feeling of continual fullness occurs and patients strain even harder at stool because they think they have not emptied the rectum of stool (the phenomenon of incomplete evacuation). Eventually the intussusception is exteriorized. One problem with this hypothesis is that some patients with complete rectal prolapse have no abnormalities of puborectal or external anal sphincter innervation and no incontinence.

CLINICAL FEATURES

The true incidence of rectal prolapse in the general population is unknown. In adults, the condition occurs much more frequently in women, the incidence varying from three to ten times that in men. In women, the incidence increases with age, peaking in the sixth and seventh decades, but in men the incidence does not increase after the age of 40.[12] In the past, multiparity was proposed as a possible etiologic factor. However, a higher incidence is actually seen in nulliparous women.[13] The rates of nulliparity in rectal prolapse vary from 39% to 58%,[14–16] rates which are much higher than would be expected in the general population.

Several additional factors predispose to the development of rectal prolapse. Poor bowel habits, notably chronic constipation with long-standing laxative abuse, associated with prolonged straining at stool, are frequently a factor. Such straining may be the consequence of an underlying disorder of the pelvic floor which might have led to the prolapse in the first place, or may be caused by the prolapse itself. Ihre and Seligson[17] studied 90 patients with rectal intussusception and found that 61% had obstructed defecation, 33% had pain on defecation, 34% had bleeding, and diarrhea was present in 18%.

Diseases of the nervous system, such as multiple sclerosis, tabes dorsalis, and lesions of the cauda equina may contribute.[18] Patients in psychiatric hospitals and nursing homes are commonly afflicted. Rectal prolapse may also be a consequence of a number of anorectal surgical procedures, but it is important to distinguish between true prolapse and mucosal prolapse. Injury to the puborectalis muscle during anal fistulotomy or pull-through operations may predispose to either mucosal or true prolapse. Uterine prolapse is commonly found coincident with rectal prolapse.[12]

The most frequent primary complaint of patients with rectal prolapse is referable to the prolapse itself: three fourths of patients complain of the protrusion.[19] Problems with bowel regulation and continence are also prominent presenting symptoms. Feelings of incomplete evacuation after bowel movements and fecal incontinence are nearly always present.[18–20] Constipation with straining is associated with prolapse in about half of the patients.[19]

Incontinence becomes increasingly likely the longer the protrusion is present and the larger it becomes. Early, the patient may have internal intussusception and the sensation of incomplete evacuation, fullness, or obstruction in the rectum. Most patients suffer long-standing constipation and spend up to several hours per day forcibly straining to have a bowel movement.[3] The application of manual perineal or intravaginal pressure or digital removal of stool to achieve evacuation is frequently reported.[3,19] Later in the course, protrusion may be present only with straining at stool or when lifting heavy objects. In time, the rectum may prolapse when simply assuming an upright position or walking. Attempts by the patient to reduce the prolapse manually become increasingly futile until finally the rectum protrudes continuously.[18] At this point, a constant mucoid discharge, fecal incontinence, and frequent bleeding from irritation of the exposed mucosa are present.

Evaluation

Usually the diagnosis of complete rectal prolapse is easy to make; protrusion of the rectum occurs while straining. Therefore, examination of the patient with suspected rectal prolapse should begin with the patient sitting on the toilet and straining. Inspection of the protruding rectum reveals concentric rings of mucosa. Both walls of the prolapsed bowel are palpated by the examiner and the lumen of the protrusion is centrally located (Fig. 15-3). The tip of the prolapse is usually displaced posteriorly. The mucosal surface is edematous and hyperemic and superficial ulcerations may be seen. Excoriation and irritation of the perineal skin resulting from fecal soiling and mucous discharge is often present. Reduction of the rectal prolapse reveals a patulous anus and weak anal sphincters. Since complete rectal prolapse is a clinical diagnosis, studies to document this are obviously not necessary. However, it is appropriate to ensure that the rectum and proximal colon do not harbor concomitant abnormalities. Sigmoidoscopy is indicated to exclude a neoplasm acting as a lead point for the intussusception, and biopsies should be performed if suspicious lesions are seen. A barium enema (or colonoscopy) should be performed to assess the possible association of another disease process which may modify the treatment recommended (i.e., neoplasm, inflammatory bowel disease, or diverticular disease). If clinically suspected, radiographs of the lumbar spine and pelvis should be obtained to provide clues of neurological disease (i.e., spina bifida occulta).

Anorectal manometry is performed to quantify the function of the internal anal sphincter and external anal sphincter. Documentation of the pre- and postrepair resting and squeeze pressures should probably be performed. Sphincter pressures vary widely in patients with either complete or occult rectal prolapse. Incontinent patients with complete rectal prolapse have lower resting and squeeze pressures than do controls.[21] However, most patients with complete prolapse who are continent have normal pressures. Interestingly, overall, patients with occult rectal prolapse have pressures that are the same as controls. However, resting pressures differ among patients with occult rectal prolapse *who are incontinent;* resting pressures are lower in incontinent patients. It has been proposed that occult prolapse may reduce resting pressure by reflexively inhibiting the internal sphincter (constant presence of the rectal anal sphincter inhibition response). This hypothesis is supported by Holmstrom and colleagues,[22] who found that rectopexy improves continence and increases resting pressure in patients with occult rectal prolapse. The even lower resting pressures seen in patients with complete rectal prolapse may be caused by primary damage to the pudendal nerve with resulting external anal sphincter denervation.[23]

In patients with a history of severe chronic constipation, colon transit studies are also performed preoperatively to identify those with idiopathic slow transit constipation; such patients may be candidates for an aggressive colon resection concomitant with repair of the prolapse.

The diagnosis of occult rectal prolapse is more difficult on physical exam. Perineal bulging with effacement of the anus with straining is seen classically but not invariably. Digital rectal examination often reveals the intussuscepting mass of rectal wall on straining, but this is unreliable. In patients in whom occult rectal prolapse is suspected, a defecating proctogram (cinedefecography) is the only definitive way of making the diagnosis. If occult prolapse is present, a circumferential fold 6 cm to 8 cm above the anal canal is seen within the rectum[24] (Fig. 15-2). This circular fold forms the apex for the intussusception, which with straining fills the rectal ampulla, thereby blocking the anal canal. Interpretation of defecating proctograms should be made with great care; fully 50% of healthy young people without defecatory complaints have a mild to moderate rectal intussusception on straining.[25]

Differential Diagnosis

A protruding complete rectal prolapse is easy to diagnose. At times, however, it may be difficult to distinguish it from mucosal prolapse or prolapsed third-degree internal hemorrhoids. Although it may appear that the entire rectal wall is protruding, the mucosal folds are arranged in a radial fashion to the level of the anal skin in patients with mucosal prolapse. With prolapsed hemorrhoids, edema and thrombosis may give the impression of complete rectal prolapse; however, radial grooves are usually present between the masses of hemorrhoidal tissue, down to the anal skin (Fig. 15-1). In true rectal prolapse, concentric rings of intact mucosa are evident throughout the circumference of the protruding mass (Fig. 15-3). A complete rectal prolapse protrudes for varying distances but usually for more than 4 cm to 5 cm from the anus. It is rare for mucosal prolapse to protrude more than 1 cm to 2 cm. The protruding mass in mucosal prolapse is very thin, consisting only of a double layer of mucosa.

Rarely, a villous polyp or carcinoma of the rectum may intussuscept and protrude through the anus. Differentiation is usually easy after reduction of the prolapse and visualization of the lesion with sigmoidoscopy.

SYNDROMES RELATED TO RECTAL PROLAPSE

Two clinical syndromes have features suggesting a relationship to rectal prolapse: solitary rectal ulcer (SRU) and colitis cystica profunda (CCP). Most investigators believe that the SRU is a distinct clinical inflammatory manifestation that is associated with rectal prolapse and the preprolapse condition.[19] Defecating proctography frequently reveals occult rectal prolapse in patients with SRU. Another possible mechanism is the failure of inhibition of puborectalis muscle contraction during defecation straining.

The diagnosis of SRU and CCP requires inspection and biopsy of the rectal mucosa. Solitary rectal ulcer is actually a spectrum of disease; patients may have no ulcers, a single or multiple ulcers, or single or multiple polypoid masses.[26] Physical examination classically reveals an ulcer with hyperemic edges and surrounding induration. A combination of ulcerating and polypoid lesions are often noted on the anterior rectal wall, usually at a level 6 cm to 8 cm from the anus.[19] CCP is either localized on the anterior rectal wall or is diffuse. The localized type occurs at the same site as solitary rectal ulcer, and may protrude slightly into the lumen of the bowel as a polypoid mass.[19]

There are a number of characteristic histological features which allow the pathologist to distinguish SRU and CCP from other lesions. SRU is defined histologically as the obliteration of the lamina propria of the rectum by fibroblasts, which are generally arranged at right angles to the muscularis mucosa.[19,26] CCP is a nonneoplastic condition characterized by the presence of submucosal mucous cysts, deep to the muscularis mucosa and usually confined to the sigmoid and rectum.[19,26]

When solitary rectal ulcer or colitis cystica profunda is associated with prolapse, as demonstrated by clinical examination or more definitively by defecography, good results can be expected from repair of the complete rectal prolapse.[26] Such procedures are generally not successful when the prolapse is occult.

COMPLICATIONS OF RECTAL PROLAPSE

Serious complications of complete rectal prolapse are rare, but prompt recognition is essential to prevent morbidity and mortality. Irreducibility (incarceration) of the rectal prolapse may produce progressive edema and subsequent strangulation of the extruded bowel. This situation requires urgent surgical intervention. Strangulation may produce necrosis and perforation of the bowel, with subsequent sepsis and even death. Bleeding caused by extensive ulceration of the exteriorized mucosa is sometimes seen.[18] Rupture of the cul-de-sac with evisceration of small intestine through the anus has also been reported.[27]

TREATMENT FOR COMPLETE RECTAL PROLAPSE

Nonoperative Treatment

Nonoperative treatment is not effective in adults with repeated episodes of complete rectal prolapse. These episodes usually occur more frequently with time and may result in incontinence. Surgical intervention is indicated in patients with complete rectal prolapse.

The appropriate timing of surgery in patients with a single or at least infrequent episodes of complete prolapse is not as obvious. In these patients, a trial of high residue diet and reeducation of bowel habits to prevent straining may control the problem.[24,28] However, the longer the prolapse exists the more likely the development of incontinence. At present, there is no known method for predicting the onset of incontinence in patients with complete prolapse. If conservative therapy is recommended, anal sphincter function should be assessed regularly to ensure that there is no deterioration of pressures. If deterioration is detected, surgical intervention must be undertaken.[24,28]

For patients who are unwilling or unable to undergo surgery, some nonoperative methods have been employed in addition to a vigorous bowel program to prevent constipation. These include adhesive strapping of the buttocks, manual anal support during defecation, perineal strengthening exercises, electronic stimulation, injection of sclerosing agents, and rubber band ligation. These palliative measures may provide occasional relief in some patients.

OPERATIVE TREATMENT

Once the diagnosis of complete, progressive rectal prolapse is established in an adult who is an acceptable surgical risk, operative intervention is indicated. Numerous approaches have been described, and are classified accordingly as transabdominal, perineal, or transsacral procedures (Box 15-2). Transabdominal procedures utilizing pelvic floor repairs have been largely abandoned because of technical difficulties and high recurrence rates. They will be briefly described

---

Box 15-2
Operation for Complete Rectal Prolapse

I. Transabdominal Procedures
  A. Repair of pelvic floor defects
    Obliteration of the pouch of Douglas (Moschcowitz)
    Restoration of the pelvic floor (Graham)
    Abdominoperineal levator repair (Hughes)
  B. Suspension or fixation of the rectum
    Sigmoidopexy (Pemberton-Stalker)
    Presacral suture proctopexy (Cutait)
    Presacral fascia lata proctopexy (Orr)
    Ivalon sponge implant (Wells)
    Anterior Teflon sling rectopexy (Ripstein)
    Puborectalis sling rectopexy (Nigro)
  C. Rectal wall stenting
    Rectal plication (Devadhar)
    Ivalon stint (Wedell)
  D. Rectosigmoid resection
    Low anterior resection (Muir)
    Anterior resection with proctopexy (Frykman-Goldberg)
II. Perineal Procedures
  A. Anal encirclement (Thiersch and modifications)
  B. Perineal rectopexy (Wyatt)
  C. Mucosal sleeve resection (Delorme)
  D. Perineal rectosigmoidectomy (Miles, Altemeier)
  E. Graciloplasty (Atri)
III. Transsacral Procedures
  A. Transsacral resection and fixation (Thomas)

---

here. The most commonly performed transabdominal procedures are rectal suspension operations with or without foreign material and anterior resection.

Perineal and transsacral procedures result in higher rates of recurrence than transabdominal procedures. Their principal advantage is that they are better tolerated by elderly or debilitated patients in whom laparotomy or general anesthesia would entail prohibitive risks.

TRANSABDOMINAL PROCEDURES

Repair of Pelvic Floor Defects

Obliteration of the pouch of Douglas (cul-de-sac) was the operation advocated by Moschcowitz in 1912,[4] based on his theory that complete rectal prolapse was a form of sliding hernia. The abnormally deep cul-de-sac, which usually is present with complete prolapse, constitutes the hernial sac; Moschcowitz believed repair of the pelvic floor and obliteration of the cul-de-sac would eliminate the hernia and therefore the prolapse. He felt this was best accomplished via a transabdominal approach using concentric purse-string sutures to obliterate the cul-de-sac and reestablish the pelvic floor. However, high recurrence rates of 50% to 63%[7,8] along with the subsequent work of Broden and Snellman[6] led to the rejection of this theory for the etiology of rectal prolapse and this operation.

Graham[29] proposed that in order to prevent prolapse, the widely separated levator ani muscles must be reapproximated with sutures anterior to the rectum; this maneuver would force the rectum back into the hollow of the sacrum. For additional support, the lateral rectal walls were sutured to the fascia overlying the levatores, and the pelvic floor reperitonealized with obliteration of the cul-de-sac. Goligher[30] modified the Graham procedure to include complete posterior mobilization of the rectum. These operations have been abandoned, however, due to high recurrence rates (27%).[31]

Hughes in 1957[17] described a combined abdominoperineal approach, thus modifying the Graham-Goligher procedure; his recurrence rate was 1.8%. However, from a practical standpoint, this procedure was too technically complex to gain wide acceptance.

Suspension or Fixation of the Rectum

Probably the most common operation for treating rectal prolapse in the United States today is the Teflon sling repair, described by Ripstein in 1965 (Fig. 15-6).[32]

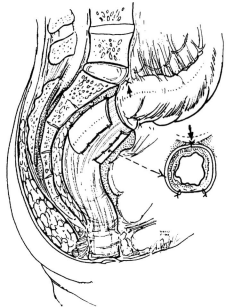

Fig. 15-6 Diagram of the Ripstein procedure. A sling of teflon mesh is used to fix the posteriorly mobilized rectum to the presacral fascia. In early operations, this sling enveloped the rectum. In later procedures (shown here), the sling was wrapped such that the anterior aspect of the rectum remained uncovered. The upper arrow points to the sacral fixation of the sigmoid colon at the level of the promontory. Note the suture in the inset which fixes the rectum to the sacrum.

Earlier, however, Pemberton and Stalker[33] pioneered suspension-fixation procedures in the treatment of complete rectal prolapse and emphasized the importance of complete posterior mobilization of the rectum.

Pemberton and Stalker[33] believed that an abnormally loosely attached rectum, the result of a developmental defect, was the most important predisposing anatomic defect in the development of rectal prolapse. Their approach was to fully mobilize the rectum posteriorly in the presacral space to the level of the coccyx. The sigmoid and rectum were then gently pulled taut. The elevated bowel was fixed by attaching it to itself, to the uterus, and to the walls of the pelvis. The rectum would become firmly and permanently scarred to the sacrum and this would prevent recurrences of incontinence. Their initial report[33] consisted of 6 cases without recurrence. However, later follow-up by Theuerkauf and colleagues[7] revealed a recurrence rate of 32% in 68 patients.

Presacral proctopexy by simple suture was first advocated by Cutait in 1959.[34] This procedure is simple and effective if the sigmoid redundancy is not severe; again, success lies in complete posterior mobilization of

the rectum with adequate fixation of its lateral peritoneal attachments to the presacral fascia.[18] Blatchford and colleagues[35] reported a 2% recurrence rate at a mean of 28 months in a recent series of 43 patients undergoing simple posterior suture rectopexy. Graham and coworkers[36] had no recurrence in 23 patients managed in a similar fashion.

The use of foreign material to aid in the suspension and fixation of the rectum to the sacrum was initially proposed by Orr in 1947.[37] Orr's technique involved the use of strips of autogenous fascia lata, which were sutured superiorly to the presacral fascia and inferiorly along the lateral aspects of the rectum, thereby suspending the rectum. The cul-de-sac was obliterated using sutures placed across the pelvis, and a fold of pelvic peritoneum was sutured to the rectum on each side to cover the fascial strips. Loygue and coworkers[38] modified the Orr procedure by using strips of nylon to laterally suspend the rectum, with a recurrence rate of only 4.3%.

Ripstein in the U.S. and Wells in the U.K. developed variations of the suspension-fixation technique which have become the most commonly used procedures for complete rectal prolapse in their respective countries (Fig. 15-6). Ripstein first reported on 4 successful cases in 1952[39] and Wells on 15 cases in 1959.[40] In the Ripstein procedure,[41] a T-shaped sling of Teflon mesh, 2 inches wide, was used as an anterior sling to fix the posteriorly mobilized rectum to the presacral fascia. No attempt was made to repair the pelvic floor. Recurrence following the Ripstein procedure has ranged from 5% to 13%.[8] Furthermore, a survey by Gordon and Hoexter[42] of 1111 cases managed by this technique disclosed a 17% complication rate and a 4% reoperation rate. The drawbacks to the Ripstein procedure include postoperative sepsis, rectal stenosis, sling obstruction, and fecal impaction. Bowel management problems ranging from episodic cramping abdominal pain to fecal impaction to sling obstruction were reported between 7% and 33% of patients following the Ripstein procedure.[18,42] In patients with long-standing rectal prolapse and chronic constipation, bowel management problems were often not improved by the Teflon sling repair; on the contrary, the constipation became more severe.[43]

Wells[40] described the use of a rectangular sheet of Ivalon sponge (polyvinyl alcohol) sutured to the sacrum and partially wrapped posteriorly about the rectum. The anterior 20% to 25% of the rectal circumference was left free, and this probably accounted for the lower rates of stenosis, fecal impaction, and sling obstruction compared to the Ripstein procedure.[18,19,44] The Ivalon sponge was selected because it induced an intense fibrotic reaction which fixed the rectum to the sacrum. However, the Ivalon sponge tends to fragment and infection in the presence of Ivalon is a serious problem requiring its removal.[18] This is not easy. Recurrence of complete rectal prolapse following the Wells procedure ranges from 0 to 20%.[18,19] Ivalon is not currently approved for use in the United States.

Due to the potential problems of infection with Ivalon rectopexy, Keighley and colleagues[45] have utilized inert Marlex mesh for posterior rectopexy. Of 100 patients who underwent this procedure, none developed recurrence of rectal prolapse during a 2-year follow-up period and none had intraabdominal infection around the Marlex mesh.

Another approach to the suspension of the rectum was developed by Nigro.[46] He designed an intraabdominal sling of Teflon mesh that suspended the rectum from the pubis. The sling was sutured posteriorly to the lower rectum and anteriorly to the pubic tubercles. Using this technique, Greene[47] reported on 15 patients, 8 with fecal incontinence. None of the patients had recurrent prolapse 6 months to 4 years later, and none had incontinence. Correction of both the prolapse and incontinence was attributed to re-creation of the puborectal sling (anorectal angle). Importantly, this teflon sling procedure is not widely employed because dissection along the anterior pelvis puts vital urinary and genital structures in jeopardy, and if performed in a woman of child-bearing age, subsequent pregnancies will require cesarean section.[19] In male patients, impotence is much more likely to be a complication than if a more conventional operation is used.[19] Its theoretical advantage with respect to restoration of fecal continence is probably overrated as well.

Rectal Wall Stenting

Devadhar[5] believed that rectal prolapse was caused by rectorectal intussusception. He noted that the site of the intussusception or "crucial point" could be palpated at surgery. He then constructed a "reverse intussusception" at this point by plicating the proximal rectum over the distal rectum with anterior purse-string and Lembert sutures and lateral longitudinal plicating sutures. These lateral sutures shorted the rectum and splinted the rectal wall to discourage intussusception. No mobilization was necessary posteriorly. Devadhar performed this operation on 28 patients, 10 of whom had been observed for 5 years without recurrence.

Stenting of the rectal wall to prevent intussusception

was also performed by Wedell and colleagues.[48] They reported on five patients with complete rectal prolapse who underwent rectal mobilization and placement of an Ivalon sponge partially around the rectum to stent the rectal wall. This differs from the Wells procedure because no sacral fixation was performed. Though the follow-up interval was quite short, none of the patients had a recurrence.

Rectosigmoid Resection

The use of rectosigmoid resection in the treatment of complete rectal prolapse was first reported in 1951 by Stabins[49] but was really popularized by Muir in 1954.[50] The success of this operation was due to the formation of firm fibrous adhesions between the site of the anastomosis and the underlying sacrum. The rectum was initially fully mobilized anteriorly and posteriorly to the levator ani muscles and then divided, leaving a short stump of about 3 inches above the levator floor. A suitable site on the sigmoid was selected, which removed any unnecessary slack but avoided tension at the low anterior anastomosis. The peritoneum was also mobilized and relaid to form fresh attachments. All of Muir's eight original patients had no recurrence of rectal prolapse.

Frykman and Goldberg[51] modified the method of rectosigmoid resection to include a rectopexy and performance of a high rectal anastomosis (Fig. 15-7). This abdominal procedure proceeds initially by fully mobilizing the rectum anteriorly and posteriorly but preserving the lateral stalks. The freed rectum is drawn up into the abdomen and the lateral stalks are sutured to the sacral periosteum to hold the rectum firmly in this elevated position. The left colon is mobilized to the splenic flexure and a sufficient amount of colon is resected so that the anastomosis can be accomplished without tension, but completely eliminating the redundancy. Any convenient site may be selected for the anastomosis. Sixty-seven patients were treated by Frykman and Goldberg[51] in this fashion with no evidence of recurrence, no mortality, and little morbidity.

Schlinkert and colleagues[52] compared the results of low anterior versus high anterior resection for patients with complete rectal prolapse. They found that low anterior resection, with the anastomosis in the deperitonealized portion of the rectum, was associated with increased morbidity without significantly decreasing recurrence when compared to high anterior resection. Of the patients undergoing high anterior resection, 19% had a complication, as opposed to 52% of those under-

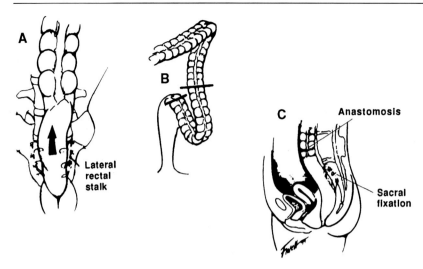

Fig. 15-7 Diagram of the Frykman, Goldberg procedure for rectal prolapse. This consists of **A**, fixation of the lateral stalks after complete elevation of the rectum; **B**, resection of redundant sigmoid colon, and **C**, sacral fixation. (Reprinted from Henry MM, Swash M, *Coloproctology and the Pelvic Floor: Pathophysiology and Management*, London: Butterworths; 1985, with permission.)

going low anterior resection. Nine percent of the 113 patients experienced recurrence of complete rectal prolapse.

PERINEAL PROCEDURES

Perineal approaches in patients with complete rectal prolapse have long been recognized as being less strenuous on the general health and recovery of the patient than abdominal methods of repair.[53] This has led to the use of perineal procedures on high-risk patients. In general, perineal operations are designed to treat the prolapse by accomplishing one (or a combination) of the three following goals: narrowing of the anal outlet through anal encirclement, suspension or fixation of the rectum, and resection of the redundant bowel comprising the prolapse.

Anal Encirclement

Thiersch introduced the concept of anal encirclement for the treatment of rectal prolapse in 1891.[54] Silver wire was used to encircle the anus and narrow its orifice and provide mechanical support and contain the prolapse (Fig. 15-8). The wire caused little fibrotic reaction and when left in place for prolonged periods of time, complications inevitably occurred.[10] These were due to wire breakage or ulceration, or fecal impaction secondary to interference with the passage of stool through the narrowed anal orifice.

Modifications of the Thiersch procedure involve the

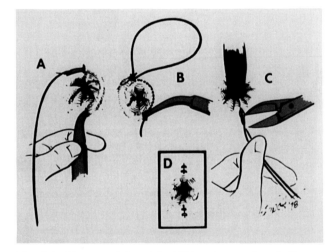

Fig. 15-8 Diagram of the original Thiersch operation. A silver wire is passed about the anal orifice and snugged tightly. This approach was largely abandoned in favor of the operation depicted in Fig. 15-9. Incisions are made posteriorly and anteriorly at the level of the anal verge through which a silver wire is passed, **A**, first to the patient's right and then **B**, to the left. **C**, The surgeon's finger determines the caliper of the anus as the wire is tied. **D**, Final appearance of the anus.

use of material other than the silver wire; silk, fascia, tendon, nylon, polypropylene mesh or suture, Teflon, Dacron, and even Angelchik prostheses[2,55,56] (Fig. 15-9) The great advantage of this procedure and its variations is the minimal degree of surgical trauma. It can be performed under local, spinal, or general anesthesia. Two small incisions are made, one anterior and the other posterior to the anal orifice, just outside the anal verge. The encircling material is passed around the anus in the subcutaneous layer through these incisions and fastened to narrow the outlet.

The main drawbacks of the anal encirclement procedure is that the prolapse is not in fact cured, it merely is changed to an occult or hidden rectal prolapse. Difficult bowel management problems often remain following the procedure. The clinical application of this procedure is therefore very limited.

Perineal Fixation and Resection Procedures

Perineal rectopexy involves securing the rectum to the sacrum through a posterior approach, the coccyx being removed in some patients to facilitate exposure. Wyatt[57] modified the Wells procedure by using the perineal approach to suspend and fixate the rectum to the sacrum by means of a Mersilene mesh which is fixed by sutures or staples to the presacral fascia. The mesh is then partially wrapped about the rectum. Wyatt[57] reported one recurrence in 22 patients, but the large scope of this procedure makes it much more difficult than similar abdominal rectopexy operations.

Mucosal sleeve resection for the treatment of complete rectal prolapse was originally described by Delorme in 1900[58] (Fig. 15-10). Only the mucosa of the redundant segment is resected, beginning 1 to 2 cm proximal to the dentate line. Following excision of a tube of mucosa, the proximal cut edge is sutured to the distal cut edge. During placement of each suture, multiple bites are taken in the intervening bared muscular wall of the rectum, thus pleating the muscle like an accordion as the two mucosal edges are drawn together. The plication of the rectal muscular wall forms a "supralevator donut" that has a pessary effect in preventing further prolapse.[59] The recurrence rate following the Delorme procedure is low, varying from 7% to 17%[58–60] and there is minimal morbidity.

Perhaps the most popular perineal operation for the treatment of complete rectal prolapse is the perineal rectosigmoidectomy, originally described by Miles in 1933.[62] In the United States, the operation is associated with Altemeier and coworkers.[63,64] The operation involves incising the full thickness of the outer layer of prolapsed bowel 2 cm proximal to the dentate line (Fig. 15-11). After unfolding the prolapse, the mesorectum is serially divided and ligated and the inner layer of bowel is transected. The cut edges are sutured or stapled together.[65] The excised specimen comprises 15 to 25 cm of rectosigmoid.

In Altemeier's hands, perineal rectosigmoidectomy had a very low rate of recurrence, approximately 3%.[63] However, in other series, the rates of recurrence of 35%

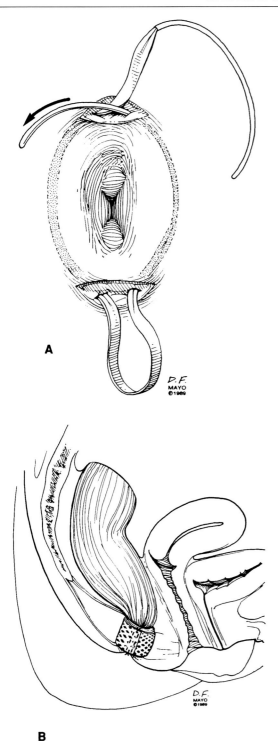

Fig. 15-9 Diagram of the modified Thiersch procedure for rectal prolapse. **A,** A 2 cm wide sling of dacron mesh is wrapped around the anal orifice via anterior and posterior incisions at the anal verge. **B,** The width of the sling and its depth of placement is appreciated in this diagram. (Reprinted from Dietzen[53] with permission.)

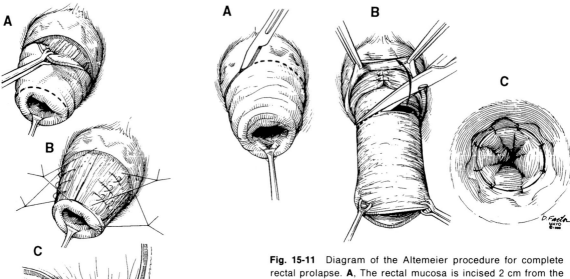

Fig. 15-10 Diagram of the Delorme procedure for complete rectal prolapse. **A**, The mucosa is incised about 1 cm from the dentate line and dissected from the underlying rectal muscularis for a varying distance, depending on mobility of the rectum. **B**, Plicating sutures are placed between the cut end of the rectal mucosa near the dentate line *(top)* and the prolapsed rectum *(bottom)*. **C**, Note how the rectal muscularis is plicated to form a "supra levator donut" which acts like a pessary, preventing further prolapse. (Reprinted from Dietzen[53] with permission.)

Fig. 15-11 Diagram of the Altemeier procedure for complete rectal prolapse. **A**, The rectal mucosa is incised 2 cm from the dentate line. **B**, The prolapse is unfolded, the mesentery serially ligated, and the bowel divided. **C**, The cut edges are sutured together 2 cm above the dentate line. (Reprinted from Dietzen[53] with permission.)

TRANSSACRAL PROCEDURES

The transsacral approach to the treatment of complete rectal prolapse has remained unpopular despite the reported success by Thomas and coworkers.[68,69] The rectum is approached posteriorly following disarticulation and removal of the coccyx as well as the lower two sacral segments. The procedure then involves resection of redundant rectosigmoid with primary anastomosis, followed by suture fixation of the rectum to the periosteum of the anterior surface of the sacrum. Anterior approximation of the levators is also accomplished. Davidian and Thomas[69] reported on 30 patients followed for 1 to 11 years with no mortality and no recurrence of prolapse. This approach has not achieved widespread popularity due to the unfamiliar operative approach for most surgeons, and a morbidity rate which approaches 38%, mainly due to wound infections and anastomotic leaks.[7]

POSTOPERATIVE ANORECTAL FUNCTION

Perhaps the greatest disappointment in the operative treatment of complete rectal prolapse is the high incidence of persistent fecal incontinence despite anatomic correction of the prolapse. A high percentage of patients are incontinent preoperatively, from 26% to 81%.[70] Approximately half of those patients who are incontinent improve following a transabdominal repair

to 60%[10,66] were higher than for anterior resection or the Ripstein procedure via the abdominal approach. For this reason, the perineal rectosigmoidectomy is usually reserved for elderly, debilitated patients who are at high operative risk for abdominal surgery.

Another innovative perineal approach to complete rectal prolapse was introduced by Atri in 1980.[67] He described the use of graciloplasty (transposition of the gracilis muscles) to form a "neosphincter" in 15 patients with complete prolapse. Follow-up on 10 patients showed no recurrence or mortality in a period of at least 6 months. The author claimed that all of these patients experienced improvement in defecation frequency and all regained complete continence after graciloplasty. Despite these favorable very short-term results, there are no other reports in the literature on this approach.

of the prolapse, but this may require 6 to 12 months.[2,18,70] Following perineal rectosigmoidectomy, incontinence improves in only 6% to 20% of the patients and, in this respect, the functional results of transabdominal procedures are superior to the perineal rectosigmoidectomy.[18]

For a long time it was believed that mechanical stretching of the anal sphincter by the protruding prolapsed segment caused the incontinence associated with rectal prolapse. However, electromyography and biopsy studies confirmed Parks and other's theory[71] that incontinence was the result of abnormal perineal descent, which led to a traction injury of the pudendal and perineal nerves, resulting in denervation of the pelvic floor musculature and sphincters. Fortunately, preoperative anal manometry sometimes can predict which patients with preoperative incontinence will regain acceptable levels of continence following correction of the prolapse[72]; if patients can generate a squeeze pressure, they will fare better than patients who cannot.

Postoperative regulation of bowel habits by use of a high fiber diet, bulk agents, and correction of mucosal prolapse, if present, will correct minor degrees of incontinence. The value of physiotherapy and perineal exercises following anatomic correction of the prolapse are probably useful but data are not available. Operative correction of persistent incontinence by postanal repair or plication sphincteroplasty has been generally unrewarding in these patients.

Solitary Rectal Ulcer Syndrome

Most patients with solitary rectal ulcer syndrome present with rectal bleeding, mucous discharge, tenesmus, and rectal pain. Those patients who have this syndrome in association with complete rectal prolapse or internal intussusception are effectively treated by operative correction of the prolapse, either by anterior resection or abdominal rectopexy.[26,73,74] Perineal rectosigmoidectomy is contraindicated in these patients.

Patients with solitary rectal ulcer refractory to conservative measures (i.e., high-fiber diet, bulk agents, avoidance of straining at defecation) and who do not have prolapse or intussusception are very difficult to manage. For these patients, pelvic floor retraining, using biofeedback techniques, has been shown to have some benefit and may be a promising advance.[26]

Colitis Cystica Profunda

Localized colitis cystica profunda that does not respond to conservative measures after 6 months and is not associated with complete rectal prolapse or internal intussusception may be treated with local excision. This local approach achieves relief of symptoms in 70% to 79% of patients.[26] If complete rectal prolapse or internal intussusception accompanies colitis cystica profunda, therapy is directed toward repair of the prolapse. The risk of recurrence of colitis cystica profunda parallels that of the prolapse.[26]

Internal Intussusception of the Rectum

Internal intussusception of the rectum usually presents as a functional outlet obstruction with chronic constipation and excessive straining at stool. Success with transabdominal fixation procedures for complete prolapse led to the application of various transabdominal fixation procedures for internal intussusception as well. Unfortunately, this frequently resulted in worsening constipation despite correction of the internal intussusception.[75] In the same series, however, patients with internal intussusception associated with fecal incontinence showed significant improvement in continence following Ripstein rectopexy.

Although patients with internal intussusception and incontinence may be functionally improved by anterior resection or transabdominal rectopexy, alternative modes of treatment are required in those patients with associated constipation. Nonoperative management with high-fiber diet and bulking agents targeted toward decreasing straining at defecation may be useful. Berman and others[76] have advocated the use of the Delorme procedure in this setting, with symptomatic relief in 70% of otherwise refractory constipated patients. This is not substantiated by any other reported experience in the literature. The use of pelvic floor retraining measures utilizing biofeedback techniques is also currently being evaluated at our own institution in this subset of patients.

Anterior Resection

The operation we prefer in patients with complete rectal prolapse is anterior resection (Fig. 15-12). For patients who are in poor general health and therefore at high operative risk for abdominal surgery, a perineal approach is advocated. In this circumstance, we favor performing a perineal rectosigmoidectomy (Altemeier procedure).

Anterior resection for rectal prolapse has been performed at the Mayo Clinic since 1952, and our current technique will be described in detail. Following a me-

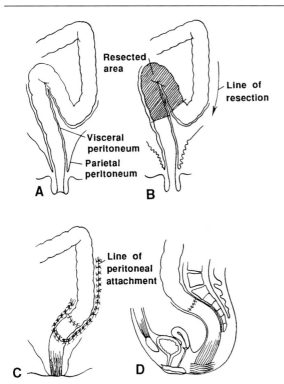

Fig. 15-12 Diagram of the anterior resection operation for complete rectal prolapse. **A,** The peritoneum is incised as shown. The rectum is mobilized posteriorly to the coccyx, anteriorly to the mid-vagina (or prostate) and laterally; the lateral stalks are loosened but not divided. **B,** The redundant sigmoid colon is resected. **C,** A "high" anterior resection is performed so that when the rectum is replaced in the pelvis **D,** it assumes the curve of the sacrum and is not taut.

chanical and antibiotic bowel preparation, a midline laparotomy is performed.

After freeing the sigmoid colon from any developmental lateral abdominal wall attachments, the "white line" is incised and the gonadal vessels and underlying left ureter are swept laterally. Then, by firmly elevating the sigmoid loop, the inferior mesentery artery is placed on stretch, making identification of the superior hemorrhoidal artery easier. With the forceps, the tissue clinging to the superior hemorrhoidal artery (superior rectal artery) is swept directly posteriorly, opening a window in the sigmoid mesentery immediately below the superior hemorrhoidal artery at the level of the aortic bifurcation. The tissue separated from the superior hemorrhoidal artery by this maneuver contains the aortic plexus and the origin of the presacral nerve and its left hypogastric nerve branch.

The arch of the superior hemorrhoidal artery is followed forward towards the rectum which, by strong upward traction, is oriented in an anterior and posterior direction. Again, using the forceps or scissors, the tissue behind the superior hemorrhoidal artery is pushed downward and once across the promontory, the presacral space is easily entered. Using the scissors, this space is developed sharply downward to about S_3 and then downward and forward to the rectal sacral fascia, at the level of S_4. If easily seen, the retrosacral fascia is then sharply incised. If not, the posterior dissection is carried laterally by sweeping hand motions which loosen the perirectal areolar tissue. Transecting the retrosacral fascia then allows safe, blunt finger dissection to the level of the levator raphe. By using this technique to enter the pelvis behind the rectum, the hypogastric nerves, and the hypogastric plexus are protected throughout their course.

The peritoneum on both sides of the rectum is incised such that the incisions meet in the midline, over the rectum, in the retrovesical or vaginal pouch. Then, sweeping hand motions from posterior to lateral are made on each side of the rectum, loosening and elevating the perirectal tissue. There are no nerves or vessels in this plane as they lie on the sidewalls near the ureters. By elevating the rectum out of the pelvis, the lateral ligaments can be better identified.

After incising the peritoneum over the retrovesical or retrovaginal pouch, sharp dissection is carried posteriorly toward the rectum, thus incising Denonvilliers' fascia. The dissection proceeds sharply between the rectum and Denonvilliers' fascia to the level of the low prostate or middle vagina. The periprostatic plexus is adjacent to this dissection, but its fibers are sent to the genitalia and prostate above Denonvilliers' fascia; they should, therefore, be protected by staying close to the rectum.

Only after anterior and posterior dissections are complete can the lateral ligaments be adequately defined and mobilized. This is because traction of the rectum does not tent the ligaments if the posterior and anterior rectal attachments are present. It is important to remember that the pelvic plexus of nerves is quite lateral, being adjacent to the pelvic sidewalls, such that even relatively aggressive mobilization of the lateral ligaments should not result in nerve damage.

The anastomosis should be performed at the level of the abdominal wall. This is accomplished by tenting the rectum firmly out of the pelvis and transecting it flush with the abdominal wall. The point of transection of the sigmoid/descending colon is likewise determined by stretching the colon out of the abdomen firmly and transecting it flush with the abdominal wall. In this way, the redundant sigmoid colon is resected. The anastomosis is then performed, usually by hand. Because the levels of transection were determined as outlined above, when the anastomosis is dropped back to the pelvis, the rectum will lie in the natural curve of the pelvis without tension. This type of anastomosis is a "high" anterior anastomosis. Postoperative fibrosis in the pelvis and at the site of the anastomosis will fix the rectum to the sacrum. Recurrence with this method is low, with 3% recurring at two years, 6% at five years, and 14% at ten years.[52] The morbidity in this group of 52 patients treated by high anterior resection was 19%.

Patients identified as having idiopathic slow transit constipation by preoperative colon transit studies require consideration of abdominal colectomy and ileorectostomy for treatment of their complete rectal prolapse. Correction of the prolapse by anterior resection of the rectosigmoid will not alleviate the problem of slow colonic transit; in fact, it may worsen postoperatively. Rather, by removing the entire dysfunctional colon and performing an ileorectostomy, both the prolapse and constipation are effectively treated simultaneously.

Perineal Rectosigmoidectomy

Perineal rectosigmoidectomy for rectal prolapse (Fig. 15-11) is particularly useful in high-risk patients or in patients presenting with strangulation. This procedure may be performed in the lithotomy or prone positions. The lithotomy position is associated with fewer ventilatory problems and is generally favored. The choice of anesthesia for perineal rectosigmoidectomy may be either local, spinal, or general, depending on the particular clinical situation. A mechanical and antibiotic bowel preparation should always be performed except in patients requiring urgent surgery for incarceration or strangulation of the prolapsed segment.

After positioning the patient and administering anesthesia, a circumferential incision about 2 cm proximal to the dentate line is made through the outer bowel layer of the prolapsed segment (Fig. 15-11). This creates a two layer thick tube of large bowel. The cut edge of the proximal bowel is grasped and the prolapsed segment is gently unfolded. The blood supply to the exposed bowel is ligated and divided near its entry from the mesorectum and mesosigmoid. Continued gentle traction allows the entire redundant segment to be pulled out through the anus and resected. The peritoneum is commonly entered anteriorly via the cul-de-sac; suture of the peritoneum to the bowel serosa closes the defect.

After the redundant rectosigmoid is removed, the proximal and distal ends of the bowel are anastomosed with absorbable sutures or a circular stapling device. The anastomosis is performed with good exposure outside of the anus. It then retracts back into the pelvis with manual assistance.

Complications with this perineal approach to complete rectal prolapse are infrequent. Altemeier and colleagues[63] reported only three recurrences in 106 patients with no mortality, although other series report considerably higher recurrence rates of up to 60%.[9,15]

We generally do not perform a posterior rectopexy and levator repair at the time of perineal rectosigmoidectomy as described by Prasad and coworkers.[77] Fecal incontinence may improve with or without these additional maneuvers, which significantly increase the potential for serious presacral hemorrhage.

SUMMARY

Rectal prolapse is an uncommon problem whose etiology still remains incompletely understood. Our current concept of rectal prolapse evolving as a rectorectal intussusception has helped to explain the high recurrence rates which resulted from earlier operative approaches. Although a number of abdominal and perineal approaches are presently used to treat rectal prolapse, *the common goal is to achieve fixation of the rectum to the sacrum by means of postoperative fibrosis or rectopexy.* Persistent incontinence and constipation following anatomic correction of the prolapse remain the major sources of postoperative disability and patient dissatisfaction.

REFERENCES

1. Mann CV. Rectal prolapse. In: Morson BC, ed. *Diseases of the Colon, Rectum and Anus.* New York: Appleton-Century-Crofts; 1969:238–250.
2. Wassef R, Rothenberger DA, Goldberg SM. Rectal prolapse. *Curr Prob Surg.* 1986;23:398–451.
3. Theuerkauf FJ, Kodner IJ, Hoffman MJ, Fry RD. Rectal prolapse and internal intussusception of the rectum: diagnosis and surgical treatment. In: Kodner IJ, Fry RD, Roe JP, eds. *Colon, Rectal, and Anal Surgery: Current Techniques and Controversies.* St. Louis: CV Mosby Co; 1985:76–90.
4. Moschcowitz AV. The pathogenesis, anatomy, and cure of prolapse of the rectum. *Surg Gynecol Obstet.* 1912;15:7–21.
5. Devadhar DSC. A new concept of mechanism and treatment of rectal procidentia. *Dis Colon Rectum.* 1965;8:75–77.
6. Broden B, Snellman B. Procidentia of the rectum studied with cineradiography: a contribution to the discussion of causative mechanism. *Dis Colon Rectum.* 1968;11:330–347.
7. Theuerkauf FJ, Beahrs OH, Hill JR. Rectal prolapse: causation and surgical treatment. *Ann Surg.* 1970;171:819–835.
8. Nigro ND. An evaluation of the cause and mechanism of complete rectal prolapse. *Dis Colon Rectum.* 1966;9:391–398.

9. Porter NH. A physiological study of the pelvic floor in rectal prolapse. *Proc Roy Soc Med.* 1962;55:1090.

10. Parks AG, Swash M, Urich H. Sphincter denervation in anorectal incontinence and rectal prolapse. *Gut.* 1977;18:656–665.

11. Rutter KRP. Electromyographic changes in certain pelvic floor abnormalities. *Proc Roy Soc Med.* 1974;64:53–56.

12. Kupfer CA, Goligher JC. One hundred consecutive cases of complete prolapse of the rectum treated by operation. *Br J Surg.* 1970;57:481–487.

13. Goligher JC. *Surgery of the Anus, Rectum, and Colon.* 5th ed. London: Bailliere-Tindall; 1984;246–284.

14. Jurgeleit HC, Corman ML, Coller JA. Procidentia of the rectum: teflon sling repair of rectal prolapse, Lahey Clinic experience. *Dis Colon Rectum.* 1975;18:464–467.

15. Boutsis C, Ellis H. The Ivalon-sponge-wrap operation for rectal prolapse: an experience with 26 patients. *Dis Colon Rectum.* 1974;17:21–37.

16. Hughes EJR. Discussion on prolapse of the rectum. *Proc Roy Soc Med.* 1949;42:1007–1011.

17. Ihre T, Seligson U. Intussusception of the rectum-internal procidentia: treatment and results in 90 patients. *Dis Colon Rectum.* 1975;18:391–396.

18. Schoetz DJ, Veidenheimer MC. Rectal prolapse: pathogenesis and clinical features. In: Henry MM, Swash M, eds. *Coloproctology and the Pelvic Floor: Pathophysiology and Management.* London: Butterworths; 1985;303–339.

19. Corman ML. Rectal prolapse. In: Corman ML, ed. *Colon and Rectal Surgery.* 2nd ed. Philadelphia: JB Lippincott Co; 1989:209–247.

20. Corman ML, Veidenheimer MC, Coller JA. Managing rectal prolapse. *Geriatrics.* 1974;29(10):87–93.

21. Bartolo DCC. Pelvic floor disorders: incontinence, constipation, and obstructed defecation. In: Schrock TR, ed. *Perspectives in Colon and Rectal Surgery.* St. Louis: Quality Medical Publishing; 1988:1–24.

22. Holmstrom B, Broden G, Dolk A, Frenckner B. Increased and resting pressure following the Ripstein operation. A contribution to continence? *Dis Colon Rectum.* 1986;29:485–487.

23. Neill ME, Parks AG, Swash M. Physiological studies of the anal sphincter musculature in fecal incontinence and rectal prolapse. *Br J Surg.* 1981;68:531.

24. Buls JG. Rectal prolapse. In: Fazio VW, ed. *Current Therapy in Colon and Rectal Surgery.* Toronto: Decker Inc; 1990:92–97.

25. Pemberton JH. Rectal prolapse: pathogenesis and diagnosis. *Endoscopy Rev.* June 1990:50–53.

26. Nelson H, Pemberton JH. Solitary rectal ulcer. In: Fazio VW, ed. *Current Therapy in Colon and Rectal Surgery.* Toronto: Decker, Inc; 1990:98–102.

27. Wrobleski DE, Daily TH. Spontaneous rupture of the distal colon with evisceration of the small intestine through the anus: report of two cases and review of the literature. *Dis Colon Rectum.* 1979;22:569–572.

28. Lowry AC, Goldberg SM. Internal and overt rectal procidentia. *Gastroenterol Clin N Am.* 1987;16:47–70.

29. Graham RR. The operative repair of massive rectal prolapse. *Ann Surg.* 1942;115:1007–1014.

30. Goligher JC. The treatment of complete prolapse of the rectum by the Roscoe Graham operation. *Br J Surg.* 1958;45:323–333.

31. Kuijpers JHC, Lubbers EJC. The Roscoe Graham-Goligher procedure in the treatment of complete rectal prolapse. *Neth J Surg.* 1983;35:24–26.

32. Ripstein CB. Surgical care of massive rectal prolapse. *Dis Colon Rectum.* 1965;8:34–38.

33. Pemberton JdeJ, Stalker LK. Surgical treatment of complete rectal prolapse. *Ann Surg.* 1939;109:799–808.

34. Cutait D. Sacro-promontory fixation of the rectum for complete rectal prolapse. *Proc Roy Soc Med.* 1959;52(suppl):105.

35. Blatchford GJ, Perry RE, Thorson AG, Christenson MA. Recto-

pexy without resection for rectal prolapse. *Am J Surg.* 1989;158:574–576.

36. Graham W, Clegg JF, Taylor V. Complete rectal prolapse: repair by a simple technique. *Ann Roy Coll Surg Engl.* 1984;66:87–89.

37. Orr TG. A suspension operation for prolapse of the rectum. *Ann Surg.* 1947;126:833–840.

38. Loygue J, Nordlinger B, Cunci O, Malafosse M, Huguet C, Parc R. Rectopexy to the promontory for the treatment of rectal prolapse: report of 257 cases. *Dis Colon Rectum.* 1984;27:356–359.

39. Ripstein CB. Treatment of massive rectal prolapse. *Am J Surg.* 1952;83:68–71.

40. Wells C. New operation for rectal prolapse. *Proc Roy Soc Med.* 1959;52:602–603.

41. Ripstein CB, Lanter B. Etiology and surgical therapy of massive prolapse of the rectum. *Ann Surg.* 1963;157:259.

42. Gordon PH, Hoexter B. Complications of the Ripstein procedure. *Dis Colon Rectum.* 1978;21:277–280.

43. Lescher TJ, Corman ML, Coller JA, Veidenheimer MC. Management of late complications of Teflon sling repair for rectal prolapse. *Dis Colon Rectum.* 1979;22:445–447.

44. Morgan CN, Porter NH, Klugman DJ. Ivalon (polyvinyl alcohol) sponge in the repair of complete rectal prolapse. *Br J Surg.* 1972;59:841–846.

45. Keighley MRB, Fielding JWL, Alexander-Williams J. Results of Marlex mesh abdominal rectopexy for rectal prolapse in 100 consecutive patients. *Br J Surg.* 1983;70:229–232.

46. Nigro ND. A sling operation for rectal prolapse. *Proc Roy Soc Med.* 1970;63:106–107.

47. Greene FL. Repair of rectal prolapse using a puborectal sling procedure. *Arch Surg.* 1983;118:398–401.

48. Wedell J, Zueissen PM, Fielder R. A new concept for the management of rectal prolapse. *Am J Surg.* 1980;139:723–725.

49. Stabins SJ. A new surgical procedure for complete rectal prolapse in the mentally ill patient: case report. *Surgery.* 1951;29:105.

50. Muir EG. Rectal prolapse. *Proc Roy Soc Med.* 1954;48:33–44.

51. Frykman HM, Goldberg SM. The surgical treatment of rectal procidentia. *Surg Gynecol Obstet.* 1969;129:1225–1230.

52. Schlinkert RT, Beart RW, Wolff BG, Pemberton JH. Anterior resection for complete rectal prolapse. *Dis Colon Rectum.* 1985;28:409–412.

53. Dietzen CD, Pemberton JH. Perineal approaches for the treatment of complete rectal prolapse. *Neth J Surg.* 1989;41:140–144.

54. Goligher JC. *Surgery of the Anus, Rectum, and Colon.* 4th ed. New York: Macmillan; 1980:224–258.

55. Ladha A, Lee P, Berger P. Use of Angelchik anti-reflux prosthesis for repair of total rectal prolapse in elderly patients. *Dis Colon Rectum.* 1985;28:5–7.

56. Lomas MI, Cooperman H. Correction of rectal procidentia by use of polypropylene mesh (Marlex). *Dis Colon Rectum.* 1972;15:416–419.

57. Wyatt AP. Perineal rectopexy for rectal prolapse. *Br J Surg.* 1981;68:717–719.

58. Corman ML. Classic articles in colonic and rectal surgery: Edmond Delorme. *Dis Colon Rectum.* 1985;28:544–553.

59. Uhlig BE, Sullivan ES. The modified Delorme operation: its place in surgical treatment for massive rectal prolapse. *Dis Colon Rectum.* 1979;22:513–521.

60. Houry S, Lechaux JP, Huguier M, Molkhou JM. Treatment of rectal prolapse by Delorme's operation. *Int J Colorect Dis.* 1987;2:149–152.

61. Christiansen J, Kirkegaard P. Delorme's operation for complete rectal prolapse. *Br J Surg.* 1981;68:537–538.

62. Miles WE. Rectosigmoidectomy as a method of treatment for procidentia recti. *Proc Roy Soc Med.* 1933;26:1445–1447.

63. Altemeier WA, Culbertson WR, Schwengerdt C, Hunt J. Nineteen years experience with the one-stage repair of rectal prolapse. *Ann Surg.* 1971;173:993–1006.

64. Altemeier WA, Culbertson WR. Technique for perineal repair of rectal prolapse. *Surgery.* 1965;58:758–764.

65. Vermeulen FD, Nivatvongs S, Fang DT, Balcos EG, Goldberg SM. A technique for perineal rectosigmoidectomy using autosuture devices. *Surg Gynecol Obstet.* 1983;156:85–86.

66. Friedman R, Muggia-Sulam M, Freund HR. Experience with the one-stage perineal repair of rectal prolapse. *Dis Colon Rectum.* 1983;26:789–791.

67. Atri SP. The treatment of complete rectal prolapse by graciloplasty. *Br J Surg.* 1980;67:431–432.

68. Jenkins SG, Thomas CG. An operation for the repair of rectal prolapse. *Surg Gynecol Obstet.* 1962;114:381–383.

69. Davidian UA, Thomas CG. Transsacral repair of rectal prolapse. *Am J Surg.* 1972;123:231–235.

70. Watts JD, Rothenberger DA, Buls JG, Goldberg SM, Nivatvongs S. The management of procidentia: 30 years' experience. *Dis Colon Rectum.* 1985;28:96–102.

71. Parks AG, Swash M, Urich H. Sphincter denervation in anorectal incontinence and rectal prolapse. *Gut.* 1977;18:656–665.

72. Yoshioka K, Hyland G, Keighley MRB. Anorectal function after abdominal rectopexy: parameters of predictive value in identifying return of continence. *Br J Surg.* 1989;76:64–68.

73. Keighley MRB, Shouler P. Clinical and manometric features of the solitary rectal ulcer syndrome. *Dis Colon Rectum.* 1984;27:507–512.

74. Schweiger M, Alexander-Williams J. Solitary rectal ulcer syndrome of the rectum: its association with occult rectal prolapse. *Lancet.* 1977;i:170–171.

75. Holmstrom B, Broden G, Dolk A. Results of the Ripstein operation in the treatment of rectal prolapse and internal rectal procidentia. *Dis Colon Rectum.* 1986;29:845–848.

76. Berman IR, Harris MS, Rabeler MB. Delorme's transrectal excision for internal rectal prolapse: patient selection, technique and three-year follow-up. *Dis Colon Rectum.* 1990;33:573–580.

77. Prasad ML, Pearl RK, Abcarian H, Orsay CP, Nelson RL. Perineal proctectomy, posterior rectopexy, and postanal levator repair for the treatment of rectal prolapse. *Dis Colon Rectum.* 1986;29:547–552.

CHAPTER 16

Rectocele, Descending Perineal Syndrome, Enterocele

J. Thomas Benson

INTRODUCTION

The portion of the pelvic floor relating to the perineal body encompasses the rectovaginal septum, the levator plate, and the uterosacral cardinal attachments. Defects in this area of the pelvic floor lead to rectocele, descending perineum, and enterocele which will be discussed in this chapter, with emphasis on diagnostic as well as therapeutic measures for each.

RECTOCELE

Derived from the Greek *kele,* meaning hernia, rectocele, by definition, is protrusion or herniation of the posterior vaginal wall by the anterior wall of the rectum through the vagina.

The definition itself leads to difficulty. Throughout the years, the diagnosis and management of rectocele has been an uncomfortable arena for the pelvic surgeon. The results have been disappointing and in many places rectocele repair has given rise to more dissatisfaction than satisfaction, and the procedure has been abandoned. Greater understanding of the diagnosis, pathogenesis, and treatment of rectocele can lead to a high degree of satisfaction among patients with this disturbing disorder.

By definition, *rectocele* is the anterior rectal wall prolapsed with the posterior vaginal wall. In actuality, the two structures are quite separate. The rectal-vaginal space in the normal patient is a true space allowing complete separation of vaginal and rectal function and independence of one from the other. When a patient presents with a protrusion of the posterior vaginal wall, it is assumed that the anterior rectal wall is in continuity with this protrusion, but this is frequently incorrect. When examined clinically, a rectal finger is used to push on the anterior rectal wall and the effects of this on the posterior wall of the vagina are observed. The impression will virtually always be that the two are herniating together. Defecography, however, has shown a remarkable degree of variance. Many patients who present with prolapsing of the posterior vaginal wall have no anterior rectal wall defect demonstrable on defecography. In fact, this point of separation can become exaggerated, so that in some patients presenting with complete uterovaginal prolapse (vaginal vault prolapse) defecography reveals that the rectum may remain in its completely normal anatomic position (see Chapter 13D, Fig. 7).

Other patients who, on examination, have little defect in the posterior vaginal wall will, on defecography, have a remarkably large rectocele which empties poorly with defecation (Fig. 16-1). Such patients do have symptoms of defecation disorder that correlate well with the defecography findings, even though it does not correlate with the clinical findings.

Because of the great disparity in findings on clinical examination and defecography, and the disparity of the physical findings with the patient's symptoms, and be-

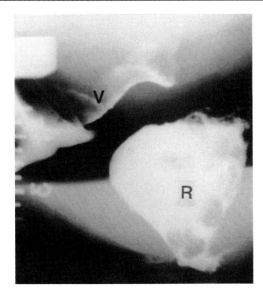

Fig. 16-1 Pronounced nonemptying rectocele seen on defecography in patient with negative clinical examination. *V* = vagina, *R* = nonemptying rectocele.

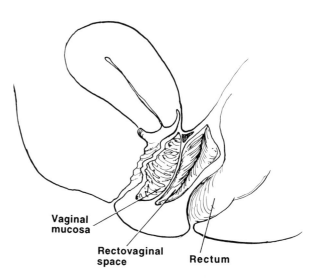

Fig. 16-2 Diagrammatic representation of the rectovaginal space in a normal patient. The space is a true space allowing functional separateness of vagina and rectum.

cause the surgical therapy depends on knowledge of what is indeed happening with the anterior rectal wall during the process of defecation, we now routinely require defecography as part of the preoperative evaluation prior to rectocele surgery. This is especially helpful if the patient's clinical findings and symptomatology are inconsistent.

Pathogenesis

It is helpful from a functional and a prognostic standpoint to generalize the pathogenesis of rectocele into two types: (1) the rectocele that occurs secondary to traumatic change, usually as a result of obstetrical delivery, and (2) rectocele that develops in response to long-standing defecation disorder.

Obstetric injuries involving tearing of the firm rectovaginal septum (Denonvilliers' fascia) may lead to rectocele. When the rectovaginal septum is torn from its attachment to the perineal floor, rectoceles occur in the lower vagina. Weakening and tearing of the rectovaginal septum in the posterior wall of the vagina may lead to mid or even high rectocele locations. Attenuation of the posterior vaginal wall, as described for the pulsion cystocele on the anterior vaginal wall, may occur with pulsion type posterior vaginal wall protrusion. Whether or not the rectum is involved in this process is best determined by defecography. The rectal wall involvement with the process may be secondary to the loss of

functional separateness of the vagina and the rectum by adhesive processes occurring in the rectovaginal space (Fig. 16-2). Here, adhesive processes associated with thinning and attenuation of the posterior vaginal wall allow the anterior rectal wall to accompany the posterior vaginal wall in its pulsion defect.

In the secondary types of rectocele, rectal dysfunction, primarily constipation, is the predisposing factor. In constipation, arbitrarily defined as straining more than 25% of the total time of defecation, repeated Valsalva maneuver efforts lead to observable physiologic changes. Ultrasound studies (Fig. 16-3) may show hypertrophy of internal rectal sphincter in many cases of chronic constipation. Continual weakening of the actual anterior rectal wall can occur in such conditions which are, in effect, attempts to void against obstruction. Many patients demonstrate failure of puborectalis relaxation in association with Valsalva maneuver (anismus), and this may be demonstrated by electromyography needle techniques (Figs. 16-4 and 16-5). Such studies must be cautiously interpreted, as false positive reactions may occur in the laboratory setting. Typically, these patients may have development of symptomatic rectocele, which is observable on defecography, whereas the posterior vaginal wall may have relatively less defect clinically observable.

Further supporting the concept of secondary rectocele development are those cases associated with congenital neuropathy seen in spina bifida occulta. Other

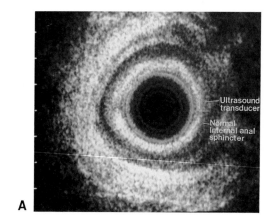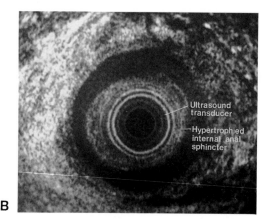

Fig. 16-3 Anal ultrasound studies in **A**, normal and **B**, constipated patient. Note hypertrophy of internal anal sphincter in **B**. (Courtesy of C. Bartram, St. Mark's Hospital, London.)

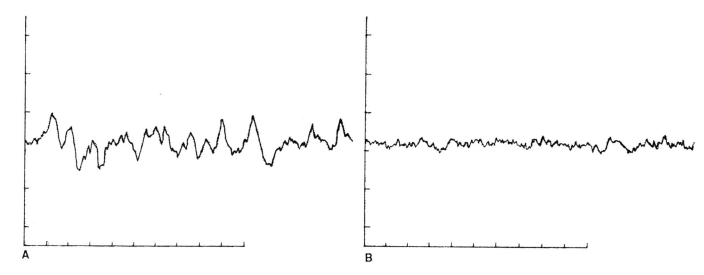

Fig. 16-4 Needle EMG study of the puborectalis muscle in normal subject with squeeze **A**, and strain **B**. Note diminished puborectalis activity with Valsalva in **B**.

patients with primary cauda equinal defects have constipation disorders also, and may eventually develop rectocele findings. The component of neurologic injuries and its effect on defecation disorders is only now recognized, the study of which is just beginning.

DESCENDING PERINEAL SYNDROME

As noted by Henry,[1] this pelvic floor disorder was first recognized by Parks and his colleagues in 1966 while investigating rectal prolapse. Initially defined ra-

diologically by the relationship of the anal rectal angle to the pubococcygeal line, the syndrome can now be clinically defined when the plane of the perineum (led by the anal verge) extends beyond the ischial tuberosities during Valsalva maneuvers, a movement usually of more than 2 cm (see Chapter 6). A perineometer is used to measure such movement.[2]

Some authors consider descending perineum as a symptom rather than a syndrome, but in our experience the symptomatology is linked frequently enough to justify its definition as a syndrome. The symptomatology is, first and foremost, a pronounced difficulty with defecation leading to prolonged straining efforts. It is postu-

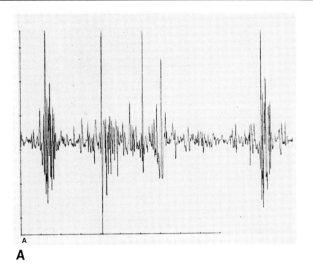

A

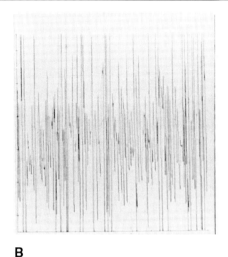

B

Fig. 16-5 Needle EMG study in patient with failure of relaxation of the puborectalis muscle with Valsalva (anismus). **A**, relaxed; **B**, squeeze; **C**, strain.

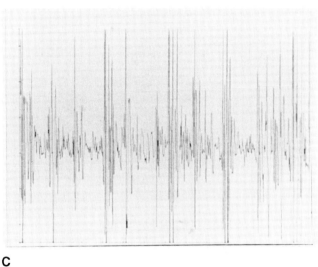

C

lated that the sensation of full rectum may be in part caused by prolapsing mucosa, which leads to mucous discharge and, frequently, rectal bleeding.

Pain can be a highly problematic component of the syndrome. It is a poorly localized deep discomfort precipitated by prolonged standing and relieved by lying down or sleep. It is not related to defecation. Treatment of this pain is extremely difficult to manage regardless of the method of treatment used.

Many patients with perineal descent having the same electrophysiologic abnormalities that are recorded in patients with fecal incontinence[2,3] show that irreversible nerve damage occurs when nerves are stretched by as little as 12%. In these patients the pelvic floor is moving 2 to 3 cm. The terminal portion of the pudendal nerve in the adult is approximately 9 cm, so 20% to

30% stretch may occur with this distal segment of the nerve.

The neurologic damage may, in time, lead to anal incontinence. Thus, an element of treatment is to avoid prolonged stretching of the nerve. Attempts to correct this nonsurgically include explaining the situation to the patient. Defecation through a hole in a board is a way to reduce the amount of perineal descent, although most patients find this method of treatment unsatisfactory. Surgical treatment with retrorectal levatoplasty in an attempt to prevent further damage to the nerve may be a consideration, and levatoplasty should strongly be considered in conjunction with posterior colporrhaphy when perineal descent is present. Attempting to do levatoplasty with a posterior colporrhaphy whereby the levator musculature is brought together anterior to the rectum and not through the retrorectal space makes for a nonanatomic repair. Such a repair frequently leads to dyspareunia and has little effect on the perineal descent.

Because these patients are at risk for developing fecal incontinence, they frequently maintain continence only by dependence on the normal internal sphincter. Therefore, attempts to treat the constipation or voiding dysfunction by manual dilation or other internal sphincterotomies may result in severe fecal incontinence.

Classification of Rectocele

Rectoceles are typically classified as low, mid, and high depending on their location. As described above, defecography is extremely useful and, perhaps, necessary to establish the actual diagnosis. Based on defecography findings during the actual act of defecation, the rectocele sides may be measured and, when the vagina is outlined with radiopaque dye, the actual relative location of the rectocele to the vagina is described radiologically. Therefore, this method may be better for defining size and location of the rectocele.

The high rectoceles are characteristically related to enteroceles, and preoperative recognition of enterocele is helpful for proper planning of pelvic floor restorative surgery. The relation to perineal defects must also be appreciated preoperatively to plan appropriate perineorrhaphy repair when indicated. Therefore, the classification of rectocele should include size, location, and the related pelvic floor defects.

Symptomatology

The symptomatology is quite variable and is not a simple single symptom of manual assistance required for defecation. Rectoceles that develop as a result of obstetric defect may frequently have this symptom, but, as indicated above, the clinical and radiologic findings are quite variable. Rectoceles developing secondary to anal dysfunction indeed require manual assistance for defecation and may additionally have other colonic symptoms. The manual assistance required varies with the pathophysiology. Manual assistance to elevate the perineum posterior to the anus is frequently associated with some degree of perineal descent and levator plate weakness. Manual assistance anterior to the rectum is classically seen with anterior rectocele and is sometimes seen with the anal flap anterior mucosal prolapse associated with descending perineum.

Many patients have been seen whose colonic function is characterized by delay. Arbitrarily, patients who defecate fewer than two times a week are classified as having constipation in this definition. Radiologic studies that involve following the transition of markers (see Chapter 7A1) may be helpful with this. In patients whose marker accumulation is in the area of the rectocele, improvement in the transit time has followed rectocele repair. There have been no well-conducted studies on this association, but there may indeed be a more significant relationship of rectocele to colonic function than has been assumed.

SURGICAL CORRECTION

Posterior Colporrhaphy

The principle of posterior colporrhaphy attempts to maintain functional independence of the posterior vaginal wall and anterior rectal wall. The decision to incorporate an associated perineorrhaphy must be made prior to beginning the operation, as the incision for the rectocele with, versus without, perineorrhaphy differs. The effective repair must always begin proximal to the point of weakness in the posterior vaginal wall. And as always, associated pelvic floor defects must be carefully sought for, recognized, and repaired simultaneously.

Posterior Colporrhaphy with Perineorrhaphy

Allis clamps are placed at the posterior introitus at a width which, when approximated, still allows coital functioning. Thus, two or three fingers should be admissable with the Allis clamps approximated, as this tissue will be approximated at the conclusion of the procedure. A third Allis clamp is placed above the anal verge and a triangular segment of skin overlying the perineum is removed between these three Allis clamps. With the operator's finger in the rectum, a sagittal incision is made in the posterior wall of the vagina after ascertaining the highest level to which the incision will go to encompass the entire rectocele. Once the rectovaginal space is entered successfully, Allis clamps are placed on the full thickness of the posterior vaginal wall. Straight Mayo scissors are used to incise the complete vaginal wall on a sagittal line extending through the complete posterior vaginal wall defect. Any adhesions in the rectovaginal space are lysed and the space is completely opened. At the superior aspect of the open rectovaginal space, careful inspection for enterocele is made and appropriate repair carried out if enterocele is present (see section under enterocele repair). Usually, by blunt dissection the rectum can be freed from its attachments. At this point the decision is made as to imbrication of the anterior rectal wall. This decision is based on defecography findings as well as symptomatology, and is necessary in cases of nonemptying rectocele on defecography. The ballooning defect in the anterior rectal wall is corrected by one or more layers of locked 2-0 polyglycolic absorbable suture running the entire length of the rectal wall (Fig. 16-6). When such imbrication is created by firm, running, interlocking sutures, healing involves a degree of apparent mucosal sluffing as the imbricated mass decreases.[4] The surgeon's finger is kept in the rectum during this procedure so that the suture goes into the muscularis but not into the rectal mucosa. Even when a large defect exists, imbrication is preferred over resection of the anterior rectal wall. Occasionally two or even three layers are employed.

Denonvilliers' fascia and the entire vaginal wall thickness is now trimmed to an area that, when reapproximated, does not create any transverse ridges. A single layer of the absorbable suture utilized for the rectal wall repair is then used to close the trimmed posterior vaginal wall. The cranial margin is fixed by the suture to the tissue of the rectal vaginal septum and the closure is completed to the point of the musculature of the urethrovaginal sphincter and compressor urethrae and transverse perineal musculature. Standard perineorrhaphy is then performed. The suture closing Denonvilliers' fascia is approximated to the perineal musculature. If the Denonvilliers' fascia is closed by separate continuous suture, a second suture closes the remaining vaginal wall in a similar running manner. If there is a large, attenuated pulsion defect in the posterior vaginal wall, the wall is dissected from the recto-

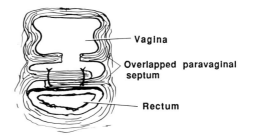

Fig. 16-7 Overlapping closure of rectovaginal septum during posterior colporrhaphy.

vaginal septum, which is then overlapped and closed in a multilayer fashion (Fig. 16-7).

Posterior Colporrhaphy without Perineorrhaphy

This procedure differs from the above only in the initial incision and in that the perineal musculature is not addressed. The initial incision enters the rectovaginal space and may be either transverse or longitudinal. The incision should be done with the operator's finger in the rectum to avoid rectal wall injury and should be made delicately until the rectovaginal space is encountered, at which time the incision may be extended with relative ease. A diamond-shaped removal of the full thickness of the vaginal wall is conducted in a manner similar to the one previously described. Again, rectal wall imbrication depends on the defecography findings.

Rectocele repair from the rectal approach is advocated by some. It is wise not to attempt simultaneous vaginal and rectal approach, as this is associated with the infrequent but serious complication of rectovaginal fistula.

Enterocele

Enterocele, by definition, is a hernia of the intestine through the vagina. The location of such herniation is typically posterior to the uterus and anterior to the rectum in the pouch of Douglas. In the absence of the uterus, herniation may occur at the vaginal apex, and rarely after hysterectomy, an anterior enterocele may occur which is actually between the bladder and anterior wall of the vagina.[5] Lateral vaginal defects have been described also.[6] Other than location, they may be further classified as congenital, iatrogenic, pulsion, and traction.

Fig. 16-6 Imbricating suture on rectal wall during posterior colporrhaphy.

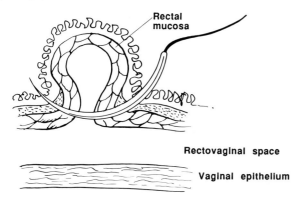

Pathogenesis for Congenital Enterocele

When the Müllerian ducts fuse with the urogenital sinus in embryologic development, the cul-de-sac peritoneum is located deep between the rectum and the developing vagina. Thus, it is very possible for the cul-de-sac to be congenitally deep with failure of normal fusion of its anterior and posterior peritoneum. Certainly not all deep cul-de-sacs are occupied by small intestine. Nichols[6] makes the point that for small bowel to occupy a deep cul-de-sac there must be an abnormally lengthened mesentery, and whether the long bowel mesentery precedes or follows the enterocele sac is unknown. Certainly it is true that for many years vaginal cuffs were left open when performing vaginal hysterectomy, and the occurrence of enterocele through the open vaginal cuff was uncommon.

Congenital enteroceles characteristically present posterior to the vaginal vault and may not be associated with vaginal inversion.

Pulsion Enterocele

Pulsion enterocele is the type produced by increased abdominal pressure inverting of the apical portion of the vagina. When the inversion continues far enough, an associated vault prolapse becomes evident. Vault prolapses may occur without enterocele, and pulsion enterocele may occur without significant vault inversion, but most commonly the two are associated. When the process continues long enough, a secondary eversion of the lower portion of the vagina may occur with the development of cystocele and rectocele following that of the pulsion enterocele.

Traction Enterocele

When uterovaginal descent occurs there is progressive pulling of the anterior cul-de-sac wall through the levator hiatus. Secondary development of herniation of small bowel with this type of process is referred to as traction enterocele.

Iatrogenic Enterocele

Iatrogenic enteroceles may be thought of as those occurring when pelvic floor surgery displaces vectors of forces. For example, in anterior urethropexy, especially with Burch-type colposuspension, but also with needle suspension, there is a change in the vector of forces increasing the tendency to enterocele development, thus

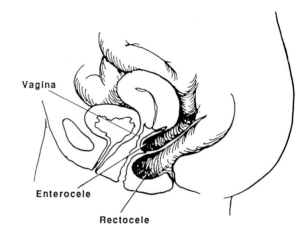

Fig. 16-8 Enterocele

constituting one form of iatrogenic enterocele (see Chapter 11D2, Fig. 1). Anterior enteroceles are virtually always secondary to hysterectomy, with defects occurring between the area of bladder pillars, allowing small bowel herniation in this area.

Diagnosis

Enterocele is best diagnosed clinically and does not always require radiologic evaluation as does rectocele. However, to make the clinical diagnosis in a preoperative mode a patient must be examined in a standing position while doing the Valsalva maneuver. Simultaneous examination of the rectum and vagina is required so that the herniating bowel may be palpable (Fig. 16-8). Occasionally, the prolapsing mass may be transluminated by cystoscopy to distinguish cystocele from enterocele. Defecography may be helpful when simultaneous painting of the vagina with radiopaque substance shows increased rectovaginal distance (Fig. 16-9A). Small bowel opacification can then show the enterocele (Fig. 16-9B). Rectoceles may be misdiagnosed clinically as an enterocele, and defecography may correct this error (Fig. 16-10). The examination also may be aided by ultrasound guidance to distinguish bladder and bowel components.

Surgical Management

The important consideration and principle is that enterocele is frequently associated with other separate disorders of the pelvic floor, and each requires surgical repair to achieve satisfactory results. Disorders that

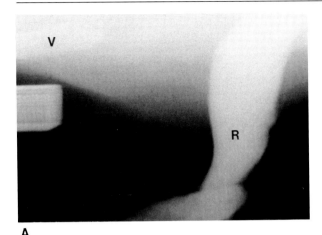

A

B

Fig. 16-9 Defecography showing abnormally large space between vagina *(V)* and rectum *(R)* in **A**. Small bowel opacification *(S)* is shown in **B**, demonstrating enterocele.

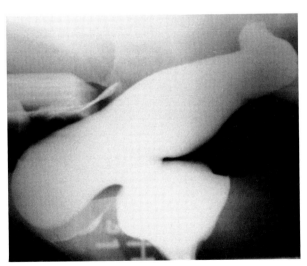

Fig. 16-10 Prolapsed high rectocele diagnosed on defecography and clinically confused with enterocele.

may be associated include cystocele, rectocele, vaginal vault prolapse, and levator hiatal defects. The surgical approach to these repairs may be either abdominal or vaginal. If cystocele is associated, the defect leading to the cystocele must be appreciated as to whether it is lateral, central, or both, and proper repair performed (see Chapter 12). Associated rectocele is repaired by the vaginal approach (Chapter 16). Vaginal vault defect repaired as described in Chapter 13D, either from abdominal or vaginal route, and levatoplasty (see Chapter 14D2) must be performed when levator hiatus is so attenuated and wide that the repaired vault defect has no supportive base. Consideration of the repair of each of these leaves the enterocele principles to be considered as a separate isolated surgical entity. Again, it is emphasized that to attempt repair separately when the other conditions coexist does not lead to an effective solution.

The principles of the enterocele repair are excision of the hernial sac, high ligation of the hernial sac, and adequate supporting structure support.

Abdominal Approach

Recognition of the hernia sac abdominally allows the appreciation of the deep cul-de-sac of Douglas. Closure of this cul-de-sac is performed by using permanent suture interrupted in anterior-posterior direction (see Fig. 16-11). This effectively closes the pouch of Douglas and prevents descent of small bowel into the area. The anterior-posterior sutures prevent two problems that occur with the traditional Moschcowitz purse-string sutures. The Moschcowitz procedure tends to pull the lateral cul-de-sac too far medially and may lead to ureteral obstruction. Also, the upper purse-string stitches can become sufficiently loosened to permit small bowel herniation through them, causing possible bowel obstruction. Both of these objections are overcome by using anterior-posterior interrupted sutures to close the cul-de-sac. Associated vaginal deficiencies must be treated concurrently and abdominal colposacral suspension employed when significant vaginal vault inversion is associated with the enterocele (see Chapter 13D).

Vaginal Route

The vaginal therapy for enterocele involves opening the rectovaginal space to the vaginal apex. At this point, using blunt and sharp dissection, the enterocele sac is dissected free. Frequently, confusion exists regarding the enterocele sac and cystocele. Helpful maneuvers to demonstrate the cystocele at this juncture may be to

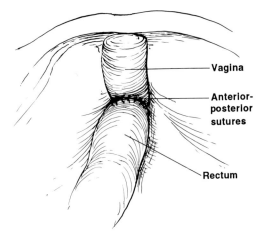

Fig. 16-11 Abdominal approach to enterocele repair. Anterior-posterior (Halban) sutures are used to close the cul-de-sac.

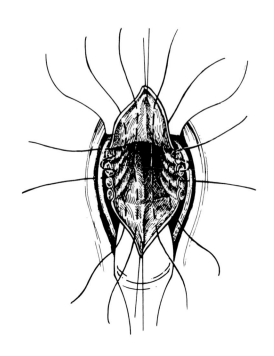

Fig. 16-12 Vaginal approach to enterocele repair. Closure of the cul-de-sac is performed with anterior-posterior sutures. (Reprinted from Nichols DH, Randall CL, *Vaginal Surgery,* 3rd ed, Baltimore: Williams & Wilkins Co; 1989:324, with permission.)

insert a probe into the bladder to palpate the extent of the bladder, or to transluminate the bladder with the cystourethroscope so that the extent of the bladder is seen separately from the enterocele. When the enterocele sac is dissected free, high ligation is performed, usually with permanent suture of gortex, and a pursestring closure made and the sac resected distal to the closure.

Attending fascial support is the next step in the procedure. As mentioned, if associated vault descensus is present, it is corrected with bilateral sacrospinous suspension, as described in Chapter 13D. If the enterocele is isolated and there is no significant vault descensus, then the uterosacral cardinal complex is adequate and can be utilized in a fascial repair. It is important at this juncture to realize that closing the defect might lead to vaginal shortening, which may be prevented by doing the closure as described by McCall.[7] The cul-de-sac may be closed by a sagittal obliteration using interrupted anterior-posterior stitches as described from the abdominal approach (Fig. 16-12). However, if a shortened vagina is a concern, then the McCall colpoplasty (Figs. 16-13A to C) may be employed. The principles underlying this repair is that a spot on the posterior vaginal wall that provides the longest length possible is arbitrarily selected, and a suture is incorporated through this into uterosacral ligaments, then through the peritoneum to close the hernia sac, resulting in a closed hernia sac occupying an anterior position on the vagina which is not at the vaginal apex. This modification is one way to provide fascial support for the closed hernia sac without shortening the vagina. Again, it is

stressed that this type of closure is useful only when the uterosacral cardinal complex is adequately strong, that is, when there is no associated vault inversion. When the latter exists, it must be handled separately and concurrently to provide fascial support to the hernia defect, such as with bilateral sacrospinous fixation (Chapter 13D).

In summary, small congenital enteroceles may be treated with excision of the sac and high ligation and approximation of the uterosacral ligaments, or by abdominally closing the cul-de-sac.

Pulsion enteroceles with associated vaginal vault inversion require sacrospinous fixation or sacrocolpopexy in addition. If the pulsion defect occurs without significant inversion of the vaginal vault and the patient has adequately strong cardinal uterosacral complements, then these components may be utilized in the fascial repair. Modified colpoplasty should be considered to avoid vaginal shortening.

Traction enteroceles usually have associated cystocele and rectocele, so they require the same considerations as a pulsion cystocele. In addition, these require

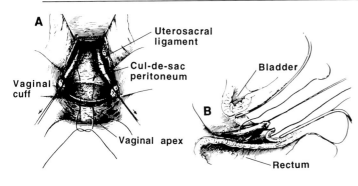

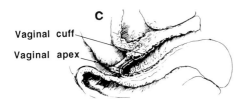

Fig. 16-13 McCall colpoplasty: the preferred closure when a shortened vagina is a consideration. Note the apex of the vagina is now posterior and cranial to the opened cuff. **A**, Sutures through uterosacral ligament, cul-de-sac, peritoneum, and posterior vaginal wall. **B**, Sagittal drawing of sutures placed in **A**. **C**, Sagittal drawing showing vaginal apex supported and cranial and posterior to vaginal cuff. (Reprinted from Nichols DH, Randall CL, *Vaginal Surgery*, 3rd ed, Baltimore: Williams & Wilkins Co; 1989:223, with permission.)

repair of the cystocele and rectocele. In iatrogenic cystoceles the principles of excising or obliterating the sac and restoring the normal vaginal axis become impera-tive. These may frequently be accomplished by sac obliteration from either abdominal or vaginal route with careful attention to restoration of vaginal vault if descensus and attenuation of the uterosacral cardinal ligament complex is present.

SUMMARY

Defects in the perineal compartment of the pelvic floor leading to rectocele, perineal descent, and enterocele are commonly associated with other pelvic floor defects. Modern diagnostic aids employing radiologic, ultrasound, and electrodiagnostic modalities are helpful in understanding the pathophysiology. Surgical repairs performed in a manner that restores normal anatomic relationships serve best to improve surgical success.

REFERENCES

1. Henry MM. Descending perineum syndrome. In: Henry MM, Swash M, eds. *Coloproctology and The Pelvic Floor*. London: Butterworths; 1985:299.
2. Henry MM, Parks AG, Swash M. The pelvic floor musculature in the descending perineum syndrome. *Br J Surg*. 1986;69:470–472.
3. Sunderland S. *Nerves and Nerve Injuries*. 2nd ed. Edinburgh: Churchill Livingstone; 1978:62–66.
4. Block IR. Transrectal repair of rectocele using obliterative suture. *Dis Colon Rect*. 1986;29:707–711.
5. Wilensky AV, Kaufman PA. Vaginal hernia. *Am J Surg*. 1940:49; 31–41.
6. Nichols DH. Types of enterocele and principle underlying the choice of operation for repair. *Obstet Gynecol*. 40:257–263.
7. McCall ML. Posterior culdoplasty; surgical correction of enterocele during vaginal hysterectomy: a preliminary report. *Obstet Base Gynecol*. 1957;10:595.

CHAPTER 17

Rectovaginal Fistulae

Tiffany J. Williams

INTRODUCTION

A rectovaginal fistula is a communication between the rectum and the vagina, irrespective of the location of the fistulous tract or the cause of the defect (congenital, inflammatory, traumatic, iatrogenic, or neoplastic). Because this definition refers to the rectum, the fistula must be located above the dentate line; defects below this line would be anovaginal fistulae or perineal defects. However, a large defect may include communication of perineal or sphincteric defects as well as the rectum itself within the vagina.

This chapter discusses the situations that might result in a rectovaginal fistula, the criteria that might be of help in diagnosis, treatment, and preoperative and postoperative management, as well as consideration of complications and results. A concise overview has been published by Stern and Dreznik.[1]

HISTORY

Rectovaginal fistulae have been a condition of concern since antiquity, occurring subsequent to intercourse, conception, parturition, or tearing of the rectovaginal septum. Indeed, some Egyptian mummies display the presence of a cloaca secondary to trauma of delivery, with tearing not only of the rectovaginal septum but also of the vesicovaginal septum.

In the early days, treatment was based on postural and philosophic measures. Binding the legs in apposition, an inverted position, confinement to bed for 6 weeks (or use of both binding and positioning), or use of unguents and foments all were tried, but to little avail unless spontaneous healing from approximation occurred.

Attempts at surgical treatment apparently were initiated in the 16th century by Guillemeau, a student of Paré. Subsequently, Mauriceau and Smellie, in the 17th and 18th centuries, recommended operation and repair.

Barton[2] was the first to cure a rectovaginal fistula by a surgical procedure in 1840. Multiple procedures were described during the early part of the 19th century, with attempts at freshening, excising, and approximating the fistulous defect; yet, surgical treatment still was considered a last resort in the repertoire of management.

The advent of anesthesia with the use of chloroform allowed better anatomic reconstruction. Use of diet, bowel care (with medications to delay intestinal motility), permanent sutures, and bacteriostatic sutures, such as silver, all were tried with varying degrees of success. The ultimate aim of these techniques was to provide comfort to the patient bothered by continual leakage of bowel content through the vagina and the lack of control of feces and flatus.

ETIOLOGY

The etiologic processes that create a rectovaginal fistula may be divided into congenital, inflammatory, traumatic, and neoplastic types; each of these will be considered separately.

Congenital

A rectovaginal fistula may arise embryologically when the müllerian ducts migrate to the perineum to join with the urogenital sinus.[3] During this time, the müllerian tubercles may incorporate the rectum as a rectovaginal fistula in the back wall of the vagina. Such a condition is uncommon and is likely to be associated with anal agenesis and other urogenital abnormalities. In these instances, the vagina and hymen may appear to be entirely normal.

However, in addition there may be a longitudinal vaginal defect so that the potential exists for a tripartite vagina and communications with both intestinal and urologic systems. Because of the descent of the müllerian tubercles, the fistula generally is located posteriorly and has an oblique entry. There usually is some degree of a cloacal formation even though there may be urethral, vaginal, and rectal separation within this vaginal cloaca. Unfortunately, in many instances it is difficult to describe accurately what has occurred because most patients have undergone one or more surgical procedures—by pediatric, colorectal, or gynecologic surgeons—often with little attention to the embryologic development and the need for appropriate correction. The review by Lescher and Pratt[4] suggests that 12% of rectovaginal fistulae are related to a congenital situation (primarily imperforate anus) and attempts at surgical correction.

Inflammatory

Inflammatory conditions involving the rectovaginal septum were the most common cause found at the Mayo Clinic, being 22% of those reported.[4] Usually, these patients had chronic ulcerative colitis, although extensive Crohn's disease with involvement of the rectum and perineum might well be included in this category.

When one considers a process such as Crohn's disease, an incidence of fistulization between 2% and 4% may be noted.[1] The importance of an accurate history and attention to gastrointestinal symptoms is paramount when considering etiologic possibilities and the opportunity for appropriate surgical correction.

Traumatic

Traumatic injuries to the rectovaginal septum were another early cause of this debilitating injury. These injuries generally were obstetric although, more recently, traumatic injury, as from automobile accident, subsequent irradiation for malignancy, and, currently, surgical misadventure after attempts at reparative surgery, are other possibilities.

Injury

Actual injury from a fall, an accident, or the like was not mentioned in the experience from the Mayo Clinic reported by Lescher and Pratt[4]; however, erosion from a foreign body such as a pessary has been reported, as well as erosion from the use of vaginal stents in reconstructive surgery. Although infrequent, a proctoscope or rectosigmoidoscope may perforate the vagina; however, such gross traumatic damage is infrequent and is unlikely without prompt recognition and care. Hibbard's report[5] in 1978 described such trauma. Reports by others do not include this cause in their incidence data.

Obstetric

Obstetric injuries seem to account for about 10% of rectovaginal damage reported in the current literature worldwide. In the developing countries, such obstetric injuries are more common than iatrogenic, surgical, or treatment complications. It appears to be irrelevant whether these defects are subsequent to obstetric laceration or to the attempts at preventing such laceration by an extended episiotomy or episiorectotomy that failed to heal. In these underdeveloped countries with poor obstetric care and prolonged and difficult attempts at vaginal delivery, there is a higher percentage of obstetric injury and also more extensive damage.

Given reported[6] obstetric injury as being responsible in nearly 40% of rectovaginal fistulae. Hibbard's data[5] are even more impressive: 92% of cases were secondary to obstetric injury.

Surgical

A surgical cause appears to be increasing in frequency and significance in the current gynecologic literature. Surgical trauma as a cause is most common with attempts at repair of symptomatic pelvic relaxation. Such operations for benign disease accounted for 11% of the fistulae reported by Lescher and Pratt.[4] These complications were not noted in Hibbard's report,[5] whereas Given[6] reported 9 (24%) of 38 cases being related to an operative procedure, either posterior repair or hysterectomy.

Irradiation

In regard to rectovaginal fistula, it often is difficult to distinguish between the effects of the malignancy and the effects of the treatment of it. Irradiation for carcinoma of the cervix, endometrium, vagina, rectum, bladder, or urethra may eventuate in fistulization. Such defects require the use of neovascularized tissue for appropriate repair, and it is important to be sure that no tumor is present. Unfortunately, vascular obliteration and subsequent tissue damage may be ongoing in the tissue even after the occurrence of the fistula.

Neoplastic

Neoplastic tumors that eventuate in rectovaginal fistulae may arise from either the vagina or the rectum, although the treatment (either surgery or irradiation) may be the paramount etiologic factor. In this age of patient awareness, a primary fistula developing in an untreated malignant condition is uncommon, because the patient's symptoms of rectal or vaginal bleeding or presence of tumor, mass, or inflammatory reaction would prompt treatment prior to the development of symptoms from the fistula.

DIAGNOSIS

The diagnosis of rectovaginal fistula usually is simplified by the history that can be obtained from the patient, and this generally relates to an episode of trauma—actual damage from an accident, obstetric complication, or surgical misadventure (the technique or complications subsequent to it). One should pay careful attention to a history of intestinal symptoms because inflammatory bowel disease may be a significant factor.

Symptoms

The most common symptom is passage of fecal material through the vagina. Shieh and Gennaro[2] reported this in 77% of their cases in an experience covering 11 years. The second most common symptom, the passage of gas through the vagina, accounted for nearly 30% of complaints in their series. Other symptoms were diarrhea, tenesmus, urinary frequency, abdominal cramps, and rectal bleeding. A burning sensation in the perineum and back pain also were noted.

However, some patients may have absolutely no complaints, and the fistula is an incidental finding during examination. A small rectovaginal fistula may have so little leakage or seepage that it is not detectable by the patient.

Clinical symptoms may be related to the size of the fistulous defect. When the fistula is large, the problems of passage of flatus or feces or vaginal discharge and fecal odor are more likely to occur. These symptoms appear to be common during diarrhea. A history of diseases known to promote diarrhea is important.

Examination

Physical examination would be expected to detect the communication between the rectum and the vagina. The presence of fecal material within the vagina or granulation or inflammatory tissue at the site of the fistula is to be anticipated. Digital palpation should reveal the presence of induration or scarring in the suspected area.

When the fistula is large and its location is low, the opening may be easily visualized during vaginal examination and observation through the speculum. Fecal material within the vagina should be obvious and, when the fistula is large enough, visualization of the rectum itself is possible with the distinct difference between the dark red mucosa of the rectum and the lighter pink of the vaginal mucosa.

A small fistula may be extremely difficult to detect. A small dimple may be the site of the defect, and a silver probe sometimes may be easily passed into the rectum, where it is palpated. If the patient's history is strongly suggestive, despite what would appear to be an absence of findings at the time of examination, additional tests may be required. In the majority of cases, vaginal, rectal, and combined rectovaginal examination should suffice for making or confirming the diagnosis of rectovaginal fistula. Manipulation of the tissues may allow expression of material into the vagina, which further confirms the patient's complaints and facilitates the diagnosis.

Endoscopy

If simple observation and palpation of the vagina and rectum do not detect a fistula, even with a suggestive history, endoscopic evaluation may be helpful. Anoscopy and rectoscopy are not usually available in the gynecologist's office but can be useful in detecting the intestinal component of the defect. Scarring and dimpling may indicate the area of the communication. Rectoscopy was able to diagnose rectovaginal fistula in 59% of the series reported by Shieh and Gennaro.[2]

The use of magnification in the vagina may be helpful and, although the tangential view of the vagina is a problem with use of colposcopy, such optical magnification may delineate the site of communication more clearly.

Radiologic Diagnosis

If simpler methods of diagnosis are not successful, radiologic contrast studies may be of use, such as vaginography, rectography, or, among current techniques, computed tomography (CT)[7] and magnetic resonance imaging (MRI). The latter usually are not necessary, and plain contrast studies generally provide adequate documentation, not only of the presence of the fistula but also of the site(s) and number of communications. Some type of pressure may be required to dilate the fistulous tract adequately for diagnosis. Shieh and Gennaro[2] reported diagnosis by barium enema in 63.6% of their series.

Careful evaluation is necessary to be sure that there is only one communication and to rule out the possibility that there are several that may require correction, particularly when there is an inflammatory condition.

The injection of contrast medium into the vagina under pressure with an occlusive balloon may be required to confirm the diagnosis of a rectovaginal fistula.[8] This is particularly true when contrast studies are initiated through the rectum because pressure may be required to open the communicating defect. Such tests are recommended to determine the number of communications present. The use of a thinner contrast medium is suggested rather than the standard medium for barium enema.

Both MRI and CT, particularly with contrast medium, allow accurate documentation of the diagnosis of rectovaginal fistula. Simpler methods, however, should be used first. These more expensive techniques are considered only as a last resort when confirmation is not possible with more economical means.

Contrast Media

Other simpler techniques using various contrast media without radiation may be helpful. Air, water, and various dyes all have been suggested at one time or another. Even with examination under anesthesia, a small fistula may be difficult to detect. Carey[9] reported that after application of a soap solution in the vagina followed by distention of the rectum with air, the presence of vaginal bubbles confirms the diagnosis and identifies the site of the communication. He recommended anal obstruction by a Foley catheter bulb so that the positive pressure could be suitably applied. Marking of the fistula was recommended if surgery was not planned

at the time of diagnosis. Air injected into the rectum with any fluid present in the vagina should create bubbles with or without a soap solution.

Injection of a fluid such as water or even a dye solution into either the vagina or the rectum may allow visualization of the site of communication when the opposite viscus is observed. Methylene blue is commonly recommended but, because this is a supravital stain, any spillage is likely to be an obfuscating factor by staining adjacent tissue. Tampons may be inserted into either the vagina or rectum when the dye is placed in the opposite organ. It is recommended that the patient be up and moving about during this period so that, if position is important, this will have a chance to cause staining when movement has opened the fistulous tract. These tests may facilitate detection of the site of the fistula by virtue of the area of staining on the tampon itself. When methylene blue is injected into the vagina, proctoscopic visualization is helpful and probably superior to attempts at using a rectal tampon. However, Shieh and Gennaro[2] reported that the methylene blue test was diagnostic in only 9% of their patients.

COMMENT

One can generally anticipate that the history will be of paramount significance in reaching the appropriate diagnosis. Physical examination with visualization and palpation of the rectovaginal septum are most likely to be the confirmatory diagnostic procedures. Proctoscopy and vaginoscopy, particularly when utilized with various dyes, may be useful. However, radiologic confirmation is best in that it documents the site of the communication as well as the number of tracts that are present.

TREATMENT

Observation

If a rectovaginal fistula is small and the symptoms minor, no therapy may be necessary. Unless the passage of gas or feces is noxious to the patient, it is unlikely that such passage is of any significance to her health. Unless a surgical procedure is needed to improve the patient's comfort, whether mental or physical, there is little need for an operation. A small, asymptomatic fistula does not require therapy just because it is present.

Intestinal symptoms such as diarrhea may accentuate the patient's symptoms and then become an indication for therapy. Unfortunately, if such diarrhea is secondary to an underlying bowel disease, correction of this disease itself may be required before the symptoms are eliminated. Such cases are uncommon, and generally the patient's presentation is itself an indication that she has enough difficulty to justify correction. A colon transit study with radiopaque markers may be helpful in assessing the intestinal motility and its effect on the symptoms of rectovaginal fistula.

Even though the history may be characteristic for rectovaginal fistula, an examination under anesthesia may be required before the diagnosis is confirmed. It is obvious that documentation of the defect is required before surgical correction may be accomplished. Although the patient may complain of passage of gas via her vagina, this does not necessarily mean that there is a rectovaginal communication. With minimal symptoms and only diarrhea present, just correction of the intestinal problem may be efficacious. This decision is one in which the patient must consider her discomforts and annoyances relative to the risks and results of an operative procedure.

In general, observation would seem appropriate when the fistula is very small and causing minimal symptoms. Obviously, observation is required when, despite an appropriate history, the diagnosis cannot be confirmed.

Medical

When such defects are of minimal size and consequence, medical manipulations may be appropriate. These include the use of antibiotics if an infection is present and modification of the diet to change intestinal motility and stool quality. If the patient has symptoms only when she has diarrhea, use of low-residue diets and stool bulk enhancers may be appropriate. Changes in frequency of feeding and type of food ingested may be useful with the small, relatively asymptomatic fistulous communication.

A history of inflammatory disease indicates use of antibacterial therapy. However, there is the risk of complications from the treatment itself, such as pseudomembranous colitis. It is recommended that antibiotic therapy be given only when there is a clinical manifestation of an infection.

Surgical

It generally is expected that, when the patient has symptoms of sufficient severity to cause her to seek medical advice, the condition is significant enough to require correction. It is considered uncommon that a fistula of such size as to be diagnosed at routine examination would not cause symptoms. Medical therapy is not expected to be permanently successful but may be useful in those rare instances of intermittent symptoms.

There is strong belief that when the fistula is secondary to an underlying bowel disease, this disease process itself requires correction. Such correction is mandatory prior to expectation of a successful surgical reconstruction. Although some reports[10,11] indicate that surgical correction may be accomplished, the results are likely to be temporary, and it is my opinion that underlying bowel disease per se is a contraindication to an attempt at surgical repair of a rectovaginal fistula caused by the intestinal tract itself.

If repair of the fistula is to be attempted at the patient's insistence, it is important she understands that the results may be temporary and that complete correction of the underlying bowel disease is required before permanent success can be anticipated. Therefore, it is recommended that all primary bowel disease be successfully managed, medically or surgically, prior to definitive attempts at correction of rectovaginal fistulae related to that bowel disease. When such control is achieved, surgical correction may be planned after appropriate tissue healing, generally between 4 and 6 months later. Repeated and unnecessary early attempts at correction are doomed to failure.

Surgical correction of the fistula is related to the size, the position relative to the vaginal location, and the cause (i.e., obstetric, surgical, or radiologic).

Operative Possibilities

A rectovaginal fistula may be repaired through the vagina or the rectum. Gynecologists have preferred to operate through the vagina, and there are several surgical techniques that provide satisfactory results. Three types of procedures generally are considered: (1) layer-by-layer anatomic reconstruction, (2) Warren-flap type of operation, and (3) rectovaginal technique of anterior rectal wall advancement. Repair procedures may be accomplished transvaginally as described by Noble[12] and subsequently Mengert and Fish[13] or through the rectum as described by Rothenberger and Goldberg[14] and others.[15–17] Simple incision of the fistula allowing healing by secondary intention may also result in a satisfactory outcome and fecal control.

Preoperative Management

Once the diagnosis of rectovaginal fistula is confirmed, one must decide on the recommended therapy. The possibilities are: the fistula may heal spontaneously; the symptoms may be so minimal that they do not require surgical correction; or anatomic surgical reconstruction may be required because of the symptoms.

Generally, enough time has elapsed since the trauma that caused the fistula so attempted immediate repair is not a feasible option. However, when the diagnosis is made within 24 hours after a surgical insult, the condition should be amenable to immediate direct correction. Otherwise, attempts at definitive repair should be delayed until tissue healing has become complete. Ordinarily, this would require at least 3 months, and the recommended time between occurrence of the fistula and possible surgical correction is 4 to 6 months to avoid incomplete healing and inflammatory reaction. Although surgery may be desired by the patient, such an attempt may be doomed to failure.

When there is significant inflammatory reaction, subsequent either to the initiating bowel disease or to the fistulization itself, delay in reconstruction is of paramount importance. Indeed, a short-circuiting type of procedure such as colostomy may be recommended to minimize the inflammation and to enhance healing. Such procedures generally are not necessary for a low-lying rectovaginal fistula. However, when there has been antecedent inflammatory bowel disease or significant inflammation related to the fistulization, the possibility of colostomy must be considered and discussed with the patient and her family. If colostomy is decided upon, prompt scheduling of the procedure is wise to allow cleansing of the defect and minimization of the patient's symptoms.

A loop-type colostomy, in either the transverse or descending colon, has the advantage of easier reconstruction and the disadvantage of possible contamination of the distal defect despite the presence of the colostomy. Complete isolation between the ostomy and the distal end will minimize problems of contamination but make subsequent reconstruction more difficult than closure of a loop colostomy. Consideration of these factors and what is best for the patient will facilitate selection of the type of colostomy. Generally, at least 3 months should be allowed for tissue healing after colostomy formation. Similarly, 3 to 4 months should be allowed after reconstruction before consideration of colostomy closure.

Bowel Preparation

Preoperative bowel preparation is recommended in all instances in which entry into, or involvement of, the intestinal lumen is anticipated. It is recommended that preoperative bowel preparation be accomplished prior to fistula closure. The scheduling of this procedure may be facilitated by hospital admission to ensure its accomplishment. Serum electrolyte values may be monitored;

Table 17-1

Standard Laxative Enema/Antibiotic Preoperative Bowel Preparation.

Two Days Preop	One Day Preop	Day of Operation
Minimum residue diet	Clear liquid diet	NPO after midnight
Two tapwater 1000-ml enemas after admission	Three tapwater 1000-ml enemas in morning, three tapwater 1000-ml enemas in afternoon; enemas until clear, up to 8	No enemas
Phosphosoda, 15 ml orally on admission and 4 hours later	Phosphosoda, 15 ml orally at 8:00 AM	No rectal aspirations
	Neomycin, 1 g orally at 1:00 PM, and erythromycin base, 1 g orally at 11:00 PM	

this may be significant with some types of bowel preparations and in patients who have other fluid-balance problems.

A standard laxative enema/antibiotic preoperative bowel preparation appears in Table 17-1. Physical activity is important. The patient should be encouraged to take numerous walks during bowel preparation.

An additional type of preparation recently recommended is the GoLYTELY type. This preparation is shown in Table 17-2.

Procedures

A strongly held belief is that when a primary intestinal disease causes fistula formation, satisfactory and permanent correction of the fistula is not accomplished until the bowel disease is treated successfully. The persistence of diseased intestine eventually will cause another fistula, and permanent repair cannot be expected until all of the disease is removed.

As suggested by Beecham,[11] Bandy and coworkers,[10] and others,[18,19] it may be reasonable to attempt correction of a fistula even though granulomatous bowel disease persists. Should this be considered, it is important that the patient understand that correction may be of only temporary benefit in the absence of diversion or extirpation of the diseased intestine.

Table 17-2
GoLYTELY Preparation

One Day Preop	Day of Operation
Clear liquid diet beginning at noon	Weigh patient at 6:00 AM
No laxatives	NPO from previous 12:00 midnight
GoLYTELY lavage
Drink 4–6 L of GoLYTELY from 12:00 noon to 6:00 PM (need not drink all 6 L if bowel return is clear and remains clear before 6:00 PM). (Keofeed feeding tube may be needed.)
Neomycin, 2 g, 6:00 PM–11:00 PM.
Metronidazole, 2 g, 6:00 PM –11:00 PM (after GoLYTELY is finished)	

However, it is recommended that a definitive single operation be planned for correction of a fistula when the intestinal disease is adequately treated. Once that disease is treated, spontaneous healing of the fistula may occur, obviating the necessity for a specific rectovaginal fistula repair.

The selection of the operative technique is modified by the disease that caused the fistula and by the location of the fistulous tract. A high rectovaginal fistula may require an abdominal approach with separation of the rectum and vagina. Subsequently, each viscus is separately closed in an inverted fashion. Transposition of peritoneum or omentum between the suture lines separates them satisfactorily and improves the opportunity for healing of both rectum and vagina without subsequent refistulization.

Rosenshein and colleagues[20] developed a classification system based on anatomic location to help decide on the type of operative procedure best suited for the patient. A high rectovaginal fistula may be treated through the vagina by using a Latsko-type closure[21] in which the tract is dissected free and closed and the vagina itself is obliterated in its upper portion with several layers of sutures to create broad tissue apposition without tension (Fig. 17-1). Fistulae in the middle or lower vagina appear to be best managed transvaginally. A small fistula in the lower or middle vagina may be repaired after the preoperative preparation. Under suitable anesthesia and with the patient in the dorsolithotomy position, a pack is placed in the upper vagina to minimize genital tract contamination if the uterus is

still present. A circumcising incision may be made through the vaginal mucosa around the fistulous opening. Dissection is then continued laterally beneath the vaginal mucosa away from the fistula until healthy tissues are reached (Fig. 17-2).

Such small fistulae may be closed by a purse-string suture inverting into the rectum. When fistulae are small, it is recommended that the tract not be excised but merely inverted. Such techniques minimize the extent of the dissection that is required as well as limit the size of the rectal defect. A 3-0 chromic catgut or a nonreactive polyglycolic acid type suture works very satisfactorily. A second purse-string suture may be placed, and even a third if deemed appropriate. After this, the submucosa and muscularis may be approximated with either continuous or interrupted sutures of the same material; size 2-0 or 0 is recommended for these subsequent layers. The mucosa then may be approximated with a continuous suture, which may be locked or not, of 2-0 or 0 material.

When the rectovaginal fistula is larger (Fig. 17-3) a more complete dissection is necessary so that the edges may be approximated without tension and there is adequate mobilization of both rectal and vaginal walls to allow closure without tension. Once the tissues are dissected free, the defect may be closed by whichever method creates the least tension. It is my preference to utilize a continuous suture for the first layer in the submucosal portion of the intestine. A second layer of interrupted or mattress type sutures into the muscularis completes the intestinal portion of the reconstruction. It is suggested that the edges of the defect be inverted into the intestinal lumen and that the subsequent sutures further invert the preceding ones. After the bowel is closed with this two-layer technique, the overlying pararectal tissues may be approximated with 0 or 2-0 interrupted sutures. Further plication of the puborectalis component of the levatores may add support to the reconstruction. The vaginal mucosa then may be closed in a longitudinal fashion with a continuous suture locking it for better hemostasis. It is recommended that dead space be obliterated with additional sutures if required.

When the defects are lower, as commonly seen with obstetric laceration, an anatomic layered reconstruction may be preferable (Fig. 17-4). In these instances, an incision is made around the scarred defect between the rectum and the vagina. When there is a complete perineal laceration, the excision should be extended laterally and deeply enough into the perineum so that the ends of the sphincter muscle are located and approximated. An incision upward into the vagina frequently is required for adequate dissection, this being in the

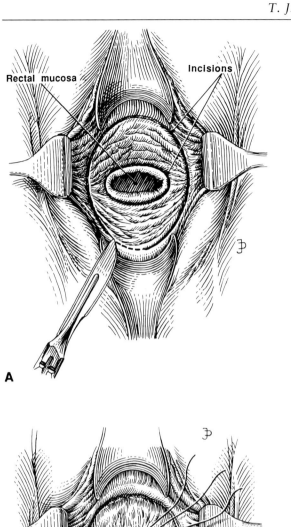

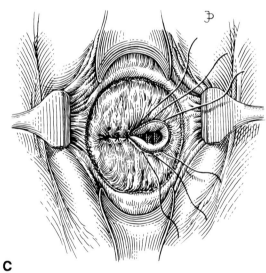

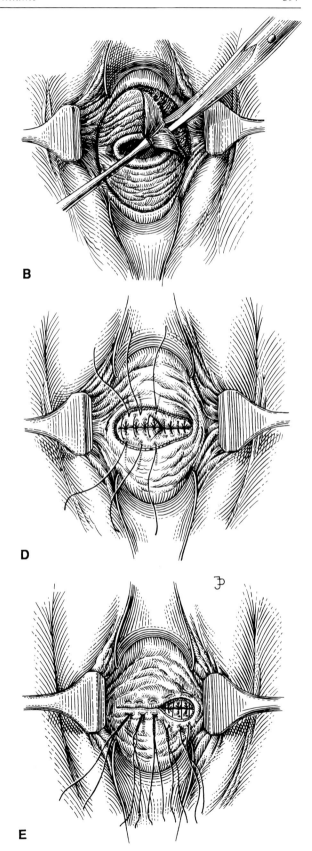

Fig. 17-1 Closure of rectovaginal fistula by Latzko technique. **A**, Incisions around margins of fistula. **B**, Excision of mucosa from anterior and posterior vaginal walls. **C**, The first line of sutures is placed, inverting the edge into the rectal lumen. **D**, The first line of sutures has been placed and tied. The second line of sutures is being placed into the rectal musculature and fascia. Note horizontal mattress sutures in the second layer. **E**, Vertical or horizontal mattress sutures of delayed-absorbable suture form the third layer of closure. (Reprinted from Mattingly and Thompson[21] with permission.)

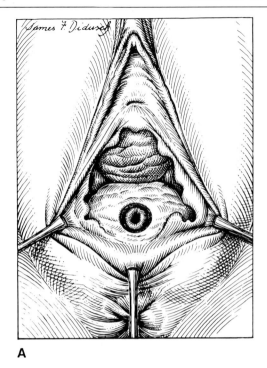

A

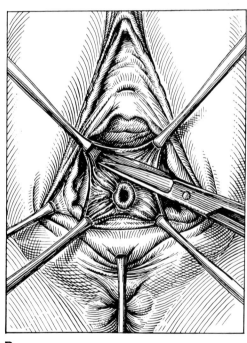

B

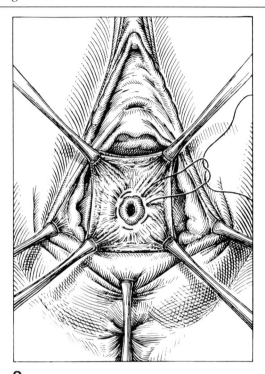

C

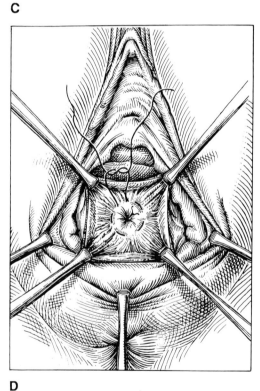

D

Fig. 17-2 Repair of small rectovaginal fistula. **A**, Circular incision through the vaginal mucosa is made about the fistulous opening. **B**, Flaps of vaginal mucosa are dissected free for about 2 cm from the margin of the fistulous opening. **C**, A 3-0 delayed absorbable material purse-string suture is placed about the fistulous opening. **D**, The first purse-string is tied, inverting the fistulous opening. The second purse-string is placed and is about to be tied. **E**, The second purse-string is tied, and a third is placed. **F**, Submucosal-muscularis tissues are approximated with 2-0 continuous or interrupted delayed absorbable sutures. **G**, The mucosa is closed with a continuous lock stitch of 2-0 suture. (Reprinted from Mattingly and Thompson[21] with permission.)

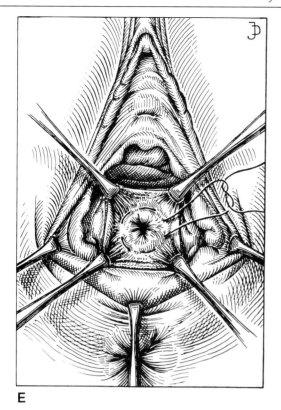

E

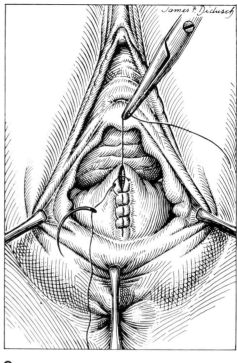

G

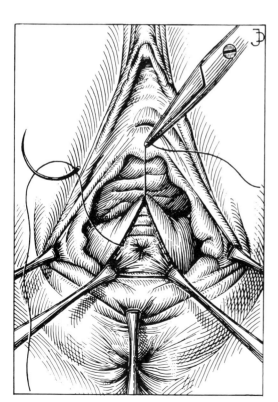

F

form of an inverted "Y." It is recommended that scar tissue be excised from the margins and that the dissection continue cephalad and laterally so that tissue approximation is accomplished with broad surfaces and no tension. After completing dissection the anorectal mucosa and submucosa are approximated by full-thickness suturing if a submucosal suture is not feasible. These sutures should tend to invert the mucosa into the intestinal lumen and then be supported by an additional layer in the muscularis of the rectum or anus.

Once intestinal closure is accomplished, sphincter repair may be carried out. Although the ends of the sphincter may be difficult to locate, this can generally be accomplished by locating the ends with an Allis clamp in the region of the dimple where retraction has occurred. Use of nerve stimulators facilitates identification of the anal sphincter at the beginning of the operation and documents its integrity at the end. Interrupted mattress type sutures, either long-acting resorbable or permanent, are satisfactory.

Our preference is to use a permanent nonreactive suture of size 0; three or four sutures may be required. The continuity of the sphincter may be tested with a regloved finger so that, if additional sutures are needed, they may be placed prior to proceeding to the perineal reconstruction. The puborectalis should be approx-

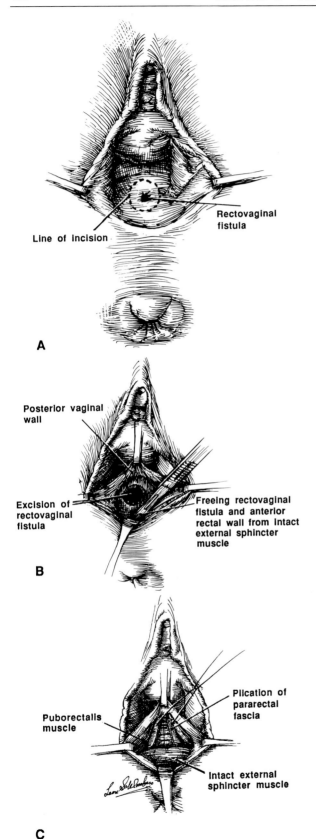

Line of incision

Rectovaginal fistula

A

Posterior vaginal wall

Excision of rectovaginal fistula

Freeing rectovaginal fistula and anterior rectal wall from intact external sphincter muscle

B

Puborectalis muscle

Plication of pararectal fascia

Intact external sphincter muscle

C

Fig. 17-3 Repair of large rectovaginal fistula. **A**, Opening of the fistula in the posterior vaginal wall. The incision is indicated by the dotted line. **B**, A broad flap of vaginal mucosa is dissected away from the margin of the fistula. **C**, Interrupted inverting sutures are placed in the margin of the fistula. When these sutures are tied, the fistulous opening will be inverted. The pararectal fascia is plicated over the rectal wall to support the initial suture layers. The puborectalis muscle should be plicated to add further support to the anal canal and perineal body. (Reprinted from Mattingly and Thompson[21] with permission.)

imated as well as the pararectal tissues, further supporting the repair, obliterating dead space, and increasing the size of the perineal body.

Dead space should be avoided and constriction of the vagina must be considered if the sutures are placed too far cephalad. Subsequent closure of the vaginal mucosa may be accomplished after the excision of any redundant tissue that is present. The perineal reconstruction is more comfortable if the last layer of sutures is placed in a subcuticular fashion rather than through-and-through sutures.

An earlier operation was recommended by John Warren of Harvard and is known as the Warren-flap technique.[22] In this procedure, a curved incision is made 2 cm to 3 cm into the vaginal mucosa above the scarred defect and continued down laterally in an inverted "U" fashion to the ends of the sphincter muscle (Fig. 17-5). The full thickness of the vaginal wall is then dissected downward until the ends of the sphincter are located; the dissected vagina then forms the flap that becomes the anterior wall of the rectum. Subsequently, the sphincter end may be approximated with interrupted or mattress sutures of permanent or delayed resorbable material. The pararectal tissues and levator components are approximated, dead space is obliterated, and the vaginal mucosa is closed in a longitudinal fashion. This then leaves the flap, which may further serve as an "apron" to protect the vaginal reconstruction from fecal contamination. It is recommended that trimming of apparent excess tissue be delayed to avoid possible retraction and to allow healing that may obviate additional tissue excision. It is important to avoid "buttonholing" into the rectal mucosa during the dissection of the flap, but the procedure has the definitive advantage of avoiding suture and dissection into the rectal mucosa, the repair being completed entirely from the vaginal side of the defect.

With an inflammatory condition, it is important to ascertain whether multiple fistulae are present. In such instances, all of them must be resected or appropriately closed because any communication with the intestinal

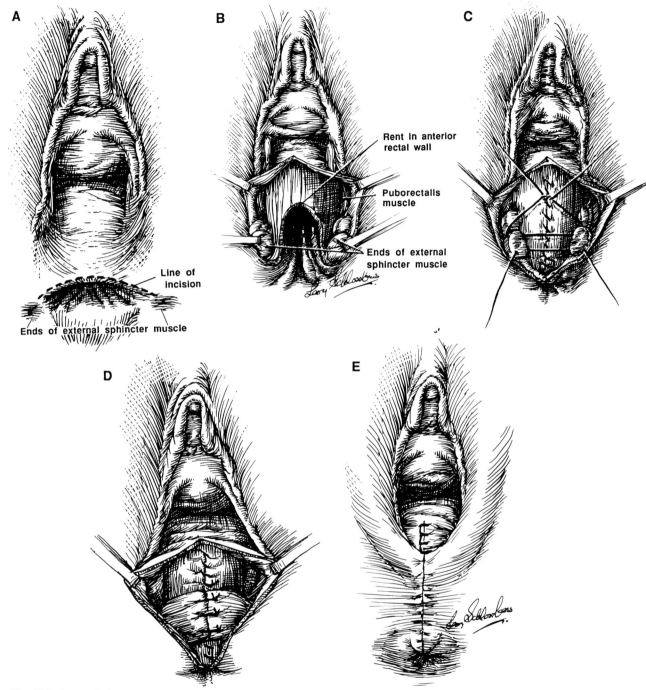

Fig. 17-4 Layered closure of a complete third-degree perineal laceration with anal extension. **A**, A small transverse incision is made at the junction of the vaginal and rectal mucosa. Toward the ends of the sphincter, which are seen as dimples, is the remnant of the perineum. A midline incision is made in the mucosa of the lower one half of the posterior vaginal wall. **B**, The ends of the lower portion of the anal sphincter are identified and grasped with Allis clamps. **C**, The rent in the anal mucosa is closed with a continuous 3-0 delayed absorbable suture. A second, supporting layer of interrupted sutures is placed in the submucosa and inner muscularis to invert the mucosal edges into the bowel lumen. **D**, After approximating the base loop and possibly the intermediate loop of the external anal sphincter with two or three delayed absorbable or permanent sutures as shown in **C**, the puborectalis muscles are brought together with deep interrupted 0 or 1 sutures. **E**, The vaginal mucosa is closed with a continuous lock stitch of 2-0 delayed absorbable suture which is continued subcuticularly to approximate the perineal skin. (Reprinted from Mattingly and Thompson[21] with permission.)

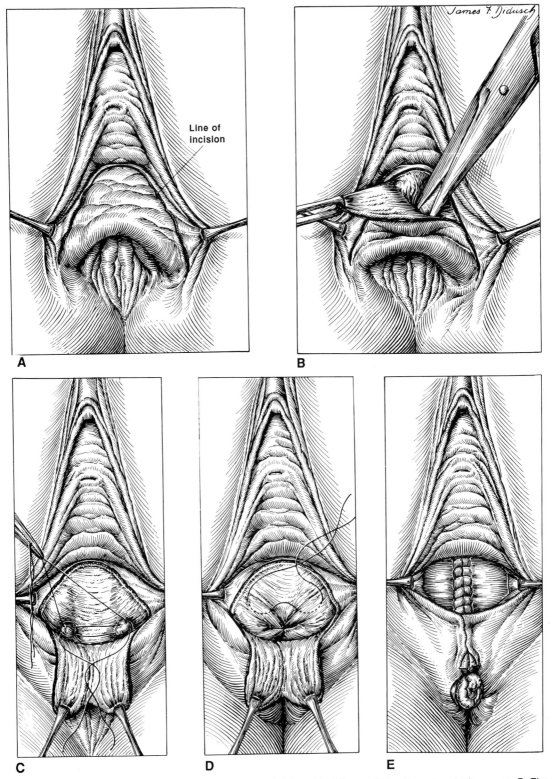

Fig. 17-5 Warren-flap operation for complete third-degree tear. **A**, Line of incision, outlining flap of vaginal mucosa. **B**, The flap is dissected free and turned back. **C**, The flap is retracted downward. The ends of the sphincter are delivered and are sutured with delayed absorbable sutures. **D**, The sphincter ends are united, and the puborectalis muscles are approximated in the midline with 0 sutures. **E**, The vaginal incision is closed with a continuous lock stitch that is continued subcuticularly over the perineum. The margins of the flap are included in the continuous suture, which may create a peaked appearance, temporarily, to the perineal skin. If redundant, it may be trimmed. (Reprinted from Mattingly and Thompson[21] with permission.)

lumen allows possible fecal and bacterial contamination with subsequent infection, abscess formation, and breakdown of an otherwise well-executed operation.

An additional technique that may be considered as ancillary to the above-described methods is the use of the paradoxic incision. Described by Miller and Brown,[23] this attempted to improve the success of rectovaginal fistula repair and to avoid the long immobilization recommended with previous techniques. They reasoned that relief of tension on the reconstructed sphincter would allow better healing; indeed, this raises the question of sphincterotomy as an initial step to facilitate approximation of the sphincter. Although their study reported no controls, they did document an improvement with restoration of function in 87% of the patients with paradoxic incision compared to 71% without paradoxic incision. They recommended the incision be made in the posterior quadrant at about the 4 to 5 o'clock position, and specifically pointed out that an immediate posterior incision was not likely to be useful. They further recommended the use of the flap type procedure as opposed to that described by Noble[12] or the layered technique.

Mengert and Fish[13] repopularized the operation described by Noble[12] in 1902, which consisted of an advancement of the anterior anorectal wall (Fig. 17-6). This has the advantage of not having the suture lines from the repairs of the rectum and vagina in close approximation to each other. The procedure is initiated with an inverted "Y" incision at the edges of the defect, with the base of the "Y" continuing cephalad into the vagina. Dissection is then continued between the rectovaginal septum and the bowel wall. As the rectum is freed, it is advanced downward toward the edges of the sphincter, which is then located and approximated over the advanced rectal wall. After completion of the approximation of the levatores and the pararectal tissue, the vaginal mucosa is closed, as is the perineum, and the operation is completed with approximation of the anal mucosa to the adjacent perineal skin. When closed, the incision has the appearance of an inverted "Y." Interrupted sutures may be utilized in the vagina and perineum but are likely to be more uncomfortable than a subcuticular technique in the perineum itself.

More complicated rectovaginal fistulae, such as those caused by irradiation, are unlikely to be cured by the above conventional techniques. The factors of paramount importance are wide tissue apposition, closure without tension, obliteration of dead space, and good blood supply along with appropriate hemostasis. In the case of an irradiation-induced defect, there is poor blood supply and significant scarring. Accordingly, correction of such defects requires the addition of new tissue and new blood supply.[23–31]

A technique that is most useful is the bulbocavernous transplant, or Martius flap. Boronow,[25] Aartsen and Sindram,[24] and others reported success with this technique. Indeed, Boronow[25] was able to accomplish successful closure in nearly 85% of rectovaginal fistulae cases without mortality or significant surgical morbidity. Colostomy was not required. The technique involves excision of scar tissue and attention to the tenets previously described. With wide dissection, adequate mobilization, freshened edges, and inverting closure, the use of chromic or delayed resorbable sutures is appropriate. Adequate visualization may require an episiotomy or Schuchart-type incision. After the rectal defect is closed, a vulvar incision is placed and dissection is carried down to the bulbocavernosus muscle and fat pad. This pad is then dissected free and, in the case of a rectovaginal fistula, the blood supply is kept intact through the posterior pedicle from the external pudendal vessels. A tunnel is then made beneath the vulva and vaginal mucosa to the area of the fistula repair. The pad is sutured in place over the repair of the rectal wall. Subsequently, the tissues between the rectum and the vagina may be approximated; then the vaginal mucosa and the vulvar defect are closed. It is suggested that a drain be left in place at the dependent portion of the vulvar incision.

An additional modification is the use of a full-thickness vulvar flap. This technique requires excision of the vaginal mucosa and rotation of an "island" flap (full-thickness vulvar skin and underlying fatty tissue). This flap is then sutured in place, approximating the vulvar skin to the vaginal mucosa. A further modification includes a combination of the Martius flap and vulvar skin,[28] again providing additional blood supply and tissue to allow approximation without tension.

Additional operations may be accomplished from the abdominal route by using bowel with its own blood supply to form an interpositioning flap type reconstruction as described by Bricker and coworkers.[27]

POSTOPERATIVE MANAGEMENT

General Aspects

Postoperative management follows the basic rules that apply after any operative procedure. The postoperative analgesia and fluid and electrolyte monitoring are as with any postoperative patient. Immobilization is not required, and the patient generally is allowed bathroom

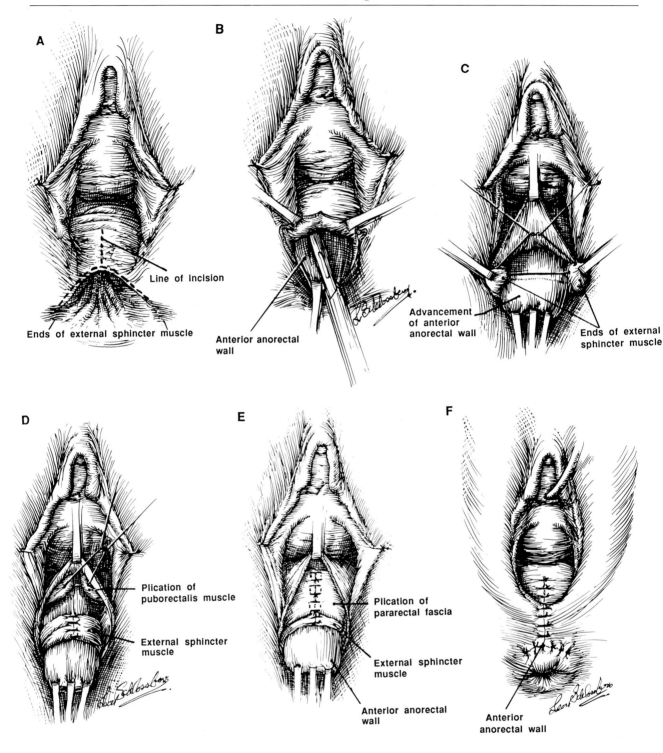

Fig. 17-6 Noble-Mengert procedure. **A**, An initial linear incision is made in the margin of rectovaginal septum. **B**, The anal wall is widely separated laterally from vagina by using Metzenbaum scissors or a medium-blade scalpel. **C**, The rectal wall is withdrawn outside the site of the anal orifice, and the lower loops of the external anal sphincter are dissected free and approximated with deeply placed delayed absorbable or Tycron sutures. **D**, Plication of puborectalis muscle is continued after ligatures are tied in external sphincter. **E**, The anal wall is drawn outside the anal orifice and the pararectal fascia is plicated. **F**, The vaginal mucosa and perineal skin are closed and the anal mucosa is sutured to the perianal skin. (Reprinted From Mattingly and Thompson[21] with permission.)

privileges unless a urethral catheter is required to monitor fluid balance or because of limited mobility.

It is generally recommended that nothing be given by mouth until there is resumption of intestinal activity after the effects of anesthesia are gone. Progression through liquid, soft, and full diet is to be expected, as tolerated by the patient. However, it is recommended that a low-residue diet be considered. The use of constipating medication has been part of the past treatment, but is not now thought to have any advantage, and was discontinued in our institution some years ago.

Other medical management of intestinal motility, bulk, and quality may be considered. Hard stool and straining should be avoided and, for these reasons, softeners and bulk enhancers such as Metamucil may be helpful once the patient has resumed full diet and activity. Laxatives containing oil or those that promote looseness of the stool are best avoided, as they penetrate the suture line and allow infection with subsequent breakdown.

Antibiotic coverage during the operation and the subsequent 48 hours is appropriate if there is significant infection present. Resumption of activity from the standpoint of diet, fluids, and mobilization need not be modified. Prolonged hospitalization is not required, although it is preferred that the patient have a bowel movement prior to dismissal so that the early results can be assessed objectively.

Postoperative rectal examination and enemas should be avoided, and it is important to stress this to the patient so that she knows that she is not to have an enema, whether or not this order is specifically written and discussed with the nursing staff.

Complications

Infection

Contamination of the incision with bowel contents, either at operation or by a flare-up of an occult infection in unhealed tissues, is a primary concern. Antibiotic coverage during the operation is preferred; it need not be continued past 48 hours postoperatively unless there is clinical evidence of an active inflammatory process.

If infection does occur, appropriate management is required. The use of warm, dry heat is helpful with all patients. With infection, moist heat is useful, and sitz baths may help allow drainage away from the operative site so that the repair maintains its integrity. If an abscess develops, drainage is required, and this should be placed as far from the operative site as is feasible.

Breakdown

Breakdown is unlikely to occur unless there is infection. However, patients who have been on long-term steroid therapy may have poor or delayed healing. In these instances, additional permanent through-and-through sutures may be advantageous for minimizing tissue separation unrelated to infection. Breakdown is nearly always related to infection, and sitz baths are recommended with intermittent use of dry heat. Even if there is infection, once breakdown and drainage have occurred, further treatment with antibiotics is rarely necessary. Methods to facilitate healing, such as use of moist and dry heat, are recommended with the goal of avoiding recurrence of the fistula. Hospitalization is generally not prolonged because home care is satisfactory during the healing process.

Recurrence

The fistula may recur after infection and breakdown. Should this happen, techniques to promote healing are appropriate. Other than drainage of an abscess, no other surgical approach is required. However, with inflammatory bowel disease, colostomy may be indicated if the inflammatory disease is the cause. This should be performed as soon as possible to minimize the patient's morbidity, to promote healing, and to facilitate earlier subsequent reconstruction.

If the fistula recurs late, this generally is related to incomplete removal of fistulous tract or abscess areas or the presence of inflammatory bowel disease. With a recurrent fistula, more consideration is given to the use of colostomy prior to subsequent attempts at reconstruction.

RESULTS

Miller and Brown[23] were able to restore function in 87% of their patients with primary operation using a paradoxic incision; the procedure most commonly used was the Warren flap. Lescher and Pratt[4] reported healing in 82% of their patients; only two patients had a colostomy. Mengert and Fish[13] reported complete healing in all of their patients after the Noble-type procedure. Noble[12] himself reported satisfactory results in all of his five patients. In irradiated patients Boronow[25] was able to achieve 84% satisfactory results with the use of additional new tissue and blood supply. Hibbard[5] reported satisfactory healing with no further complications in 49 of 51 patients.

Thus, the operative techniques currently available

allow satisfactory repair of rectovaginal fistulae. It is important that the fistula be symptomatic, the diagnosis be complete, and inflammatory granulomatous bowel disease be excluded. If satisfactory tissue healing is allowed with appropriate bowel preparation to avoid contamination and an appropriate surgical technique is used, satisfactory results in more than 90% of cases can be anticipated.

SUMMARY

Adequate diagnosis and appropriate delay in surgical attempts are necessary so healing is complete and inflammation is minimized. Bowel diversion or adequate cleansing or both along with appropriate surgical technique are important. Such surgical techniques involve broad tissue apposition, suturing without tension, avoidance of dead space, good blood supply, meticulous hemostasis, and avoidance of leakage with subsequent contamination and infection. These characteristics may be accomplished by the layered closure, by the Warren-flap procedure, or by the Noble-Mengert rectal advancement.[12,13] Paradoxic incision[23] is not required, but if there are irradiation-induced changes, new tissue and blood supply are necessary for satisfactory results.

REFERENCES

1. Stern HS, Dreznik Z. Rectovaginal fistula. *Adv Surg*. 1987;21: 245–262.
2. Shieh CJ, Gennaro AR. Rectovaginal fistula: a review of 11 years experience. *Int Surg*. 1984;69:69–72.
3. de Vries PA. High, intermediate, and low anomalies in the female. *Birth Defects*. 1988;24:73–98.
4. Lescher TC, Pratt JH. Vaginal repair of the simple rectovaginal fistula. *Surg Gynecol Obstet*. 1967;124:1317–1321.
5. Hibbard LT. Surgical management of rectovaginal fistulas and complete perineal tears. *Am J Obstet Gynecol*. 1978;130:139–141.
6. Given FT Jr. Rectovaginal fistula: a review of 20 years' experience in a community hospital. *Am J Obstet Gynecol*. 1970;108:41–46.
7. Kuhlman JE, Fishman EK. CT evaluation of enterovaginal and vesicovaginal fistulas. *J Comput Assist Tomogr*. 1990;14:390–394.
8. Arnold MW, Aguilar PS, Stewart WRC. Vaginography: an easy and safe technique for diagnosis of colovaginal fistulas. *Dis Colon Rectum*. 1990;33:344–345.
9. Carey JC. A new method of diagnosing rectovaginal fistula: a case report. *J Reprod Med*. 1988;33:789–790.
10. Bandy LC, Addison A, Parker RT. Surgical management of rectovaginal fistulas in Crohn's disease. *Am J Obstet Gynecol*. 1983; 147:359–363.
11. Beecham CT. Recurring rectovaginal fistulas. *Obstet Gynecol*. 1972;40:323–326.
12. Noble GH. A new operation for complete laceration of the perineum designed for the purpose of eliminating danger of infection from the rectum. *Tr Am Gynec Soc*. 1902;27:357–363.
13. Mengert WF, Fish SA. Anterior rectal wall advancement: technic for repair of complete perineal laceration and rectovaginal fistula. *Obstet Gynecol*. 1955;5:262–267.
14. Rothenberger DA, Goldberg SM. The management of rectovaginal fistulae. *Surg Clin North Am*. 1983;63:61–79.
15. Jones IT, Fazio VW, Jagelman DG. The use of transanal rectal advancement flaps in the management of fistulas involving the anorectum. *Dis Colon Rectum*. 1987;30:919–923.
16. Hoexter B, Labow SB, Moseson MD. Transanal rectovaginal fistula repair. *Dis Colon Rectum*. 1985;28:572–575.
17. Lowry AC, Thorson AG, Rothenberger DA, Goldberg SM. Repair of simple rectovaginal fistulas: influence of previous repairs. *Dis Colon Rectum*. 1988;31:676–678.
18. Cohen JL, Stricker JW, Schoetz DJ Jr, Coller JA, Veidenheimer MC. Rectovaginal fistula in Crohn's disease. *Dis Colon Rectum*. 1989;32:825–828.
19. Francois Y, Descos L, Vignal J. Conservative treatment of low rectovaginal fistula in Crohn's disease. *Int J Colorectal Dis*. 1990; 5:12–14.
20. Rosenshein NB, Genadry RR, Woodruff JD. An anatomic classification of rectovaginal septal defects. *Am J Obstet Gynecol*. 1980;137:439–442.
21. Mattingly RF, Thompson JD, *Te Linde's Operative Gynecology*, 6th ed. Philadelphia: JB Lippincott; 1985;669–686.
22. Warren JC. A new method of operation for the relief of rupture of the perineum through the sphincter and rectum. *Trans Am Gynecol Soc*. 1882;7:322–330.
23. Miller NF, Brown W. The surgical treatment of complete perineal tears in the female. *Am J Obstet Gynecol*. 1937;34:196–209.
24. Aartsen EJ, Sindram IS. Repair of the radiation-induced rectovaginal fistulas without or with interposition of the bulbocavernosus muscle (Martius procedure). *Eur J Surg Oncol*. 1988;14:171–177.
25. Boronow RC. Repair of the radiation-induced vaginal fistula utilizing the Martius technique. *World J Surg*. 1986;10:237–248.
26. Gorenstein L, Boyd JB, Ross TM. Gracilis muscle repair of rectovaginal fistula after restorative proctocolectomy: report of two cases. *Dis Colon Rectum*. 1988;31:730–734.
27. Bricker EM, Johnston WD, Patwardhan RV. Repair of postirradiation damage to colorectum: a progress report. *Ann Surg*. 1981;193:555–564.
28. Falandry L, Lahaye F, Marara C. Le lambeau pédiculé cutanéograisseux de la grande lèvre dans le traitement des fistules vésicovaginales complexes: a propos de 11 cas. *J Urol (Paris)*. 1990;96: 97–102.
29. Elkins TE, DeLancey JOL, McGuire EJ. The use of modified Martius graft as an adjunctive technique in vesicovaginal and rectovaginal fistula repair. *Obstet Gynecol*. 1990;75:727–733.
30. Falandry L. La double autoplastie de la grande lèvre dans la cure des fistules vésico-recto-vaginales d'origine obstétricale: a propos de dix-sept cas. *J Chir (Paris)*. 1990;127:107–112.
31. Anderl H. Refinements in closure of radiation induced rectovaginal fistula. *J Plast Surg*. 1989;12:183–185.

CHAPTER 18

Constipation

Geoffrey K. Turnbull

INTRODUCTION

When patients complain of constipation they may mean many things. The first responsibility of the clinician is to determine what the patient means by the term "constipation."[1-2] Many definitions are used, varying from stool weight, stool frequency, and even stool consistency. A useful guideline that is generally accepted as a normal range of bowel frequency is 3 times per day to 3 times per week.[1-7] Therefore, patients moving their bowels twice a week or less would fit a diagnosis of constipation.[2,4,5] Many patients who complain of constipation, however, have a bowel frequency that falls within the "normal" range, yet find that the associated symptoms they have with the change in bowel habit is significant enough to complain to a physician about. The most common associated symptoms are a feeling of having to strain at stool, abdominal pain or abdominal bloating, and an awareness of dissatisfaction or feeling of incomplete rectal emptying after passing stool. All these symptoms may be of prime importance and are important to clarify when a patient presents with constipation.

During the investigation and treatment of a constipated patient, an understanding of the many causes of constipation is required. There are many secondary causes and primary or "idiopathic" colonic causes of constipation that must be considered but successful treatment of constipation most often results if a secondary or "dietary" cause of constipation is found and corrected. Because of the widely held belief that bowel frequency has to be daily to be "healthy,"[1] it is important to clarify whether a patient actually is suffering any associated symptoms with an infrequent bowel habit. Many women have a normal bowel frequency less than once a day[2,5] and are quite normal at three times a week. Patient reassurance is most important along with the avoidance of laxative use to increase an otherwise normal bowel frequency.

To begin, the causes of constipation are reviewed along with a synopsis of normal colonic and anorectal function. Then the clinical features and therapeutic measures are reviewed that may alleviate the constipation and its associated symptoms.

PATHOGENESIS

The causes of constipation can be varied or multifactorial in some patients. Constipation is only a symptom that may be due to a number of underlying disorders. There are three broad categories of disorders that cause constipation: systemic factors that affect normal colonic and rectal function, primary colonic and anorectal factors (including disorders in pelvic floor function), and finally psychological factors. All can affect colonic function resulting in constipation (Box 18-1).

Box 18-1
Causes of Constipation

1. Primary (Idiopathic)
   Hereditary
2. Secondary
   A. Inadequate dietary fiber
   B. Drug therapy
   C. Metabolic/endocrine
      Hypothyroidism
      Diabetes
      Hypercalcemia
      Hyperparathyroidism
      Hypokalemia
   D. Infiltrative
      Scleroderma
      Amyloidosis
   E. Neurologic
      CNS
         Frontal lobe disease
         Multiple sclerosis
      Peripheral
         Pudendal neuropathy
         Pelvic parasympathetic damage
      Intestinal
         Chaga's disease
3. Psychological factors
   Irritable bowel syndrome

SYSTEMIC FACTORS

Metabolic and Endocrine Factors

Hypothyroidism, diabetes, and all causes of hypercalcemia, including hyperparathyroidism, can cause constipation. Any severe electrolyte abnormality such as hyponatremia or hypokalemia can cause colonic neuromuscular dysfunction and be manifest with constipation.[8]

Diabetes warrants special mention, as constipation is a very common symptom. Constipation is often present early in the disease with the exact cause being unclear, but is probably multifactorial. Diet may play a role, but a diabetic diet should be high in fiber when refined carbohydrates are removed from the diet. A recent study[9] implicated hyperglucagonemia as a cause for delayed small bowel transit even before any changes of autonomic neuropathy develop. Diabetic patients with long-standing disease may have autonomic neuropathy as a contributing factor to the constipation.

Hypothyroidism frequently presents with constipation. This appears to be caused by a delay in intestinal transit[10] which is reversed by thyroid replacement. Hyperparathyroidism, by causing hypercalcemia, also causes constipation, presumably through a direct effect of the elevated calcium concentration on normal intestinal muscle function with delayed intestinal transit.

Systemic Diseases Causing Changes in Colonic Function

Diseases that cause structural changes in the intestine frequently result in constipation. These are rare but include diseases such as scleroderma and amyloidosis, where the intestinal muscle and nerves are gradually destroyed. These diseases can affect both the small and large bowel with widespread effects on intestinal function, usually leading to intestinal pseudoobstruction.[11] Some patients with scleroderma may present with diarrhea, and in these patients there is a reduction in the normal compliance of the rectosigmoid colon.[12]

Neurologic Disorders

Neurologic abnormalities are frequently associated with constipation. These can be divided into two groups: those diseases that affect primarily the central nervous system[13–16] and those diseases that affect the peripheral nerve innervation of the colon, particularly the sacral outflow tract.[17–20] Any central neurologic disease may be associated with constipation. The symptom of the constipation may be caused by the reduced physical activity of patients with severe central nervous system disorders, yet the effect of exercise on colonic transit can be quite variable.[21,22] There is mounting evidence that patients with spinal cord diseases such as multiple sclerosis have constipation as a frequent symptom.[14] It is not uncommon for constipation to be a very disabling symptom in paraplegic and quadriplegic patients.[15,16]

The parasympathetic sacral outflow tract is particularly vital for normal colonic function.[17,19] Methods of assessing the integrity of the sacral outflow tract are still limited, but new data from implanted stimulators in patients who are paraplegic or quadriplegic suggests there is some direct influence of the sacral outflow tract on the frequency of colonic motor activity.[18] There is evidence for both autonomic and somatic pelvic neuropathy in some constipated patients (see Chapter 5).

Miscellaneous

Other systemic factors that may have constipation associated with them are severe disability due to cardiorespiratory disease, presumably caused by impaired blood supply, oxygenation, or both to the colon; and the lack of physical activity or drugs used to treat the disease.

Anorexia nervosa, a disorder that affects primarily young women, is frequently associated with constipation. Most evidence indicates that this is caused by the severe disorder in diet of these patients,[24] but there may be intrinsic changes secondary to the neuropsychiatric dysfunction in anorexia nervosa that can contribute to constipation. One study found that patients with anorexia nervosa and bulimia nervosa had prolonged gut transit which was hypothesized to contribute to the eating disorder by making patients feel "bloated"[25] and possibly by causing rectal distention which has been shown to delay gastric emptying.[26]

Drug therapy is probably the most common cause of constipation following inadequate dietary fiber. Many drugs cause constipation, and a careful drug history of both prescription and over-the-counter medications must be tabulated to identify drugs taken that may cause constipation. Box 18-2 lists some common drugs that are associated with constipation as a side effect, but most drugs have the ability to aggravate constipation in some patients.

Box 18-2
Drugs Commonly Associated with Constipation

Prescription Medications
Anticholinergics
Antidepressants
Beta blockers
Calcium channel blockers
Cholestyramine
Diuretics
Narcotic analgesics
Phenothiazines
Sucralfate

Over-the-Counter Medications
Aluminum-containing antacids
Kaopectate
Loperamide

COLONIC FACTORS

The colon remains poorly understood because of the difficulty in studying normal colon function. This is because of the difficulty identifying normal colonic manometric or myoelectric patterns, and the colon normally contains solid as well as liquid material, complicating the study of colonic transit. The colon (unlike the stomach and small intestine) is active infrequently, often with predictable cyclic activity only every 24 hours.[27,28] The exact correlation of colonic function as far as stool output with manometric and myoelectric activity has not been clearly elucidated. New techniques have been developed to look at disorders in colonic function[24] but most of the methods still require colonic intubation and do not facilitate prolonged recordings. Recent reports of ambulant monitoring[29] may help clarify and improve our knowledge of colonic function (see Chapter 8B). The anorectum is most easily accessed for ambulant monitoring and a review of normal anorectal function is presented in Chapter 5.

Normal Colonic Function

An overview of normal colonic function is beneficial before describing the abnormalities found in constipated patients. The colon is two organs functionally, with the right colon having a different role from the left colon.[30] There are differences in the right colon compared with the left colon in smooth muscle responsiveness to stretch.[31] When colonic transit is evaluated by scintigraphic techniques, storage of feces with delayed progression of the radiolabel is seen in the transverse colon,[32] although delay in right colonic transit on a solid diet[33] may shift this storage site toward the ascending colon and cecum, depending on the content of the diet. If segmental colonic transit is evaluated by radiopaque markers, there appears to be an equal transit time through the right, left and rectosigmoid colon of between eleven to thirteen hours for each segment with the longer time of transit in the rectosigmoid.[34]

Studies comparing colonic motor activity with electrical activity and colonic transit report marked differences in the responses of the right colon compared with the left colon.[35–38] The electrical activity of the colon consists of two types: short spike bursts of about 10 bursts/min, associated with rhythmic colonic muscle contractions, and long spike bursts that can propagate orally or aborally and are associated with mass movements of colonic content[36–39] (Fig. 18-1). The movement of colonic material is determined by pressure

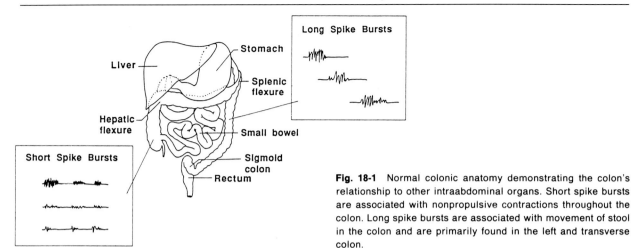

Fig. 18-1 Normal colonic anatomy demonstrating the colon's relationship to other intraabdominal organs. Short spike bursts are associated with nonpropulsive contractions throughout the colon. Long spike bursts are associated with movement of stool in the colon and are primarily found in the left and transverse colon.

gradients between different colonic segments, and again data shows frequent orad movement of material post-prandially into the transverse colon from the descending colon.[38] Long spike bursts are rarely seen during sleep, although the short spike bursts may continue[36] producing the infrequent contractions seen during sleep.[27] Colonic motor and electrical activity is most active on awakening,[27,36] after meals[27,35–40] and under stress.[41] When long spike bursts are propagated aborally over long distances in the colon into the rectosigmoid, then an urge to defecate,[27,40] or an awareness of cramping[27,39] results. Most colonic motility is not associated with symptoms in normal subjects.

Colonic Abnormalities

The myenteric plexus that regulates colonic motor function may be abnormal in some constipated patients. Smith[42] first described this and reported similar changes in mice fed stimulant laxatives. Other reports have shown widespread abnormalities in the myenteric plexus of some constipated patients.[43–45] Some of these patients have widespread gastrointestinal dysmotility with alterations in esophageal and gastric function as well.[44,45] These patients may also have a lack of sigmoid colon response to Bisacodyl as described by Preston and others.[46] An immunostaining technique using a monoclonal antineurofilament antibody showed lack of staining of axons in both the myenteric and submucosal plexus.[47] Van Tilburg and others[48] also defined a defect in some constipated patients having a low Na^+-dependent ileal bile acid transport, resulting in a low fecal bile acid loss which would reduce the amount of colonic fluid secretion. The converse was true for some patients with ileal disease and diarrhea.

There may be an inherited tendency to constipation as well. One study found 59 of 676 twin children to be constipated but the monozygotic twins were almost four times as likely as the dizygotic twins to be concordant for constipation. Constipation was also more likely to be found in the twins if another member of the family (parent, sibling, or twin) also had constipation.[49]

Gut Hormones and Neurotransmitters

Many gut hormones function as neurotransmitters, and several of these hormones are abnormal in some constipated patients. Experiments in rats and guinea pigs show that vasoactive intestinal peptide (VIP) mediates descending relaxation in the colonic peristaltic reflex with the VIP neurons coupled to cholinergic neurons.[50] Two studies[51,52] identified reduced VIP levels in the colon in constipated patients, and it might be postulated that this reduction in VIP may lead to impairment in the inhibition of colonic muscle, which could explain the paradoxic hypermotility observed in the sigmoid colon of constipated patients.[28,53–57] This is supported by the increased sensitivity of distal colonic circular muscle to VIP compared with the proximal colon.[58]

Other gut hormones reported to be abnormal in constipation include low levels of substance P[59], motilin, pancreatic polypeptide, and gastrin.[60] Thyrotropin-releasing hormone (TRH) appears to be important in increasing both colonic transit and contractility in the rat and opioids appear to delay colonic transit.[61,62] However, naloxone accelerates transit,[62] suggesting endogenous opioids may play an inhibitory role in human colonic function, and this is supported by the need for opiate receptors (along with cholinergic neurons) to produce a gastrocolonic response.[63] Neurotensin also may be involved in normal colon function because it immediately increases right colon contractions followed by an increase in rectosigmoid contractions.[64] The neurotransmitter serotonin or 5-hydroxtryptamine (5-HT) are increased in the mucosa and circular muscle of the sigmoid colon in constipated patients,[65] yet a recent report showed that a selective 5-HT$_3$ receptor antagonist slows colonic motility without significant effect on other gut hormones.[66] Further studies should clarify this apparent paradox of increased 5-HT and serotonin in colons of constipated patients, yet the 5-HT$_3$ antagonist Ondansetron slows colonic transit in healthy individuals.

Women suffer from constipation more often than men[2,4–6] so several studies have looked at the effect of sex hormones on colonic and intestinal function. Although orocecal transit is reported to be delayed in pregnancy,[67] no difference was found between normal and constipated women in the luteal or follicular phase of menstruation[68] and Kamm and coworkers[69] could find no effect of menstrual cycle on whole gut transit. Adrenal hormones were found to be abnormal in women with constipation[70] and a higher frequency of hyperprolactinemia[71] was reported. A more recent study did not confirm the hyperprolactinemia in women with severe constipation, but found reduced follicular phase progesterone, testosterone, and cortisol with reduced estradiol and cortisol and testosterone in the luteal phase of the menstrual cycle.[72]

Intestinal Transit and Motility

A subgroup of patients with constipation have delayed whole gut transit, termed "slow transit"[73] constipation. Two types of delayed transit were found: a delay in the entire colon, sometimes termed *colonic "inertia,"* and a distal hold-up in the rectosigmoid colon.[74–76] It is thought that patients with slow transit constipation may have a disorder of the myenteric plexus[46] but some patients respond to a high fiber diet,[76] so care must be exercised to ensure an adequate fiber intake is taken by the patient before colonic transit is measured.

Patients with delay in rectosigmoid transit may have hyperactive motility at the rectosigmoid junction,[77] but its function in constipation is unclear, because normal subjects also have been shown to have this hyperactive segment.[36] Manometric studies of the colon show decreased mass movements and a reduced urge to defecate with mass movements[28] in constipated patients and concomitant studies with radiolabelled transit markers confirmed some patients with constipation have impaired movement of colonic material after meals[57] or after taking Bisacodyl.[78] Patients with colonic "pseudoobstruction" may overlap patients with slow transit constipation, as they have reduced lower bowel motility along with marked gaseous distention of the colon.[79] One patient was described with delayed right colon transit and absent propagating electrical activity.[80] Autonomic neuropathy was found in some patients with constipation[75,81,82] as another cause for delayed colonic transit. A recent study using the acetylcholine sweat spot test identified even more frequent abnormalities in slow transit constipation,[83] confirming the likelihood of an autonomic neuropathy in some of these patients.

There appears to be abnormalities in small bowel function in patients with the irritable bowel syndrome, many of whom complain of constipation. One study reported a delay in orocecal transit in irritable bowel patients with predominantly constipation[84] but another study failed to show significant orocecal delay in constipated female patients.[68] Small bowel transit was reported to be delayed by painless rectal distention,[26] a condition that might be expected in some chronically constipated patients. Other reports suggest that the cramping abdominal pain reported by patients with an irritable bowel is associated with propulsive ileal motility on small bowel manometric recordings,[85–87] or duodenal phase 3 intestinal contractions seen during fasting.[88]

Urologic abnormalities were described in which constipated patients have an increased capacity and reduced sensitivity of the bladder[85] and more frequently report hesitancy in initiating the urinary stream.[73] These findings suggest that there may be a diffuse defect in smooth muscle in these patients that causes the constipation and the smooth muscle abnormalities in the lower urinary tract.

Diet

Constipation cannot be mentioned without discussing dietary fiber, and since Burkitt's hypothesis[90] regarding fiber in normal bowel function was popularized, there have been conflicting results of investigations. Fiber may shorten delayed transit, increase stool weight, and delay short whole gut transit in some patients.[91–95] However, increasing dietary fiber in constipated patients has had limited success.[92,95–99] One problem in studying the effects of fiber on symptoms in constipation is the high placebo response rate of 50% to 60%,[96,97,99] often similar to the treatment response with fiber. Constipated patients do not seem to respond as well to fiber as other subjects[93–95] and the form of fiber may play a role.[92,100] A small proportion of irritable bowel patients, some of whom may complain of constipation, can have symptoms aggravated by certain foods, the most common food being wheat (the usual source of bran fiber).[101] Other variables aside from dietary fiber may have an even greater role in stool output. Although dietary fiber does correlate with stool output in one study, this had a greater effect in men than in women.[102] Personality may be even more important than fiber, since an increase in fiber predicted only an increase in stool weight but not stool frequency, and individuals who described themselves in "favorable terms" produced more frequent stools.[103]

DISORDERS OF DEFECATION

Many constipated patients (who do not have deficient fiber in their diet or a secondary cause for constipation) appear to have dysfunction in the act of defecation. Before discussing these abnormalities, a review of normal defecation is appropriate. It appears from studies of the rectum with evacuation proctography that there are no active rectal contractions[104] during defecation, but rather stool is delivered into the rectum, and a sensation of a desire to defecate is experienced that initiates a normal reflex relaxation of the internal anal sphincter. The external anal sphincter and puborectalis muscles (striated muscles under voluntary control) contract. This contraction is followed by "voluntary" muscle relaxation if it is socially appropriate to empty the rectum (Fig. 18-2) and then when intraabdominal pressure increases, rectal contents are expelled through the open anal canal. The anorectal abnormalities that interfere with normal defecation can be divided into three types: patients with dilatation of the rectum and/or colon, such as megarectum or megacolon; patients with local anorectal abnormalities; and an idiopathic group of constipated patients who have no structural anorectal abnormality to explain their defecation difficulties.

Megacolon patients can be divided into those who have loss of the normal myenteric plexus ganglion cells (which is diagnostic of Hirschsprung's disease) and idiopathic megacolon. Hirschsprung's disease usually presents in childhood or early adulthood[105–107] and the age at which it presents depends on the length of the aganglionic segment. The segment of bowel without ganglion cells is chronically contracted due to absence of the inhibitory neurons of the myenteric plexus leading to hyperexcitability of the muscle in the aganglionic segment.[108] The normal bowel proximal to the aganglionic segment becomes dilated.[109] Hirschsprung's disease is

ANORECTAL FUNCTION DURING DEFECATION

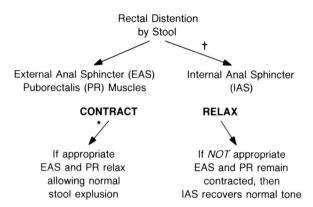

Fig. 18-2 A diagram of what happens to the anal sphincters during defecation. * identifies the defect in anismus where the EAS and PR do NOT relax to allow stool expulsion. + identifies where the IAS does not relax in Hirschsprung's disease.

congenital and one report suggested that it is caused by ischemia in utero due to fibromuscular dysplasia in the adventitia of the involved segment of intestine.[110] Acquired causes of megacolon have been described; most of these cases occur in other countries, such as Chagas' disease in Brazil and "East African megacolon,"[111] but there are cases of idiopathic acquired hypoganglionosis[112] and disorders in the myenteric plexus of some patients.[79] Hypoganglionosis is still difficult to diagnose, and even after surgery standard histopathological techniques may not be able to make this diagnosis.

Some adults have very short segments of aganglionosis (Hirschsprung's disease) and present later in life, although often on history, these patients have had longstanding defecation problems.[106] With time the progressive dilatation of the normal proximal rectum and colon causes the patient enough symptoms to seek medical advice. All patients with Hirschsprung's disease require surgical correction due to the structural blockage caused by the loss of the normal myenteric ganglion fibers.[106,107]

Most constipated patients presenting with an enlarged rectum have "idiopathic megacolon."[109] These patients do not appear to have a disorder of the myenteric plexus and have a normal rectoanal inhibitory reflex,[114] where rectal distention causes a reflex relaxation of the internal anal sphincter muscle (see Fig. 18-2). They present with dilatation of the rectum or colon and an inability to move their bowels regularly. Because the internal anal sphincter relaxes normally to rectal distention, the constipation is often associated with stool seepage, particularly with onset in childhood.[115,116] The cause is unclear but many megacolon patients who have been studied have contraction of the puborectalis and external anal sphincter muscles on straining at stool.[117] This causes progressive retention of feces in the rectum with impaction and eventual "overflow" diarrhea and seepage of feces. Therefore, at presentation these patients may not complain of constipation, but for therapy to be successful the constipation must be recognized and treated.

Local structural abnormalities that may present with constipation are rectal prolapse or rectal intussusception where the outlet to the rectum is blocked by the prolapse.[118] Many of these patients present with a history typical of prolapse. Sometimes if the prolapse does not protrude through the anus the patient may not be able to feel the prolapse, and further investigation is usually necessary to confirm this. Proctosigmoidoscopy, along with evacuation proctography, are the best methods by which a rectal intussusception can be diagnosed. One must be careful not to overinterpret normal fold patterns seen during evacuation of barium from the rectum on evacuation proctography, and guidelines for identifying these have been published[104,119] (see Chapter 7A1). Finally, local anal pathology such as anal fissures or other painful anal conditions give rise to pain and potential obstruction to normal stool passage. The influence of hemorrhoids in constipation is controversial, as a recent study showed differences in the epidemiologic data comparing the incidence of hemorrhoids with constipation[120] and another study found few constipated patients actually have hemorrhoids.[121] Therefore, hemorrhoids appear to be an unlikely cause of constipation but may worsen symptoms in a patient already suffering with a constipated bowel habit.

Pelvic Floor and Anorectal Abnormalities

Constipated patients with no structural abnormality to the anorectum may have dysfunction of the pelvic floor musculature. Although some patients with constipation and a normal anorectum have slowed colonic transit, a subgroup of patients with constipation (almost all of whom are women) appear to have difficulty emptying the rectum.[122–127] Some patients who manifest a delay in transit through the colon have also been identified as having impaired rectal emptying on dynamic studies, such as evacuation proctography.[124,126,128] Electromyography and anal canal manometry have identified anal sphincter musculature

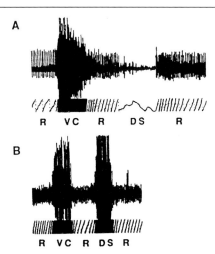

Fig. 18-3 Electromyography (EMG) of the puborectalis. **A,** A normal EMG tracing of the puborectalis showing the normal resting (R) EMG activity with an increase in activity on voluntary contraction (VC) and a normal decrease or relaxation of EMG activity on defecation straining (DS). **B,** An example of a patient with anismus showing the paradoxic contraction and increased EMG activity in the puborectalis on defecation straining (DS).

contraction on attempted defecation which blocks the anal canal[122,125–127] (see Fig. 18-3). These patients have a disorder in which the anus fails to open due to contraction rather than relaxation of the anal sphincter muscles on attempted defecation (Fig. 18-4). This has been termed *anismus*,[122] and pelvic floor dysynergia, a condition that blocks normal rectal emptying by causing an "outlet" obstruction to the colon. This disorder may explain why some patients fail to respond to increased dietary fiber and laxatives due to the obstruction to rectal emptying, sometimes even to liquid stool.[126,129] The incidence of anismus or a spastic pelvic floor in constipated patients has varied, but difficulty in emptying the rectum can be quantified by evacuation proctography or dynamic proctography using Technetium-labelled artificial stool.[130] Increasing delay in colonic transit along with impairment to rectal emptying was noted in a group of 58 patients referred for constipation,[131] and a more recent study found 25% of constipated patients demonstrated failure of relaxation of the puborectalis muscle at evacuation proctography.[132] Other studies of constipated patients identified a frequency of 15% to 38%[133–135] of anismus by evacuation proctography and/or electromyography. Klauser and others[136] showed that voluntary inhibition of stool passage by healthy men to simulate rectal outlet obstruction does delay segmental colonic transit in both the rectosigmoid and right colon. The true significance of

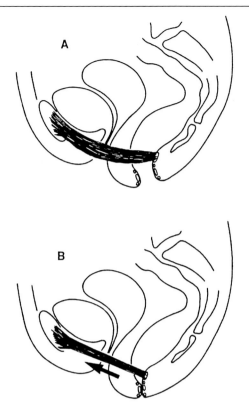

Fig. 18-4 Puborectalis muscle function. **A,** The puborectalis muscle is relaxed allowing the anal canal to open. **B,** On contraction, the puborectalis muscle sling pulls forward toward the pubic bone *(arrow)* and closes the proximal anal canal, thus obstructing rectal emptying.

this finding of paradoxic contraction of the puborectalis muscle on defecation is controversial, as some "normal" subjects have been reported who also manifest this abnormality.[125,135,137] Jones and colleagues[135] concluded that since they found this disorder in 48% of their patients with idiopathic perineal pain, this abnormality can be found without "constipation," but no evaluation of rectal emptying was performed. Our experience in treating these constipated patients using a combined therapeutic approach of anal sphincter biofeedback and relaxation therapy shows that the symptoms of constipation can improve without altering the anismus,[138] thus further suggesting that anismus alone is not the cause of their symptoms. Another study reported no correlation between the electromyographic evidence of anismus with impaired rectal emptying and the presence of delayed colonic transit.[139] Therefore, care must be exercised to avoid overdiagnosing anismus,[140] but impairment to rectal emptying is a common finding in severely constipated patients,[131] and this may

explain why some patients practice digital evacuation of the rectum to assist defecation.[126,129,131]

Many constipated patients (the majority of whom are women[129]) have reduced awareness of rectal distention often, with a reduction in the inhibition of the resting anal sphincter tone.[124,125,137,140–145] This may be an effect of constipation, because rectal sensitivity was more reduced in those patients with prolonged whole gut transit.[143] But it probably is a cause of constipation because the delivery of stool into the rectum was impaired in these women.[142] A more recent study using ambulant manometry confirmed the reduced delivery of stool into the rectum, suggesting there may be a motor neuropathy in the rectum of women with constipation.[144] The lack of awareness of rectal distention may be secondary to a sensory neuropathy of the rectum[146]. Further evidence of an autonomic neuropathy was found in some constipated women with an impaired urethrovesical reflex,[137] but the majority of these women also had evidence of anismus and impaired rectal awareness to distention. Others have demonstrated impaired urinary flow along with rectal outlet obstruction, indicating a diffuse pelvic floor disorder of obstruction in the anismus patients.[147] In addition, damage to the pudendal nerves was found in constipated women with chronic defecation straining,[148] and an impaired sacral reflex with stimulation of the dorsogenital nerve.[137,149] Perineal descent may result from chronic defecation straining and contribute to the pudendal neuropathy,[148] but the role of perineal descent as a cause for constipation seems unlikely since there is no difference between control subjects and constipated patients when perineal descent is evaluated by evacuation proctography.[131]

IRRITABLE BOWEL SYNDROME

Psychologic Factors

Constipation is a frequent symptom in patients with the irritable bowel syndrome (IBS) and a growing body of evidence has been evaluating the effect of psychologic factors on patients with IBS and constipation. The use of the criteria of Manning and colleagues[150] (Box 18-3) to diagnose the presence of an irritable bowel have been recently validated[151] as highly predictive for IBS when all six criteria are present. Other noncolonic symptoms such as fatigue, backache, and frequency of urination have been reported to be increased in irritable bowel patients as well.[152] However, another study showed

---

Box 18-3
Manning Criteria* for Irritable Bowel
Syndrome

1. Abdominal pain eased with defecation
2. Looser stools at onset of abdominal pain
3. More frequent stools at onset of pain
4. Abdominal distention (often worse later in day)
5. Mucus in stool
6. Sensation of incomplete rectal emptying after
   defecation

*Adapted from Manning[150] with permission.

---

poor correlation of the Manning criteria with the irritable bowel syndrome in men, but confirmed that these criteria were a good predictor for women with an irritable bowel.[153] Population studies suggest that irritable bowel symptoms are quite common in healthy people not seeking medical attention, with the frequency of constipation as a symptom in 15% to 45% of nonpatient groups.[154–157] From 6% to 8% of these patients have constipation as their main symptom[154,155] and constipation (following abdominal pain) was the second most significant factor in determining if a patient sought medical attention. Women are more than three times more likely than men and whites are five times more likely than blacks to report a self-diagnosis of irritable bowel.[158] A recent study reported that an irritable bowel is the seventh most common diagnosis in general practice in the United States with 5% to 11% of these patients complaining of constipation.[159] Irritable bowel is common in women having diagnostic laparoscopy or hysterectomy, with these women often doing less well, especially since their pain persisted after surgery. Between 30% to 35% of women presenting for laparoscopy or hysterectomy had constipation, versus 19% for the control population.[160]

A recent report found 44% of women with functional bowel complaints had a history of childhood sexual and physical abuse.[161] The women who had suffered sexual abuse had more abdominal and pelvic pain complaints and were more likely to have had surgery. Only 17% of these women had told their doctors of the abuse. This study suggests that childhood sexual abuse contributes to functional bowel complaints and that this history may not be evident on the initial clinical assessment.

Several studies show that the psychologic status of patients often determine whether or not they seek advice about irritable bowel symptoms.[162–165] This is termed "illness behavior" and best predicts those people who complain to doctors with their symptoms.[163] In patients attending a gastroenterology clinic, depression was a common symptom among patients without organic disease, often presenting with irritable bowel symptoms or abdominal pain,[166] and in another study 72% of patients with a diagnosis of IBS had a psychiatric illness, usually hysteria or depression.[167] Another study screening constipated patients before surgery reported the constipated patients to have more depression than matched controls.[168] When patients with irritable bowel symptoms are followed for 2 years their symptoms persist, although the symptoms often improve, particularly if the depression improves.[169] A recent review summarizes the present status of stress and the irritable bowel,[170] but a definite link is still elusive.

Personality factors may be as important as dietary fiber in predicting stool frequency[103] and high sources of psychologic distress were found in constipated patients without delayed colonic transit versus slow transit constipation patients.[171] Another study found that in constipated women with delayed colonic transit, the transit time in the ascending colon correlated with the level of anxiety.[172] Many women also have variation in their bowel function with menses[68,69] but this does not appear to be related to any psychologic changes during menstruation, although patients with IBS had increased symptoms of bowel gas during menstruation.[173]

Symptoms

The association of increased symptoms of abdominal pain and bloating in patients with IBS does not appear to be a result of lactose malabsorption in these patients, but swallowed gas may be the source of the abdominal gas causing bloating.[174] A recent study of 20 bloated irritable bowel patients by computed tomography could not identify excess intestinal gas, however, and it was postulated that the abdominal bloating may be due to changes in intestinal muscle motility or tone.[175]

Abdominal pain seems to be caused by distention of the colon[176] with reproduction of abdominal pain and extraabdominal sites of pain including right shoulder, right sacroiliac joint, right lower ribs, and right loin with right-sided colonic distention and left thigh, perineal, or left sacroiliac pain with left-sided colonic distention.[176] Patients with IBS have reduced tolerance to rectosigmoid distention yet are not different[177] or have a greater pain tolerance to other painful stimuli[178] when compared with normal subjects. Lack of tolerance to rectosigmoid distention did not correlate with any measurable psychologic traits either.[177] A recent study has suggested the abnormality causing irritable bowel symptoms is in the visceral afferents of the central nervous system processing this information, thus resulting in the symptoms and abnormal gut function seen in irritable bowel patients.[179] These studies suggest that patients with IBS have some alteration in colonic sensitivity which results in symptoms of abdominal pain and bloating with normal physiologic stimuli.

CLINICAL FEATURES

Constipation in adults is a symptom suffered primarily by women.[5] Women may be more prone to constipation due to the observation that women have less frequent bowel actions normally.[2] It is clear that there are many causes of constipation and that constipation is just a symptom that may indicate deficiency in dietary fiber, colonic motor dysfunction, drug ingestion, or other systemic diseases causing constipation. Women are much more likely than men to have dysfunction in the pelvic floor muscles[131] with anismus as one manifestation of this.[122] Anismus can obstruct the colon and lead to increased symptoms and unresponsiveness to other forms of therapy.[124–129,131] Constipated women may also have impaired awareness of rectal distention[125,142–144] and impaired colonic transit[73] contributing to their symptoms.

Abdominal pain and bloating are often of more concern to the patient than the reduced stool frequency. Although individuals who do not complain of their irritable bowels, and even "normal" female subjects frequently have abdominal pain and bloating, these symptoms are more frequent and severe in irritable bowel patients seen in gastrointestinal clinics.[180] The association between the abdominal symptoms and stool frequency (or lack thereof) reinforces a desire to effect a normal stool frequency, but an increase in stool frequency does not always eliminate the abdominal symptoms associated with the constipation.[181] This abnormal symptom generation is part of the irritable bowel symptom complex (Box 18-3) and it appears that abnormal small bowel[85–87] and colonic sensitivity[174–178] produces the symptoms in these patients.

An approach to deciding when further investigations should be performed in a patient presenting with constipation is outlined in Box 18-4. The dietary history is extremely important because many patients do not eat enough fiber and do not drink enough liquids to facilitate fiber action in the bowel. Most patients with constipation can improve their stool frequency with fiber even

> **Box 18-4**
> Indications for Investigations in Constipated Patients
>
> 1. Lack of response to increased dietary fiber
> 2. Lifelong constipation
> 3. Symptoms of obstructed defecation
> 4. Rectal bleeding
> 5. Dilation of the rectum and/or colon

though they may continue to have abdominal symptoms related to the underlying irritable bowel.[93–95] Since low fiber intake causes constipation in otherwise healthy adults,[90,91] attention to an adequate dietary fiber intake avoids unnecessary testing in otherwise normal patients.

Constipated patients with lifelong symptoms are likely to have anorectal or colonic disorders causing their constipation. Symptoms of difficult defecation and obstruction to the passage of stool (with or without the need to manually assist defecation) predicts patients most likely to have anorectal dysfunction as a cause for their symptoms. Rectal bleeding is not a symptom of uncomplicated constipation, and particularly in patients over the age of 40 years, investigations to exclude obstructing malignancy of the colon must be performed before attempting to increase dietary fiber or other therapy. If investigations (particularly barium enema or sigmoidoscopy) suggest the presence of rectal dilatation, further anorectal testing is necessary to exclude Hirschsprung's disease.

The author's approach to assessing a patient with constipation is as follows. A detailed history is required with particular emphasis on the onset of the constipation, weekly stool frequency, and methods used by the patient to assist stool passage. Clarification about any sense of rectal prolapse or need to assist rectal emptying is important, and any associated symptoms should be documented. Past history including previous abdominal operations, details of childbirth and any difficulties with the deliveries, other medical problems, and medications presently in use should be inquired about. It is surprising how many patients present with "constipation" who are taking Codeine or other narcotic analgesics for chronic pain and do not recognize the association between their symptoms and these drugs. It is worthwhile identifying when each drug was introduced and the time association with any worsening of symptoms. Most drugs are reported to cause constipation in some patients, and Box 18-2 only serves as a list of the more common drugs associated with constipation.

On physical examination, evidence for other diseases, particularly hypothyroidism or neurologic abnormalities, must be sought. The presence or absence of any abdominal abnormalities must be noted, and further investigations planned when abnormalities are found. On perineal exam, perineal descent below the plane of the ischial tuberosities when the patient strains downward should be recorded. Perianal sensation should be tested. On digital rectal exam, abnormalities in anal canal tone or function can be assessed with the patient contracting the sphincter voluntarily and making a defecatory effort to assess for paradoxic anal sphincter contraction on straining. An excellent description of a systematic approach to examination of the anorectum was recently published.[182]

Proctosigmoidoscopy should be performed to exclude any mucosal disease and exclude rectal prolapse, while asking the patient to strain to expel the proctoscope. Laboratory screening tests should include a complete blood count, electrolytes, and thyroid function studies. Other tests would be dictated by the findings on examination.

Reassurance at the initial interview helps the patient to understand the source of her symptoms, and in most young adults, extensive testing is not required if bowel function normalizes with increases in dietary fiber. As many tests of colonic and anorectal abnormalities are unpleasant and time consuming, they should be reserved for patients with evidence of significant bowel dysfunction as outlined above.

TREATMENT

Medical Treatment

The treatment of constipation is determined by the cause of the constipation. Dietary fiber intake must be optimized. This does not mean that patients should have excessive fiber; giving a patient too much fiber will aggravate many symptoms, particularly abdominal bloating and pain. It is best to gradually introduce fiber into the diet of patients who have not been ingesting enough fiber. A reasonable aim would be to try to achieve 30 g of fiber per day. To help patients achieve this they should eat a concentrated source of fiber in the morning, usually a high fiber breakfast cereal, and then choose high fiber food alternatives for their other meals

during the day. Adequate fluid intake must be stressed and the usual guideline is 6 to 8 eight ounce (250 ml) glasses per day. The majority of patients with unresponsive constipation improve with a gradual introduction of fiber with high fluid intake. Reports of IBS patients with food intolerance and reproduction of symptoms makes dietary adjustment difficult for some patients, but a recent large study found no particular association with foods precipitating symptoms in constipated subjects,[183] although wheat was a commonly reported food that aggravated other IBS symptoms. Ispaghula husk fiber may be better tolerated by the gut with fewer symptoms[184,185] but there are no good clinical trials comparing different fibers in the treatment of IBS[186] or constipation.

The aggravation of abdominal symptoms by the use of fiber can be controlled sometimes with the use of antispasmodic medication[187] and peppermint oil may also work by decreasing colonic contractility,[188] although studies assessing abdominal pain and colonic motility have not shown any correlation.[99,177] Antidepressants provide significant improvement in IBS patients with diarrhea, but the anticholinergic effects seem to worsen symptoms in constipated IBS patients.[189]

Laxative therapy is sometimes necessary and some patients achieve good results with episodic dosing with laxatives. It is best to avoid the use of stimulant laxatives and osmotic laxatives containing magnesium salts, lactulose, or sorbitol are usually preferred. Unfortunately, many constipated patients do not tolerate these laxatives because of nausea or an increase in abdominal pain that may be caused by an exaggerated colonic response in these patients to endogenous cholecystokinin, which is released by magnesium (particularly magnesium sulphate).[190] Lactulose may be poorly tolerated by patients due to the increased colonic gas produced by bacterial fermentation of the lactulose with increased abdominal pain and bloating.[174,191] If a stimulant laxative is to be used, bisacodyl, cascara, or the senna derivatives are preferred over phenolphthalein or danthron, since phenolphthalein can cause allergic reactions and danthron has been implicated in causing liver disease.[192]

Enemas and suppositories are sometimes necessary, as some patients with outlet constipation may be improved by liquifying the stool to assist rectal emptying, but some of these patients cannot even empty liquid stool from the rectum normally.[126] A new prokinetic motility agent, Cisapride, may be beneficial for some patients since it does decrease orocecal transit and decrease the time of colonic transit[193] with increased stool frequency in constipated patients,[194] but has no significant effect on stool weight and frequency[193] in normal subjects. Thompson's overview of treatment strategies in the medical management of IBS patients is recommended,[195] along with a summary report from an international workshop on the management of constipation, for further reading.[196]

The other abdominal symptoms associated with constipation may not be relieved even if stool frequency is normalized.[181] Newer approaches using behavioral and biofeedback techniques to treat constipated patients suggest that stool frequency may be increased along with a reduction in other abdominal symptoms.[197–200] Further studies show that patients with anismus may improve with biofeedback training to teach appropriate relaxation of the pelvic floor muscles during straining to allow more normal defecation.[200–204] Follow-up of a group of children taught to relax the pelvic floor muscles showed only 50% recovered from their constipation.[205] Biofeedback techniques may also have an effect through their ability to induce a "relaxation response" in some patients.[206] Unfortunately, a recent large study in IBS patients showed little change in constipated patients after relaxation training.[207] The time commitment for the clinician and the psychologist can be excessive, so psychologic approaches to therapy should be reserved for patients unresponsive to dietary and other lifestyle therapeutic approaches.[208]

The treatment of idiopathic megacolon/megarectum deserves special mention. Some reports show biofeedback therapy to be successful in some children with a megarectum and fecal soiling.[202,203,209] However, the first line of therapy is to empty the fecal bolus distending the rectum, then to administer daily laxatives in a dose which will keep the stool loose, with a frequency of two to three per day.[210] Osmotic laxatives are better tolerated by adults, but frequently children are treated with mineral oil or osmotic laxatives with good results. The success of therapy appears to be predicted by the severity of the constipation and the degree of outlet obstruction at presentation, and not psychologic factors.[211,212]

A nonsurgical approach that is reported to successfully treat anismus is the use of injectable botulinum A toxin[213] into the striated muscles of the anal sphincter. Unfortunately, this treatment can cause muscle damage and care must be exercised to avoid injecting too much toxin. Two of the seven patients initially receiving this treatment had fecal incontinence after the therapy[213] but over time most recover the lost muscle tone. This treatment requires repeated injections to maintain the benefit, often at 3 to 4 month intervals.

Finally, a study of 4 women with "debilitating" functional bowel complaints with constipation as one of their symptoms were treated with leuprolide acetate (Lupron®).[214] Although all the patients relapsed in 3–5 days upon withdrawal of this gonadotropin-releasing hormone analog, they had been symptomatically controlled for as long as 15 months when the study was reported. Again, concern about prolonged therapy with leuprolide acetate will limit the usefulness of this approach.

Surgical Treatment

Constipated patients who do not respond to medical therapy and have severe symptoms may be candidates for surgical intervention. It is still unclear how best to predict those patients who will do well with surgery, but patients with slow transit through the colon without evidence of anismus are the candidates one would expect to do well with an ileorectal anastomosis following a subtotal colectomy.[215,216] Other operations with only partial colonic resections or a cecorectal anastomosis are not as successful and reoperation[140,217,218] may be necessary for continued constipation. If an ileorectal anastomosis is to be done, the colonic resection must be down to the pelvic brim since patients having more proximal resections with an ileosigmoid anastomosis frequently continue to be constipated.[217]

Several reports have been published recently of the long term therapeutic result of subtotal colectomy and ileorectal anastomosis in constipated patients.[181,219–221] Stool frequency is increased in the majority of patients (50% to 100%) but abdominal pain, abdominal bloating, and the need to continue taking laxatives or straining at stool continued in the majority of patients (69% to 82%)[181,219,220] but Zenilman and colleagues[221] reported 92% "excellent" results at 24 months of follow-up in their patients. Some patients with evidence of outlet obstruction do not respond to a subtotal colectomy[126,181,220] but it was not possible to predict outcome from preoperative studies.[181,219,220] Therefore, surgery is only recommended after all other therapeutic modalities are exhausted[215,216] and patients should be warned that many of their symptoms may persist and they could experience episodic diarrhea and/or fecal incontinence.[181,219,220] Subtotal colectomy with an ileorectal anastomosis is the preferred operation for constipated patients with idiopathic magarectum who have failed medical therapy.[222]

Specific surgical treatments for anismus and "outlet obstruction" have been reported. Initial reports of resection of part of the puborectalis muscle suggested this operation was highly successful[223,224] but recent reports of posterior division[225,226] and lateral division of the puborectalis muscle[227] have not been very successful. As well, an initial response to surgery has not always resulted in long-term improvement.[140] Some patients may be left with reduced fecal continence following the above surgery, but usually they remain continent for solid stool.[227]

SUMMARY

Constipation and its associated symptoms can be one of the more intractable bowel complaints the clinician encounters. This chapter has attempted to provide an overview of the many causes of constipation and to outline what is known about normal colonic and anorectal function, and what has been shown to be abnormal in patients complaining of constipation.

The clinical features of constipation were reviewed and therapy, both medical and surgical, are summarized. The approach to the constipated patient is best achieved by a multidisciplinary team including a gastroenterologist, dietician, surgeon, and psychologist to achieve the best clinical outcome. Patients with anismus or pelvic floor dyssynergia on attempting defecation are usually female and are best treated by biofeedback therapy. Surgery at present is reserved for patients unresponsive to other therapy or with a defined, treatable cause amenable to surgery.

REFERENCES

1. Moore-Gillion V. Constipation: what does the patient mean? *J Roy Soc Med*. 1984;77:108–110.
2. Sandler RS, Drossman DA. Bowel habits in young adults not seeking health care. *Dig Dis Sci*. 1987;32:841–845.
3. Wyman JB, Heaton KW, Manning AP, Wicks ACB. Variability of colonic function in healthy subjects. *Gut*. 1978;19:146–150.
4. Drossman DA, Sandler RS, McKee DC, Lovitz AJ. Bowel patterns among subjects not seeking health care. *Gastroenterology*. 1982;83:529–534.
5. Everhart JE, Go VLW, Johannes RS, Fitzsimmons SC, Roth HP, White LR. A longitudinal survey of self-reported bowel habits in the United States. *Dig Dis Sci*. 1989;34:1153–1162.
6. Sonnenberg A, Koch TR. Physician visits in the United States for constipation: 1958 to 1986. *Dig Dis Sci*. 1989;34:606–611.
7. Sonnenberg A, Koch TR. Epidemiology of constipation in the United States. *Dis Colon Rectum*. 1989;32:1–8.
8. Wrenn K. Fecal impaction. *N Eng J Med*. 1989;321:658–662.

9. Chesta J, Debnam ES, Srai SKS, Epstein O. Delayed stomach to cecum transit time in the diabetic rat. Possible role of hyperglucagonaemia. *Gut*. 1990;31:660–662.
10. Shafer RB, Prentiss RA, Bond JH. Gastrointestinal transit in thyroid disease. *Gastroenterology*. 1984;86:852–855.
11. Colemont LJ, Camilleri M. Chronic intestinal pseudo-obstruction: diagnosis and treatment. *Mayo Clin Proc*. 1989;64:60–70.
12. Whitehead WE, Taitelbaum G, Wigley FM, Schuster MM. Rectosigmoid motility and myoelectric activity in progressive systemic sclerosis. *Gastroenterology*. 1989;96:428–432.
13. Weber J, Delangre T, Hannequin D, Beuret-Blanquart F, Denis P. Anorectal manometric anomalies in seven patients with frontal lobe brain damage. *Dig Dis Sci*. 1990;35:225–230.
14. Hinds JP, Eidelman BH, Wald A. Prevalence of bowel dysfunction in multiple sclerosis. *Gastroenterology*. 1990;98:1538–1542.
15. Glick ME, Meshkinpour H, Haldeman S, Hoehler F, Downey N, Bradley WE. Colonic dysfunction in patients with thoracic spinal cord injury. *Gastroenterology*. 1984;86:287–294.
16. Glick ME, Meshkinpour H, Haldeman S, Bhatia NH, Bradley WE. Colonic dysfunction in multiple sclerosis. *Gastroenterology*. 1982;83:1002–1007.
17. Devroede G, Arhan P, Duguay C, Tetreault L, Akoury H, Perey B. Traumatic constipation. *Gastroenterology*. 1979;77:1258–1267.
18. MacDonagh RP, Sun WM, Smallwood R, Read NW. Sacral anterior root stimulation and defecation: new hope for paraplegics? *Gastroenterology*. 1990;98:A373.
19. Bouvier M, Grimaud J-C, Abysique A. Effects of stimulation of vesical afferents on colonic motility in cats. *Gastroenterology*. 1990;98:1148–1154.
20. Devroede G, Lamarche J. Functional importance of extrinsic parasympathetic innervation to the distal colon and rectum in man. *Gastroenterology*. 1974;66:273–280.
21. Bingham SA, Cummings JH. Effect of exercise and physical fitness on large intestinal function. *Gastroenterology*. 1989;97:1389–1399.
22. Meshkinpour H, Kemp C, Fairshter R. Effect of aerobic exercise on mouth-to-cecum transit time. *Gastroenterology*. 1989;96:938–941.
23. Oettle GJ. Effect of moderate exercise on bowel habit. *Gut*. 1991;32:941–944.
24. Waldholtz BD, Andersen AE. Gastrointestinal symptoms in anorexia nervosa. *Gastroenterology*. 1990;98:1415–1419.
25. Kamal N, Chami T, Anderson A, Rosell FA, Schuster MM, Whitehead WE. Delayed gastrointestinal transit times in anorexia nervosa and bulimia nervosa. *Gastroenterology*. 1991;101:1320–1324.
26. Youle MS, Read NW. Effect of painless rectal distention on gastrointestinal transit of solid meal. *Dig Dis Sci*. 1984;29:902–906.
27. Narducci F, Bassotti G, Gaburri M, Morell A. Twenty-four hour manometric recording of colonic motor activity in healthy man. *Gut*. 1987;28:17–25.
28. Bassotti G, Gaburri M, Imbimbo BP, et al. Colonic mass movements in idiopathic chronic constipation. *Gut*. 1988;29:1173–1179.
29. Kumar D, Waldron D, Williams NS, Browning C, Hutton MRE, Wingate DL. Prolonged anorectal manometry and external anal sphincter electromyography in ambulant human subjects. *Dig Dis Sci*. 1990;35:641–648.
30. Sandle GI, Willis NK, Alles W, Binder HJ. Electrophysiology of the human colon: evidence of segmental heterogeneity. *Gut*. 1986;27:999–1005.
31. Gill RC, Cote KR, Bowes KL, Kingma YJ. Human colonic smooth muscle: spontaneous contractile activity and response to stretch. *Gut*. 1986;27:1006–1013.
32. Krevsky B, Malmoud LS, D'Ercole F, Maurer AH, Fisher RS.

Acknowledgments: Supported in part by MRC of Canada Grant No. MA-10371. I wish to thank Ms. R. Klatt for typing the manuscript.

Colonic transit scintigraphy. *Gastroenterology.* 1986;91:1102–1112.

33. Kaufman PN, Richter JE, Chilton HM, et al. Effects of liquid versus solid diet on colonic transit in humans. *Gastroenterology.* 1990;98:73–81.

34. Metcalfe AM, Phillips SF, Zinsmeister AR, McCarty RL, Beart RW, Wolff BG. Simplified assessment of segmental colonic transit. *Gastroenterology.* 1987;92:40–47.

35. Kerlin P, Zinsmeister AR, Phillips S. Motor responses to food of the ileum, proximal colon, and distal colon of healthy humans. *Gastroenterology.* 1983;84:762–770.

36. Frexinos J, Bueno L, Fioramonti J. Diurnal changes in myoelectric spiking activity of the human colon. *Gastroenterology.* 1985;88:1104–1110.

37. Dapoigny M, Trolese J-F, Bommelaer G, Tournut R. Myoelectric spiking activity of right colon, left colon, and rectosigmoid of healthy humans. *Dig Dis Sci.* 1988;33:1007–1012.

38. Moreno-Osset E, Bazzocchi G, Lo S, et al. Association between postprandial changes in colonic intraluminal pressure and transit. *Gastroenterology.* 1989;96:1265–1273.

39. Schang JC, Devroede G. Fasting and postprandial myoelectric spiking activity in the human sigmoid colon. *Gastroenterology.* 1983;85:1048–1053.

40. Holdstock DJ, Misiewicz JJ, Smith T, Rowlands EN. Propulsion (mass movements) in the human colon and its relationship to meals and somatic activity. *Gut.* 1970;11:91–99.

41. Narducci F, Snape WJ Jr, Battle WM, Landon RL, Cohen S. Increased colonic motility during exposure to a stressful situation. *Dig Dis Sci.* 1985;30:40–44.

42. Smith B. Effect of irritant purgatives on the myenteric plexus in man and the mouse. *Gut.* 1968;9:139–143.

43. Krishnamurthy S, Schuffler MD. Pathology of neuromuscular disorders of the small intestine and colon. *Gastroenterology.* 1987;93:610–639.

44. Krishnamurthy S, Schuffler MD, Rohrmann CA, Pope, CE. Severe idiopathic constipation is associated with a distinctive abnormality of the colonic myenteric plexus. *Gastroenterology.* 1985;88:26–34.

45. Reynolds JC, Ouyang A, Lee CA, Baker L, Sunshine AG, Cohen S. Chronic severe constipation: prospective motility studies in 25 consecutive patients. *Gastroenterology.* 1987;92:414–420.

46. Preston DM, Lennard-Jones JE. Pelvic motility and response to intraluminal Bisacodyl in slow-transit constipation. *Dig Dis Sci.* 1985;30:289–294.

47. Kluck P, Kate FJW, Schouten WR, et al. Efficacy of antibody NF2F11 staining in the investigation of severe long-standing constipation. *Gastroenterology.* 1987;93:872–875.

48. van Tilburg AJP, De Rooij FWM, van Blankenstein M, van den Berg JWO, Bosman-Jacobs EP. Na⁺-dependent bile acid transport in the ileum: the balance between diarrhea and constipation. *Gastroenterology.* 1990;98:25–32.

49. Bakwin H, Davidson M. Constipation in twins. *Amer J Dis Child.* 1971;121:179–181.

50. Grider JR, Makhlouf GM. Colonic peristaltic reflux: identification of vasoactive intestinal peptide as mediator of descending relaxation. *Am J Physiol.* 1986;251:640–645.

51. Koch TR, Carney JA, Go L, Go VLW. Idiopathic chronic constipation as associated with decreased colonic vasoactive intestinal peptide. *Gastroenterology.* 1988;94:300–310.

52. Milner P, Crowe R, Kamm MA, Lennard-Jones JE, Burnstock G. Vasoactive intestinal polypeptide levels in sigmoid colon in idiopathic constipation and diverticular disease. *Gastroenterology.* 1990;99:666–675.

53. Connell AM. The motility of the pelvic colon II: paradoxical motility in diarrhea and constipation. *Gut.* 1962;3:342–348.

54. Sullivan MA, Cohen S, Snape WJ Jr. Colonic myoelectrical activity in irritable bowel syndrome. *N Engl J Med.* 1978;298:878–883.

55. Frieri G, Parisi F, Corazziari E, Caprilli R. Colonic electromyography in chronic constipation. *Gastroenterology.* 1983;84:737–740.

56. Meunier P. Physiologic study of the terminal digestive tract in chronic painful constipation. *Gut.* 1986;27:1018–1024.

57. Bazzocchi G, Ellis J, Villanueve-Meyer J, et al. Postprandial colonic transit and motor activity in chronic constipation. *Gastroenterology.* 1990;98:686–693.

58. Burleigh DE. Motor responsiveness of proximal and distal human colonic muscle layers to acetylcholine, noradrenaline, and vasoactive intestinal peptide. *Dig Dis Sci.* 1990;35:617–621.

59. Goldin E, Karmeli F, Selinger Z, Rachmilewitz D. Colonic substance P-levels are increased in ulcerative colitis and decreased in chronic severe constipation. *Dig Dis Sci.* 1989;34:754–757.

60. Preston DM, Adrian TE, Christofides ND, Lennard-Jones JE, Bloom SR. Positive correlation between symptoms and circulating motilin, pancreatic polypeptide and gastrin concentrations in functional bowel disorders. *Gut.* 1985;26:1059–1064.

61. Tache Y, Garrick T, Raybould H. Central nervous system action of peptides to influence gastrointestinal motor function. *Gastroenterology.* 1990;98:517–528.

62. Kaufman PN, Kreusky B, Malmud LS, Maurer AH, Somers MB, Siegel JA, Fisher RS. Role of opiate receptors in the regulation of colonic transit. *Gastroenterology.* 1988;94:1351–1356.

63. Sun EA, Snape WJ Jr, Cohen S, Renny A. The role of opiate receptors and cholinergic neurons in the gastrocolonic response. *Gastroenterology.* 1982;82:689–693.

64. Thor K, Rosell S. Neurotensin increases colonic motility. *Gastroenterology.* 1986;90:27–31.

65. Lincoln J, Crowe R, Kamm MA, Burnstock G, Lennard-Jones JE. Serotonin and 5-hydroxyindoleacetic acid are increased in the sigmoid colon in severe idiopathic constipation. *Gastroenterology.* 1990;98:1219–1225.

66. Talley NJ, Phillips SF, Haddad A, et al. GR 38032F (Ondansetron), a selective 5-HT₃ receptor antagonist, slows colonic transit in healthy man. *Dig Dis Sci.* 1990;35:477–480.

67. Wald A, Van Thiel DH, Hoechstetter L, et al. Effect of pregnancy on gastrointestinal transit. *Dig Dis Sci.* 1982;27:1015–1018.

68. Turnbull GK, Thompson DG, Day S, Martin J, Walker E, Lennard-Jones JE. Relationships between symptoms, menstrual cycle and orocecal transit in normal and constipated women. *Gut.* 1989;30:30–34.

69. Kamm MA, Farthing MJG, Lennard-Jones JE. Bowel function and transit rate during the menstrual cycle. *Gut.* 1989;30:605–608.

70. Kamm MA, Lennard-Jones JE, Farthing MJG, McLean A, Perry L, Chard T. Adrenal hormones are abnormal in women with severe idiopathic constipation. *Gastroenterology.* 1989;96:A246.

71. Preston DM, Rees LH, Lennard-Jones JE. Gynecological disorders and hyperprolactinemia in chronic constipation. *Gut.* 1983;24:A480.

72. Kamm MA, Fathing MJG, Lennard-Jones JE, Perry LA, Chard T. Steroid hormone abnormalities in women with severe idiopathic constipation. *Gut.* 1991;32:80–84.

73. Preston DM, Lennard-Jones JE. Severe chronic constipation of young women: "idiopathic slow transit constipation." *Gut.* 1986;27:41–48.

74. Ducrotte P, Rodomanska B, Weber J, et al. Colonic transit time of radiopaque markers and rectoanal manometry in patients complaining of constipation. *Dis Colon Rectum.* 1986;29:630–634.

75. Wald A. Colonic transit and anorectal manometry in chronic idiopathic constipation. *Arch Intern Med.* 1986;146:1713–1716.

76. Chaussade S, Khyari A, Roche H, et al. Determination of total and segmental colonic transit time in constipated patients. *Dig Dis Sci.* 1989;34:1168–1172.

77. Chowdhury AR, Dinoso VP, Lorber SH. Characterization of a hyperactive segment at the rectosigmoid junction. *Gastroenterology.* 1976;71:584–588.

78. Kamm MA, Lennard-Jones JE, Thompson DG, Sobnack R, Garvie NW, Granowska M. Dynamic scanning defines a colonic defect in severe idiopathic constipation. *Gut.* 1988;29:1085–1092.

79. Loening-Baucke VA, Anuras S, Mitros FA. Changes in colorectal function in patients with chronic colonic pseudo-obstruction. *Dig Dis Sci.* 1987;32:1104–1112.

80. Likongo Y, Devroede G, Schang J-C, et al. Hind gut dysgenesis as a cause of constipation with delayed colonic transit. *Dig Dis Sci.* 1986;31:993–1003.

81. Watier A, Devroede G, Duranceau A, et al. Constipation with colonic inertia. *Dig Dis Sci.* 1983;28:1025–1033.

82. Camilleri M, Fealey RD. Idiopathic autonomic denervation in eight patients presenting with functional gastrointestinal disease. *Dig Dis Sci.* 1990;35:609–616.

83. Altomare DF, Pilot MA, Waldron D, Scott M, Williams NS. Detection of subclinical autonomic neuropathy in patients with slow transit constipation by the acetylcholine sweat spot test. *Gut.* 1990;31:A606.

84. Cann PA, Read NW, Brown C, Hobson N, Holdsworth CD. Irritable bowel syndrome: relationship of disorders in the transit of a single solid meal to symptom patterns. *Gut.* 1983;24:405–411.

85. Kellow JE, Phillips SF. Altered small bowel motility in irritable bowel syndrome is correlated with symptoms. *Gastroenterology.* 1987;92:1885–1893.

86. Kellow JE, Phillips SF, Miller LJ, Zinsmeister AR. Dysmotility of the small intestine in irritable bowel syndrome. *Gut.* 1988;29:1236–1243.

87. Kellow JE, Gill RC, Wingate DL. Prolonged ambulant recordings of small bowel motility demonstrate abnormalities in the irritable bowel syndrome. *Gastroenterology.* 1990;98:1208–1218.

88. Kellow JE, Eckersley GM, Jones MP. Enhanced perception of physiological intestinal motility in the irritable bowel syndrome. *Gastroenterology.* 1991;101:1621–1627.

89. Bannister JJ, Lawrence WT, Smith A, Thomas DG, Reid NW. Urological abnormalities in young women with severe constipation. *Gut.* 1988;29:17–20.

90. Burkitt DP, Walker ARP, Painter NS. Effect of dietary fiber on stools and transit times, and its role in the causation of disease. *Lancet.* 1972;ii:1408–1412.

91. Payler DK, Pomare EW, Heaton KW, Harvey RF. The effect of wheat bran on transit time. *Gut.* 1975;16:209–213.

92. Graham DY, Moser SE, Estes MK. The effect of bran on bowel function in constipation. *Am J Gastroenterol.* 1982;77:599–603.

93. Jenkins DJA, Peterson RD, Thorne MJ, Ferguson PW. Wheat fiber and laxation: dose response and equilibration time. *Am J Gastroenterol.* 1987;82:1259–1263.

94. Muller-Lissner SA. Effect of wheat bran on weight of stool and gastrointestinal transit time: a meta analysis. *Br Med J.* 1988;296:615–617.

95. Hamilton JW, Wagner J, Burdick BB, Bass P. Clinical evaluation of methylcellulose as a bulk laxative. *Dig Dis Sci.* 1988;33:993–998.

96. Longstreth GF, Fox DD, Youkeles L, Forsythe AB, Wolochow DA. Psyllium therapy in the irritable bowel syndrome. *Ann Intern Med.* 1981;95:53–56.

97. Soltoft J, Gudmand-Hoyer E, Krag B, Kristensen E, Wulff HR. A double-blind trial of the effect of wheat bran on symptoms of irritable bowel syndrome. *Lancet.* 1976;i:270–272.

98. Manning AP, Heaton KW, Harvey RF. Wheat fiber and irritable bowel syndrome. *Lancet.* 1977;ii:417–418.

99. Cook IJ, Irvine EJ, Campbell D, Shannon S, Reddy SN, Collins SM. Effect of dietary fiber on symptoms and rectosigmoid motility in patients with irritable bowel syndrome. *Gastroenterology.* 1990;98:66–72.

100. Ritchie JA, Truelove SC. Comparison of various treatments for irritable bowel syndrome. *Br Med J.* 1980;281:1317–1319.

101. McLaughlan P, Shorthouse M, Workman E, Hunter JO. Food intolerance: a major factor in the pathogenesis of irritable bowel syndrome. *Lancet.* 1982;ii:1115–1117.

102. Davies GJ, Crowder M, Reid B, Dickerson JWT. Bowel function measurements of individuals with different eating patterns. *Gut.* 1986;27:164–169.

103. Tucker DM, Sandstead HH, Logan GM, Jr, Klevay LM, Mahalko J, Johnson LK, Inman L, Inglett GE. Dietary fiber and personality factors as determinants of stool output. *Gastroenterology.* 1981;81:879–883.

104. Bartram CI, Turnbull GK, Lennard-Jones JE. Evacuation proctography: an investigation of rectal expulsion in 20 subjects without defecatory disturbance. *Gastrointest Radiol.* 1988;13:72–80.

105. Ikawa H, Kim SH, Hendron H, Donahoe PK. Acetylcholinesterase and manometry in the diagnosis of the constipated child. *Arch Surg.* 1986;121:435–438.

106. Wheatley MJ, Wesley JR, Coran AG, Polley TZ. Hirschsprung's disease in adolescents and adults. *Dis Colon Rectum.* 1990;33:622–629.

107. Luukkonen P, Heikkinen M, Huikuri K, Jarvinen H. Adult Hirschsprung's disease. Clinical features and functional outcome after surgery. *Dis Colon Rectum.* 1990;33:65–69.

108. Seidel ER, Woods J, Eikenberg BE, Johnson LR. Muscarinic cholinergic receptors in the piebald mouse model for Hirschsprung's disease. *Gastroenterology.* 1983;85:335–338.

109. Earlam R. (ed.) A vascular cause for Hirschsprung's disease. *Gastroenterology.* 1985;88:1274–1279.

110. Taguchi T, Tanaka K, Ikeda K. Fibromuscular dysplasia of arteries in Hirschsprung's disease. *Gastroenterology.* 1985;88:1099–1103.

111. Lennard-Jones JE. Constipation: pathophysiology, clinical features, and treatment. In: Henry MM, Swash M, eds. *Coloproctology and the Pelvic Floor: Pathophysiology and Management,* London: Butterworth & Co. Ltd.; 1985;350–375.

112. Matsui T, Iwashita A, Iida M, Kimek, Fujishima M. Acquired pseudoobstruction of the colon due to segmental hypoganglionosis. *Gastrointest Radiol.* 1987;12:262–264.

113. Preston DM, Lennard-Jones JE, Thomas BM. Towards a radiologic definition of idiopathic megacolon. *Gastrointest Radiol.* 1985;10:167–169.

114. Verduron A, Devroede G, Bouchoucha M, et al. Megarectum. *Dig Dis Sci.* 1988;33:1164–1174.

115. Callaghan RP, Nixon HH. Megarectum: physiologic observations. *Arch Dis Childh.* 1964;39:153–157.

116. Meunier P, Mollard P, Marechal J-M. Physiopathology of megarectum: the association of megarectum with encopresis. *Gut.* 1976;17:224–227.

117. Porter NH. Megacolon: a physiologic study. *Proc Roy Soc Med.* 1961;54:1043–1047.

118. Roe AM, Bartolo DC, Martensen NJ. Techniques in evacuation proctography in the diagnosis of intractable constipation and related disorders. *J R Soc Med.* 1986;79:331–333.

119. Shorvon PJ, McHugh S, Diamant NE, Somers S, Stevenson GW. Defecography in normal volunteers: results and implications. *Gut.* 1989;30:1737–1749.

120. Johanson JF, Sonnenberg A. The prevalence of hemorrhoids and chronic constipation. *Gastroenterology.* 1990;98:380–386.

121. Gibbons CP, Bannister JJ, Read NW. Role of constipation and anal hypertonia in the pathogenesis of hemorrhoids. *Br J Surg.* 1988;75:656–660.

122. Preston DM, Lennard-Jones JE. Anismus in chronic constipation. *Dig Dis Sci.* 1985;30:413–418.

123. Barnes PRH, Lennard-Jones JE. Balloon expulsion from the rectum in constipation of different types. *Gut.* 1985;26:1049–1052.

124. Kuijpers HC, Bleijenberg G. The spastic pelvic floor syndrome: a cause of constipation. *Dis Colon Rectum.* 1985;28:669–672.

125. Read NW, Timms JM, Barfield LJ, Donnelly TC, Bannister JJ.

Impairment of defecation in young women with severe constipation. *Gastroenterology.* 1986;90:53–60.

126. Turnbull GK, Lennard-Jones JE, Bartram CI. Failure of rectal expulsion as a cause of constipation: why fiber and laxatives sometimes fail. *Lancet.* 1986;i:767–769.

127. Shouler P, Keighley MRB. Changes in colorectal function in severe idiopathic chronic constipation. *Gastroenterology.* 1986;90:414–420.

128. Womack NR, Williams NS, Holmfield JH, Morrison JF, Simpkins KC. New method for the dynamic assessment of anorectal function in constipation. *Br J Surg.* 1985;72:994–998.

129. Editorial. Constipation in young women. *Lancet.* 1986;i:778–779.

130. Ambroze WL, Pemberton JH, Bell AM, Brown ML, Zinsmeister AR. The effect of stool consistency on rectal and neorectal emptying. *Dis Colon Rectum.* 1991;34:1–7.

131. Turnbull GK, Bartram CI, Lennard-Jones JE. Radiologic studies of rectal evacuation in adults with idiopathic constipation. *Dis Colon Rectum.* 1988;31:190–197.

132. Wald A, Caruana BJ, Freimanis MG, Bauman DH, Hinds JP. Contributions of evacuation proctography and anorectal manometry to evaluation of adults with constipation and defecatory difficulty. *Dig Dis Sci.* 1990;35:481–487.

133. Goei R. Anorectal function in patients with defecation disorders and asymptomatic subjects: evaluation with defecography. *Radiology.* 1990;174:121–123.

134. Felt-Bersma RJF, Luth WJ, Janssen JJWM, Meuwissen SGM. Defecography in patients with anorectal disorders: which findings are clinically relevant? *Dis Colon Rectum.* 1990;33:277–284.

135. Jones PN, Lubowski DZ, Swash M, Henry MM. Is paradoxical contraction of puborectalis muscle of functional importance? *Dis Colon Rectum.* 1987;30:667–670.

136. Klauser AG, Voderholzer WA, Heinrich CA, Schindlbeck NE, Muller-Lissner SA. Behavioral modification of colonic function: can constipation be learned? *Dig Dis Sci.* 1990;35:1271–1275.

137. Kerrigan DD, Lucas MG, Sun WM, Donnelly TC, Read NW. Idiopathic constipation associated with impaired urethrovesical and sacral reflex function. *Br J Surg.* 1989;76:748–751.

138. Turnbull GK, Ritvo PG, Woolnough J. Biofeedback treatment for constipation: is "sham" biofeedback as effective? *Gastroenterology.* 1991:100:A503.

139. Miller R, Duthie GS, Bartolo DCC, Roe AM, Locke-Edmunds J, Mortensen NJM. Anismus in patients with normal and slow transit constipation. *Br J Surg.* 1991;78:690–692.

140. Pemberton JH. Anorectal and pelvic floor disorders: putting physiology into practice. *J Gastroenterol Hepatol.* 1990;1(suppl):127–143.

141. Martelli H, Devroede G, Arhan P, Duguay C. Mechanisms of idiopathic constipation: outlet obstruction. *Gastroenterology.* 1978;75:623–631.

142. Waldron D, Bowes KL, Kingma YJ, Cote KR. Colonic and anorectal motility in young women with severe idiopathic constipation. *Gastroenterology.* 1988;95:1388–1394.

143. De Medici A, Badiali D, Corazziari E, Bausano G, Anzini F. Rectal sensitivity in chronic constipation. *Dig Dis Sci.* 1989;34:747–753.

144. Waldron DJ, Kumar D, Hallan RI, Wingate DL, Williams, NS. Evidence for motor neuropathy and reduced filling of the rectum in chronic intractable constipation. *Gut.* 1990;31:1284–1288.

145. Prior A, Maxton DG, Whorwell PJ. Anorectal manometry in irritable bowel syndrome: differences between diarrhea and constipation predominant subjects. *Gut.* 1990;31:458–462.

146. Kamm MA, Lennard-Jones, JE. Rectal mucosal electrosensory testing—evidence for a rectal sensory neuropathy in idiopathic constipation. *Dis Colon Rectum.* 1990;33:419–423.

147. MacDonald A, Shearer M, Paterson PJ, Finlay IG. Relationship between outlet obstruction constipation and obstructed urinary flow. *Br J Surg.* 1991;78:693–695.

148. Snooks SJ, Barnes PRH, Swash M, Henry MM. Damage to the innervation of the pelvic floor musculature in chronic constipation. *Gastroenterology.* 1985;89:977–981.

149. Varma JS, Smith AN. Neurophysiological dysfunction in young women with intractable constipation. *Gut.* 1988;29:963–968.

150. Manning AP, Thompson WG, Heaton KW, Morris AF. Towards positive diagnosis of the irritable bowel. *Br Med J.* 1978;2:653–654.

151. Talley NJ, Phillips SF, Melton LF, Mulvihill C, Wiltgen C, Zinsmeister AR. Diagnostic value of the Manning criteria in irritable bowel syndrome. *Gut.* 1990;31:77–81.

152. Maxton DG, Morris J, Whorwell PJ. More accurate diagnosis of irritable bowel syndrome by the use of "non-colonic" symptomatology. *Gut.* 1991;32:784–786.

153. Smith RC, Greenbaum DS, Vancouver JB, Henry RC, Reinhart MA, Greenbaum RB, Dean HA, Mayle JE. Gender differences in Manning criteria in the irritable bowel syndrome. *Gastroenterology.* 1991;100:591–595.

154. Thompson WG, Heaton KW. Functional bowel disorders in apparently healthy people. *Gastroenterology.* 1980;79:283–288.

155. Sandler RS, Drossman DA, Nathan HP, McKee DC. Symptom complaints and health care seeking behavior in subjects with bowel dysfunction. *Gastroenterology.* 1984;87:314–318.

156. Whitehead WE, Crowell MD, Bosmajian L, et al. Existence of irritable bowel syndrome supported by factor analysis of symptoms in two community samples. *Gastroenterology.* 1990;98:336–340.

157. Talley NJ, Zinsmeister AR, Van Dyke C, Melton LJ. Epidemiology of colonic symptoms and the irritable bowel syndrome. *Gastroenterology.* 1991;101:927–934.

158. Sandler RS. Epidemiology of irritable bowel syndrome in the United States. *Gastroenterology.* 1990;99:409–415.

159. Everhart JE, Renault PF. Irritable bowel syndrome in office-based practice in the United States. *Gastroenterology.* 1991;100:998–1005.

160. Longstreth GF, Preskill DB, Youkeles L. Irritable bowel syndrome in women having diagnostic laparoscopy or hysterectomy. *Dig Dis Sci.* 1990;35:1285–1290.

161. Drossman DA, Leserman J, Nachman G, et al. Sexual and physical abuse in women with functional or organic gastrointestinal disorders. *Ann Intern Med.* 1990;113:828–833.

162. Drossman DA, McKee DC, Sandler RS, et al. Psychosocial factors in the irritable bowel syndrome. *Gastroenterology.* 1988;95:701–708.

163. Whitehead WE, Bosmajian L, Zonderman AB, Costa PT Jr., Schuster MM. Symptoms of psychologic distress associated with irritable bowel syndrome. *Gastroenterology.* 1988;95:709–714.

164. Smith RC, Greenbaum DS, Vancouver JB, Henry RC, Reinhart MA, Greenbaum RB, Dean HA, Mayle JE. Psychologic factors are associated with health care seeking rather than diagnosis in irritable bowel syndrome. *Gastroenterology.* 1990;98:293–301.

165. Nicolai JJ. Psychologic factors in peptic ulcer disease and irritable bowel syndrome. *Scand J Gastroenterol.* 1989;24(suppl 171):126–132.

166. Rose JDR, Troughton AH, Harvey JS, Smith PM. Depression and functional bowel disorders in gastrointestinal outpatients. *Gut.* 1986;27:1025–1028.

167. Young SJ, Alpers DH, Norland CC, Woodruff RA. Psychiatric illness and the irritable bowel syndrome. *Gastroenterology.* 1976;70:162–166.

168. Fisher SE, Breckon K, Andrews HA, Keighley MRB. Psychiatric screening for patients with fecal incontinence or chronic constipation referred for surgical treatment. *Br J Surg.* 1989;76:352–355.

169. Bleijenberg G, Fennis JFM. Anamnestic and psychological features in diagnosis and prognosis of functional abdominal complaints: a prospective study. *Gut.* 1989;30:1076–1081.

170. Camilleri M, Neri M. Motility disorders and stress. *Dig Dis Sci.* 1989;34:1777–1786.

171. Wald A, Hinds JP, Karuana BJ. Psychological and physiological

characteristics of patients with severe idiopathic constipation. *Gastroenterology.* 1989;97:932–937.

172. Devroede G, Girard G, Bouchoucha M, et al. Idiopathic constipation by colonic dysfunction: relationship with personality and anxiety. *Dig Dis Sci.* 1989;34:1428–1433.

173. Whitehead WE, Cheskin LJ, Heller BR, et al. Evidence for exacerbation of irritable bowel syndrome during menses. *Gastroenterology.* 1990;98:1485–1489.

174. Haderstorfer B, Psycholgin D, Whitehead WE, Shuster MM. Intestinal gas production from bacterial fermentation of undigested carbohydrate in irritable bowel syndrome. *Am J Gastroenterol.* 1989;84:375–378.

175. Maxton DG, Martin DF, Whorwell PJ, Godfrey M. Abdominal distention in female patients with irritable bowel syndrome: exploration of possible mechanisms. *Gut.* 1991;32:662–664.

176. Swarbrick ET, Hegarty JE, Bat L, Williams CB, Dawson AM. Site of pain from the irritable bowel. *Lancet.* 1980;ii:443–446.

177. Whitehead WE, Holtkotter B, Enck P, et al. Tolerance of rectosigmoid distention in irritable bowel syndrome. *Gastroenterology.* 1990;98:1187–1192.

178. Cook IJ, van Eeden A, Collins SM. Patients with irritable bowel syndrome have greater pain tolerance than normal subjects. *Gastroenterology.* 1987;93:727–733.

179. Mayer EA, Raybauld HE. Role of visceral afferent mechanisms in functional bowel disorders. *Gastroenterology.* 1990;99:1688–1704.

180. Heaton KW, Ghosh S, Braddon FEM. How bad are the symptoms and bowel dysfunction of patients with the irritable bowel syndrome? A prospective, controlled study with emphasis on stool form. *Gut.* 1991;32:73–79.

181. Kamm MA, Hawley PR, Lennard-Jones JE. Outcome of colectomy for severe idiopathic constipation. *Gut.* 1988;29:969–973.

182. Rosen L. Physical examination of the anorectum: a systematic technique. *Dis Colon Rectum.* 1990;33:439–440.

183. Nanda R, James R, Smith H, Dudley CRK, Jewell DP. Food intolerance and the irritable bowel syndrome. *Gut.* 1989;30:1099–1104.

184. Ritchie JA, Truelove SC. Treatment of irritable bowel syndrome with lorazepam, hyoscine butylbromide, and ispaghula husk. *Br Med J.* 1979;1:376–378.

185. Ritchie JA, Truelove SC. Comparison of various treatments for irritable bowel syndrome. *Br Med J.* 1980;281:1317–1319.

186. Klein KB. Controlled treatment trials in the irritable bowel syndrome: a critique. *Gastroenterology.* 1988;95:232–241.

187. Narducci F, Bassotti G, Granata MT, et al. Colonic motility and gastric emptying in patients with irritable bowel syndrome: effect of pretreatment with Octylonium bromide. *Dig Dis Sci.* 1986;31:241–246.

188. Rees WDW, Evans BK, Rhodes J. Treating irritable bowel syndrome with peppermint oil. *Br Med J.* 1979;2:835–836.

189. Greenbaum DS, Maybe JE, Vanegeren LE, et al. Effects of desipramine on irritable bowel syndrome compared with atropine and placebo. *Dig Dis Sci.* 1987;32:257–266.

190. Harvey RF, Read AE. Effects of oral magnesium sulphate on colonic motility in patients with the irritable bowel syndrome. *Gut.* 1973;14:983–987.

191. Rumessen JJ, Gudmand-Hoyer E. Functional bowel disease: malabsorption and abdominal distress after ingestion of fructose, sorbitol, and fructose-sorbitol mixtures. *Gastroenterology.* 1988;95:694–700.

192. Tolman KG, Hamman S, Sannella JJ. Possible hepatotoxicity of Doxidan. *Ann Intern Med.* 1976;84:290–292.

193. Edwards CA, Hodden S, Brown C, Read NW. Effect of Cisapride on the gastrointestinal transit of a solid meal in normal human subjects. *Gut.* 1987;28:13–16.

194. Muller-Lissner SA, et al. Treatment of chronic constipation with Cisapride and placebo. *Gut.* 1987;28:1033–1038.

195. Thompson WG. A strategy for management of the irritable bowel. *Am J Gastroenterol.* 1986;81:95–100.

196. Whitehead WE, Chaussade S, Corazziari E, Kumar D. Report of an international workshop on management of constipation. *Gastroenteral Int.* 1991;4:99–113.

197. McCubbin JA, Surwit RS, Mansbach CM. Sensory discrimination training in the treatment of a case of chronic constipation. *Behavior Ther.* 1987;18:273–278.

198. van Baal JG, Leguit P, Brummelkamp WH. Relaxation biofeedback conditioning as treatment of a disturbed defecation reflex. *Dis Colon Rectum.* 1984; 27:187–189.

199. Neff DF, Blanchard EB. A multicomponent treatment for irritable bowel syndrome. *Behavior Ther.* 1987;18:70–83.

200. Turnbull GK, Ritvo PG. Anal sphincter biofeedback relaxation treatment for women with intractable constipation symptoms. *Dis Colon Rectum.* 1992. In press.

201. Bleijenberg G, Kuijpers HC. Treatment of the spastic pelvic floor syndrome with biofeedback. *Dis Colon Rectum.* 1987;30:108–111.

202. Webber J, Ducrotte PH, Touchais JY, Roussingnol C, Denis PH. Biofeedback training for constipation in adults and children. *Dis Colon Rectum.* 1987;30:844–846.

203. Emery Y, Descos L, Meunier P, Louis D, Valancogne G, Weil G. Constipation terminale par asynchronisme abdomino-pelvien: analyse des donees etiologiues, cliniques, manometriques, et des resultats therapeutiques apres reeducation par biofeedback. *Gastroenterol Clin Biol.* 1988;12:6–11.

204. Kawimbe BM, Papachrysostomou M, Binnie NR, Clare N, Smith AN. Outlet obstruction constipation (anismus) managed by biofeedback. *Gut.* 1991;32:1175–1179.

205. Loening-Baucke V. Persistence of chronic constipation in children after biofeedback treatment. *Dig Dis Sci.* 1991;36:153–160.

206. Benson H. Hypnosis and the relaxation response. *Gastroenterology.* 1989;96:1609–1611.

207. Guthrie E, Creed F, Dawson D, Tomenson B. A controlled trial of psychological treatment for the irritable bowel syndrome. *Gastroenterology.* 1991;100:450–457.

208. Creed F, Guthrie E. Psychological treatments of the irritable bowel syndrome: a review. *Gut.* 1989;30:1601–1609.

209. Keren S, Wagner Y, Heldenberg D, Golan M. Studies of manometric abnormalities of the rectoanal region during defecation in constipated and soiling children: modification through biofeedback therapy. *Am J Gastroenterol.* 1988;83:827–831.

210. Barnes PRH, Lennard-Jones JE. Constipation and Megacolon: II Adults. In: Misiewicz JJ, Pounder RE, Venables CW, eds. *Diseases of the Gut and Pancreas.* Oxford: Blackwell Scientific Publications; 1987:922–932.

211. Loening-Baucke V, Cruikshank B, Savage C. Defecation dynamics and behavior profiles in encopretic children. *Pediatrics.* 1987; 80:672–679.

212. Loening-Baucke V. Factors determining outcome in children with chronic constipation and fecal soiling. *Gut.* 1989;30:999–1006.

213. Hallan RI, Williams NS, Melling J, Waldron DJ, Womack NR, Morrison JFB. Treatment of anismus in intractable constipation with botulinum A toxin. *Lancet.* 1988;ii:714–716.

214. Mathias JR, Ferguson KL, Clench MH. Debilitating "functional" bowel disease controlled by leuprolide acetate, gonadotropin-releasing hormone (GnRH) analog. *Dig Dis Sci.* 1989;34:761–766.

215. Keighley MRB. Surgery for constipation. *Br J Surg.* 1988;75:625–626.

216. Henry MM. Surgery for constipation. *Br Med J.* 1989;298:346.

217. Preston DM, Hawley PR, Lennard-Jones JE, Todd, IP. Results of colectomy for severe idiopathic constipation in women. *Br J Surg.* 1984;71:547–552.

218. Beck DE, Jagelman DG, Fazio VW. The surgery of idiopathic constipation. *Gastro Clin N Am.* 1987;16:143–156.

219. Leon SH, Krishnamurthy S, Schuffler MD. Subtotal colectomy for severe idiopathic constipation. *Dig Dis Sci.* 1987;32:1249–1254.

220. Yoshioka K, Keighley MRB. Clinical results of colectomy for severe constipation. *Br J Surg.* 1989;76:600–604.

221. Zenilman ME, Dunnegan DL, Soper NJ, Becker JM. Successful surgical treatment of idiopathic colonic dysmotility. *Arch Surg.* 1989;124:947–951.

222. Stabile G, Kamm MA, Hawley PR, Lennard-Jones JE. Colectomy for idiopathic megarectum and megacolon. *Gut.* 1991;32:1538–1540.

223. Wasserman IF. Puborectalis syndrome. *Dis Colon Rectum.* 1964;7:87–98.

224. Wallace WC, Madden WM. Experience with partial resection of the puborectalis muscle. *Dis Colon Rectum.* 1969;12:196–200.

225. Keighley MRB, Shouler P. Outlet syndrome: is there a surgical option? *J Roy Soc Med.* 1984;77:559–563.

226. Barnes PRH, Hawley PR, Preston DM, Lennard-Jones JE. Experience of posterior division of the puborectalis muscle in the management of chronic constipation. *Br J Surg.* 1985;72:475–477.

227. Kamm MA, Hawley PR, Lennard-Jones JE. Lateral division of the puborectalis muscle in the management of severe constipation. *Br J Surg.* 1988;75:661–663.

INDEX

Numerals in *italics* indicate a figure, "t" following a page number indicates tabular matter.